Textbook of
Head Injury

FOURTH EDITION

Textbook of
Head Injury

FOURTH EDITION

AK Mahapatra
Raj Kamal

Textbook of
Head Injury

FOURTH EDITION

AK Mahapatra MS, MCh, DNB

Director
All India Institute of Medical Sciences
Bhubaneswar, Odisha

Raj Kamal MS, MCh

Additional Director
Department of Neurosurgery
Fortis Escorts Hospital
Amritsar, Punjab

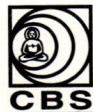

CBS

CBS Publishers & Distributors Pvt Ltd

New Delhi • Bengaluru • Chennai • Kochi • Kolkata • Mumbai
Hyderabad • Nagpur • Patna • Pune • Vijayawada

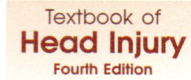

Textbook of
Head Injury
Fourth Edition

ISBN: 978-81-239-2358-1

Copyright © Authors and Publishers

Fourth Edition	**2014**
Reprint	2016
First Edition	1999
Second Edition	2001
Third Edition	2005

Published by Satish Kumar Jain and produced by Varun Jain for
CBS Publishers & Distributors Pvt Ltd
4819/XI Prahlad Street, 24 Ansari Road, Daryaganj, New Delhi 110 002, India.
Ph: 23289259, 23266861, 23266867   Fax: 011-23243014   Website: www.cbspd.com
                                                                                e-mail: delhi@cbspd.com; cbspubs@airtelmail.in.
Corporate Office: 204 FIE, Industrial Area, Patparganj, Delhi 110 092
Ph: 4934 4934   Fax: 4934 4935   e-mail: publishing@cbspd.com; publicity@cbspd.com

Branches

- **Bengaluru:** Seema House 2975, 17th Cross, K.R. Road, Banasankari 2nd Stage, Bengaluru 560 070, Karnataka
  Ph: +91-80-26771678/79   Fax: +91-80-26771680   e-mail: bangalore@cbspd.com
- **Chennai:** No. 7, Subbaraya Street, Shenoy Nagar, Chennai 600 030, Tamil Nadu
  Ph: +91-44-26680620, 26681266   Fax: +91-44-42032115   e-mail: chennai@cbspd.com
- **Kochi:** Ashana House, 39/1904, AM Thomas Road, Valanjambalam, Ernakulam 682 016, Kochi, Kerala
  Ph: +91-484-4059061–65,67   Fax: +91-484-4059065   e-mail: kochi@cbspd.com
- **Kolkata:** No. 6/B, Ground Floor, Rameswar Shaw Road, Kolkata-700014 (West Bengal)
  Ph: +91-33-2289-1126, 2289-1127, 2289-1128   e-mail: kolkata@cbspd.com
- **Mumbai:** 83-C, Dr E Moses Road, Worli, Mumbai-400018, Maharashtra
  Ph: +91-22-24902340/41   Fax: +91-22-24902342   e-mail: mumbai@cbspd.com

Representatives

- **Hyderabad** 0-9885175004   • **Nagpur** 0-9021734563   • **Patna**   0-9334159340
- **Pune**   0-9623451994   • **Vijayawada** 0-9000660880

Printed at HT Media, Noida, UP

to

*Our Respected Parents
and Teachers*

Contributors

Aditya Gupta MCh
Consultant Neurosurgeon
Medanta, Gurgaon

Amandeep Jagdevan MCh
Senior Resident
Department of Neurosurgery
All India Institute of Medical Sciences
New Delhi

Anupam Jindal MCh
Consultant Neurosurgeon
NINS Brain and Spine Hospital
Chandigarh

Ashis Patnaik MS
Assistant Professor
Trauma ad Emergency Medicine
All India Institute of Medical Sciences
Bhubaneswar

Ashok Kumar Mahapatra MS, MCh, DNB
Director
All India Institute of Medical Sciences
Bhubaneswar, Odisha

Atul Kapoor MD, MNAMS
Chief, Department of Radiology
Advanced Diagnostics
Amritsar, Punjab

Avijit Sarkari MS, MCh
Resident
All India Institute of Medical Sciences
New Delhi

Brig HS Bhatoe VSM, MCh
Consultant Neurosurgeon
Command Hospital
Chandimandir, Chandigarh

Chitra Sarkar MD
Professor
Department of Pathology
All India Institute of Medical Sciences
New Delhi, India

Deepak Agrawal MS, MCh
Additional Professor
Department of Neurosurgery
AIIMS, New Delhi

Deepak K Gupta MCh
Additional Professor
Department of Neurosurgery
All India Institute of Medical Sciences
New Delhi

GD Satyarthee
Associate Professor
Department of Neurosurgery
All India Institute of Medical Sciences
New Delhi

Himanshu Verma MBBS
IIIrd Professor
Christian Medical College and Hospital
Ludhiana

K Nagarajan MD (RD), DM (Neuroradiol)
Assistant Professor, Radiology
All India Institute of Medical Sciences
Bhubaneswar, Odisha

Kanwaljeet Garg MS
Resident, Neurosurgery
All India Institute of Medical Sciences
New Delhi

MC Sharma MD
Additional Professor, Department of Neurology
All India Institute of Medical Sciences
New Delhi

Navanil Barua MS, MCh
Director, Department of Neurosurgery
Guwahati Neurological Research Center
Guwahati

P Sarat Chandra MCh
Professor, Department of Neurosurgery
All India Institute of Medical Sciences
New Delhi

PK Gupta MS, MCh, FRCS
Consultant
Department of Neurosurgery
Bahrain

Rajesh Arora
Senior Consultant
Department of Anesthesia
Fortis Escorts Hospital, Amritsar

Raj Kamal MS, MCh
Additional Director
Department of Neurosurgery
Fortis Escorts Hospital
Amritsar, Punjab

Rajinder Kaur MD
Consultant, Department of Anesthesia
Fortis Escorts Hospital, Amritsar

Rana Patir
Director, Neurosurgery
Fortis Hospital
Gurgaon

RR Sharma MS, MCh
Consultant
Department of Neurosurgery
Khoula Hospital, MUSCAT
Sultanate of Oman

RV Devadas MCh
Specialist
Department of Neurosurgery, UAE

Sanjay Kumar MS, MCh, DNB
Chief Consultant Neurosurgeon
AR Ansari Memorial Weavers' Hospital
Apollo Hospitals Group, Ranchi

SD Lal MS, MCh
Consultant
Department of Neurosurgery
Khoula Hospital, MUSCAT
Sultanate of Oman

SJ Pawar MS, MCh
Neurosurgeon
Department of Neurosurgery
Consultant Neurosurgery, Rubby Hall, Pune

Shejoy P Joshua MCh
Senior Resident
AIIMS, New Delhi

Sumit Sinha MCh
Additional Professor
Department of Neurosurgery
All India Institute of Medical Sciences
New Delhi

Sunila Kapila MD
Consultant
Department of Anesthesia
Fortis Escorts Hospital, Amritsar

Suruchi Chopra MD
Chief Consultant
Department of Radiology
Fortis Escorts Hospital, Amritsar

V Pushkarna MD
Senior Resident
Department of Anesthesia
Frotis Escorts Hospital
Amritsar

Vinay Goyal MD, DM
Professor, Department of Neurology
All India Institute of Medical Sciences
New Delhi

Vineet Sehgal MD, DM
Consultant Neurology
Fortis Escorts Hospital
Amritsar

Vipul Gupta MD
Head, Interventional Neuroradiology
Medanta Hospital
Gurgaon

Foreword to Fourth Edition

The fourth edition of *Textbook of Head Injury* has maintained the high standards that were set in the previous editions. It has always been difficult for textbooks about head injury to remain up-to-date but this one has started off and continued in the right direction. The senior author's wide and long clinical experience has ensured a good balance between the practical advice and the science of modern medicine. The authors have an excellent grasp of the English language, which makes these chapters easy to read and to remember. These chapters cover the whole patient journey from injury prevention through acute treatment and care and onto rehabilitation and reintegration into society. The writings will, therefore, be of interest and usefulness to all medical and allied practitioners. It should also prove a source of inspiration to patients, their relatives and carers, who will be able to understand the clear text and high quality illustrations. Medical students will also find this an excellent first-read on the subject. By entering its fourth edition, this book will become one of the classic tomes on the subject of head injury. The subject is complicated by the different case mix of patients with brain injury: small rural hospitals treat many mild injuries and large regional centres tend to receive the more serious injuries. In these chapters the authors have got the balance right so that the subject matter will be relevant to all patients from the mildest to the most severe; from the rural setting to the urban. No one is immune to injury! Hopefully, this book will help to improve the understanding of head injury, and by so doing, improve the outcome for all such afflicted patients.

A David Mendelow MD
Newcastle General Hospital
Neurosurgery
Newcastle upon Tyne
England

Foreword to First Edition

This *Textbook on Head Injury* is well brought out and contains a wealth of information. India is a large country with a staggering population of 950 millions. Yet the roads are not well developed and only 3% of Indian roads are up to international standards. Vehicular population in India has increased 700 times compared to what existed in 1947, when India gained Independence. During this Golden Jubilee year we have nothing to boast about roads or road accidents. But our country records the largest number of road accidents. The manufacturers of two-wheelers find in India the best market. Many models of two-wheelers, particularly the Japanese models, have really conquered the Indian roads. Pathetically, the rule to enforce the wearing of crash helmets by the two-wheeler drivers is yet to be implemented. All told with a rising trend in road accidents contributing to head injuries, the theme of the book is of topical significance, so that the doctors working in the rural areas as well as the specialists can get good information from this textbook. At least the knowledge obtained would be beneficial in ameliorating the morbidity and reducing the mortality amongst the accident victims.

This well written textbook will certainly contribute to the better understanding and appreciation of the problem of head injuries. The chapters are well categorised and the language used is simple and intelligible. This book will be of immense use to undergraduates, postgraduates and all specialists. This book is a welcome addition to all libraries and would be of positive help to neuroscientists.

I wish the editors every success.

M Sambasivan
Chairman, Neurotrauma Committee of India
Vice-Chairman, Neurotrauma (World Federation of Neurological Surgeons)
Senior Consultant Neurosurgeon, Cosmopolitan Hospitals (P) Ltd
Pattam, Thiruvananthapuram 695004
Kerala, India

Preface to Fourth Edition

The first edition of *Textbook of Head Injury* was written by us 14 years back. This book was instant hit with the undergraduates, postgraduates (MS and MCh) and practising neurosurgeons. Head injury continues to be a major problem worldwide. Globally over five million people sustain head injuries every year. Mortality and morbidity rates are still very high. During the last two decades there have been major advances in the understanding of pathophysiology of severe brain injury. This understanding facilitates the neurosurgeon to monitor and prevent secondary injuries to the brain. Prevention of secondary injuries is the key to success in treating traumatic brain injury. We took almost one year in revising this book. We have made all efforts to include recent advances in respective field in head injury.

Advances in molecular and cellular pathophysiology have been incorporated to understand cellular behaviour of neuroglial cells following trauma. Proper emphasis is given to the modes of neuronal cell death following head injury. Also, advances in neurocritical care and development of treatment guidelines are definitely improving the medical care we provide to the head-injured patients. In the early chapters, we have discussed the mechanisms and patho-physiology of brain injury.

The later chapters deal with the latest development in the monitoring, management, prevention and other specific problems in head injury. All radiological photographs (CT scans, MRI scans) are from patients treated by us. Monitoring of head-injured patients is the key in management. We have discussed in detail about monitoring of these patients in neuro ICU.

We hope that this book will serve as a reference and guidance in the management of all types of head injury.

AK Mahapatra
Raj Kamal

Preface to First Edition

Globally over five million people sustain head injuries every year. India with its one billion plus population has a large share of this. Surprisingly, there is hardly anything which is taught to undergraduate medical students in India. This is by and large due to lack of neurosurgery department in large number of medical colleges in India. Not surprisingly, the situation is not much different for the postgraduates in general surgery. Even today a few of our neurosurgical centres do not admit head or spinal injury patients as a policy and send the MCh and DNB students to another neurosurgical centres for a few months training. This has raised a big question about the quality of head injury care in the country.

Currently there are less than 1000 neurosurgeons in India and among them over 75% are working in large cities. Hence, there is little scope of having neurosurgery department in many peripheral/private medical colleges. For years to come, we would expect head injury to be managed by general surgeons. Realising India's vast population and are, it is impossible to think of neurosurgeon in each district hospital. Hence, our aim should be to expose MBBS and MS (General Surgery) students adequately to manage head injury, even though we do not expect them to operate. At this stage it is important to realise that 90% head injuries are minor and patients do not require neither neurosurgical intervention nor ICU care, what they really need is primary care, proper observation and assurance for confidence building. Doctors and paramedics also should know prehospital care including transport of severely head injured patients. Thus, there is a vital role for the doctors to play in the periphery.

In our previous edition, we had included 34 chapters, which we considered important that time. Over the years we realised that the book did not deal with many aspects of head injury, also for the existing chapters need to be updated. In addition to what we had written in previous edition, we have added 16 more chapters. Some important aspects of new additions are, a fluid and electrolyte management. This is especially important as large number of severely head injury patients develop metabolic and electrolyte disturbances and need meticulus management. Secondly, endocrinal problems are hardly ever realised by the neurosurgeons. Endocrine problems not only occur in severely injured patients, minor head-injured patients do develop short-term or long-term problems which adversely affect their outcome. Thirdly, infective complications like, meningitis and brain abscess are not uncommon and required to be highlighted. Coagulopathies are major problem in head injury patients, which play an important role in management of head injury. Some rare aspects like, post-traumatic basal ganglia haematoma, traumatic cerebellar haematoma and dural sinus thrombosis are also included. Thus in this edition we have tried to widen the horizon of readers in management of head injury.

AK Mahapatra
Raj Kamal

Acknowledgements

I am grateful to my great teachers, Prof AK Banerjee, Prof VS Mehta, Prof AK Mahapatra and Prof T Kawase for their inspirational support.

I would like to thank my wife Seema for standing beside me throughout my career and writing this book. She has been my inspiration and motivation for continuing to improve my knowledge and move my career forward. I also thank my wonderful children, Shivam and Satyam, for making everything worthwhile.

I wish to thank my parents for their undivided support and encouraged me to go my own way. A special thanks of mine to my colleagues and friends, Dr HP Singh, Dr AK Chopra, Dr D Kapila and Dr A Kapoor, who appreciated and inspired me.

I thank my old friends, Prof Chandan Guha, Prof SS Kale, Prof Subhobrata Das and S Pushpinder Singh for motivational support.

I would like to express my gratitude to Mr Ashish Bhatia, COO Fortis Hospital, for his support in writing this book. Special thanks to Col H Chehal, Dr Gurbir Singh and Dr Pinak Moudgil for providing professional support.

I take this opportunity to acknowledge the help provided by Mr SK Jain, Managing Director, editorial–production team of CBS Publishers & Distributors, Mr YN Arjuna, Mrs Ritu Chawla, Mrs Jyoti Kaur, and all those who collaborated in producing this book.

Finally, I thank Lord Krishna who made all the things possible.

Raj Kamal

Contents

Abbreviations

AAMVA	American Association of Motor Vehicle Administrators		**BZR**	Benzodiazepine receptor
AANS	American Association of Neurological Surgeons		**CAPT**	Combined Anterior Pituitary Test
			CNG	Compressed Natural Gas
ABG	Arterial Blood Gas		**CBF**	Cerebral Blood Flow
ACA	Anterior Central Artery		**CCF**	Caroticocavernous Fistula
ADH	Antidiuretic Hormone		**CCT**	Central Conduction Time
AMPA	Alpha Amino-3-Hydroxyl-3-Methyl-4-Isoxasol		**CG**	Ciliary Ganglion
			CI	Confidence Interval
ANP	Atrial Natriuretic Peptide		**CMRO$_2$**	Cerebral Metabolism Rate of Oxygen
APB	Amino Ethoxy Diphenyl Borate		**COAD**	Chronic Obstructive Airway Disease
AP View	Anterior Posterior View		**CPP**	Cerebral Perfusion Pressure
APP	Amyloid Precursor Protein		**CRASH**	Corticosteroid Randomization after Significant Head Injury
APTT	Activated Partial Thromboplastin Time			
ARDS	Adult Respiratory Distress Syndrome		**CS**	Cavernous Sinus
ATLS	Acute Trauma Life Support		**CSF**	Cerebrospinal Fluid
ARAS	Ascending Reticular Activating System		**CSWS**	Cerebral Salt Wasting Syndrome
ASPEN	American Society for Parenteral Nutrition		**CT**	Computerised Tomography
			CVP	Central Veins pressure
AVDO$_2$	Arteriovenous Desaturation of Oxygen		**CVR**	Cerebral Vascular Resistance
AVM	Arteriovenous Malformation		**DAI**	Diffuse Axonal Injury
APOE4	Apolipoprotein 4		**DCS**	Dorsal Column Stimulation
APP	Amyloid Precursor		**DDAVP**	1-Deamino 8-D Arginine Vasopressin
AQP4	Aquaporin 4		**DECRA**	Decompressive Craniectomy
AUC	Area Under Concentration		**DI**	Diabetes Insipidus
AVS	Acute Vegetative State		**DIC**	Disseminated Intravascular Coagulation
BAEP	Brainstem Auditory Evoked Potential			
BBB	Blood–Brain Barrier		**DMSO**	Dimethyl Sulfoxide
BMI	Body Mass Index		**DNA**	Deoxyribonucleic Acid
BISIG	Brain Injury Interdisciplinary Special Interest Group		**DSA**	Digital Subtraction Angiography
			DSI	Day Since Injury
BNP	Brain Natriuretic Peptide		**DST**	Dural Sinus Thrombosis
BSH	Brainstem Haematoma		**DTI**	Diffuse Tensor Imaging
BTF	Brain Trauma Foundation		**DTPA**	Diethylene Triamine Penta-acetic Acid

DVT	Deep Vein Thrombosis	**IMPACT**	International Mission for Prognosis and Analysis of Clinical Trials in TBI
DWI	Diffusion Weighted Images		
EAA	Excitatory Amino Acid	**IONTS**	International Optic Nerve Trauma Study
EACA	Epsilon Aminocaproic Acid		
ECA	External Carotid Artery	**IP3**	Inositol Triphosphate
ECD	Ethylene Cysteine Dimer	**ITT**	Insulin Tolerance Test
ECF	Extracellular Fluid	**IVH**	Intraventricular Haemorrhage
EDH	Extradural Haematoma	**LED**	Light Emitting Diode
EEG	Electroencephalography	**LGB**	Lateral Geniculate Body
EGF	Epidermal growth factor	**LOS**	Length of Stay
EO	Evidence of	**LP**	Lumbar Puncture
EP	Evoked Potential	**MAM**	Moderate Acute Malnutrition
EPTS	Early Post-traumatic Seizures	**MAP**	Mean Arterial Pressure
ESBL	Extended-spectrum Beta-lactamase	**MCA**	Middle Cerebral Artery
ETCO$_2$	End Tidal CO_2	**MCTC**	Metrizamide Computed Tomography Cisternography
EVD	External Ventricular Drainage		
FDP	Fibrin Degradation Product	**MD**	Mild Disability
FFA	Free Fatty Acid	**MLF**	Medial Longitudinal Fasciculus
FFP	Fresh Frozen Plasma	**MOFS**	Multiple Organ Failure Syndrome
FIB	Fibrinogen Assay	**MMP**	Matrix Metalloproteinases
fMRI	Functional MRI	**MP**	Methyl Prednisolone
FSH	Follicular Stimulating Hormone	**MRC**	Medical Research Council
FV	Flow Velocity	**MRC**	Magnetic Resonance Cisternography
GH	Growth Hormone	**MRI**	Magnetic Resonance Imaging
GABA	Gamma-aminobutyric Acid	**MRS**	Magnetic Resonance Spectroscopy
GCS	Glasgow Coma Scale	**MRSA**	Methicillin Resistant *Staphylococcus aureus*
GDC	Guglielmi Detachable Coils		
GOS	Glasgow Outcome Scale	**NCCU**	Neurocritical Care Unit
GR	Good Recovery	**NHDS**	National Hospital Discharged Survey
GRH	Gonadotrophin Releasing Hormone	**NIH**	National Institute of Health
HU	Hounsfield Units	**NMDA**	N-Methyl-D-Aspartate
HIF	Hypoxia Induced Factor	**NOS**	Nitric Oxide Synthetase
HTS	Hypertonic Saline	**NSE**	Neuron Specific Enolase
ICF	Intracellular Fluid	**NSI**	Neurological Society of India
ICAM1	Intercellular Adhesion Molecule 1	**PCA**	Posterior Cerebral Artery
ICH	Intracerebral Haematoma	**PCS**	Post-concussion Syndrome
ICP	Intracranial Pressure	**PCP**	Phencyclidine
ICU	Intensive Care Unit	**PDS**	Paroxysmal Depolarization Shift
IDSA	Infectious Diseases Society of America	**PEEP**	Positive End Expiratory Pressure

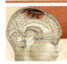

PEG	Polyethylene Glycol	**SIADH**	Syndrome of Inappropriate ADH Secretion
PET	Positron Emission Tomography	**SO**	Suggestive of
PFEDH	Posterior Fossa Extradural Haematoma	**SOV**	Superior Ophthalmic Vein
PGCS	Pediatric Glasgow Coma Scale	**SPECT**	Single Photon Emission Computed Tomography
PGD	Prostaglandin	**SSS**	Superior Sigittal Sinus
PKC	Protein Kinase C	**STITCH**	Surgical Trial in Traumatic Intracerebral Hemorrhage
PI	Pulsatility Index	**SWI**	Susceptibility Weighted Images
PPRF	Paramedian Pontine Reticular Formation	**TBGH**	Traumatic Basal Ganglia Haematoma
PT	Prothrombin Time	**TBI**	Traumatic Brain Injury
PTA	Post-traumatic Amnesia	**TCD**	Transcranial Doppler
PTE	Post-traumatic Epilepsy	**TPN**	Total Parenteral Nutrition
PTH	Post-traumatic Hydrocephalus	**TCDB**	Traumatic Coma Data Bank
PTHP	Post-traumatic Hypopituitarism	**TCT**	Thrombin Clotting Time
PTN	Pretectal Nucleus	**TDAI**	Traumatic Diffuse Axonal Injury
PTT	Partial Thromboplastin Time	**TH**	Therapeutic Hypothermia
PVI	Pressure Volume Index	**THAM**	Tris (Hydroxymethyl) Aminomethane
PVS	Persistent Vegetative State	**TIA**	Transient Ischaemic Attack
RAS	Reticular Activating System	**TICH**	Traumatic Intracerebral Hemorrhage
RBC	Red Blood Corpuscle	**TLE**	Temporal Lobe Epilepsy
RCT	Randomised Controlled Trials	**TNF-α**	Tumor Necrosis Factor Alpha
REM	Resting Metabolic Expenditure	**TON**	Traumatic Optic Neuropathy
RESCUEicp	Randomised Evaluation of Surgery with Craniectomy for Uncontrollable Elevation of Intracranial Pressure	**TPFL**	Traumatic Posterior Fossa Lesion
		tSAH	Traumatic Subarachnoid Hemorrhage
RGC	Retinal Ganglionic Cell	**TSH**	Thyroid Stimulating Hormone
RIA	Radioimmune Assay	**TT**	Thrombin Time
RLAS	Rancho Los Amigos Scale	**VBR**	Ventricular Brain Ratio
RN	Red Nucleus	**VEGFA**	Vascular Endothelial Growth Factor A
SAFE	Saline versus Albumin Fluid Evaluation	**VOC**	Voltage Operated Channel
SAH	Subarachnoid Haemorrhage	**VOR**	Vestibulo-ocular Reflex
SAM	Severe Acute Malnutrition	**VSCC**	Voltage Sensitive Calcium Channel
SD	Severe Disability	**VP**	Ventriculoperitoneal
SDH	Subdural Haematoma	**VS**	Vegetative State
SEP	Sensory Evoked Potential	**WHO**	World Health Organization

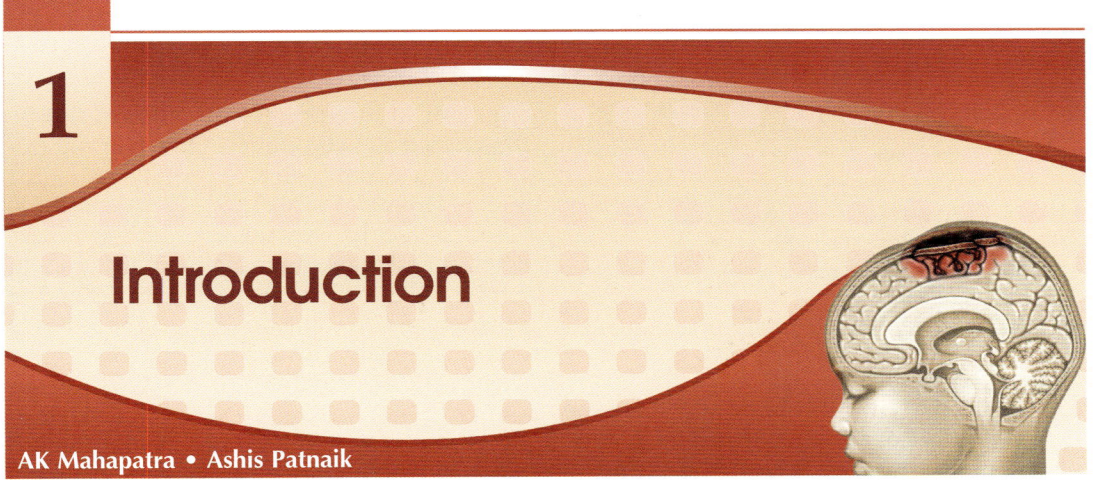

Introduction

AK Mahapatra • Ashis Patnaik

Head injury continues to be a challenge, not only for the public but also for the neurosurgeon. It is an important cause of high morbidity and mortality, particularly in young and productive age group patients. In spite of marked improvements in pre-hospital care, operative skills and overall management of head injuries, mortality/morbidity of severe head injury has not changed over the last 30 years due to urbanisation, industrialisation and increase in vehicular population.[1] In India, the condition has rather deteriorated, due to meagre availability of specialised neurotrauma centres as well as trained neurosurgeons to manage these life threatening cases. The number of head injuries are expected to increase further. While in developed countries like US, Australia or in Japan, head injury incidence has fallen significantly.

Over 5.56 million accidents occur worldwide per year with 1.2 million death annually and 3400 death/day. India has the distinction of having the highest rate of head injury in the world. In 1980, 24,600 people were killed in road traffic accidents, which increased to 80,000 in 1990. This figure is now approaching 150,000 deaths per year in 2011 (Table 1.1). Another 1 million suffer from serious head injuries. Pedestrians and motorcyclists are the most common victims of road traffic accidents in India. 1 out of 6 trauma victims die in India, while in the United States this figure is 1 out of 200 (Table 1.2). This is because of the fact that India, although has the highest incidence of head injuries in the world, has essentially no infrastructure for rapid response and treatment. This number of deaths and injuries are expected to continuously escalate, as the number of vehicles increase along with the increasing adoption of fast life by Indians. It

Table 1.1: Epidemiology of head injury in India due to road traffic accident

- More than 1 million accidents per year
- Over 150,000 deaths/year (as per 2011)
- Overall, 1 accident per minute and 1 death in every 4–5 minutes; will be every 3 minutes by 2020
- Nearly 350 people die due to road traffic accident in India per day (as compared to 3400 deaths in world daily)
- Per 1 million km driven there are 6 deaths in India, In US 1 death per 1.6 million km driven
- 60 percent of all head injury caused by road traffic accidents
- Fatality rate: 70 per 10,000 vehicles
- Fatality rate 30 times higher than of US
- Alcohol involvement: 15–20 percent of head injuries, cause by road traffic accident
- Most of those who are injured in road traffic accidents are considered "vulnerable road users": pedestrians (25 percent of those injured), motorcyclists (17 percent), four-wheel vehicle operators (15 percent), and pedal cyclists (10 percent)
- Of the victims classified as "severely injured" in road traffic accidents, 76 percent suffer head injuries

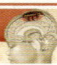

Table 1.2: Head injury profile in USA (as per 2004)
• 1 accident per minute
• 1 death every 5 minutes
• 50,000 deaths every year
• 80,000–90,000 lose their job
• 50–60% patients with minor head injury develop cognitive problems
• 1 head injury maintaining cost $4 million/year.

is expected that by 2050, India will have the highest number of automobiles on the planet, overtaking the United States. Half of those who die from head injuries, do so within the first two hours of injury caused by the primary insult to the brain **(primary injury)**. Rest of the patients die due to the progressive damage to the brain following initial insult and initiated by the primary injury **(secondary injury)**. It is this secondary injury which can be treated and modified to decrease the overall morbidity and mortality. Consequently, the early and appropriate management of head injuries is critical to the survival of these patients. In India, 90 to 95% of trauma victims who survive the primary injury, do not receive optimal care during the initial **"golden hour"** after an injury is sustained, which grossly increases the subsequent morbidity and mortality. The outcome of head injury is drastically correlated to the quality of pre-hospital care and the rapidity with which they are transferred to a specialised center, where they can be managed promptly and effectively. Near about, 30% of those who currently die from head injuries could be saved if quality care is available to them in time. Most of the road traffic accident victims are young and are in their 20s to 40s. These persons are usually the lone or main bread-earners of the family, whose death or disability in the accident leads to economic crisis of the entire family. Again the persons involved in head injuries are usually professionals or skilled and unskilled workers, whose loss is irreparable to the society.

Head injury defines an injury both to the head and brain. Hence, injury to head which does not involve the brain, should not be considered as head injury. However, neuro-surgeons often get emergency calls for management of simple scalp lacerations, bleeding scalp wounds or skull fracture without any brain abnormality in CT scan. In setting of conscious, oriented patients and in absence of neurological signs, these cases should be ideally treated by general surgeons, without over burdening the work of the neurosurgeons. This occurs due to lack of awareness, even among the primary health care providers, without knowing what actually a head injury is. Although it occurs mostly in rural, primary health centres, but it may occur in large hospital and even in medical colleges and institutions like AIIMS, such instances are not rare. This shows our casualness and shifting of responsibility in medicolegal cases to the neurosurgeons. Neurosurgeons, who are few in numbers to handle such large number of cases, are not always available for consultation, particularly in rural areas and small towns and the patients are made to wait or are referred to a large centre for unnece-ssary neurosurgical consultation, thereby wasting time, money and human resources. Therefore, head injury is a condition which not only all doctors should know, but even general public mustknow. Hence, when a doctor is confronted with such situations, he must know if the patient he is dealing with has or has not suffered from head injury.

Head injury is a neurosurgical problem and operation if required, should be performed by a neurosurgeon. However, the question then remains, whether we have enough neuro-surgeons so that every head injury can be seen, diagnosed and treated by a neurosurgeon? This has been possible in US, Japan and many other developed countries, where the trained personnels are available. In poor and developing countries it is not possible due to lack of facilities. For example, India with more than 1200 million people have only 1600 neurosurgeons (as of 2010). Only few numbers of 150–200 are added to this pool of neuro-surgeons through proper training each year, in a country with constantly and rapidly rising population. Again these neurosurgeons are mostly available in metropolis or Govt. Medical College-based cities. Even today large number of our medical colleges do not have basic neurosurgical facilities, to deal with head injury cases effectively. So the availability of trained neurosurgeons in district or sub-divisional hospitals does not arise. This means in India and other developing countries, head injury has to be primarily managed by general surgeons, with adequate (6 months to 1 year) training in head injury management.

In Delhi, over 2200 people died due to road accidents in 1997[2] and over 13,000 had non-fatal head injury, and the number is increasing. Recently over 2–3 years, the incidence of head injury has fallen in Delhi, 10% every year. This is basically because, strict implementation of helmet, seat belt, and banning of old vehicle on the Delhi road. What is surprising, however, in many small cities and townshelmet is not still compulsory for two wheeler driver. More interestingly small and medium towns do not implement the rules implemented at Delhi.

Large number of people die due to head injury, which does not evoke much reaction except occasional photos and write up in newspapers. School bus accidents have rocked India in last few years and there were several incidents in Delhi. People react, discuss for few days then forget, till another school bus disaster takes place. Our authorities and public have become immune to elicit any response. Unfortunately, a death occurring due to head injury outside and in rich and celebrity people get much more attention and publicity, like Raman Lamba's case, who died in Dhaka due to cricket ball injury. Many children become blind following the head injury by a cricket ball. A hit and run case killing 6 people, caused by BMW car at Lodhi road, Delhi in 1999 caught much media attention due to involvement of an influential businessman as the prime accused. All above emphasize the concern and need for proper management of head injury. Similar incident

happened which caught Indian attention was the head injury sustained by young prince of Jodhpur, Shivraj Singh, while playing polo in Jaipur, in 2005. He lost consciousness following the injury, was rushed to the SMS Hospital, Jaipur and subsequently to Bombay Hospital, Mumbai. After surgery he was taken to the United States of America for neurorehabilitation at The Mount Sinai Medical Center, New York. This incidence amazed everyone as he continued to improve almost six years following his injury, through an intensive neurorehabilitation program, supervised by rehabilitation specialists from India and abroad. Recently he also got married. This shows how an early and proper treatment can bring back severely head injured patients to almost normal, back to his life. Inspired by his experience, His Highness Maharaja Gajsingh II of Jodhpur founded The Indian Head Injury Foundation (IHIF) in February 2007, with a mission to build a comprehensive system in India for the prevention, diagnosis and treatment of traumatic brain injury, and to provide neurorehabilitation to such patients, which is of immense help.

Hence, it is important for all medical graduates and even public to have some knowledge of head injuries. Most important among that is, how to define head injury? As a head injury is synonymus with brain injury and the tell-tale evidence of head injury is loss of consciousness. Even if patient does not lose consciousness, he or she must have altered consciousness, it means patient is not fully conscious and oriented. Sometimes it may be difficult to know whether a patient had really lost consciousness or not. If a patient developed memory loss for the events following injury it is 100% certain that the patient had lost consciousness. The period following injury, when a patient fails to register the events, despite of being conscious and alert, is called post-traumatic amnesia (PTA). Thus, PTA is a sure shot evidence of head injury. After having defined head injury it is worth at this stage to classify head injury. Head injury by and large

Table 1.3a: Classification of head injury		
	Duration of unconsciousness	GCS (Glasgow Coma Scale)[4]
1. Minor or mild head injury	Less than 30 minutes	13–15
2. Moderate head injury	More than 30 minutes and less than 6 hours	9–12
3. Severe head injury	More than 6 hours	8 or less

is classified as (a) minor, (b) moderate, and (c) severe (Tables 1.3a and b). In a simple way one can say, head injury is minor when loss of consciousness is for less than 30 minutes, it is moderate, if the duration of unconsciousness is between 30 minutes and 6 hours. If the duration of unconsciousness is longer than 6 hours, head injury is categorised as severe. Fortunately 80% head injuries are minor.[3] However, it must be stated here is that "No head injury is minor enough to be neglected nor severe enough to be given up". Each head injury must be treated according to its own merit. Large number of patients, in whom there is no hope of surviving, not only survive but also become alright. Sadly enough, this situation is rare, nevertheless, few examples only remind us to do our best, even if a patient is bad and carries a small chance of survival or good recovery.

Large number of factors determine the outcome in a head injury patient. Age, initial neurological status (GCS score), intracranial pathology, intracranial pressure and associated injuries are few significant prognostic factors. Recently, genetic basis of head injury outcome is reported. Presence of Apolipoprotein E4 alleles is recognised as a poor prognostic factor. Patients who are homozygous or heterozygous for APO E4 allele have 14 times greater likely-hood of poor outcome.[5–8]

There is a tremendous degree of non-uniformity in the management of head injury, not only between general surgeons and neurosurgeons, but also the difference is apparent between neurosurgeons, depending on the experience, availability of facilities and even between non-practicing and practicing neurosurgeons. Considering all above points,

the American Association of Neurological Surgeons (AANS) and Neurotrauma Sub-committee of Neurological Society of India (NSI), decided to develop guidelines for management of head injuries, with an aim to evolve uniform policy in management of head injury[9–11] which is important both from medical and legal point of view. In India, so far head injury is a neglected field[12] and has not attracted the attention of public or authority.

Overall, with tremendous increase in number of head injury, the management of head injury has gained an important place today. There are only a few books written on head injury by Indian authors. Hence, there is the need for a comprehensive book on head injury, which would provide overall know-ledge on head injury. However, head injury is a vast subject and there is growing literature on various aspects of head injury. From this point of view, no book can provide everything on the subject, an attempt has been made to bring out this book only to provide our students and trainee an adequate knowledge on head injury management.

Table 1.3b: Classification of head injury
1. *Simple:* When there is no communication to outside, hence, no cerebrospinal fluid (CSF) leak or brain matter coming out from scalp wound. No CSF rhinorrhoea or otorrhoea
2. *Compound:* (a) Open compound and (b) closed compound
a. *Open compound:* This head injury means, brain is exposed to outside through scalp wound and skull fracture.
b. *Closed compound:* When there is CSF rhinorrhoea, CSF otorrhoea and X-ray skull or CT scan head shows intracranial air

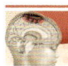
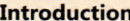

REFERENCES

1. Palmer S, Bader MK, Qureshi A, Palmer J, Shaver T, Borzatta M, et al. The impact on outcomes in a community hospital setting of using the AANS traumatic brain injury guidelines. Americans Associations for Neurologic Surgeons. J Trauma 2001;50:657–64.

2. Mahapatra AK. Management of Head Injury. Neurosciences Today 1997; 2:197–204.

3. Bagchi AK. An Introduction to Head Injury. Calcutta, Oxford University Press 1980.

4. Teasdale G, Jennett B. Assessment of coma and impaired consciousness. A practical scale. Lancet 1974,13;2:81–4.

5. Kunter KC, Evlonger Dun, Tsai J, et aL Lower Cognitive performance of older football players positive for apolipoprotein E Epsilon 4 Neurosurg 2001;47:651–7.

6. Jordan BD, Relkin NR, Ravdin LD, et al. Apolipoprotein E Epsilon 4 associated with chronic traumatic brain injury in Boxing. JAMA 1997; 278:136–40.

7. Friedman G, Froom P, Suzbon L, et al. Apolipoprotein E Epsilon 4 genotype predict poor outcome in Survivors & Traumatic brain injury. Neurology 1999;15:244–8.

8. MaCFarlane DP, Nicoll JA, Smith C, et al. APOE epsilony allele and amyloid beta protein deposition in long-term survivors of head injury. Neuroreport 1999;10:3945–8.

9. Guidelines for the management of "Severe Head Injury" A joint initiative, The Brain Trauma Foundation. The AANS and the joint section of Neurotrauma and critical care. J Neurotrauma 1996;13:641–734.

10. Ramani PS, Mahapatra AK. Basic Manual for the Management of Head and Spinal Injury, Published by Neurotraumatology Committee (NSI) Neurological Society of India, Mumbai 1996.

11. AANS news letter. Save the teen by think first society of US. April 2004.

12. Head injuries—a neglected field in India. Editorial National Medical Journal of India (NMJI) 1991;4:53–64.

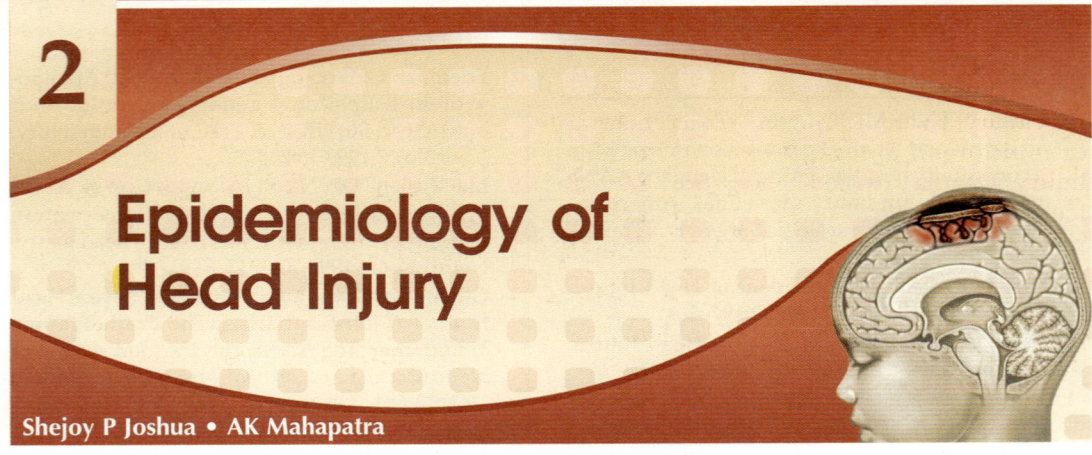

2

Epidemiology of Head Injury

Shejoy P Joshua • AK Mahapatra

Epidemiology is defined as the study of the patterns of disease occurrence in human populations and the factors that influence them.[1] Analytical epidemiology is the study of distribution of disease based on causal factors which traditionally, are divided into the *host* (characteristics intrinsic to the person), the *agent* (physical, chemical, nutritive or infectious) and the *environment* (characteristics extrinsic to the person that influence the exposure or susceptibility to the agent).

William Haddon, in late 1960s, proposed a phase-factor matrix, based on the host, agent and environment framework. He divided the time sequence into three phases: Pre-event, event and post-event. Factors in the pre-event phase determine whether the event (e.g. motor vehicle crash) will occur. Factors in the event phase determine whether an injury will occur; factors in the post-event phase influence the outcome or consequences of the injury.[2] Table 2.1 illustrates the Haddon's phase factor matrix, that contribute to injury.

Overview

Fifty percent of all deaths occur within minutes of injury. The most common cause is massive hemorrhage and severe neurologic

Table 2.1: The Haddon's phase factor matrix for injury			
	Factors		
	Host (Human)	*Agent (Vehicle)*	*Environment physical*	*Environment social*
Pre-event	Driver's age, gender, driving experience, drug or alcohol use, vision, fatigue, frequency of travel, risk taking behaviour	Vehicle speed, brakes, tyres, road holding ability	Road design, road conditions, weather, traffic flow, density and control, visibility	Speed restrictions, impaired driving laws, licensing restrictions, road rage, seat belt, helmet and child restraint laws
Event	Age, pre-existing conditions, restraint use	Vehicle speed, size, type of seat belts, airbags, interior surface hazards	Guardrails, median dividers	Enforcement of speed limits
Post-event	Age, comorbidities	Integrity of fuel system	Distance from emergency medical care	Quality of trauma care, rehabilitation and compensation

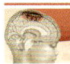
injury. An additional 30% die of neurologic dysfunction within several hours to 2 days post injury. The remaining 20% die of infection or multiorgan failure days or weeks after injury. Deaths are only the tip of the injury iceberg. Many non-fatal injuries have far reaching consequences in terms of reduced quality of life and high costs accrued to the health care system. Moreover, the loss of productivity due to temporary and permanent disability has an overall impact on society.

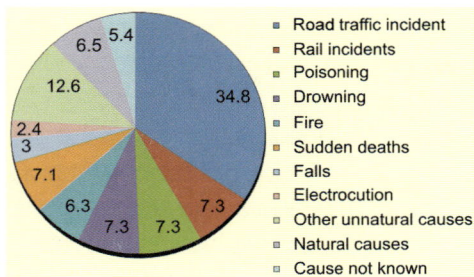

Fig. 2.1: Percentage of various of accidental deaths during 2010

Injury Patterns by Age and Gender

Majority of fatal and non-fatal injuries occur in the young. Patients under 45 years account for 61% of all injury fatalities, 62% of hospitalization and 80% of emergency department visits.

Nearly three quarters (72%) of injury deaths and over half (56%) of non-fatal injuries occur among males. In every age except very young (0–9 years), the rate of injury death for males is more than twice as high as for females. The risk of non-fatal injury in females is twice the risk of similar injuries in males in elderly age group (above 65 years).

Patterns of Injury by Mechanism and Intent

Mechanism refers to the external agent or activities that case the injury (e.g. motor vehicle, fall, firearm, poisoning, etc.). Intent is classified into unintentional, intentional (e.g. assault, homicide or suicide) and intent undetermined. Mechanism of injury can also be classified into natural and unnatural causes. Each accounts for 6.5% and 93.5% in 2010 respectively. The average percentage share of various caused of accidental deaths during 2010 have been depicted in Fig. 2.1.

Distribution of Injuries by their Nature and Severity

Head injuries are the second leading cause (after extremity injury) for injury hospitalization. Mild head injuries by and large are treated on out patient basis. Motor vehicle injury is the leading cause as mentioned in Figs 2.1 and 2.2.

Distribution of Injuries by Place

Unintentional injury deaths are more common in rural areas whereas homicides are more common in cities. Head injuries occur most often on Fridays, Saturdays and Sundays. Higher incidence in summer is noted. Alcohol and drug abuse contribute to 38% and 7%, respectively, of all cases of severe head injury.[3]

Mechanisms of Major Trauma

Two leading mechanism of major trauma: motor vehicle injury and falls are described in detail.

Motor Vehicle Injuries

Adolescent and young adult males are at highest risk of both fatal and non-fatal injuries due to motor vehicles.

Reasons for increasing accidental deaths in India

- **Infrastructural problems**
  - Poor road design
  - Poor lighting
  - Poor maintenance
  - Lack of Bi-lane system
  - Lack of safety measures-traffic control, signals
- **Vehicular problems**
  - Lack of seat belts
  - Improper braking system
  - Mixed traffic—two and four-wheelers
  - Poor vehicle standards

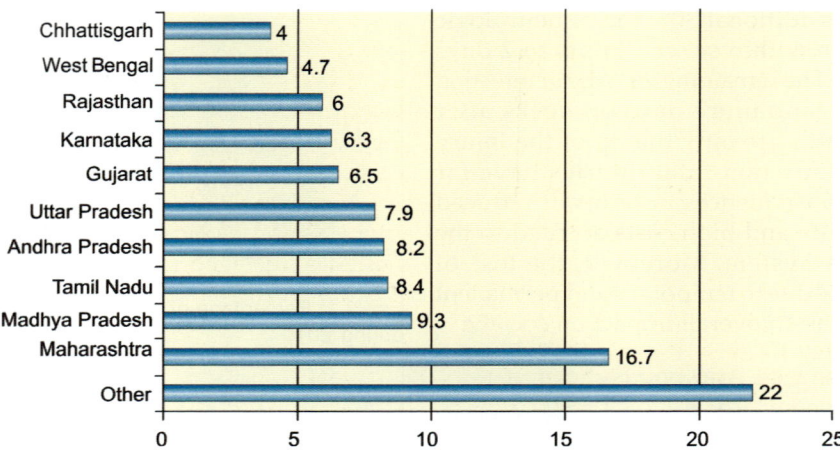

Fig. 2.2: Percentage of accidental deaths in 2010

- **Host factors**
  - Inadequate driving training
  - Non-compliance with traffic rules
  - Poor visual acuity

FALLS

Fall risk is greatest in the young children and elderly members of our society, although the severity profile of these 2 groups is quite different. In children falls are common but not severe. This age group has the highest emergency department visits for injury. Half occur at home and a quarter at school. Older children falls are associated with play and recreational activities. Fall deaths are mostly unintentional (93%). Rarely, person may commit suicide by jumping from a height. Gender ratios for injur deaths in dadults is higher for men up to 44 years. From age 45 this trend reverses. And by 65 years falls in women are 2.7 times that of men.

DISABILITY

Survivors of closed head injuries are often left with varying degrees of disability. This occurs in 10, 50 to 60% and greater than 99% survivors of mild, moderate and severe head injury.[4] The psychological and social sequelae of head injury are tremendous. Many patients experience significant depression from loss of independence. Decreased earning power due to permanent and substantial disability leads to the loss of economic status.

There are many kinds of impairments that may occur as a result of TBI. These injuries may impair:

- Cognition—concentration, memory, judgment, and mood
- Movement abilities—strength, coordination, and balance
- Sensation—tactile sensation and special senses such as vision
- TBI sometimes results in seizure disorders (epilepsy). About 1% of persons with severe TBI survive in a state of persisting unconsciousness.

PEDIATRIC HEAD INJURY

Fifty percent of the accident and emergency departments after head injury are children. They account for a third of admissions, a quarter of severe injuries, and a fifth of deaths. Head injuries account for 15% of deaths of children aged 1–15 years. Fewer than 10% have any evidence of brain damage, and most admissions are patients with mild injuries. Causes vary according to severity, road accidents accounting for fewer than 10% of attenders but for more than 70% of severe and fatal injuries. Many injuries on the road are to

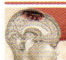

pedestrians. Fewer children need to be admitted if risk factors for complications in mild injuries are carefully assessed.[6]

INDIAN SCENARIO

Traumatic brain injuries (TBI) cause morbidity, mortality, disability and socioeconomic losses in India and other developing countries. It is estimated that nearly 1.5 to 2 million persons are injured and 1 million succumb to death every year in India. Road traffic injuries are the leading cause (60%) of TBIs followed by falls (20–25%) and violence (10%). Alcohol involvement is known to be present among 15–20% of TBIs at the time of injury. The rehabilitation needs of brain injured persons are significantly high and increasing from year to year. India and other developing countries face the major challenges of prevention, pre-hospital care and rehabilitation in their rapidly changing environments to reduce the burden of TBIs.[5]

There is a 50% increase in the incidence of accident deaths in India occurred in the year 2010 compared to 2000 even though there was only a 18.3% increase in the population. If we compare India and China in 1990, and 2010. China had 1,20000 death in 1990 as compared to India where 90,000 died in 1990. However, in 2010, in India app 1,50000 died as compared to 85,000 deaths in China. Thus China has

successfully controlled and reduced head injury deaths. The various causes have been illustrated in Fig. 2.1. Maharashtra reported the highest rate of accidental deaths (16.7%). The state wise incidence of accidental deaths has been depicted in Fig. 2.2. Delhi accounted for maximum number (1.7%) of road accident among Union territories. Over last 2 decade, Delhi has managed to decrease the incidance of injury and also the number of deaths. More males succumbed to accidents compared to females. The break up of various modes of transport involved in accident deaths has been depicted in Fig. 2.3. Two-wheelers are the most common type of vehicle involved in road accident deaths in India. Road accidents are more common during May and March months. Maximum road accidents reported during 6 to 9 pm, followed by 3 to 6 pm and least duing 12 to 3 am. However, maximum rail road accidents occurred during 6 to 9 am.

Mega cities refers to cities with population greater than 10 lakhs. Accidental deaths in such cities are higher than other cities, with maximum reported at Pune, Nasik, Indore, Meerut, Nagpur, Rajkot, Vijayawada, Jaipur, Delhi, Surat, Bengaluru, Agra, Kanpur, Jamshedpur, Amritsar, Kochi, Patna and Lucknow in decreasing order of frequency. Surprisingly, however death incidence is much lower in Mumbai and Kolkata.

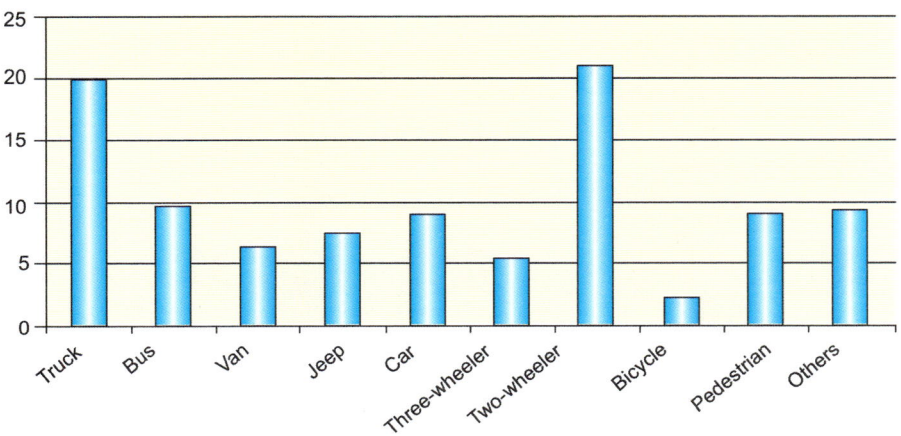

Fig. 2.3: Road accidents by type of vehicle

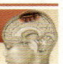

CONCLUSIONS

Epidemiology is defined as the study of the patterns of disease occurrence in human populations and the factors that influence them. The haddon phase matrix is used to identify and thereby to prevent injury. Majority of injuries occur in the middle aged and cause loss of productivity due to disability. Differences in age, gender, mechanism and intent have been noted.

REFERENCES

1. Lilienfeld AM, Lilienfeld DE. Foundations of Epidemiology. New York, Oxford University Press 1980;3–22.

2. MacKenzie EJ, Fowler C. Epidemiology. In Mattox KL, Feliciano DV, Moore EE (Ed). Trauma. New York, McGraw-Hill, 4th Ed,21–40.

3. Foulkes MA, Eisenberg HM, Jane JA, et al. The Traumatic Coma data Bank Research Group: The Traumatic Coma Data Bank: Design, methods and baseline characteristics. J Neurosurg 1991; 75:S8.

4. Kraus JF. Epidemiology of head injury. In Cooper PR (Ed). Head injury. Baltimore, Williams & Wilkins 1987;1–19.

5. Gururaj G. Epidemiology of traumatic brain injuries: Indian scenario. Neurol Res. 2002 Jan; 24(1):24–8.

6. Jennett . Epidemiology of head injury. Arch Dis Child 1998;78:403–406.

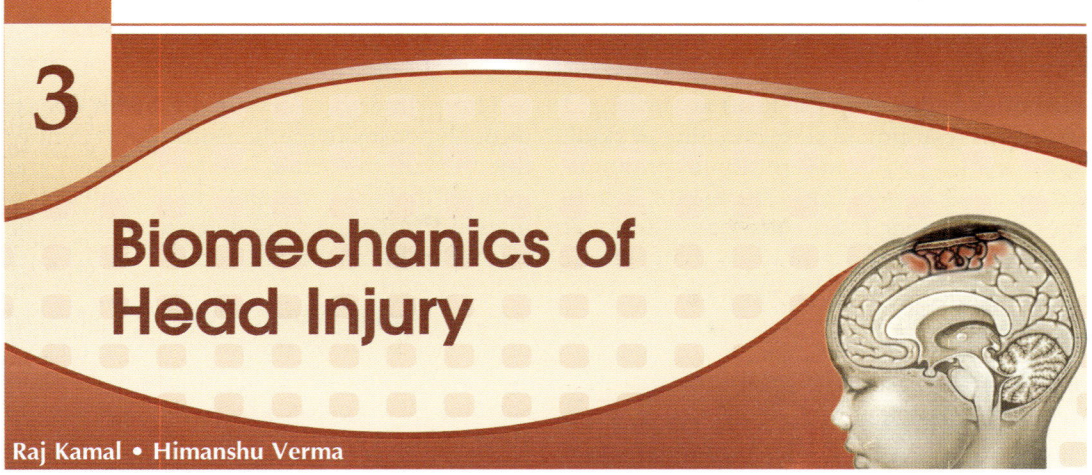

3

Biomechanics of Head Injury

Raj Kamal • Himanshu Verma

INTRODUCTION

Biomechanics is the application of the science of mechanics to the biological systems. Traumatic brain injuries can be classified according to whether the head is struck or strikes an object (contact or "impact" loading) and/or the brain moves within the skull (noncontact or "inertial" loading). The magnitude and direction of each type or combination of loading forces may predict type and severity of injury.[1] The mechanical forces can be classified (Fig. 3.1) as **dynamic or static** in nature.[1] **Dynamic loading** is more common and is defined as input force applied to the cranium in a very short time, usually less than 50 ms. There is considerable, but not perfect,

correlation between physical mechanism of injury and pathoanatomic injury type. For instance, most focal injuries, such as skull fracture, brain contusion, and epidural hematoma, result from impact loading, whereas **impulsive loading** generally causes more diffuse injuries such as concussion, subdural hematoma and diffuse axonal injury (DAI). Recently, there has been increased interest in blast mechanisms of brain injury, which are at present incompletely understood. Mechanistic classification has great utility in modeling injuries and in prevention.

Static loading is uncommon and is defined as input force applied to the load slowly in period greater than 200 ms. Typical examples of static loading are slowly moving vehicles,

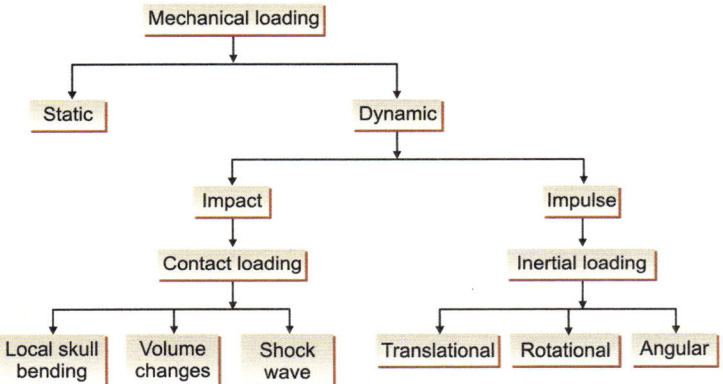

Fig. 3.1: Classification of the types of mechanical loading

11

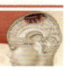

earthquakes that trap the head against rigid structures resulting in slow crushing of skull. **Static loading** will cause multiple comminuted fractures of vault or base of skull. Severe neurological deficits are uncommon and will be present only if the brain is distorted or compressed directly because of the static loading.

IMPULSIVE AND IMPACT LOADING

Impact loading and impulsive loading are two sub-types of dynamic loading. Impact load is defined as the dynamic effect on a structure, either moving or at rest, of a forcible momentary contact of another moving body. Impact loading is due to collision between two objects and is common type of dynamic loading usually a combination of contact forces and inertial forces. The quick impact force causes head to accelerate. In certain situation inertial effects are minimised when the head is immobilised following impact. Effects on intracranial structures and skull differ when head is allowed to accelerate or not in particular situation. The response of the skull to impact depends on the position of head and the object that strikes the head. This skull deformity will result in skull fracture if it exceeds the tolerance of skull. An impact will also produce contact effects on the head, such as skull deformation or fracture, with an associated risk of injury to the brain. However, in practice it appears that injury to the human brain is almost always the result of an impact to the head, or to a protective helmet, rather than an impulse transmitted through the neck.[2, 3]

Impulsive loading occurs when the head is set into motion or when the moving head arrested without its being struck or impacted. In impulsive loading there is no direct impact on the head hence no contact forces occur. The resulting head injuries are caused only by the inertial forces. A blow to the thorax or face car set head into violent motion without direct impact to the skull, e.g. fall from height or being thrown off a moving vehicle.

The primary injury to the brain occur; through two major mechanisms: Direct injuries due to skull distortion (contact injuries) and indirect that arise irrespective of skull deformation.[4,5] An impact to a given location on the head can be characterized by the impact velocity and the physical properties of the struck or striking object. There is no physical difference between the forces involved in a stationary head being hit or a moving head striking a fixed object, given that other factors such as the velocity of the impact and the characteristics of the object contacted by the head are the same. The severity of head injury depends upon the **physical properties of striking or struck object, location of the impact on brain, force of impact, response of head to impact and whether there is associated linear or angular acceleration.**[6] A concrete wall or floor is extremely hard and can cause severe head injury whereas, a thin sheet of glass is very hard on the surface but it will bend, or deflect, easily when loaded. It has a low level of stiffness, which, of course, decreases abruptly to zero when the glass breaks. Certain areas of brain, such as temporo-parietal areas require lesser force for producing skull fractures. Nahum[7] et al. (1968) estimated that for a contact area of approximately 1 square inch (6.5 cm²) the force required to produce a clinically significant skull fracture in the frontal area of the cadaver skull was twice that required in the temporoparietal area. High velocity head injury is usually very severe having both components of injury (impact and impulsive loading). For a given head impact velocity, an impact with a sheet metal panel of a car will result in a much smaller impact force, and hence lower acceleration of the head, than will an impact with a concrete floor.[6] This is because the moving head is brought to rest over a greater distance in the former case, as indicated by the considerable dent which is often seen in the panel following a head impact. However, the lower acceleration means that the impact force, albeit at a lower level, is acting on the head for a longer time. The severity of injury to the head depends on whether or not the head is free to change its velocity when struck[8] not, the skull may be crushed to a greater or lesser degree and the injury to the head, and the brain, will be directly related to the location and extent of the skull deformation. An example of such an impact would be a block falling on the head of a person lying on a concrete floor.

Contact injuries result from the forces that occur during direct impact. The direct impact results in complex mechanical events that occur both near and distant from the point of contact (contact phenomenon).

Contact injuries typically causes focal in juries, they do not cause diffuse brain injury Neural damage by this mechanism, therefore, is typically superficial and localized to the immediate vicinity of skull injury.[9,10] Since most impact set the head into motion, these injuries are associated with acceleration injuries contact forces have local and remote effects.

FOCAL EFFECTS

Effects of local contact include **depressed fractures, linear fractures, basilar skull fractures extradural hematoma and coup contusions.** Focal injuries produced by a direct impact to a localised area of the brain ranging from minor contusions (bruising) to direct penetration of the brain often associated with blunt or sharp object impacts. Cranial fractures can be produced by several different impact-loading mechanisms.

- Impact with a flat surface producing linear type fractures
- Impact with a blunt object producing localised depressed fractures
- Impact with a sharp pointed object producing depressed fractures (penetrating injuries).

Linear skull fractures[9] follows local skull bending occurring at the site of impact which exceeds the strain limit for the bone. The bone bends inwards like a cone and it breaks at inner table which forms the apex of cone. The inner table breaks first because of greater tensile strain on the inner table.

Depressed skull fractures are the result of concentrated force immediately beneath the impacting object. The area of hitting object is small enough to cause concentration of stress square and strain.

Figure 3.2 for objects larger than 2 sq inch, local skull deformation of the skull immediately beneath the point of impact. The momentum of object is bore by the localised area of skull and not to the remaining skull as in linear fractures. If the area of striking object is less than 2 square inch, the momentum may be strong enough to penetrate completely through the skull.

BIOMECHANICS OF HEAD INJURY

Forces and strains, are weaker to the tensile forces on the inner table. The fracture tends to follow the path of least resistance and splits into components thus dissipating the energy into fracture. The linear fracture is complete when the energy in the impact process is dissipated completely.

The direct impact to **mastoid and occiput** can produce basilar skull fractures in similar manner. A strong impact on facial bones can also result in basilar skull fracture.

Local bending of skull bones due to direct impact can lead to tear of dural vessels and injury to brain or pial vessels with or without fracture resulting in **epidural hematoma and coup contusions.**

High negative pressure develops when the inbent skull rapidly snaps back to its normal position which puts brain and pial vessels to a very high degree of tensile strain. This high strain can lead to disruption of pial vessels and cortical vessels resulting in localised contusion of brain.

REMOTE CONTACT EFFECTS

Remote contact effects are the result of skull distortion and stress waves. If the impacting object is broad and the impact occurs over a thick portion of the skull, then the remote thinner position of skull will bend due to

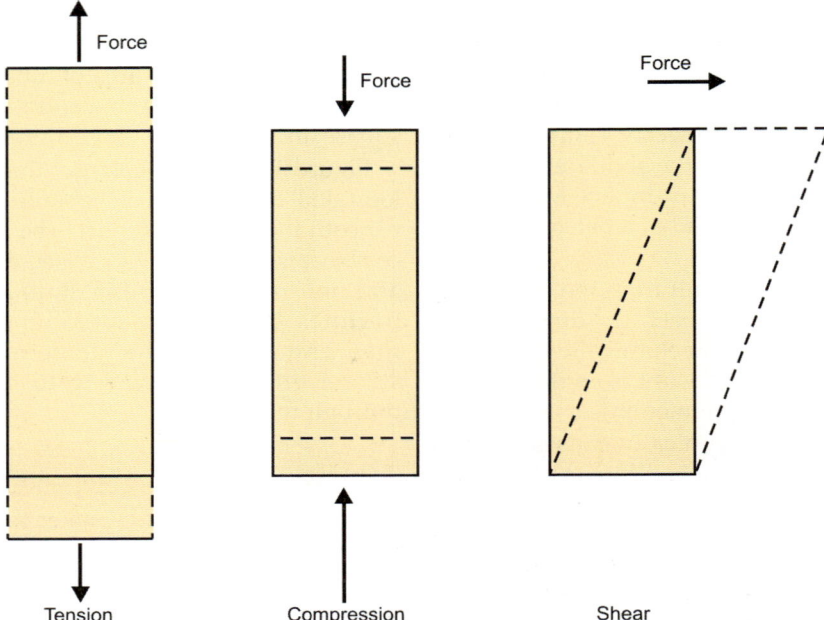

Fig. 3.2: Types of strains. Strain is the amount of deformation that tissue can undergo as a result of mechanical force

decreased tensile strength resulting in remote linear fracture.

Large broad impacts can lead to localised pressure changes and intracranial volume fluctuations. These changes are transient because of inherent elastic properties of the skull. Above mentioned events produce negative pressure at places where the skull has been pulled away from the brain (Fig. 3.3) which may result in contrecoup contusion. A sudden change in ICP can lead to brain herniations, e.g. tentorial herniation. The intracranial volume changes may explain part of distinct neurological and pathological observations found in infants and children with developing skulls that maintain a fair degree of flexibility.

Stress waves also account for the remote contact effects. Stress waves originate at the point of impact travelling at very high speed in all directions producing remote vault fractures, basilar fractures, potential hemorrhages and intracerebral hematomas.

INERTIAL INJURIES

These are commonly called acceleration and deceleration injuries. The acceleration of the head causes either a functional or structural failure of neural and vascular structures, where the severity and extent of disruption are linked to magnitude, rate, duration and type of inertial loading.[5] If the line of action (the vector) of the impact force passes through the center of gravity of the head then the head will be accelerated in a straight line. This is known as linear acceleration. However, if the force vector does not pass through the center of gravity then the head will be subjected to both linear and angular acceleration, with the latter resulting in rotation about the center of gravity.

Head motion will cause structural or functional damage by relative movement of brain in relation to dura and skull. Bridging veins may tear if the strain exceeds the vascular tolerance. The relative movement of brain away from skull creates tensile strain causing contrecoup contusions.[6]

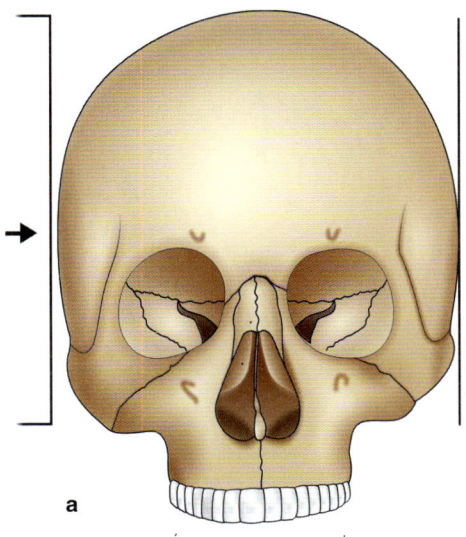
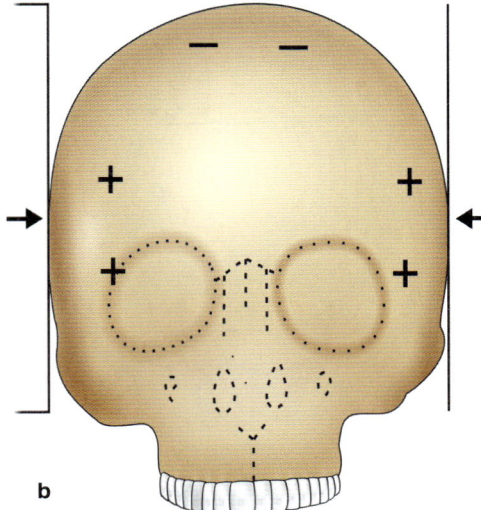

Figs 3.3a and b: Impact loading with no head motion. Note high pressure at the impact site and negative pressure at outward bending site

The head motion can produce strain in the brain parenchyma itself causing cerebral **concussion, diffuse axonal injury, deep petechial hemorrhages.**[11]

Three types of acceleration may occur (Figs 3.4a to c):

1. **Translational or linear acceleration** occurs when the brain moves in a straight line at its centre of gravity, i.e. pineal gland (Fig. 3.4a).

2. **Rotational acceleration** occurs when brain tissue moves around its static centre of gravity (Fig. 3.4b).

3. **Angular acceleration** occurs when there is movement of the centre of gravity in an angular manner. Angular acceleration is combination of both translational and rotational acceleration (Fig. 3.4c).

Angular acceleration is most commonly encountered clinically. The centre of angulation is usually mid cervical to lower cervical region. Higher the centre of angulation greater will be the rotational component. As the centre of gravity becomes lower in cervical spine, proportionately translational component increases.

Angular acceleration is most injurious and the severity depends on the amount of acceleration, its rate and duration. Angular acceleration or deceleration causes shear strain deformation, which is characterised by a change in shape without change in volume.[4,5] Shear strain forces are maximum at the junction of tissues of different density and rigidity. Shear strain develops because of differential movement of one portion of brain with respect to another portion. Neurons are highly susceptible to the shear strain forces.

Three zones (surface, intermediate, deep) of interest are encountered as acceleration duration increases at a constant acceleration.[6] At short acceleration duration, brain experiences very little strain resulting in only **surface** zone injury.

At longer acceleration duration, inertial effects are maximum and the resulting strains are able to propagate deeper into the brain. This can cause deep diffuse axonal injury. **Intermediate** zone injury occurs with acceleration duration is intermediate. Strain rate also increases if the acceleration magnitude is increased resulting in vascular tissue intolerance.

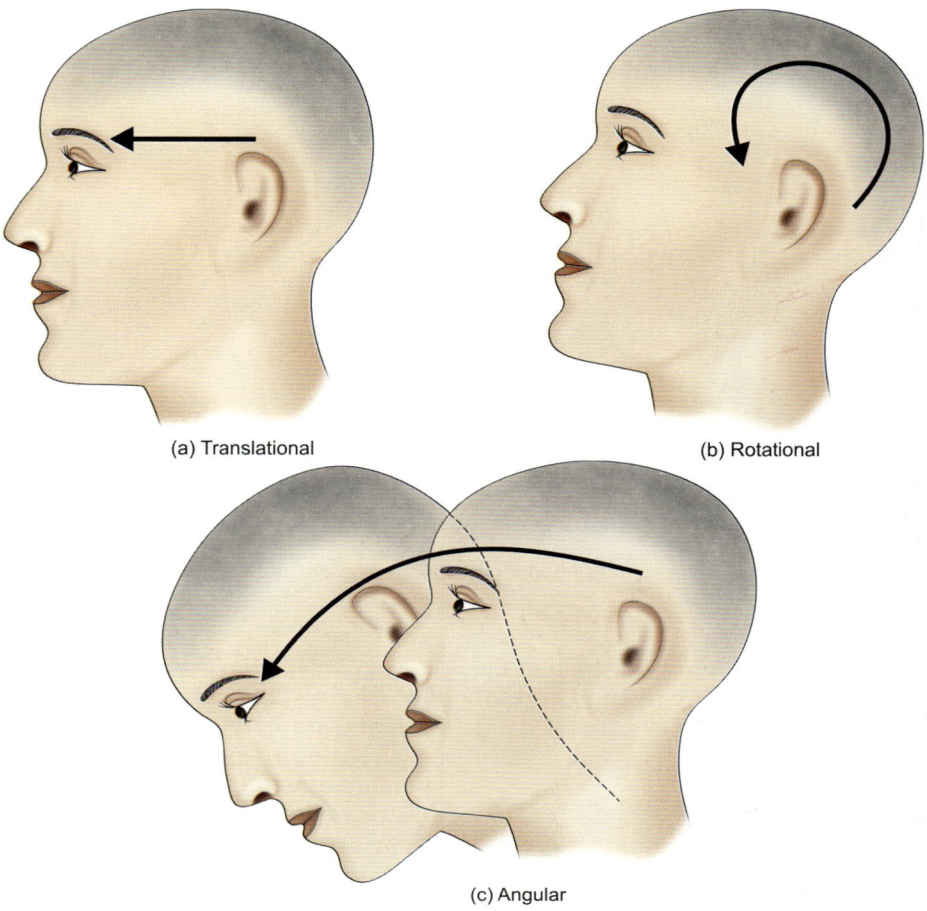

(a) Translational

(b) Rotational

(c) Angular

Figs 3.4a to c: Types of acceleration

Hence, structural damage to **superficial** vascular tissue (bridging veins and pial vessels) occurs in short acceleration duration with large acceleration magnitude whereas brain tissue injury occurs in longer duration and lesser acceleration magnitude.

Mechanism of Injuries

Skull fractures, epidural hematoma coup contusions: These are the result of contact injuries. In infants arid children, sutural diastasis may occur. The mechanisms of linear fracture, depressed fracture, basilar skull fractures, epidural hematoma and coup contusions are described above.

Contrecoup contusions: The predominant mechanism for **contrecoup contusions** is head acceleration (inertial effects). For contrecoup contusions impact is not necessary, hence the term is misnomer. In situations where the head undergoes impulsive loading, contrecoup lesions occur solely because of acceleration effects.[12]

A hard, small impact surface such as hammer blow tends to produce depressed fracture with underlying coup contusion with no contrecoup contusion. But, if the object has larger impact surface following fall then it results in a very little focal injury, more energy is converted into setting the head into motion, thus producing large contrecoup contusions.

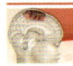

INTRACEREBRAL HEMATOMA

Intracerebral hematomas are usually associated with extensive cortical contusion in which larger and deeper vessels have been disrupted. Smaller hematomas that are not associated with contusion occurs because of stress waves concentration due to impact or acceleration induced tissue strains. Small deep hemorrhagic tensions are due to areas of strain concentration due to acceleration effects.

SUBDURAL HEMATOMA

Acute subdural hematoma is due to disruption of surface vessels, usually bridging veins. Disruption of bridging vein occurs mostly from inertial and not from contact forces.

Subdural hematoma (SDH) results from head acceleration that produce short duration, high strain ratio loading.[13] Hence subdural hematomas are usually associated with diffuse axonal injury (DAI). This explains those cases where SDH is small but associated brain damage is great.

Cerebral Concussion

Concussion refers to an immediate but transient loss of consciousness associated with a short period of amnesia. It occurs after deceleration of the frontal or occipital areas that creates sudden movement of brain within skull. Angular or rotational head motions cause transient electrophysiologic dysfunction of reticular activating system (RAS) in the upper midbrain, caused by rotation of the cerebral hemispheres on a relatively fixed brainstem. In this type of injury, most of the strain is insufficient to cause structural damage, but biochemical and ultrastructural changes such as mitochondrial ATP depletion and local disruption of the blood–brain barrier may occur. The physiological basis of amnesia is not yet clear.

DIFFUSE AXONAL INJURY

Diffuse axonal injury (DAI) considered to be severe form of concussion injury. Diffuse axonal injury is caused by angular acceleration or rotational acceleration. The extent of axonal damage depends upon magnitude, duration and rate of angular acceleration.[14] Normally, brain white matter tissue is compliant and responsive to stress, however under these strong mechanical forces, axons become stiff and brittle, making the axon far more susceptible to damage and deformation.[15] Immediately following the injury, a small subpopulation of axons is completely disconnected by shear inertial force. Diffuse axonal injury subsequently develops over a progressive pathophysiological process which occurs over the course of several hours, days, and weeks.[16] The extension of focal neuronal damage is centripetal from the cortex inward to the brainstem as the injury force increases. Almost all cases of severe DAI arise from vehicular accident in which acceleration is long. The direction of acceleration is important in the production of axonal injury. Sagittal acceleration only occasionally produces DAI of grade I. Angular acceleration is coronal plane has a high incidence of severe form of DAI.

HEAD INJURY PREVENTION

Head injury following vehicular accident could possibly be prevented through padding, load distribution and avoiding contact to an object. Head loading of impact is determined primarily by force. Most protective devices aim at reducing translational acceleration through reduction of the force acting upon the head during an impact. This also decreases rotational acceleration, thus preventing severe head injury like DAI or acute SDH. By using deformable padding materials, one expects that it will absorb forces that could injure head. An excellent example is padding of helmet. If moving head strikes an object that deforms and thereby allows a longer deceleration distance for the head, the forces generated would be lower. As a result the acceleration (deceleration) would be reduced. The extent of energy absorption depends strongly upon the material, the shape, and thickness of padding.

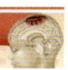

The energy absorption capabilities are increased by maximizing padding areas, padding thickness and uniformity of crushing strength of the padding material. Hence proper padding of car's interior and helmet are equally important. In addition to these mechanisms, all vehicles should be equipped with airbags and restraint systems like seat belt for head injury protection. The three point seat belt prevents head contact by restraining driver/passenger. It prevents/reduces risk of head striking the front region including steering wheel and dashboard (Fig. 3.5).

SEAT BELT AND AIRBAG (Figs 3.6a and b)

A seat belt is best protection in all types of collision. Airbags are designed to supplement seat belts, not replace them. Restrain with proper seat belts is must for airbags to be effective during unfortunate accident. Seat belts are single most important effective safety device for adults and children. Seat belts are designed to bear upon the bony structure of the body, and should be worn low across the front of the pelvis or the pelvis, chest and the shoulders.

Airbags are normally designed with the intention of supplementing the protection of an occupant who is correctly restrained with a seat belt. Most designs are inflated through pyrotechnic means and can only be operated once.

The first generation of airbags (Fig. 3.6b) followed this relatively simple deployment

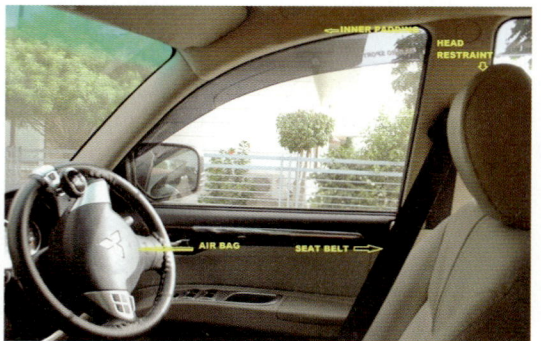

Fig. 3.5: Mandatory safety measures in a car

strategy. There is a collision severity, the deployment threshold, below which the airbags will not fire. The seat belt system provides adequate protection in such minor crashes. The vehicle's computer uses multiple criteria to judge if airbag deployment is required, thus it is not possible to give a single collision speed below which the airbags will not fire.

The chemical propellent is burnt and produces nitrogen gas, an inert component of normal air.

Risks of Airbag

Because airbag deployment happens so rapidly, it is extremely important that vehicle occupants should not be too close to the airbag modules. These are generally located in the steering wheel hub and the upper right-front dashboard. There would be significant risk of head, neck and chest injury if an occupant were to be struck by the flaps of the airbag cover as they open (punch out), or by the rapidly expanding fabric of the bag as it is inflated (membrane loading). Most agencies recommend that occupants should be at least 25 cm (10 inches) away from the airbag module. Children are at special risk (*see* next section).

Mechanism of Protection

Airbags are computer controlled. Sensors monitor the vehicle's deceleration and determine when a collision is occurring. If the crash is of sufficient severity, the computer commands the airbags to deploy. All this happens very quickly–typically in just a few hundredths of a second–faster than the blink of an eye! The airbag firing circuit is activated, the chemical propellent ignited, and the gas generated inflates the fabric of the airbag. This creates a cushion, spreading the forces of collision and allowing the occupant to avoid any hard contacts with portions of the vehicle's interior. Airbags are normally designed with the intention of supplementing the protection of an occupant who is correctly restrained with a seat belt. Most designs are inflated

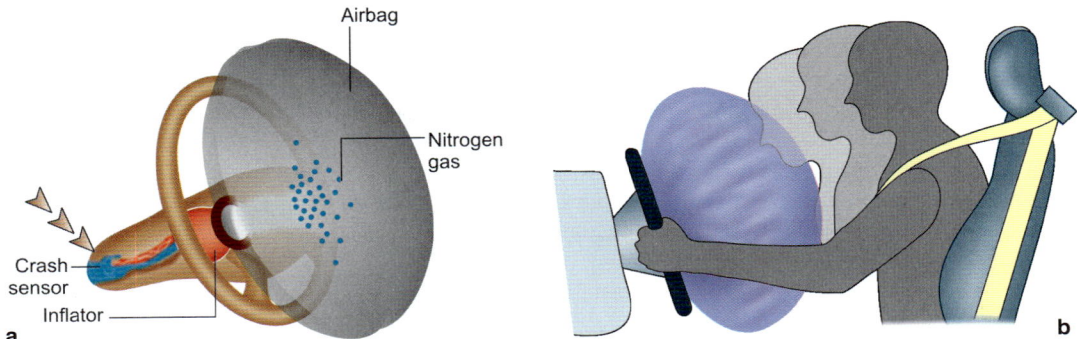

Figs 3.6a and b: Seat belt and airbag

through pyrotechnic means and can only be operated once.

The first generation of airbags followed this relatively simple deployment strategy. There is a collision severity, the deployment threshold, below which the airbags will not fire. The seat belt system provides adequate protection in such minor crashes. The vehicle's computer uses multiple criteria to judge if airbag deployment is required, thus it is not possible to give a single collision speed below which the airbags will not fire.

The chemical propellent is burnt and produces nitrogen gas, an inert component of normal air. Vehicle occupants often see "smoke" and believe that their vehicle is on fire. However, this is mostly a cloud of talcum powder coming from the folds of the airbag fabric where it is used as a lubricant to allow the bag to unfold smoothly.

Where a vehicle is equipped with dual (driver and right-front passenger) first-generation airbags, both airbags will normally be fired at the same time. But, some early-model vehicles were equipped with only a driver's airbag. Crash sensors respond to primarily frontal impacts. Consequently, airbags may very well not be deployed in rear-end collisions, side impacts, and rollovers. In angled frontal crashes deployment of the airbag is dependent on both the crash severity and the direction of the collision force (i.e. an impact more from the side than from the front may not deploy the bag).

Children and Airbags

Child passengers in the right-front seat of vehicles equipped with airbags are of particular concern. Rear-facing infant carriers should never be installed in the right-front seat when there is an airbag. This would place the child's head much too close to the passenger's airbag module. Many children have been killed or seriously injured in this manner. Similarly, most agencies recommend that children aged 12 and under should be seated in the rear of the vehicle with an age-appropriate restraint system (infant carrier, child seat, booster cushion and seat belt). Children frequently do not sit still in vehicles. They will often sit on the edge of their seat, lean forward, and may even slip their body out of the seat belt or child restraint harness. If a child were to do this in the right-front passenger's seat at the very instant that a collision occurred, they would be out of position and too close to the airbag, and this could easily result in serious injury or fatality.

CONCLUSIONS

The mechanical forces causing head injury can be classified into dynamic and static in nature. If the input force is applied to the cranium in short time (less than 50 ms) then it is called dynamic loading. Dynamic loading is further sub-classified into impact loading and impulsive loading. Direct impact results in contact injuries. Contact injuries cause skull fractures, extradural hematomas and coup contusions. Both impulsive and impact loading will result in acceleration injuries. Acceleration injuries are of 3 types (translational, rotational and angular). Acceleration produces different magnitude of strain in brain depending upon its rate and duration. Cerebral concussion, diffuse axonal injury and acute subdural hematoma are typical examples that occur following acceleration injuries.

REFERENCES

1. Gennarelli TA, Meaney DF. Cranial Trauma, Neurosurgery (ed). Wilkins RH, Rengachary SS, McGraw-Hill 1996;2611–22,.
2. McLean AJ. Brain injury without head impact? Journal of Neurotrauma 1995;12(4):621–5.
3. Tarriere C. Risk of head and neck injury if there is no direct head impact, in Proceedings of Head and Neck Injury Criteria: A Consensus Workshop, Session 1, National Highway Traffic Safety Administration, Washington, DC 1981;13–15.
4. Holbourn AHS. Mechanics of Head Injuries. Lancet 1943;2:438–41.
5. Holbourn AHS. The Mechanics of Brain Injuries. Br Med Bull 1945;3:147–9.
6. McLean AJ. Anderso RWG. Biomechanics of Closed Head Injury; In Head Injury Pathophysiology and Management, 2nd Edn (eds Reilly Pl and Bullock R). Hodder Arnold 2005; 26–40.
7. Nahum A, Gatts J, Gadd C, Danford J. Impact tolerance of the skull and face, Proc 2nd Stapp and crash conference SAE 1968;680–785.
8. Denny-Brown D and Russell WR. Experimental cerebral concussion. Brain 1941;64:93–164.
9. Row Botham GF. The mechanism of injuries to the head. In: Acute injuries of the head. (Ed) Row Botham GF, E & S Livingstone Ltd 1964;56.
10. Adams JH, Gennarelli TA, Graham DI. Brain Damage in nonmissile head injury: Observation in man and subhuman primates. In Smith W, Cavanal JB (eds). Recent advances in Neuropathology, Edin: Churchill Livingstone 1982;165–90.
11. Gennarelli TA. Head injury in man and experimental animals: Clinical aspects. Acta Neurochir (Wien) Supp 1983;32:1–13.
12. Ommaya AK, et al. Coup and contrecoup injury observations on the mechanics of visible brain injuries in the rhesus monkeys. J Neurosurg 1971;35:503.
13. Gennarelli TA, Thibault LE. Biomechanics of acute subdural hematoma, J Trauma 1982;22:680–6.
14. Adams JH, Graham DI, et al. Diffuse axonal injury due to non-missile head injury in humans; An analysis of 45 cases: Ann Neurol 1982;12:557–63.
15. Farkas O & Povlishock J. Cellular and subcellular change evoked by diffuse traumatic brain injury: a complex web of change extending far beyond focal damage. Progress in brain research 2007; 161:43–59.
16. Buki A, Okonkwo D, Wang K, Povlishock J. Cytochrome c Release and Caspase Activation in Traumatic Axonal Injury. J. Neuroscience 2000; 20:2825–34.

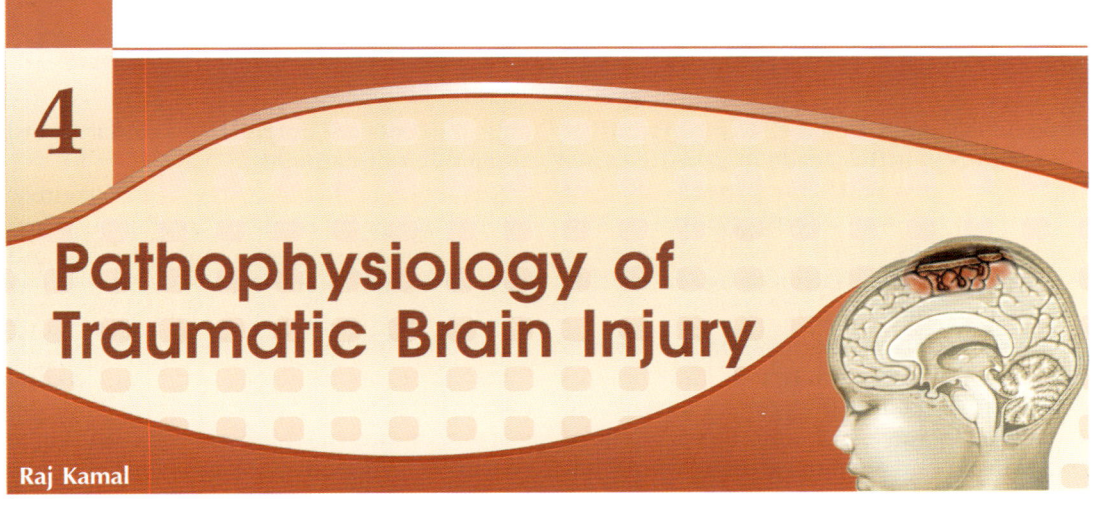

4

Pathophysiology of Traumatic Brain Injury

Raj Kamal

Traumatic brain injury (TBI) is an insult to the brain caused by an external physical force, resulting in functional disability. Falls and motor vehicle accidents are the primary causes of TBI, while sports, assaults and gunshot wounds also contribute significantly to these types of injuries. TBI is one of the leading causes of death and disability worldwide, including the developing world. Direct impact injury to brain produces parenchymal contusion and axonal injuries of brain. **Primary injuries trigger a sequence of events which result in alterations in brain metabolism, disruption of cerebral blood flow (CBF) and brain edema. These secondary alterations can produce increased intra-cranial pressure (ICP) and brain herniation.** Many casualties can be prevented by early recognition and successful treatment of these secondary derangements. In a study from the USA, traumatic coma data bank, on 716 patients hypotensional and hypoxia was associated with 150% increase in mortality rate.[1,2] Accordingly, another recent study from US, the death and disability correlate well with duration of systemic hypotension.[3,4]

Secondary changes ultimately produces cerebral ischemia and hypoxia.[5] Ischemia after head injury may result from (1) increased ICP, (2) local brain distortion secondary to clot and (3) vasoconstriction due to release of neurotransmitters. Hypoxia results from inadequate ventilation or problems of oxygen delivery.

The pathophysiology of TBI is complex and involves several pathways causing damage of the brain. **TBI has been classified into primary and secondary injury. The primary injury occurs at the time of trauma causing skull fractures, brain contusions, lacerations, diffuse axonal injuries, vascular tearing and intracranial hemorrhages. Secondary types of traumatic brain injury (TBI) are attributable to further cellular damage from the effects of primary injuries. Secondary injuries may develop over a period of hours or days following the initial traumatic assault.** Secondary neuronal damage is induced through several pathophysiologic mechanisms including raised intracranial pressure, disruption of blood–brain barrier, brain edema, decreased cerebral blood flow, altered tissue perfusion, cerebral hypoxia, ischemia and reperfusion injury.[5,6] **Furthermore, a cascade of molecular, neurochemical, cellular and immune processes contribute to secondary damage such as disruption of calcium homeostasis, oxidative stress, excitatory mediators release, cytoskeletal and mitochondrial dysfunction, inflammatory cell infiltration and neuronal cell apoptosis and death.**[7] Gene expression studies have demonstrated that several genes are implicated in the pathophysiology of secondary brain damage.[8]

Secondary damage to the brain results from intracranial hypertension and cerebral hypoxia/hypoperfusion which can lead to hypoxic-ischemic damage. **The consecutive Ca^{2+}- and Na^+-influx leads to self-digesting (catabolic) intracellular processes. Ca^{2+} activates lipid peroxidases, proteases, and phospholipases which in turn increase the intracellular concentration of free fatty acids and free radicals.**

The secondary pathophysiological events are potentially avoidable and amenable to treatment. Currently, the primary focus in the acute management of traumatic brain injury is to prevent and ameliorate these events that reduce secondary brain injury. In practice, the multimodality brain monitoring to certain extent, bears much reflection of these complex inter-related events, and hence explains the rationale of intense ICU monitoring.

MOLECULAR AND CELLULAR MECHANISMS OF SECONDARY BRAIN INJURY

Ischemia or hypoxia will cause decrease in ATP level because of anaerobic glycolysis. In presence of oxygen, pyruvate is oxidised through the reactions of Krebs cycle, generating a net 36 moles of ATP per mole of glucose by the reaction of oxidative phosphorylation. Anaerobic glycolysis produces only 2 moles of ATP per mole of glucose. The Na^+, K^+ pump uses ATP and pumps $2K^+$ into cell and $3Na^+$ out of cell across cell membrane. The Ca^{2+} pumps out $2Ca^{2+}$ out of cell per ATP (Fig. 4.1).

Secondary damage to the brain results from intracranial hypertension and cerebral hypoxia/hypoperfusion which can lead to **hypoxic-ischemic damage**. The consecutive Ca^{2+}- and Na^+-influx (Figs 4.2 and 4.3) leads to self-digesting (catabolic) intracellular processes. Ca^{2+} activates lipid peroxidases, proteases, and phospholipases which in turn increase the intracellular concentration of free fatty acids and free radicals. **Additionally, activation of caspases (ICE-like proteins, interleukin-1β converting enzyme ICE), translocases, and endonucleases initiates progressive structural changes of biological membranes and the nucleosomal DNA (DNA fragmentation and inhibition of DNA repair). The secondary pathophysio-** logical events are potentially avoidable and amenable to treatment.

Secondary brain damage is produced either by hypoxia or by ischemia/oligemia. When delivery of substrates, mainly glucose and oxygen, is inadequate to sustain cellular function, a series of inter-related biochemical reactions known as ischemic cascade is initiated. Other biochemical processes leading to a greater severity of injury include an increase in extracellular potassium, leading to edema; an increase in cytokines, contributing to inflammation; and a decrease in intracellular magnesium, contributing to calcium influx.

The cascades involved opening of **voltage dependent and agonistgated ion and calcium channels causing intracellular calcium and sodium overload and efflux of potassium** (Figs 4.2 and 4.3). Intracellular sodium overload causes cytotoxic oedema while efflux of potassium leads to peri-infarcted brain tissue depolarisation and seizures. **Influx of calcium is further promoted by the release of large amount of excitatory amino acids particularly glutamate. Intracellular calcium and glutamate act in a vicious circle which augments the amount of intracellular calcium.** Excess intracellular calcium can induce damage to the organelles such as mitochondria, intracellular second messengers, cellular membrane and activation of numerous intracellular enzymes system which finally lead to cell death.

MODES OF CELL DEATH

There are three types of cell death which are described for mammalian cell: **Necrosis, Apoptosis, and Autophagy,** each of which exhibits a distinct histologic and biochemical signature.[11] Necrosis is nonprogramed cell death in response to overwhelming stress that is incompatible with cell survival. But recent evidences suggest that necrosis can also be tightly regulated. Apoptosis, or programed cell death, plays an important role in both physiologic and pathologic conditions. **Autophagy** or **autophagocytosis**, is a catabolic process involving the degradation of a cell's

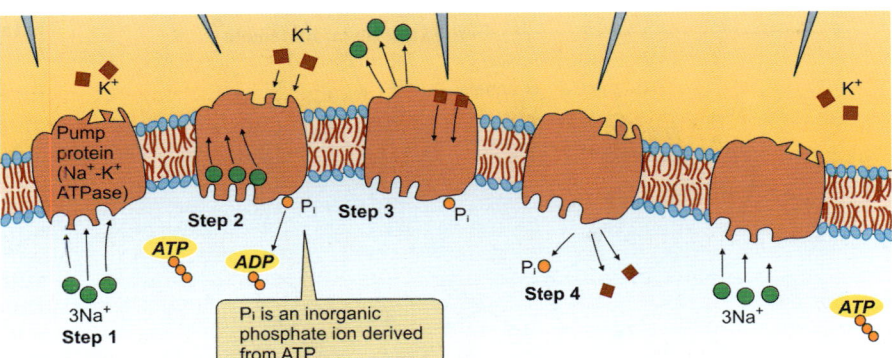

Fig. 4.1: Na+-K+ ATPase pump; physiology. **Step1:** Three Na+ ions bind to the ATPase under conditons of low Na+ concentrations because ATP and the transport protein has a high affinity for Na+. This means the protein will bind Na+ ions even when the Na+ concentration is low. Mg++ bind to the protein, **Step 2:** The transport protein cleaves ATP into ADP and phosphate ion. The phosphate ion becomes covalently bonded to the protein. The phosphorylated of the protein is unstable and the protein changes conformation. The shift in conformation of the protein in some manner causes the Na+ to travel across the protein and they are released from the protein on the other side of the membrane because the protein now has a low affinity for Na+, **Step 3 and 4:** K+ ions bind to the protein even it there is a low K+ concentration because in this conformation the protein has a high affinity for K+ ions. The covalently bound phosphate group is cleaved from the protein which causes the protein to undergo another conformational shift. This conformational shift causes the K+ to be in some manner transported across the protein and released on the other side of the membrane. The K+ ion is released because now the protein has a low affinity for K+ ions. The protein is restored to the ordinal conformation of the protein and the process starts again

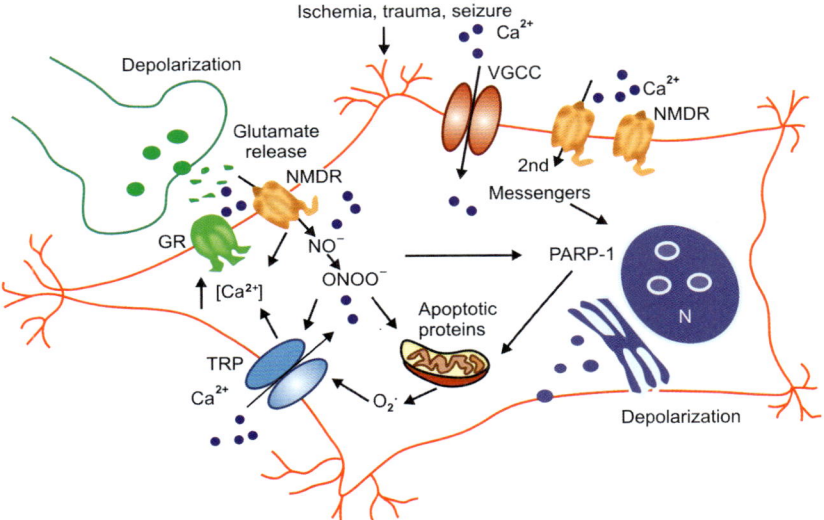

Fig. 4.2: Excitotoxicity due to glutamate release; Over-activation of glutamate receptors (GR) in an excitatory synapse leads to Ca^{2+} influx (dark circles, Ca^{2+}) in the postsynaptic neuron, via N-methyl-D-aspartate receptors (NMDR), voltage-gated Ca^{2+} channels (VGCC) and non-specific cation conductances via transient receptor potential (TRP) channels. TRP is one of the hundreds of channels that broker the passage of charged ions across impermeable lipid bilayers. Ca^{2+} entering, in particular via NMDARs activates neurotoxic signaling cascades. During acute neuronal injury, excess nitric oxide can result in the formation of peroxynitrite, a toxic free radical that causes direct damage to cellular structures

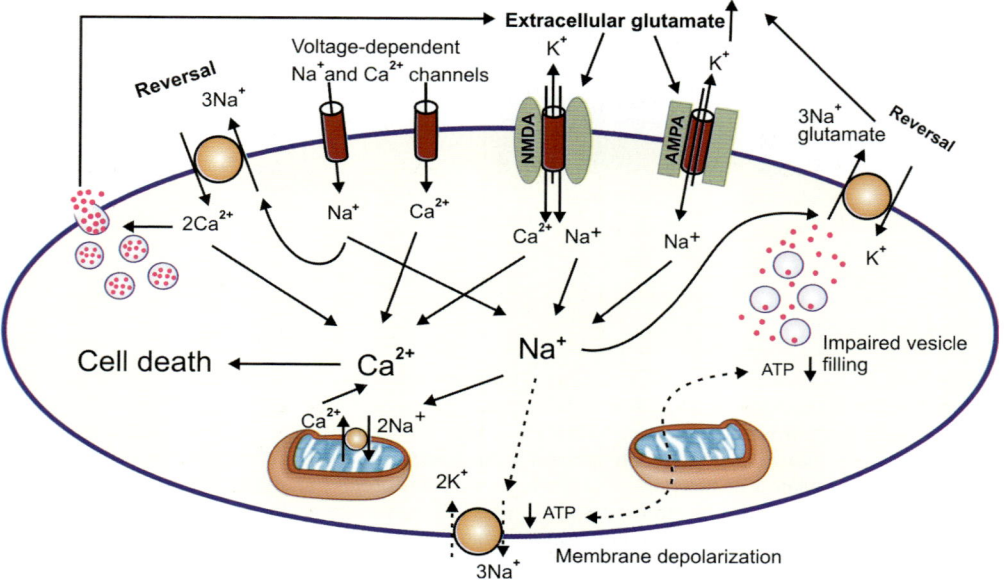

Fig. 4.3: Cell death due to excess intracellular calcium ion

own components. Autophagy is a tightly regulated process that is essential to embryonic development and cell survival, helping recycling of cellular products.

Cell Death; Excitotoxicity and Apoptosis

Necrotic cell death is morphologically characterized by cell swelling, that culminates in the rupture of the plasma memebrane, swelling of the mitochondria and other organelles. The nucleus exhibits pyknosis and irregular clumping of the chromatin. The initial stages of cerebral injury after TBI are characterized by direct tissue damage and impaired regulation of CBF and metabolism. This 'ischemia-like' pattern leads to accumulation of lactic acid due to anaerobic glycolysis, increased membrane permeability, and consecutive edema formation. Since the anaerobic metabolism is inadequate to maintain cellular energy states, the ATP-stores deplete and failure of energy-dependent membrane ion pumps occurs. The second stage of the pathophysiological cascade is characterized by terminal membrane depolarization along with

excessive release of excitatory neurotransmitters (i.e. glutamate, aspartate), activation of N-methyl-D-aspartate, α-amino-3-hydroxy-5-methyl-4-isoxazol-propionate, and voltage-dependent Ca^{2+}- and Na^+-channels (Figs 4.2 and 4.3). This process is commonly known as **excitotoxicity**. Excitotoxicity is not a single event but rather a cascade of events.

Excitatory amino acids (EAAs), including glutamate and aspartate, are significantly elevated after a TBI.[12] EAAs results in influx of chloride and sodium, leading to acute neuronal swelling. EAAs can also cause an influx of calcium, which is linked to delayed damage. Increased calcium influx, activates nitric oxide (NO) synthases leading to a toxic production of NO (Figs 4.2 and 4.3). Moreover, after TBI, free radicals are highly produced and participate to a deleterious oxidative stress. **Evidence has showed that the major toxic effect of NO comes from its combination with superoxide anion leading to peroxynitrite formation,** a highly reactive and oxidant compound (Fig. 4.4). Indeed, peroxynitrite mediates nitrosative stress and is a

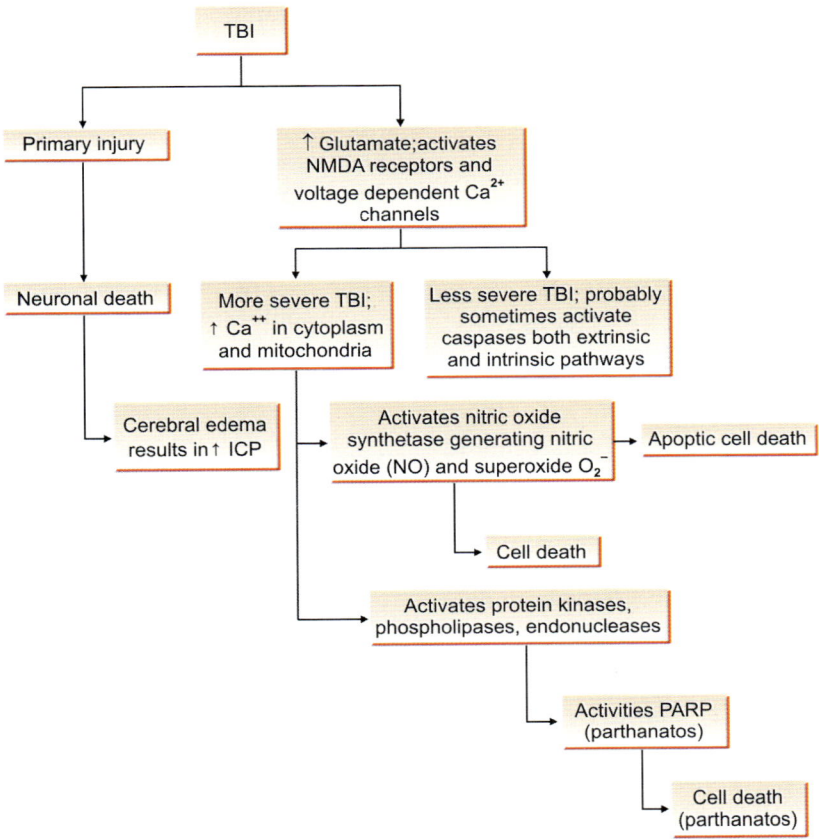

Fig. 4.4: Cascade of chemical and macroscopic events depicting necrotic/apoptic cell death following TBI. Parthanatos is due to overactivity of PARP [Poly(ADP-ribose) polymerase]

potent inducer of cell death through its reaction with lipids, proteins and DNA.[13]

Another critical pathway is activation of poly-ADP-ribose polymerase (PARP). PARP-1 is a nuclear enzyme implicated in DNA repair. In response to excessive DNA damage, massive PARP activation leads to energetic depletion and finally to cell death. David et al[14] coined the term parthanatos after thanatos, the personification of death in Greek mythology, to refer to PAR-mediated cell death.

Glutamate acting on N-methyl-D-aspartate (NMDA) receptors induces neuronal injury following stroke, through activation of poly (ADP-ribose) polymerase-1 (PARP-1) and

generation of the death molecule poly(ADP-ribose) (PAR) polymer. Andrabi et al.[15] identified Iduna, a previously undescribed NMDA receptor-induced survival protein that is neuroprotective against glutamate NMDA receptor-mediated excitotoxicity both *in vitro* and *in vivo* and against stroke through interfering with PAR polymer-induced cell death **(parthanatos)** (Fig. 4.4). Along with N-methyl-D-aspartate receptor agonists, which also contribute to increased calcium influx, EAAs may decrease high-energy phosphate stores (adenosine 5'-triphosphate, or ATP) or increase free radical production. EAAs can cause astrocytic swellings via volume-activated anion channels (VRACs). Tamoxifen is a potent inhibitor of VRACs and potentially could be of therapeutic value.

Apoptosis, or programed cell death, is regulated by Caspases. Caspases are a family of cysteine proteases and are executioners of cell death. In response to CNS injury, microglia become active and induce detrimental neurotoxic effects by releasing a diverse set of cytotoxic substances, including proinflammatory cytokine TNF-α.[23, 24] TNF-α plays a key role in many physiological and pathological processes including acute and chronic inflammation, and apoptosis.[25] Accordingly, TNF-α produced by microglia is generally thought to induce sequential activation of caspases ultimately resulting in the apoptosis.[26,27] Amongst caspases, activated caspase-3 is directly linked to the neuronal cell death following TBI.[28] Programed cell death (which is often referred to as apoptosis although strictly speaking this refers to the distinct morphological changes after programed cell death) is a genetic mechanism by which cells are eliminated during development and is the physiological mechanism by which cells are normally removed in the adult animal.[19] Following TBI there is increased expression of two main sets of genes which are genes encoding for the caspase family of **cysteine proteases [interleukin-1α converting enzyme (ICE) and CPP32]** (cysteine protease protein 32) **and a family of genes that are homologous to the oncogene Bcl-2** that either promote or suppress cell death. **The Bcl-2 gene family controls both caspase dependent and independent apoptosis.**[19, 21–23] The endpoint of all these steps is fragmentation of cellular DNA with collapse of the nuclear structure, followed by the formation of membrane-wrapped apoptotic bodies, cleared by macrophages.[24]

Apoptosis is now recognised as an important factor in secondary brain injury.[25] Following TBI, two different types of cells are visible; type 1 and 2 cells. The type 1 cells show a classic necrotic pattern (this follows the primary brain injury) and type 2 cells show a classic apoptotic pattern on microscopy.[19,25] Cells undergoing apoptosis die without membrane rupture and therefore elicit less inflammatory reactions. This is in contrast to the cells undergoing necrosis.[26] There is therefore a suggestion that neuronal apoptosis after TBI may be a protective response by the brain in order to remove injured tissue cells whilst having little effect on remaining brain tissue.[27] Apoptotic cells have been identified within contusions in the acute post-traumatic period and in regions remote from the site of injury days and weeks after trauma.

Oxidative Stress

Oxidative stress is due to production of **ROS (reactive oxygen species, also known as free radicals).** Free radicals can cause membrane damage through peroxidation of unsaturated fatty acids in the phospholipids making up the cell membrane.[37] The ROS particularly responsible in oxidative stress are nitric oxide (NO) and superoxide radical anion (O_2^-).[36] The toxicity of ROS can be farther increased by the reaction between the two ROS to form peroxynitrite $(ONOO^-)$, a molecule that causes oxidation and nitration of tyrosine residues on proteins. Low quantity of ROS are controlled by endogenous antioxidant systems that include superoxide dismutase (SOD), glutathione peroxidase, catalase and antioxidant vitamins.[36] However, large quantity of **ROS can cause damage of membrane lipids, peroxidation of docosahexaenoic acid, cleavage of DNA during the hydroxylation of guanine and methylation of cytosine.**[36] **ROS can also block mitochondrial respiration by inhibiting complex enzymes involved in the electron transport chain.**[38]

Associated Inflammation

The BBB is disrupted after TBI resulting in invasion of neutrophils, monocytes and lymphocytes from the periphery and activation of microglia and other resident cells and thus initiating a potent inflammatory response. The initiation, progression and resolution of inflammation in TBI is multifaceted involving

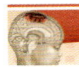

leukocyte infiltration, activation of resident immune cells and secretion of inflammatory mediators such as pro- and anti-inflammatory cytokines, chemokines, adhesion molecules, complement factors, reactive oxygen species and other factors. Several lines of evidence support a dual role for the neuroinflammation either detrimental or beneficial depending on the extent, time and site of induction. Elucidation of the inflammatory cascade in the injured brain would offer the possibility of novel therapies. Inflammation after TBI is believed to be triggered by several factors such as extravasated blood products, tissue debris, intracellular components, complement fragments, prostaglandins, reactive oxygen and nitrogen species. A biphasic BBB breakdown after TBI has been reported with a first opening occurring immediately after the primary impact reaching a maximum permeability within a few hours and then being declined. A second-delayed opening as a result of secondary injury cascades was found to peak around 3–7 days following TBI and can last from days to years.[34, 35]

Acidosis

Failure of Na^+, K^+ pump and Ca^{2+} pump following non-availability of ATP will result in (1) increase in intracellular Na^+, (2) increase in intracellular accumulation of Ca^{2+} and (3) intracellular acidosis. Acidosis further inhibits glycolysis. Thus a vicious cycle is established. Acidosis alters protein function, displacing Ca^{2+} from intracellular binding sites. So acidosis and Ca^{2+} pump failure leads to significant increase in intracellular Ca^{2+}, which activates Ca^{2+} dependent proteases, causing proteolysis and breakdown of cell membrane. Phospholipases are also activated by intracellular Ca^{2+}, which causes release of FFA. Free fatty acids disrupt the lipid portion of cell membranes.

CBF is closely coupled with the cerebral metabolism (Table 4.1). Following severe traumatic brain injury relationship between metabolism and cerebral blood flow (also called metabolism-CBF coupling) has been

Table 4.1: The relationship between brain activity $CMRO_2$ and CBF[37]

		$CMRO_2$ ml/100 g/min	CBF
Unconscious	Epilepsy	9	150
		8	125
	Delirium	7	
	Anxiety	6	100
	Excitation	5	
Conscious	Alertness	4	75
	Sleep	3	50
		2	
Unconscious		1	25
	Death	0	0

found to be abnormal. CBF is often normal in presence of low metabolism (relative hyperemia) or high CBF in relation to normal metabolism (absolute hyperemia. Continuous jugular venous bulb's oxygen saturation measurements have been used to estimate $CMRO_2$/CBF ratio.[9] **Metabolic demands can be reduced by barbiturate induced coma by increasing the availability of O_2 in ischemic cortex provided mean arterial pressure is maintained.**[10]

Brain Edema

Brain edema is defined as a net increase in the water content of cerebral tissue that leads to an increase in overall brain mass. Brain swelling refers to increase in brain volume, caused by increase in intracranial blood volume and brain edema.

Classically, two major types of traumatic brain edema exist: "vasogenic" due to blood–brain barrier (BBB) disruption resulting in extracellular water accumulation and "cytotoxic" due to sustained intracellular water collection.[35] Characteristics of the BBB are depicted in Fig. 4.5. Rarely, after TBI do we encounter a "interstitial" brain edema related to an obstruction of cerebrospinal fluid outflow. Following TBI, various mediators are released which enhance vasogenic and/or cytotoxic brain edema. These include glutamate, lactate, H^+, K^+, Ca^{2+}, nitric oxide, arachidonic acid and

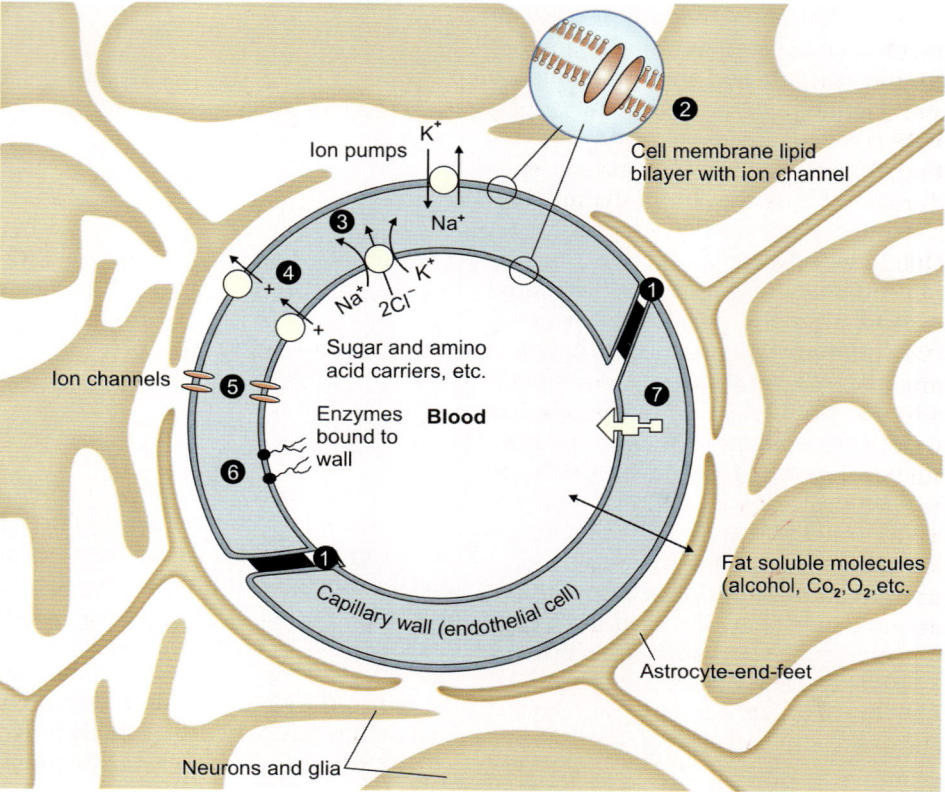

Fig. 4.5: Characteristics of the blood–brain barrier (BBB) are indicated: (1) tight junctions that seal the pathway between the capillary (endothelial) cells; (2) the lipid nature of the cell membranes of the capillary wall which makes it a barrier to water-soluble molecules; (3), (4) and (5) represent some of the carriers and ion channels; (6) the 'enzymatic barrier' that removes molecules from the blood; (7) the efflux pumps which extrude fat-soluble molecules that have crossed into the cells

its metabolites, free oxygen radicals, histamine and kinins.[35] (Also, *refer* to Chapter 6: Traumatic Brain Edema.)

Vasogenic edema refers to the influx of fluid and solutes into the brain through incompetent blood–brain barrier (BBB).

The fluid resultant from BBB disruption is usually protein rich, having more characteristics of blood ultrafilterate. **Vasogenic edema** extends preferentially through white matter. The spread of vasogenic edema compromises local microcirculation, adding further ischemic insult to edematous area. Clinically, vasogenic edema is demonstrated by hypodensity of the white matter on computed tomography (CT).

In **cytotoxic edema** cellular swelling occurs. BBB remains intact. Following severe head injuries astrocytic swelling was seen three hours to three days after injury. Breakdown of cell membrane following traumatic brain injury is the cause of cytotoxic edema. As discussed above, cell membrane breakdown results from ischemia which causes failure of Na^+-K^+ pump and Ca^{2+} pump, release of free fatty acids (FFA) and free radicals. Cellular swelling can produce numerous deleterious secondary effects in the cell, including membrane depolarization secondary to loss of intracellular K^+ release and decreased uptake of excitatory amino acids, as seen in astrocytes.

CBF

Cerebral blood flow is measured as volume of blood delivered to a defined mass of brain tissue per unit time, usually ml/gm/min. The mean CBF obtained in an adult male by Kety was 54 ml/100 g/min.[7] Gray matter flows are considerably higher than those in white matter, with typical relative values of 70 and 20 ml/100 g/min, respectively. CBF values are higher in children and decrease after the age of 60 years. For the entire brain, CBF amounts 750 to 900 ml/min. Cerebral tissue requires constant optimum perfusion in order to maintain adequate delivery of substrate. Although brain mass is only is 2% of body mass but it receives 15–20% of cardiac output. Cerebral perfusion pressure (CPP) provides the driving force for circulation across the capillary beds of brain. CPP represents the pressure gradient across the intracranial compartment and is defined as the mean arterial pressure (MAP) minus the ICP.

$$CPP = MAP - ICP$$

Cerebral autoregulation is defined as the maintenance of a constant level of CBF in the presence of alterations in systemic arterial pressure. Cerebral autoregulation fails below 70 mm Hg and above 150 mm Hg.

Disordered autoregulation may occur following traumatic brain injury, causing CBF to become passively dependent on mean arterial pressure (hence cerebral perfusion pressure or CPP). In absence of an autoregulatory response, moderate or transient hypotension can cause cerebral ischemia (Fig. 4.6).

Cerebral autoregulation refers to the physiologic response where by CBF remains constant over a wide range of blood pressure as a consequence of alterations of cerebrovascular resistance (CVR). The main regulator of brain blood flow is pressure-dependent activation of smooth muscle in the arterioles of the brain. The control over CBF is mainly Myogenic. The more the arteriole is stretched, the more it contracts and this lasts as long as the stretch occurs. CBF is equal to the cerebral perfusion pressure (CPP) divided by the cerebrovascular resistance (CVR):[7]

$$CBF = CPP / CVR = MAP - ICP/CVR$$

Hence CBF increases with increase in MAP (mean arterial pressure) and decrease in CVR (cerebrovascular resistance).

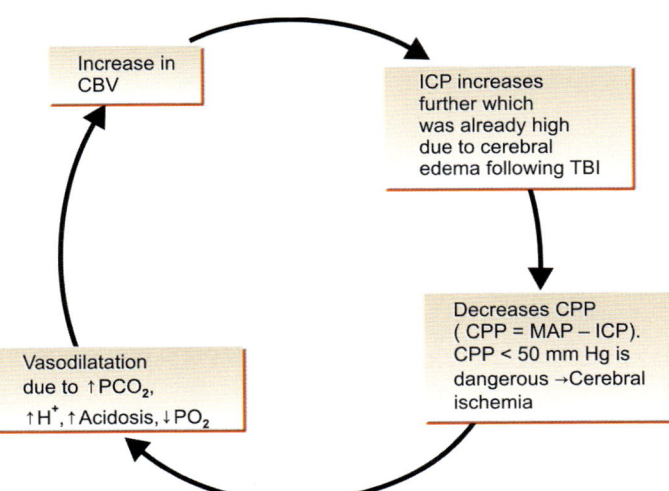

Fig. 4.6: Vicious cycle following TBI, resulting in cerebral ischemia and raised ICP. CPP: cerebral perfusion pressure, CBV: cerebral blood volume, MAP: mean arterial pressure, ICP: intracranial pressure

The Hagen-Poiseuille equation predicts that the pressure-flow relationship goes through the origin. Assuming constant CVR, CBF and CPP would be perfectly proportional, going to zero with zero CPP (Fig. 4.7). For changes in the CPP so short-lasting that cerebral autoregulation or other factors changing the caliber of the resistance vessels do not react, this theory assumes that the relationship between CPP and CBF would be a linear one illustrated by the straight lines in the figure going toward the origin. This can be described as the dynamic cerebral pressure-flow relationship. In contrast, the static cerebral pressure-flow relationship is the familiar autoregulation curve illustrated by the thick line in the figure, i.e. the horizontal portion of the pressure-flow curve. This allows CVR to change in order to compensate for variations in CPP. This is accomplished by a shift between the dynamic pressure-flow relationship lines. This model of dynamic and static changes covers both fast and slow aspects in the cerebral pressure-flow relationship. The dynamic pressure-flow curves are valid only for short time intervals when there is no change in vasomotor tone. The static pressure-flow curve, on the other hand, represents the pressure-flow relationship when sufficient time has elapsed so that the dynamic behavior of the autoregulation mechanism has settled down.

Factors which influence CBF are:
i. Arterial partial pressure of CO_2, H^+
ii. Oxygen deficiency

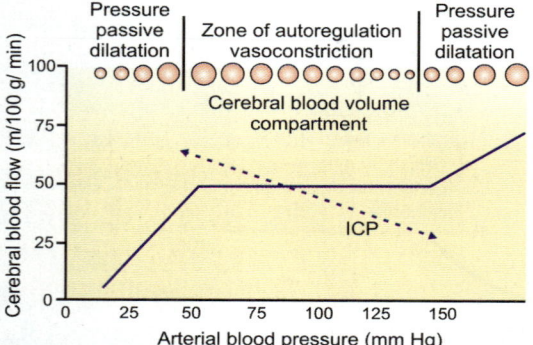

Fig. 4.7: Cerebral autoregulation

iii. Substances released from astrocytes.
iv. CPP.

i. **Carbon dioxide** is believed to increase cerebral blood flow by combining first with water in the body fluids to form carbonic acid, with subsequent dissociation of this acid to form hydrogen ions. The hydrogen ions then cause vasodilation of the cerebral vessels—the dilation being almost directly proportional to the increase in hydrogen ion concentration up to a blood flow limit of about twice normal. Other substances that increase the acidity of the brain tissue, and therefore, increase hydrogen ion concentration will likewise increase cerebral blood flow (Fig. 4.6). Such substances include lactic acid, pyruvic acid and any other acidic material formed during the course of tissue metabolism. Increased hydrogen ion concentration greatly depresses neuronal activity. Therefore, it is fortunate that increased hydrogen ion concentration also causes increased blood flow, which in turn carries hydrogen ions, carbon dioxide, and other acid-forming substances away from the brain tissues. Loss of carbon dioxide removes carbonic acid from the tissues; this, along with removal of other acids, reduces the hydrogen ion concentration back toward normal. Thus, this mechanism helps maintain a constant hydrogen ion concentration in the cerebral fluids and thereby helps to maintain a normal, constant level of neuronal activity.

ii. **Oxygen deficiency** as a regulator of cerebral blood flow.
Except during periods of intense brain activity, the rate of utilization of oxygen by the brain tissue remains within narrow limits—almost exactly 3.5 (±0.2) ml of oxygen per 100 grams of brain tissue per minute. If blood flow to the brain ever becomes insufficient to supply this needed amount of oxygen, the oxygen deficiency almost immediately causes vasodilation, returning the brain blood flow and

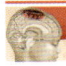

transport of oxygen to the cerebral tissues to near normal. Thus, this local blood flow regulatory mechanism is almost exactly the same in the brain as in coronary blood vessels, in skeletal muscle, and in most other circulatory areas of the body.

Experiments have shown that a decrease in cerebral tissue PO_2 below about 30 mm Hg (normal value is 35 to 40 mm Hg) immediately begins to increase cerebral blood flow. This is fortuitous because brain function becomes deranged at lower values of PO_2, especially so at PO_2 levels below 20 mm Hg. Even coma can result at these low levels. Thus, the oxygen mechanism for local regulation of cerebral blood flow is an important protective response against diminished cerebral neuronal activity and therefore, against derangement of mental capability.

iii. **Substances released from astrocytes as regulators of cerebral blood flow**

Increasing evidence suggests that the close coupling between neuronal activity and cerebral blood flow is due, in part, to substances released from astrocytes (also called astroglial cells) that surround blood vessels of the central nervous system. Astrocytes are star-shaped non-neuronal cells that support and protect neurons, as well as provide nutrition. They have numerous projections that make contact with neurons and the surrounding blood vessels, providing a potential mechanism for neurovascular communication. Gray matter astrocytes (protoplasmic astrocytes) extend fine processes that cover most synapses and large foot processes that are closely apposed to the vascular wall.

Experimental studies have shown that electrical stimulation of excitatory glutaminergic neurons leads to increases in intracellular calcium ion concentration in astrocyte foot processes and vasodilation of nearby arterioles. Additional studies have suggested that the vasodilation is mediated by several vasoactive metabolites released from astrocytes. Although the precise mediators are still unclear, nitric oxide, metabolites of arachidonic acid, potassium ions, adenosine, and other substances generated by astrocytes in response to stimulation of adjacent excitatory neurons have all been suggested to be important in mediating local vasodilation.

iv. **Cerebral perfusion** is an important factor. CPP between 60 and 70 is safe. CPP below 60–65 mm of Hg in adult or below 55 mm of Hg in child is consider critical, below which ischemic changes occur.[16,17] As autoregulation is disrupted in severe head injury, CBF is largely dependent an CPP.[17]

After TBI, CBF autoregulation (i.e. cerebrovascular constriction or dilation in response to increases or decreases in CPP) is impaired or abolished in most patients.[41–45] Defective CBF autoregulation may be present immediately after trauma or may develop over time, and is transient or persistent in nature irrespective of the presence of mild, moderate, or severe damage. Also, autoregulatory vasoconstriction seems to be more resistant compared with autoregulatory vasodilation which indicates that patients are more sensitive to damage from low rather than high CPPs.

Compared with CBF autoregulation, cerebrovascular CO_2-reactivity (i.e. cerebrovascular constriction or dilation in response to hypo- or hypercapnia) seems to be a more robust phenomenon. In patients with severe brain injury and poor outcome, CO_2-reactivity is impaired in the early stages after trauma.[41] In contrast, CO_2-reactivity was intact or even enhanced in most other patients offering this physiological principle as a target for ICP management in hyperemic states.

Hemodynamic Phases after the TBI

There is also a significant patient-to-patient variation in the hemodynamic response to

TBI. However, a pattern of three distinct hemodynamic phases can be distinguished:

Hypoperfusion phase (phase 1; day 0): The first 24 hours after TBI are characterised by cerebral hypoperfusion. Although CBF is reduced, there is a normal velocity in the middle cerebral artery (VMCA) as assessed by transcranial Doppler and a normal cerebral arteriovenous oxygen difference (AVDO$_2$). During this hypoperfusion phase, cerebral metabolic rate for oxygen (CMRO$_2$) is about 50% of normal. It has been suggested that pathological microcirculatory resistance is responsible for the reduced blood flow. Given the normal AVDO$_2$, it is also plausible that the CBF during this stage represents physiological flow-metabolism coupling. Focal or global cerebral ischemia occurs frequently after TBI. Although the total ischemic brain volume may be less than 10% on average, the presence of cerebral ischemia is associated with poor ultimate neurological outcome.[46] The frequent association between cerebral hypoperfusion and poor outcome suggests that TBI and ischemic stroke share the same fundamental mechanisms. Regional blood flow measurements early after severe head injuriy have now demonstrated that flow levels <18 ml/100 gm/min is sufficient to generate neuronal ischemic necrosis in 34 percent of sever TBI.[47, 48] CBF below this level jeopardizes the energy dependent Na$^+$/K$^+$-ATPase pump system leading to disturbed ionic homeostasis. However, reduction in CBF does not necessarily result in ischemia. The diagnosis of cerebral ischemia requires demonstration that the CBF is insufficient for a metabolic demand. The metabolic demand is reflected by substrate (oxygen and glucose) uptake and metabolite (pyruvate and lactate) production.[49] Reductions in cerebral metabolic rates common in head injury and metabolic needs may be further reduced by sedative agents. In practice, a secure diagnosis of ischemia depends upon the the demonstration of an increased oxygen extraction fraction, an increase in tissue lactate level, or a high lactate/pyruvate ratio.

Accompanying initial reduction in CBF, there is increase in OEF (oxygen extraction fraction). CMRO$_2$ is reduced somewhat initially, but falls further over few hours. With reduced CBF and declining CMRO$_2$, the initially markedly increased OEF progressively decreases.

The relationship between CBF, CMRO$_2$ and AVDO$_2$ can be summarised by the formula.

$$CMRO_2 = CBF \times AVDO_2$$

The normal values for AVDO$_2$ is approximately 6.5 ml O$_2$/100 ml blood, for CMRO$_2$ is 3.2 ml O$_2$/100g/min and for cerebral oxygenation ranges between 50 and 75%. Ischemic brain with low CBF exhibits low SjVO$_2$ reading of less than 50%, whereas for the hyperemic brain, the reading is more than 75%. Similarly, in brain dead patient where no uptake of oxygen occurred, the SjVO$_2$ would also be higher than 75%.

Hyperemia phase (phase 2; days 1 to 3): After 24 hours (days 1 to 3) the CBF increases. This is associated by a fall in AVDO$_2$ and hence a rise in the SjvO$_2$. CMRO$_2$ remains depressed. CBF is often normal in presence of low metabolism (relative hyperemia) or high CBF in relation to normal metabolism (absolute hyperemia). There is both a relative hyperemia (relative to blood flow demand during this stage) and an absolute hyperemia (CBF above the normal CBF range). VMCA begins to rise rapidly. The pathophysiological mechanism of this hyperemia is unknown. This pathology seems as detrimental as ischemia in terms of outcome because increases in CBF beyond matching metabolic demand relate to vasoparalysis with consecutive increase in cerebral blood volume and in turn increases intracranial pressure (ICP).[49–51]

It is important to note that diagnosing *hypoperfusion* or *hyperperfusion* is only valid after assessing measurements of CBF in relation to those of cerebral oxygen consumption. Both cerebral ischemia and hyperemia refer to a mismatch between CBF and cerebral metabolism. For example, low flow with normal or high metabolic rate represents an ischemic situation whereas high CBF with normal or reduced metabolic rate represents cerebral hyperemia. In contrast, low CBF with a low metabolic rate or high CBF with high metabolic rates represents coupling between flow and metabolism, a situation that does not necessarily reflect a pathological condition.[52, 53]

Vasospasm phase (phase 3, days 4 to 15) TBI may also cause spasm of large cerebral vessels similar to vasospasm induced by subarachnoid hemorrhage. VMCA rises further and CBF gradually declines. Interestingly, during the vasospasm phase the $AVDO_2$ remains low (hence the SjO_2 remains high). This is probably the result of either the persistently reduced $CMRO_2$ or cell death. Vasospasm may contribute further to cerebral ischemia.

Vasomotor paralysis by Langfitt[54, 55] postulated an acute reduction in vasomotor tone that resulted in cerebral vasodilatation, increased CBV and ICP. When arterial hypertension followed trauma, massive brain swelling occurred that was associated with both hyperemia and edema.

Of particular relevance to head injury is the related concept of "vasomotor paralysis" introduced by Langfitt and coworkers,[54, 55] to explain brain swelling and intracranial hypertension in experimental studies of cerebral compression by Lassen,[56] who described a "luxury perfusion syndrome" in patients with acute brain disorders. This syndrome is characterized by cerebral hyperemia, defined as excessive blood flow relative to the brain's metabolic requirements. Lassen argued that the hyperemia was due to impaired CBF autoregulation secondary to ischemia or hypoxia, and speculated that it could lead to disruption of the blood–brain barrier and edema formation. Since then, hyperemia has been observed in a number of acute clinical conditions and trauma. They postulated an acute reduction in vasomotor tone that resulted in cerebral vasodilatation, increased blood volume, and elevated intracranial pressure (ICP). When arterial hypertension

followed trauma, massive brain swelling occurred that was associated with both hyperemia and edema. These findings suggested that brain trauma impairs CBF autoregulation, which was subsequently confirmed.[57]

It is apparent that the concepts of luxury perfusion and vasomotor paralysis refer to different aspects of the same phenomenon; namely, an acute derangement of the cerebral circulation manifested by hyperemia and a potential for brain swelling. Although repeatedly observed in human and animal studies, the pathophysiological significance of this syndrome remains obscure, including its relevance to the management of clinical head injury. Thus, the incidence and time course of hyperemia following head injury is not fully known, nor is its relationship to intracranial hypertension. Furthermore, it is not clear whether therapy should be aimed at reducing the hyperemia. Although hyperventilation therapy has been widely used to control ICP, its effect on acute hyperemia has not been systematically evaluated.

Normal or increased CBF during coma is accompanied by a narrow $AVDO_2$ argues strongly that such flows are a luxury perfusion. High CBFs were associated with both an elevated ICP and increased jugular venous pO_2 (narrow AV difference).

If blood flow is doubled, as in some patients with absolute hyperemia, CBV might be expected to increase by 30%.

Intracranial Pressure

One of the most important complications of head injury is raised intracranial pressure due to added volume of contusions, hematomas, and progressive edema surrounding them. **Normal intracranial pressure is around 5–15 mm Hg. Raised intracranial pressure can cause severe secondary damage by decreasing cerebral perfusion pressure (CPP).** Following traumatic brain injury several compensatory mechanisms can operate to keep intracranial pressure ICP low, initiating reduction in the volume of intracranial CSF. Further increase in ICP compresses veins, thus decreasing blood volume. Till this phase, there is no change in ICP. Beyond this stage intracranial compliance decreases. Thus producing comparatively higher increase in ICP with small increase in intracranial volume. This initial phase of decompensation can be rapidly controlled with mannitol and hyperventilation.

The **Monro-Kellie hypothesis**[58] states that the cranial compartment is incompressible, and the volume inside the cranium is a fixed volume. Bony skull offers excellent protection to brain but allows little tolerance for additional volume. The intracranial volume of an adult is approximately 1500 ml, which is about 2% of total body weight. It contains three constituents: CSF, blood and brain parenchyma. The largest intracranial compartment is the incompressible brain parenchyma, which comprises about 80% of this compartment. The total CSF volume in normal conditions is about 120 to 140 ml; ventricular volume is about 40 ml, the spinal subarachnoid space contains about 30 ml, and the remaining CSF occupies the cranial sub-arachnoid space and cisterns. The total cerebral blood volume is approximately 150 ml.

The cranium and the vertebral canal, along with the relatively inelastic dura, create a state of volume equilibrium, such that the increase in any of its contents; brain, blood, or CSF, will tend to increase the ICP. In addition, any increase in one of the components must be at the expense of the other two; this relationship is known as the **Monro-Kellie doctrine** (Figs 4.8 and 4.9).[58] Small increases in brain volume do not lead to immediate increase in ICP because of the ability of the CSF to be displaced into the spinal canal, as well as the slight ability to stretch the falx cerebri between the hemispheres and the tentorium between the hemispheres and the cerebellum. However, once the ICP has reached around 25 mm Hg, small increases in brain volume can lead to marked elevations in ICP; this is due to failure of intracranial compliance.

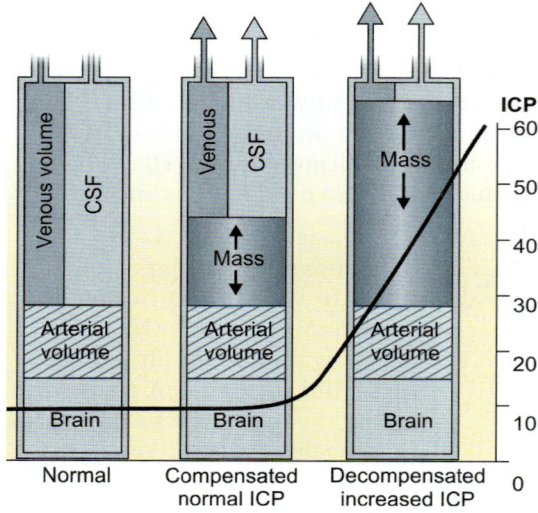

Fig. 4.8: Monro-Kellie doctrine showing relationship between volumes of intracranial contents

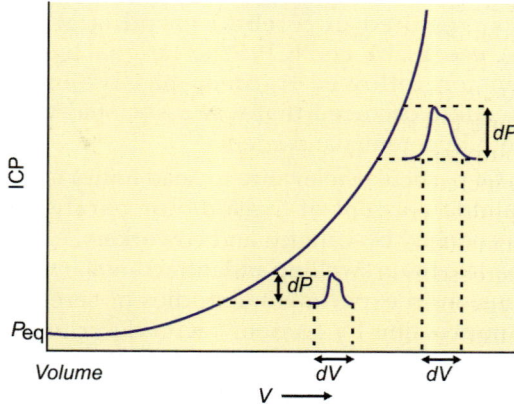

Fig. 4.9: The compliance (C) describes the volume-dependent increase of the pressure in the craniospinal space and can be used for the assessment of the cerebrospinal space reserves. Compliance is dP/dV. The inversion is termed elastance (E)

Brain parenchyma account for most of the intracranial content. A 5-year-old boy is least able to accommodate mass lesion than an elderly man. Apart from removing brain tissue or shrinking it with diuretics, the cell mass cannot be decreased.

Following traumatic brain injury several compensatory mechanisms can operate to keep intracranial pressure ICP low, initiating reduction in the volume of intracranial CSF, pressure. Further increase in ICP compresses veins, thus decreasing blood volume. Till this phase, there is no change in ICP. Beyond this stage intracranial compliance decreases. Thus producing comparatively higher increase in ICP with small increase in intracranial volume. On that part of the intracranial compliance curve where the pressure suddenly increases, a small rise in volume will cause a dramatic increase in the ICP. The pressure increase caused by volume substitution or growing of intracranial space occupying lesions occurs exponentially. This will further decrease CPP and cause cerebral ischemia, meticulous care of a patient who is around this part of the curve can be rewarding. Any small decrease in intracranial volume that can be achieved (e.g. by sitting the patient up, keeping the head straight, using mannitol and adequate sedation) can have a dramatic effect in bringing the ICP down. Minimal or no increase in ICP due to compensatory mechanisms is known as **stage 1** of intracranial hypertension. When the compensatory mechanisms are exhausted due to increase in hematoma or contusion, the ICP would increase. Any change in volume greater than 100–120 ml would mean a phenomenal increase in ICP. This is **stage 2 of intracranial hypertension.** Characteristics of stage 2 of intracranial hypertension include compromise of neuronal oxygenation and systemic arteriolar vasoconstriction to increase MAP and CPP. **Stage 3 intracranial hypertension is characterised by a sustained raised ICP, with dramatic increase in ICP with small increase in volume. In stage 3, as the ICP approaches the MAP, it becomes more and more difficult to pump blood into the intracranial space.** The body's response to a decrease in CPP is to raise blood pressure and dilate blood vessels in the brain. This results in increased cerebral blood volume, which increases ICP, lowering CPP and perpetuating this vicious cycle (Fig. 4.6). This results in widespread reduction in cerebral flow and perfusion, eventually leading to ischemia and brain infarction.

Neurologic changes seen in increased ICP are mostly due to hypoxia and hypercapnea and are as follows: decreased level of consciousness (LOC), Cheyne-Stokes respirations, hyperventilation, sluggish dilated pupils and bradycardia.

The pressure increase caused by volume substitution or growing of intracranial space occupying lesions occurs exponentially. The first part of the function takes a relatively flat course, indicating potential for compensation, while with consumption of the space reserve already small volumes may lead to an enormous pressure increase. Marmarou[59–61] demonstrated that **the non-linear craniospinal volume–pressure relationship could be described as a straight line segment relating the logarithm of pressure to volume, which implies a monoexponential relationship between volume and pressure** (Fig. 4.10). **The slope of this relationship Marmarou termed the pressure–volume index (PVI) which is the imaginary volume required to raise ICP tenfold.** Unlike elastance (change in pressure per unit change in volume dP/dV) or its inverse, compliance (change in volume per unit change in pressure dV/dP), the PVI characterizes the craniospinal volume–pressure relationship over the whole physiological range of ICP. The PVI is calculated from the

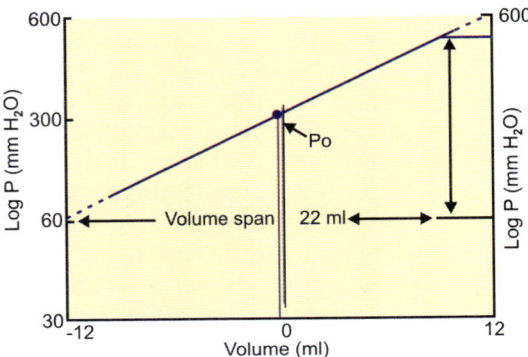

Fig. 4.10: Log intracranial pressure (ICP) *versus* intracranial volume relationship defined by Marmarou (1973). The pressure–volume index (PVI) is the notional volume (ml) which when added to the craniospinal volume, causes a tenfold rise in ICP.

pressure change resulting from a rapid injection or withdrawal of fluid. Marmarou's mathematical model developed an improved understanding not only of intracranial compliance but also of the inter-relationships of the static and dynamic processes of formation, storage and absorption mechanisms of CSF. Clearly, the balance between formation and storage is critical and if the absorption of CSF is hindered, perhaps as a result of increased CSF outflow resistance, this will result, once the storage capacity of CSF becomes exhausted, in raised ICP.[62] In general terms, causes of raised ICP can be categorized into 'vascular' and 'nonvascular' mechanisms. Vascular mechanisms would include active cerebral vasodilation due to stimuli such as increased CO_2 or decreased arterial inflow pressure (assuming intact pressure autoregulation) or passive distention of cerebral vessels in the absence of autoregulation or by venous outflow obstruction. Nonvascular mechanism include increase in cerebral edema, mass lesion, CSF pathway resistance. Any factor increasing in volume within the craniospinal axis will deplete available compensatory exchange space (decompensation), reduce compliance and eventually lead to increased intracranial pressure. Shapiro and Marmarou[64] have found a PVI reduced by 80% of control values to be predictive of raised ICP in pediatric head injury. Tans and Poortvliet,[63] also using the PVI in patients, state that the values of 10 ml and 13 ml are key values, with lower values indicating that active ICP reduction and improvement in compliance are required. 'Compliance' is defined as the ratio of the change in volume to the resulting change in pressure (dV/dP). High compliance means that large volume can be added without a much change in intracranial pressure. The pressure volume curve (Fig. 4.2) is exponential in shape.[54, 55] Hence, the compliance arid elastance, changes continuously, throughout. 'Elastance' is reciprocal of compliance (dP/dV).

Langfitt[54, 55] used an inflatable epidural balloon in monkeys and simultaneously monitored pressure in the lateral ventricle and plotted the pressure volume curve (Fig. 4.9). Compliance is high till the line is horizontal (i.e. ICP remains low even when intracranial volume is increased). As volume increases further, threshold for compensation is reached, and even small increase in volume cause very high increase in ICP. At this stage compliance is low and elastance is high. A rapidly developing hematoma is poorly tolerated than a slowly developing mass lesion because adequate time should be available for compensatory mechanisms to act. This quantity is described as cerebral capacitance. This quantity represents the rate at which the brain can accommodate changes in intracranial volume and is determined by time dependent derivatives of the same variables determining cerebral compliance.[13] Thus traumatic intracranial hematomas that grow rapidly may result in rapid increase in intracranial pressure and fatal cerebral herniation, while a meningioma in a similar location may produce a few symptoms.

Another area of research showing promise as a means of studying the effect of intracranial hypertension on craniospinal compliance and autoregulatory reserve concerns the continuous measure of transcranial middle cerebral artery (MCA) flow velocity and its correlation with CPP. Chan, et al.[65] demonstrated that, in continuously monitored head injured patients, the MCA Doppler pulsatility index (PI; systolic–diastolic/mean flow velocity), when plotted against CPP, showed a breakpoint at 70 mm Hg below which the PI increases. Simultaneous measurement of jugular venous oxygen saturation in the same patients demonstrated a fall in jugular venous saturation towards ischemic levels from the same CPP breakpoint. This data would indicate that below a CPP threshold of 70 mm Hg autoregulation in these patients was becoming exhausted. This information is useful as it provides a means of determining the optimal CPP threshold for treating raised ICP at any time during the management of head-injured patients. If there was only one 'critical CPP threshold' it would be a simple matter to treat if CPP fell below this threshold. However, there is now increasing evidence, from both clinical and experimental studies, that as a result of the varying severity of head injury and the development of the injury process with time, the critical CPP threshold changes both between patients and within patients on different days.[66-68] The development of analysis methods for detecting changes in CPP breakpoint may have a significant impact on the future management of cerebral perfusion. A similar relationship between CPP and exhaustion of autoregulation may also be identified through analysis of the ICP wave-form.

Deranged Consciousness in TBI: Causes

For maintaining consciousness, two important neurological components must function perfectly. They are **cerebral cortex and ascending reticular activating system (ARAS).** Injury to either or both of these components is sufficient to cause a patient to become comatosed. Disruption of the ARAS results in loss of consciousness and is believed to be the cause of the loss of consciousness associated with traumatic brain injury. Hence deranged consciousness can be attributed to (1) wide-spread damage to cerebral cortex due to TBI or due to hypoxia; (2) brainstem contusions/hematomas and/or brain herniation damaging ARAS (ascending reticular activating system); (3) metabolic cause, i.e. suppression of ARAS by drugs, hypoxia, hypotension, uremia, or by other metabolic derangements.

Viennese pathologist constantin von Economo[69] found during epidemic of ence-phalitis lethargica that structures in the upper brainstem and posterior hypothalamus mediate arousal.[70] Frederic Bremer later confirmed this suggestion experimentally by showing that transection of the cat's brain at the cervicomedullary junction had no effect on arousal, or on the sleep–wake cycle, while transection through the midbrain brought about a state resembling deep sleep.[71]

Bremer hypothesized that this impairment of arousal resulted from interruption of

ascending sensory pathways in the midbrain. His student Giuseppe Moruzzi, later showed that the critical areas were not, in fact, in the sensory pathways but rather in the reticular core of the upper brainstem and, probably, their thalamic targets.[72] Moreover, electrical stimulation of this region in a drowsy animal 'activated' the EEG. These observations gave birth to the concept of the 'ascending reticular activating system' (ARAS).

Experimental work in animals suggests that the following structures play key roles in the maintenance and modulation of wakefulness: cholinergic nuclei in the upper brainstem and basal forebrain; noradrenergic nuclei, in particular the locus coeruleus; a histaminergic projection from the posterior hypothalamus; and probably dopaminergic and serotonergic pathways arising from the brainstem[73] (Fig. 4.11). Much, but not all, of the influence exerted by these pathways is mediated by the thalamus, which can be regarded as the apex of the ARAS, as well as a critical synaptic relay for most sensory and many intracerebral pathways.[74] The function of these activating structures is not, of course, confined to the maintenance of wakefulness: they are of profound importance to a wide range of interrelated functions including mood, motivation, attention, learning, memory and movement.[75]

The cerebral cortex directly or indirectly in charge of all the neurological functions, from simple reflexes to complex thinking. RAS, on the other hand, is a more primitive structure in the brainstem that is tightly in connection with reticular formation (RF). The RAS area of the brain has two tracts, the ascending and descending tract. Made up of a system of acetylcholine-producing neurons, the ascending track, or ascending reticular activating system (ARAS), works to arouse and wake up the brain, from the RF, through the thalamus, and then finally to the cerebral cortex. A failure in ARAS functioning may then lead to a coma. It is, therefore, necessary to investigate the integrity of the bilateral cerebral cortices, as well as that of the reticular activating

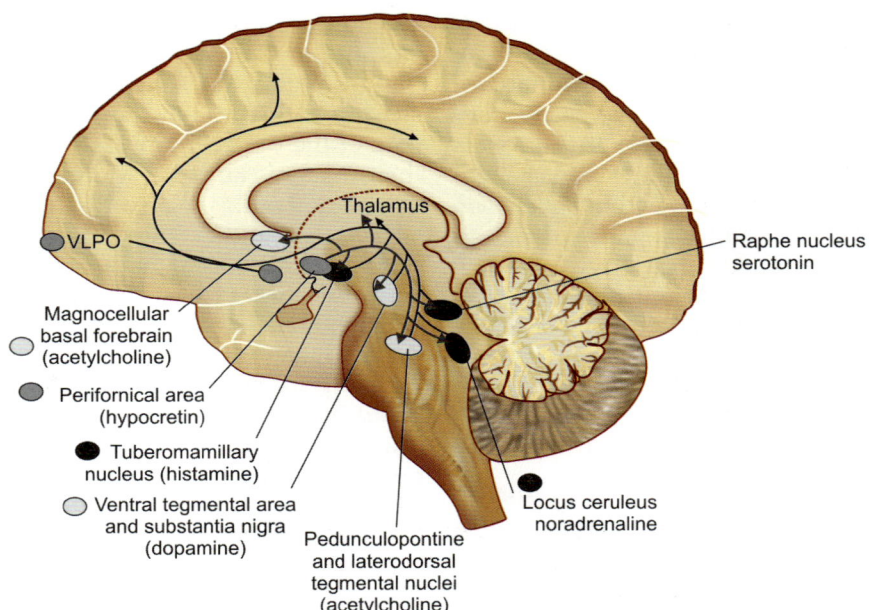

Fig. 4.11: ARAS; ascending reticular activating system, showing its dopaminergic, histaminergic and cholinergic pathways. Thalamus is regarded as apex of ARAS. VLPO; ventrolateral preoptic nucleus in hypothalamus

system (RAS) in a comatose patient neurologic unconsciousness is paralytic coma.[76] This neurologic state represents a form of brain dysfunction involving either the hemispheres or the deep structures of the brain (including the reticular activating system, which governs sleep and wake cycles[77]), or both. In the neurologic unconscious state, responses to the external world are primitive or reflexic and may be absent altogether. After severe traumatic brain injury, emergence from a coma into vegetative state does not change the fact that the individual is still unconscious, even though the eyes may be open causes tissue distortion and destruction in the early postinjury period. Clinical outcomes depend in large part on mediating the bimolecular and cellular changes that occur after the initial injury. As already discussed, these secondary injuries from traumatic brain injury lead to alterations in cell function and propagation of injury through processes such as depolarization, excitotoxicity, disruption of calcium homeostasis, free-radical generation, blood–

brain barrier disruption, ischemic injury, edema formation and intracranial hypertension.

Raised ICP and Brain Herniations

The cranial vault is divided into compartments by the dural reflections of the falx cerebri and tentorium cerebelli. Raised ICP frequently results in pressure gradients between compartments and a shift of brain structures. Many of the clinical counterparts of raised ICP are the consequence of such shifts rather than the absolute level of ICP. Three types of intracranial herniation are generally recognised: transtentorial (either lateral or central), tonsillar and subfalcine (Fig. 4.3). Patients with temporal lobe hematomas can undergo lateral **Uncal (transtentorial) herniation** is herniation of the medial temporal lobe from the middle into the posterior fossa, across the tentorial opening. The uncus of the temporal lobe is forced into the gap between the midbrain and the edge of the tentorium. This compresses the ipsilateral oculomotor nerve, causing a fixed and dilated pupil and **collapses the** ipsilateral

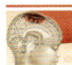
posterior cerebral artery, causing an infarct in its distribution. Cortical blindness resulting from this infarct is a false localizing sign because it gives the erroneous impression that the primary lesion is in the occipital lobe. As the herniating uncus displaces the midbrain laterally, the contralateral cerebral peduncle is compressed against the edge of the tentorium, causing paralysis on the same side as the primary lesion, another false localizing sign. Caudal displacement of the brainstem and stretching of its vessels causes a variety of hemorrhagic lesions in the midbrain and pons **(secondary brainstem hemorrhages)** that can devastate the reticular activating substance and other brainstem centers, resulting in focal neurological deficits and coma without a rise in ICP and they should be evacuated early even if they are moderate in size. **Brain herniation** can severely damage brainstem through tissue shifts and vascular compromise (e.g. PCA infarct following large temporal/parietal EDH) EDH and acute SDH are two important surgical lesions that require treatment quickly[85,86] (Figs 4.12a and b). Many of the signs associated with coma, can be due to these tissue shifts and particular clinical presentation characteristic of specific herniation. False localizing signs are typical presentation. They are due to compression of brain structures away from site of hematoma or contusion. **Uncal (transtentorial) herniation** is herniation of the medial temporal lobe from the middle into the posterior fossa, across the tentorial opening. The uncus of the temporal lobe is forced into the gap between the midbrain and the edge of the tentorium (mesencephalic cistern). This compresses the ipsilateral oculomotor nerve, causing a fixed and dilated pupil and compresses the ipsilateral posterior cerebral artery, causing an infarct in its distribution. Cortical blindness resulting from this infarct is a false localizing sign because it gives the erroneous impression that the primary lesion is in the occipital lobe. As the herniating uncus displaces the midbrain laterally, the contralateral cerebral peduncle is compressed against the edge of the tentorium,

causing paralysis on the same side as the primary lesion, another false localizing sign. Caudal displacement of the brainstem and stretching of its vessels causes a variety of hemorrhagic lesions in the midbrain and pons (secondary brainstem durets hemorrhages) that can devastate the reticular activating substance and other brainstem centers, resulting in focal neurological deficits and coma. Central transtentorial herniation is due to symmetric downward movement of thalamic medial structures through tentorial opening causing compression of upper midbrain. As compression progresses it involves pons and finally the medulla. Other forms of herniations are subfalcine and tonsillar herniation. Pressure on the posterior fossa contents from above or from within compresses the pons against the clivus and displaces the cerebellar tonsils into the foramen magnum **(tonsillar herniation)**. Compression of the pons and medulla damages vital centers for respiration and cardiac function, resulting in cardiorespiratory arrest.

Systemic Manifestations of Head Injury

Systemic abnormalities to head injury may occur immediately, over hours or days. Trauma induces catecholamine release from adrenal medulla which may cause deleterious effects on the heart, the vascular system and on metabolism.

Effect on Cardiopulmonary System

Neurogenic pulmonary edema (NPE) is not uncommon and is associated with diminished lung compliance. Alveoli are flooded by protein rich fluid. It results in decreased lung compliance. As a result severe hypoxemia develops. Pulmonary dysfunction after acute brain injury is a common but poorly understood phenomenon.[78–80] Causes of pulmonary dysfunction in patients with head injury include pneumonia, aspiration and pulmonary embolus, but seldom NPE.[81, 82] NPE is a form of pulmonary edema that develops rapidly after a cerebral injury.[78] It has been described in trauma patients as parenchymal edema,

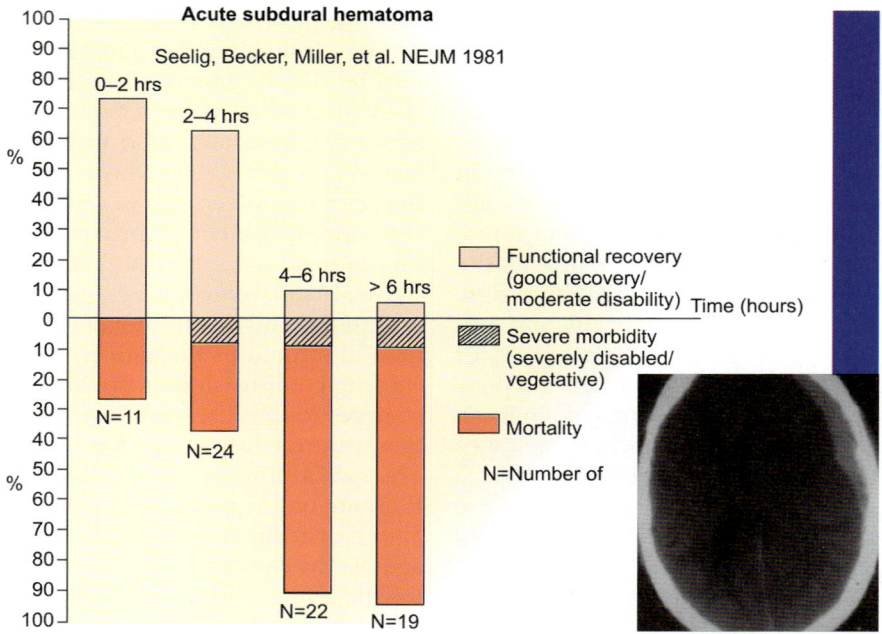

Fig. 4.12a: Acute SDH; good outcome with early evacuation

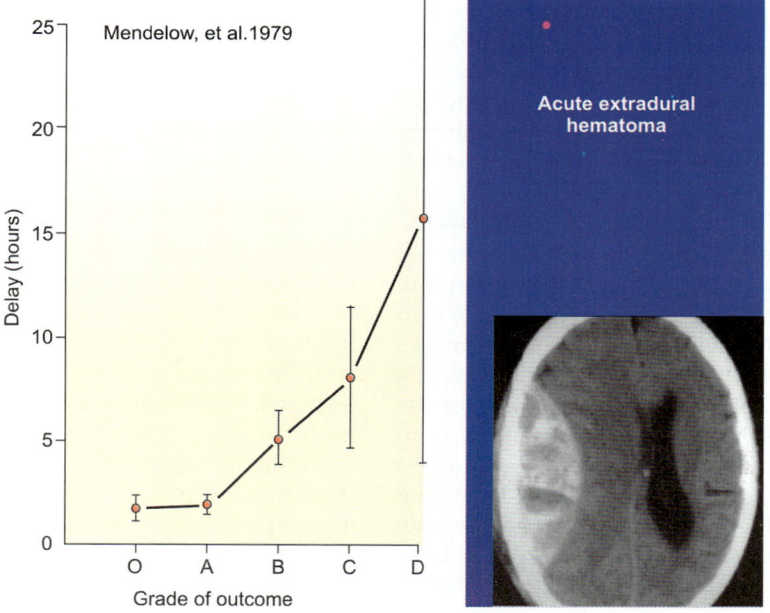

Fig. 4.12b: Acute EDH; excellent grade of outcome with early evacuation

hemorrhage and congestion without evidence of chest trauma in patients with isolated head injury.[78] Furthermore, the clinical relevance of NPE in patients with nonfatal head injury remains to be elucidated, because NPE seems to be rare in patients who survive. However, according to Rogers et al,[78] the incidence of NPE in patients with isolated head injury was 32% in patients who died at the scene and 50% in patients who died within 96 hours of the injury.

The neurogenic pulmonary edema may occur due to:

1. *Sympathetic stimulation:* Increased sympathetic stimulation on lung vasculature results in increased vascular permeability. Increased permeability as a mechanism of NPE is supported by some studies in animals that have shown high interstitial (lung lymphatic) or alveolar protein concentrations[83] and time-dependent ultrastructural changes in pneumocyte type II cells after brain injury.[84] Increased permeability may be caused by damage of the capillary endothelium or by direct neural influences on capillary permeability (the blast theory).[87, 88]

2. *Hyperdynamic state:* Increased left ventricular afterload occurs because of hypertension with increased peripheral vascular resistance. It causes increased pulmonary capillary pressure resulting in hydrostatic lung edema. This hypothesis was confirmed by experimental studies[89,90] and studies in humans.[91,92] However, pulmonary edema can occur with normal pulmonary artery wedge pressures,[93,94] suggesting a neurally mediated pressure independent of the influence on capillary permeability.

In addition to these 2 hypotheses, neurogenic pulmonary edema NPE can result from a cardiac dysfunction. In fact, the early hemodynamic changes that occur in the setting of NPE may lead to the conclusion that the pulmonary edema is of cardiac origin. Smith and Matthay[95] reported, as have others, that early analysis of NPE fluid

reveals a low fluid-serum protein ratio consistent with hydrostatic edema. In addition to the change in vascular resistance described, the pathogenesis of hydrostatic NPE may involve direct negative inotropic effects on the heart.[96]

3. *Cushings reflex:* When MAP (mean arterial pressure) is less than the intracranial pressure, a reflex called the "CNS ischemic response" is initiated by the hypothalamus in the brain. The hypothalamus activates the sympathetic nervous system, causing peripheral vasoconstriction and an increase in cardiac output. These two effects serve to increase arterial blood pressure. When arterial blood pressure exceeds the intracranial pressure, blood flow to the brain is restored. The increased arterial blood pressure caused by the CNS ischemic response stimulates the baroreceptors in the carotid bodies, thus slowing the heart rate drastically—often to the point of a bradycardia.

- Kalmer et al.[97] described the hemodynamic effects of increased intracranial pressure during endoscopic neurosurgical procedures and their respective sequence of events at high temporal resolution. Although most clinicians rely on the occurrence of bradycardia to diagnose intracranial hypertension, they found that simultaneous onset of hypertension and tachycardia is a better indicator of impaired brain perfusion. Waiting for a persistent bradycardia to alert the surgeon during endoscopic neurosurgical procedures could allow severe bradycardia or even asystole to develop. Hence, hypertension with tachycardia is an early indicator of raised ICP, which may rise further to uncontrollable levels. Cushing's triad is named after great neurosurgeon Harvey Williams Cushing (1869–1939).[98]

- Classically, the 'Cushing reflex' has been reported as the occurrence of hypertension, bradycardia and apnoea following intracranial hypertension.[99] Various animal pathophysiological studies, describing hemodynamic changes following sudden increases in intracranial pressure, refined Cushing's findings by showing an initial tachycardia associated with hypertension before the onset of bradycardia. In a clinical context, observation of increased intracranial pressure resulting in hemodynamic instability was previously limited to a phenomenon following a time course of hours, days or months depending on the underlying pathology (e.g. subdural hematoma, tumors, hydrocephalus, etc.). At the time of clinical presentation, symptoms invariably already consisted of bradycardia and hypertension.

Pathophysiology and the Concept of Neuroprotection Through Drugs

Neuroprotection is an expanding field of mainly pharmacological interventions that attempt to interrupt these processes and thus improve the outcome of TBI patients. To date, however, despite very encouraging preclinical results, almost all phase II/III clinical trials in neuroprotection have failed to show any consistent improvement in outcome for TBI patients.[1] Most of these medicines are still in experimental stage practically two pathological pathways are more certain; firstly release of excitotoxic factor glutamate and secondly, release of calcium. If one can block these processes then improvement in outcome is expected.

Glutamate Antagonists

Dizocilpine (MK-801) is an antagonist of the N-methyl-D-aspartate receptor[101–103] in the glutamate category involved with the central nervous system (CNS). NMDA receptors are key in the progression of excitotoxicity, as discussed previously in this chapter. Thus NMDA receptor antagonists including MK-801 have been extensively studied for use in treatment of diseases with excitotoxic components, such as stroke, traumatic brain injury.

MK-801 has shown effectiveness in protecting neurons in cell culture and animal models of excitotoxic neurodegeneration.[101,102] The administration of MK-801 protected the hippocampus from ischemia-induced neurodegeneration in the gerbil. The ED50 (effective dose 50) for neuroprotection was 0.3 mg/kg and the majority of the animals were protected against the ischemia-induced damage at doses greater than or equal to 3 mg/kg, when MK-801 was given one hour prior to the occlusion of the carotid arteries, although other studies have shown protection up to 24 hours post-insult. Excitatory amino acids, such as glutamate and aspartate, are released in toxic amounts when the brain is deprived of blood and oxygen and NMDA receptors are thought to prevent the neurodegeneration through the inhibition of these receptors.

Phencyclidine (PCP)-like compounds have been investigated for use in treating brain ischemia. PCP is an N-methyl-D-aspartate (NMDA) antagonist; thus, it blocks the action of glutamate and aspartate, excitatory amino acid CNS neurotransmitters. PCP is also highly anticholinergic in nature. They are not used nowadays because of addictive properties.[102]

Other glutamate antagonist such as *D-CPP-ene* and *CP 101-606* were tried with no benefit.

Nimodipine

Nimodipine is beneficial in the treatment of vasospasm due to spontaneous subarachnoid hemorrhage, reducing the incidence of infarction and ischemia and improving outcome. Its role in traumatic SAH seems to favor better outcome.

Head injury trials (HIT) for the calcium channel blockers in acute traumatic head injury patients shows that considerable uncertainty remains over their effects. The effect of nimodipine in a subgroup of brain injury patients with sub-arachnoid hemorrhage shows a beneficial effect, though the increase in adverse reactions suffered by the intervention group may mean that the drug is harmful for some patients.[103] A 2003 Cochrane review reported improved outcome with nimodipine in these patients; however, because the results of head injury trial (HIT) 4 were only partly presented there is still discussion whether patients with traumatic subarachnoid hemorrhage should be treated with this drug. Vergouwen et al[105] presented data from all head-injury trials, including previously unpublished results from HIT 4. In total, 1074 patients with traumatic subarachnoid hemorrhage were included. Mortality rates did not differ between nimodipine (26%) and placebo (27%) treated patients. **They interpreted that the beneficial effect of nimodipine on outcome in patients with traumatic subarachnoid hemorrhage is doubtful. In other word nimodipine is not useful in trumatic subarachnoid hemorrhage.**

Dexanabinol

Dexanabinol is a novel synthetic chemical analog of the active component of marijuana. It is not recognized by the cannabinoid receptors in the brain that mediate the intoxicating effect of marijuana. It is a non-competitive inhibitor of the NMDA receptor, a free radical scavenger and antioxidant, and an inhibitor of the pro-inflammatory cytokine TNF alpha. Dexanabinol inhibits breakdown of the blood–brain barrier, edema.[105,106] Treatment parameters (time to treatment, dose, and duration) were kept as close as possible to those established as safe and efficacious in relevant preclinical models. Thus, Dexanabinol was delivered within 6 h of injury (window of efficacy established in closed head injury and axonal crush models). The doses were derived from comparative pharmacokinetics in animal studies where effective doses in rats (2–5 mg/kg) produced peak plasma levels of < 2–5 mg/ml, and in the phase I trial.

Significant effects of the drug were seen on ICP. The drug appeared to prevent the increase of ICP over the first 2–3 days postinjury, such that mean ICP values (which were initially similar in the drug and placebo groups) rose above 15 mm Hg in the placebo group and remained consistently below 15 mm Hg in the Dexanabinol group. The percentage of time ICP was above 25 mm Hg was decreased in the Dexanabinol treated groups at all doses, and the effect was statistically significant from the second day. This stabilizing effect of Dexanabinol on ICP was achieved without lowering systolic blood pressure; conversely, the percentage of time systolic blood pressure fell below 90 mm Hg was reduced in the Dexanabinol-treated patients.

Tris (hydroxymethyl) Aminomethane (THAM)

In experimental models, tromethamine (THAM) reduces the side-effects of prolonged hyperventilation. It also decreases cerebral acidosis and ICP. In a randomized prospective clinical trial by Wolf et al,[107] THAM was studied to determine if it had beneficial effects in the early management of severe head injuries and if the adverse effects of hyperventilation could be prevented. Tromethamine was administered as a 0.3-M solution in an initial loading dose (body weight × blood acidity deficit, average 4.27 cc/kg/hr) given over 2 hours, followed by a constant infusion of 1 ml/kg/hr for 5 days. Outcome was measured at 3, 6, and 12 months postinjury. Although analysis indicated no significant difference in outcome between these two groups at 3 months, 6 months, and 1 year, there was a difference regarding ICP. The time that ICP was above 20 mm Hg in the first 48 hours postinjury was less in patients treated with THAM (p < 0.05). Also, the number of patients requiring barbiturate coma was significantly less in the THAM group (5.48% vs. 18.4%, p < 0.05). Wolf et al concluded that THAM ameliorates the deleterious effect of prolonged hyperventilation, may be beneficial in ICP control.

CONCLUSIONS

The primary injury to the brain triggers a sequence of events, which results in alteration in brain metabolism and cerebral blood flow.

Cerebral ischemia results due to increased "intracranial pressure (ICP), local brain distortion occurs secondary to clot and vaso-constriction. Hypoxia and cerebral ischemia will cause anaerobic glycolysis, intracellular acidosis, release of free radicals and high levels of extracellular K^+, glutamate, adenosine. All these factors will lead to tremendous increase in intracellular accumulation of Ca^{++}, causing breakdown of cell membranes by activating Ca^{++} dependent proteases and release of FFA.

Autoregulation is deranged following head injury. The relationship between metabolism ($CMRO_2$) and cerebral blood flow (CBF) has been found to be abnormal. Head trauma results in cytotoxic edema, brain swelling and hence intracranial hypertension.

Mechanisms of cell death is important in understanding pathophysiology of head injury. New drugs which block receptors to prevent cell death could be the future in managing TBI. Autoregulation is deranged following head injury. The relationship between metabolism ($CMRO_2$) and cerebral blood flow (CBF) have been found to be abnormal.

REFERENCES

1. Olson DA. Head Injury Medicine 2002.
2. Paul ME, Joseph V, Todd T. Management of Head Trauma (Critical review) Chest 2002;122: 699–711.
3. Rosner MJ, Rosner RD, Johnson AH. Cerebral perfusion pressure: Management protocol and clinical results. J. Neurosurg 1995;83:949–82.
4. Guidelines for cerebral perfusion pressue. J. Neurotrauma 2000;17:507–11.
5. Graham DI, Ford I, Adam JH, et al. Ischemic brain damage is still common in fatal non missile head injury. J Neurol Neurosug Psychiat, 1989;52:346–350.
6. Graham SH, Chen J, Clark RS: Bcl-2 family gene products in cerebral ischemia and traumatic brain injury. J Neurotrauma 2000;17(10):831–41.
7. Greve MW and Zink BJ, Pathophysiology of traumatic brain injury. Mt Sinai J Med 2009;76: 97–104.
8. Lei P, et al. Microarray based analysis of microRNA expression in rat cerebral cortex after traumatic brain injury. Brain Res 1284, 2009; 191–201.
9. Cohen GM. Caspases: the executioners of apoptosis. Biochem J 326, 1997;(1):1–16.
10. Majno G, Joris I Apoptosis, oncosis, and necrosis. An overview of cell death. The American Journal of Pathology 1995;146(1),3–15.
11. Kroemer G, Galluzzi L, Vandenabeele P, Abrams J, Alnemri ES, Baehrecke EH, Blagosklonny MV, El-Deiry WS, Golstein P, Green DR, Hengartner M, Knight RA, Kumar S, Lipton SA, Malorni W, Nuñez G, Peter ME, Tschopp J, Yuan J, Piacentini M, Zhivotovsky B, Melino G. Nomenclature Committee on Cell Death 2009. Classification of cell death: recommendations of the Nomenciature Committee on Cell Death 2009. Cell Death Differ 2009;16(1):3–11.
12. Ross Bullock, Alois Zauner, John J. Woodward, John Myseros, Sung C. Choi, John D. Ward, Anthony Marmarou, Harold F. Young, . Factors affecting excitatory amino acid release following severe human head injury J Neurosurg 1998;89: 507–18.
13. R Foresti, P Sarathchandra, J E Clark, C J Green, and to apoptosisR Motterlini-Peroxynitrite induces haem oxygenase-1 in vascular endothelial cells: a link to apoptosis. Biochem J 1999;339:729–36.
14. David KK, et al. Parthanatos, a messenger of death. Frontiers in Bioscience 2009;14:1116–28.
15. Shaida A Andrabi, Ho Chul Kang, Jean-François Haince, Yun-Il Lee, Jian Zhang, Zhikai Chi, Andrew B West, Raymond C Koehler, Guy G Poirier, Ted M Dawson and Valina L Dawson Iduna protects the brain from glutamate excito-toxicity and stroke by interfering with poly (ADP-ribose) polymer-induced cell death Nature Medicine 2011;17;692–9.
16. Yang E, Korsmeyer SJ. Molecular thanatopsis: a discourse on the bcl2 family and cell death. Blood 1996;88(2):386–401.
17. Kroemer G: The proto-oncogene Bcl-2 and its role in regulating apoptosis. Nat Med 1997; 3(6):614–20.
18. Kerr JF, Wyllie AH, Currie AR. Apoptosis: a basic biological phenomenon with wide-ranging implications in tissue kinetics. Br J Cancer 1972; 26(4):239–57.
19. Rink A, Fung KM, Trojanowski JQ, Lee VM, Neugebauer E, McIntosh TK: Evidence of apoptotic cell death after experimental traumatic brain injury in the rat. Am J Pathol 1995; 147(6):1575–83.

20. Tolias CM, Bullock MR: Critical appraisal of neuroprotection trials in head injury: what have we learned? NeuroRx 2004;1(1):71–9.

21. Raghupathi R: Cell death mechanisms following traumatic brain injury. Brain Pathol 2004; 14:215–222.

22. Raghupathi R, Graham DI, McIntosh TK: Apoptosis after traumatic brain injury. J Neurotrauma 2000;17(10):927–38.

23. Clark RS, Kochanek PM, Chen M, Watkins SC, Marion DW, Chen J, Hamilton RL, Loeffert JE, Graham SH. Increases in Bcl-2 and cleavage of caspase-1 and caspase-3 in human brain after head injury. FASEB J 1999;13(8):813–21.

24. Castillo J, Dávalos A, Alvarez-Sabín J, Pumar JM, Leira R, Silva Y, Montaner J, Kase CS. Molecular signatures of brain injury after intracerebral hemorrhage. Neurology 2002, **58**(4):624–9.

25. Tonny Veenith, Serena SH Goon and Rowan M Burnstein; Molecular mechanisms of traumatic brain injury: the missing link in management World Journal of Emergency Surgery 2009;4:7 doi:10.1186/1749-7922-4-7.

26. Hyman BT and Yuan J.Apoptotic and non-apoptotic roles of caspases in neuronal physiology and pathophysiology: Nature Reviews Neuroscience June 2012;13:395–406.

27. Neumann H. Control of glial immune function by neurons. Glia 2001;36(2):191–9.

28. Zhang D, Hu X, Qian L, O'Callaghan JP, Hong J . Astrogliosis in CNS pathologies: Is there a role for microglia? Mol Neurobiol 2010;41:232–41.

29. Tuttolomondo A, Di Sciacca R, Di Raimondo D, Renda C, Pinto A, et al. Inflammation as a therapeutic target in acute ischemic stroke treatment. Curr Top Med Chem 2009;9(14):1240–60.

30. Chang HY, Yang X. Proteases for cell suicide: functions and regulation of caspases. Microbiol Mol Biol Rev 2000;64:821–46.

31. Beer R, Franz G, Srinivasan A, Hayes RL, Pike BR, et al. Temporal profile and cell subtype distribution of activated caspase-3 following experimental traumatic brain injury. J Neurochem 2000;75:1264–73.

32. Halliwell B, Gulteridge JMC. Free radicals in biology and medicine. 2nd Edition. 1989. Oxford, Clarendon.

33. Yamamoto T, Maruyama W, Kato Y, et al. Slective nitration of mitochondrial complex I by peroxynitrite: involvement in mito-chondria dysfunction and cell death of dopaminergic SH-SY5Y cells. J Neural Transm 2002;109:1–13.

34. Baskaya MK, et al. The biphasic opening of the blood–brain barrier in the cortex and hippo-campus after traumatic brain injury in rats. Neurosci Lett 1997;226(1):33–62.

35. Shlosberg D, et al. Blood–brain barrier breakdown as a therapeutic target in traumatic brain injury. Nat Rev Neurol 2010;6,7:393–403.

36. Kety SS. Circulation and metabolism of the human brain in health and disease. Am J Med 1950;8:205–17.

37. Ingvar DH, Lassen NA. Regulation of cerebral blood flow. In: Himwich HE, ed. Brain metabolism and cerebral disorders. New York: Spectrum Publication 1976;181–206.

38. Hall JE. Cerebral Blood Flow, Cerebrospinal Fluid, and Brain Metabolism. Guyton and Hall; Textbook of Medical Physiology 12th Ed, 743–9.

39. Enevoldsen EM, Jensen FT. Autoregulation and CO_2 responses of cerebral blood flow in patients with acute severe head injury. J Neurosurg 1978;48:689–703.

40. Glenn TC, Kelly DF, Boscardin WJ, et al. Energy dysfunction as a predictor of outcome after moderate or severe head injury: indices of oxygen, glucose, and lactate metabolism. J Cereb Blood Flow Metab 2003;23:1239–50.

41. Hauerberg J, Xiaodong M, Willumsen L, Pedersen DB, Juhler M. The upper limit of cerebral blood flow autoregulation in acute intracranial hypertension. J Neurosurg Anesth 1998;10:106–12.

42. Hlatky R, Furuya Y, Valadka AB, et al. Dynamic autoregulatory response after severe head injury. J Neurosurg 2002;97:1054–61.

43. Inoue Y, Shiozaki T, Tasaki O, et al. Changes in cerebral blood flow from the acute to the chronic phase of severe head injury. J Neurotrauma 2005; 22:1411–8.

44. Jeager M, Schuhmann MU, Soehle M, Meixens-berger J. Continuous assessment of cerebrovas-cular autoregulation after traumatic brain injury using brain tissue oxygen pressure reactivity. Crit Care Med 2006;34:1783–8.

45. Johnston AJ, Steiner LA, Coles JP, et al. Effect of cerebral perfusion pressure augmentation on regional oxygenation and metabolism after head injury. Crit Care Med 2005;33:189–95.

46. Kelly DF, Korndestani RK, Martin NA, et al . Hyperemia following traumatic brain injury: relationship to intracranial hypertension and outcome. J Neurosurg 1996;85:762–71.

47. Bouma GJ, Muizelaar JP, Stringer WA, et al. Ultra-early evaluation of regional cerebral blood

flow in severely head-injured patients using xenon-enhanced.

48. Schroder ML, Muizelaar JP, Bullock MR, et al: Focal ischemia due to traumatic contusions documented by stable xenon-CT and ultra-structural studies. J Neurosurg 1995;82:966–971.

49. Huthinson PJ, Menon DK, Czosnyka M, Kirkpatrick PJ. Monitoring cerebral blood flow and metabolism. In; Head Injury Patho-physiology and management (eds Reilly Pl and Bullock R). Hodder Arnold 2005;215–45.

50. Bouma GJ, Muizelaar JP. Cerebral blood flow, cerebral blood volume, and cerebrovascular reactivity after severe head injury. J Neuro-trauma 1992;9:S333–48.

51. Bouma GJ, Muizelaar JP, Stringer WA, Choi C, Fatouros P, Young HF. Ultra-early evaluation of regional cerebral blood flow in severely head-injured patients using xenon-enhanced computerized tomography. J Neurosurg 1992; 77:360–8.

52. Coles JP, Fryer TD, Smielewski P, et al. Defining ischemic burden after traumatic brain injury using ^{15}O PET imaging of cerebral physiology. J Cereb Blood Flow Metab 2004;24:191–201.

53. Coles JP, Fryer TD, Smielewski P, et al. Incidence and mechanisms of cerebral ischemia in early clinical head injury. J Cereb Blood Flow Metab 2004;24:202–11.

54. Langfitt TW, Weinstein JD, Kassell NF. Cerebral vasomotor paralysis produced by intracranial-f hypertension. Neurology 1965;15:622–41.

55. Langfitt TW, Weinstem JD, Kassell NF, et al. Transmission of increased intracranial pressure within the craniospinal axis, J Neurosurg 1964;21:989–97.

56. Lassen NA, and Ingvar DH. The blood flow of the cerebral cortex determined by radioactive krypton-85. Experientia, L7: (L961) 42–45.

57. Obrist WD, Langfitt TW, Jaggi JL, et al. Cerebral blood flow and metabolism in comatose patients with acute head injury. Relationship to intra-cranial hypertension. J Neurosurg 1984; 61:241–53.

58. Monro A. Observations on the Structure and Function of the Nervous System, Creech and Johnston, Edinburgh 1783.

59. Marmarou A, Shulman K and LaMorgese J. Compartmental analysis of compliance and outflow resistance of the cerebrospinal fluid system. Journal of Neurosurgery 1975;43:523–34.

60. Marmarou A, Maset AL, Ward JD, et al. Contri-bution of CSF and vascular factors to elevation of ICP in severely head-injured patients. Journal of Neurosurgery 1987;66,883–890.

61. Marmarou A, Anderson RL, Ward JD, et al. Impact of ICP instability on outcome in patients with severe head trauma. Journal of Neuro-surgery 1991;75:S59–66.

62. Piper I. Intracranial Pressure And Elastance. In Head Injury Pathophysiology and management, 2nd Ed. (eds Reilly Pl and Bullock R). Hodder Arnold 2005;93–112.

63. Tans JT and Poortvliet DC. Intracranial volume–pressure relationship in man. Part 2: Clinical significance of the pressure–volume index. Journal of Neurosurgery 1983;59:810–816.

64. Shapiro K and Marmarou A. Clinical applications of the pressure–volume index in treatment of pediatric head injuries. Journal of Neurosurgery 1982;819–25.

65. Chan KH, Dearden NM, Miller JD, et al. Multi-modality monitoring as a guide to treatment of intracranial hypertension after severe head injury. Neurosurgery 1993;32:547–53.

66. Price DJ, Czosnyka M, Czosnyka, Z, Price, JR. Correlation of continuous measures of autoregu-lation and compensatory reserve with cerebral perfusion pressure and ICP, in Intracranial Pressure IX, (eds H. Nagai, K. Kamiya and S. Ishii), Springer-Verlag, Berlin, 1994;60–3.

67. Lewis, SB, Wong, MLH, Bannan, PE, et al. The relationship of cerebral blood flow to trans-cranial Doppler indices and cerebro-vascular waveform analysis in a sheep model. Journal of Neurotrauma 12, 414.

68. Wong FC, Signorini D, Piper IR and Miller JD. Differences in treatment thresholds of cerebral perfusion pressure in head injuries. Journal of Neurotrauma 12, 413.

69. Von Economo C. Encephalitis lethargica: its sequelae and treatment. London: Oxford University Press 1931.

70. Zeman A. Consciousness Brain 2001;124(7): 1263–89.

71. Bremer F. Cerveau 'isole' et physiologie du sommeil. C R Seanc Soc Biol 1929;102:1235–41.

72. Moruzzi G, Magoun HW. Brain stem reticular formation and the activation of the EEG. Electro-encephalogr Clin Neurophysiol 1949;1: 455–73.

73. McCarley RW. Sleep neurophysiology: basic mechanisms underlying control of wakefulness and sleep. In: Chokroverty S, editor. Sleep disorders medicine. Boston: Butterworth Heinemann 1999;21–50.

74. Jones BE. The neural basis of consciousness across the sleep-waking cycle. In: Jasper HH, Descarries L, Castelucci VF, Rossignol S, editors.

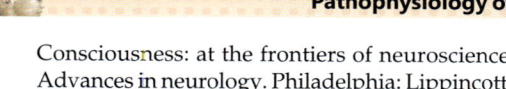

Consciousness: at the frontiers of neuroscience. Advances in neurology. Philadelphia: Lippincott-Raven 1998;77:75–94.

75. Marrocco RT, Witte EA, Davidson MC. Arousal systems. [Review]. Curr Opin Neurobiol 1994;4: 166–70.

76. Ommaya AK, Gennarelli TA. Cerebral concussion and traumatic unconsciousness: correlation of experimental and clinical observations of blunt head injuries. Brain 1974; 97:633–54.

77. Plum F, Posner JB. States of acutely altered consciousness. In: Plum F, Posner JB, editors. The Diagnosis of Stupor and Coma. 3rd ed. Philadelphia, PA: FA Davis 1982;3–5.

78. Rogers FB, Shackford SR, Trevisani GT, Davis JW, Mackersie RC, Hoyt DB. Neurogenic pulmonary edema in fatal and nonfatal head injuries. J Trauma 1995;39:860–8.

79. Fraser RG, Paré JAP. Solitary pulmonary nodules less than 6 cm. Diagnosis of Diseases of the Chest. Philadelphia, Pa: WB Saunders Co; 1970:854–60.

80. Demling R, Riessen R. Pulmonary dysfunction after cerebral injury. Crit Care Med 1990;18:768–74.

81. Helling TS, Evans LL, Fowler DL, Hays LV, Kennedy FR. Infectious complications in patients with severe head injury. J Trauma 1988;28:1575–77.

82. NIH Consensus Report. Prevention of venous thromboses and pulmonary embolism. JAMA 1986;256:744–49.

83. Kowalski ML, Didier A, Kaliner MA. Neurogenic inflammation in the airways. I. Neurogenic stimulation induces plasma protein extra-vasation into the rat airway lumen. Am Rev Respir Dis 1989;140:101–9.

84. Yildirim E, Kaptanoglu E, Ozisik K, et al. Ultrastructural changes in pneumocyte type II cells following traumatic brain injury in rats. Eur J Cardiothorac Surg 2004;25:523–529.

85. Seelig JM, Becker DP, Miller JD, et al. Traumatic acute subdural hematoma NEJM 1981;304(25): 1511–17.

86. Mendelow AD, Karmi MZ, Paul KS, Fuller GA, Gillingham FJ. Extradural hematoma: effect of delayed treatment. Br Med J 1979 May 12; 1(6173):1240–42.

87. West JB. Stress failure of pulmonary capillaries: role in lung and heart disease. Lancet 1992;340: 762–7.

88. Bachofen H, Schurch S, Weibel ER. Experimental hydrostatic pulmonary edema in rabbit lungs: barrier lesions. Am Rev Respir Dis 1993;147: 997–1004.

89. Maron MB. Analysis of airway fluid protein concentration in neurogenic pulmonary edema. J Appl Physiol 1987;62:470–6.

90. Johnston SC, Horn JK, Valente J, Simon RP. The role of hypoventilation in a sheep model of epileptic sudden death. Ann Neurol 1995; 37:531–7.

91. Wray NP, Nicotra MB. Pathogenesis of neurogenic pulmonary edema. Am Rev Respir Dis 1978; 118:783–6.

92. Mayer SA, Fink ME, Homma S, et al. Cardiac injury associated with neurogenic pulmonary edema following subarachnoid hemorrhage. Neurology 1994;44:815–20.

93. Yabumoto M, Kuriyama T, Iwamoto M, Kinoshita T. Neurogenic pulmonary edema associated with ruptured intracranial aneurysm: case report. Neurosurgery 1986;19:300–4.

94. Samuels MA. Neurogenic heart disease: a unifying hypothesis. Am J Cardiol 1987;60:15J–19J.

95. Smith WS, Matthay MA. Evidence for a hydrostatic mechanism in human neurogenic pulmonary edema. Chest 1997;111:1326–33.

96. Mabrouk Bahloul, Anis N. Chaari, Hatem Kallel, Abdelmajid Khabir, Adnène Ayadi, Hanène Charfeddine, Leila Hergafi, Adel D. Chaari, Hedi E. Chelly, Chokri Ben Hamida, Noureddine Rekik, Mounir Bouaziz. Neurogenic Pulmonary Edema Due to Traumatic Brain Injury: Evidence of Cardiac Dysfunction Am J Crit Care September 2006;15:462–70.

97. AF Kalmar, J Van Aken, J Caemaert, EP Mortier, and MMR F Struys. Value of Cushing **reflex as warning sign for brain ischemia during neuroendoscop** Br. J. Anesth 2005;94(6):791–99.

98. Cushing H: Concerning the definite regulatory mechanism of the vasomotor center which controls blood pressure during cerebral compression. **Johns Hopkins Bull** 1901;12: 290–2.

99. Fodstad H, Kelly PJ, Buchfelder M. History of the cushing reflex. Neurosurgery 2006;59(5): 1132–7; discussion 1137.

100. Narayan RK, Michael ME, The Clinical Trials in Head Injury Study Group. Clinical trials in head injury. J Neurotrauma 2002;19:503–557.

101. Mukhin AG, Ivanova SA, Knoblach SM, Faden AI (Sept 1997). "New in vitro model of traumatic

neuronal injury: evaluation of secondary injury and glutamate receptor-mediated neurotoxicity". J. Neurotrauma **14** (9): 651–63.

102. Kocaeli H, Korfali E, Oztürk H, Kahveci N, Yilmazlar S (2005). "MK-801 improves neurological and histological outcomes after spinal cord ischemia induced by transient aortic cross-clipping in rats". *Surg Neurol* **64** (Suppl 2): S22–6; discussion S27. doi:10.1016/j.surneu. 2005. 07.034

103. Langham J, Goldfrad C, Teasdale G, Shaw D, Rowan K Calcium channel blockers for acute traumatic brain injury. Cochrane Database Syst Rev 2003; (4):CD000565.

104. Vergouwen MD, Vermeulen M, Roos YB. Lancet Neurol. Effect of nimodipine on outcome in patients with traumatic subarachnoid hemorrhage: a systematic review 2006 Dec;5(12):1029–32.

105. Narayan RK, et al. Clinical trials in head injury. J Neurotrauma 2002;19:503–57.

106. Kathryn Beauchamp, Haitham Mutlak. Pharmacology of Traumatic Brain Injury: Where Is the "Golden Bullet" Mol Med. 2008 Nov-Dec; 14(11–12):731–40.

107. Wolf AL, Levi L, Marmarou A, Ward JD, Muizelaar PJ, Choi S, Young H,Rigamonti D, Robinson WL. Effect of THAM upon outcome in severe head injury: a randomized prospective clinical trial. J Neurosurg 1993;78:54–9.

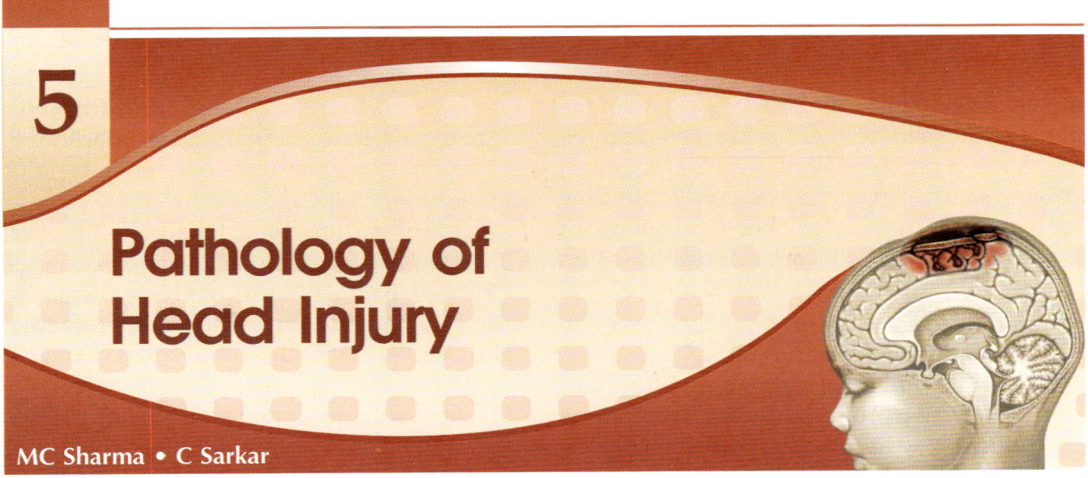

5

Pathology of Head Injury

MC Sharma • C Sarkar

INTRODUCTION

Cerebrospinal injury causing death or permanent disability remains the singlemost important public health problem encountered in industrialized society. Injuries are still responsible for more years of potential life lost than cancer and cardiovascular diseases combined. In United States, recent data shows that, on average, approximately 1.7 million people sustain a traumatic brain injury annually.[1] The head injury rate varies among different population settings for urban and rural as well as in developed and under developed countries. In America the causes of head injuries are traffic and transport accidents in 50%, gunshot in 20 to 40%, fall in 10%, and assaults in 5–10%.

Head injury is a major cause of mortality and morbidity at all ages. The death rate of head injury in children is about 10 per 100,000, five times the mortality rate of leukemia,[2] the next leading cause of death. The most common causes of head injury in childhood are falls, recreational activities, traffic accidents and child abuse.

For many years, pathologists have recognized the characteristic focal lesions found in fatal head injuries. In recent years the recognition of the diffuse lesions—**diffuse axonal injury** (DAI), ischemic brain damage and brain swelling—more fully explains the pathophysiologic abnormalities that accompany such injuries. The old concept that trauma induces immediate and irreversible injury of the central nervous system is questioned by the recent scientific studies.[3]

Types of head injuries are shown in Table 5.1.

SKULL FRACTURES

The presence of a skull fracture signifies that traumatic cranial injury had occurred. Skull fractures occur in up to 8% of fatal head injuries.[4] A number of variables will determine the case with which bone will fracture and

Table 5.1: Classification of primary head injuries		
Skull fractures	*Local injuries*	*Diffuse injuries*
Linear	Contusions	Concussion
Basilar	Coup	
	Contrecoup	
Depressed	Intermediate	
	Fracture	
Comminuted	Lacerations	Diffuse axonal injury
	Hematomas	Mild
		Moderate
		Severe
		Brain swelling
Childhood	Epidural	
	Subdural	
	Subarachnoid	
	Intracerebral	
Intraventricular		

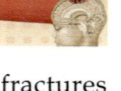

these variables include the age, sex, race of the patient, any underlying disease state and the anatomic location of the bone. Concomitant brain injuries also occur frequently, but they are by no means an invariable consequence of skull fractures.[5] Skull fractures are classified as follows:

a. *Linear fractures:* A linear fracture is a simple fracture line that tends to radiate outwards from the point of impact along with path of least resistance. A linear fracture is produced by a broadbased force such as traffic accidents and falls.

b. *Basilar skull fractures:* Basilar skull fracture may be linear, depressed or comminuted. Fracture of skull may be limited to the area of base or may spread into the base from the calvarium. Fractures of the base of skull are not reliably depicted by radiographic examination.[6] Hence, the routine removal of the dura mater from the skull is necessary to identify fractures at autopsy. Fracture line usually radiates from the impact point. Multiple interlacing fracture lines suggest that multiple blows produced the fractures at the same time or at different times.

c. *Depressed fractures:* This type of fractures are produced by forceful or heavy impacts striking the skull over a small surface area, resulting in a portion of the bone, being pushed inwards to impinge on the brain. To qualify for this, the depression should be greater than the thickness of the fractured bone. Occasionally, such fractures are referred to as **pending fracture.** If the fracture shows pending outward distal to the impact site, it is known as **bursting fracture.** When fracture separates the suture line they are called **diastatic fractures.** These fractures may be closed or open type depending upon the injuries of the overlying soft tissues and scalp.

d. *Comminuted fractures:* This type of fracture result from forceful and heavy impact striking the head over a wider area with bone breaking into multiple pieces.

e. *Compound fractures:* Compound fractures are those where overlying scalp is lacerated. They may occur with any other type of fractures.

f. *Childhood fractures:* Skull fractures of children present with a number of interesting causes. Most of the fractures of skull in children are due to abusive trauma, traffic accidents, falling from height and after devastating situations.

Hobbs[7] suggested that skull fractures after the alleged minor accident indicated abuse if one or more of the following were present.

1. Multiple and complex fractures.
2. Depressed fractures.
3. Maximum fracture width greater than 3 mm.
4. Growing fracture.
5. Involvement of more than one cranial bone.
6. Nonparietal fracture.
7. Associated intracranial injury.

Another interesting lesion is growing fracture produced by an enlarging traumatically induced leptomeningeal cyst. This cyst is lined by fibrous connective tissue and is filled by CSF. It protrudes through a tear in the underlying dura mater, enlarges the linear fracture and erodes the bone along the fracture margins. The enlargement and erosion of the bone are believed to be caused by pulsation of the brain.[8] **Growing fractures** usually occur in children less than 3 years of age and are not associated with significant injury to the brain.

Compound and basal skull fracture results in cerebrospinal fluid fistule, leading to CSF **rhinorrhea, otorrhea and meningitis.**

Lacerations: A laceration is a mechanical tear or rent in normal tissue. They result from greater force and appear at the same site as contusions. They may or may not be accompanied by skull fracture. Cerebral lacerations usually involve inferior surface of frontal lobe or temporal lobe tips. Lacerations if associated with diffuse axonal injury commonly involve **corpus callosum** and the brainstem.

Tears, lacerations or brainstem avulsion of the pontomedullary junction and cerebral

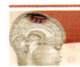

peduncles occur as a result of hyperextension.[14] They are usually seen in fatal road accidents, atlanto-occipital dislocations and high cervical fracture.

DIFFUSE AXONAL INJURY (DAI)

The diffuse axonal injury was first described by Strich[15] in 1956 as diffuse degeneration of the white matter and was thought to be essential component of post-traumatic **dementia.** Later on, some authors called it as inner cerebral trauma[16] and shearing injury.[17] The currently accepted name used to describe this entity is **diffuse axonal injury** (DAI).[18, 19]

Axonal injury is a key feature of the post-traumatic **encephalopathies** and is an important determinant of the outcome in non-missile head injuries. **DAI** is an important cause of coma, in the absence of an intracranial expanding lesion, in patients who are in vegetative state and is an important cause of disability after head injury.[20,21] **DAI** is a distinct clinicopathologic entity which may develop after mild concussion up to 24 hours of injury and is persistent for long in post-traumatic cases.[21,22]

DAI develops most frequently in patients who have been injured in vehicle accidents both occupants and pedestrians, after falls, after assaults and with child abuse. Compared with other head injury patients, patients with DAI have fewer skull fractures and a lower incidence of cerebral **contusions,** intracranial hematoma and raised intracranial pressure. Patients with moderate to severe diffuse axonal injury are rendered immediate unconscious by their injury and remain unconscious until their death. Those who survive for longer period in **vegetative** states are the patients with severely diffuse head injury but without axonal injury.[18]

In **DAI**, grossly brain may appear normal. But in most severe degree of DAI, focal lesions are seen in the **corpus callosum,** one or both dorsolateral quadrants of the **rostral brainstem.** In the early stage of injury, the lesions are hemorrhagic and appear as **petechial** size hemorrhages, streaks of hemorrhages or as small intraparenchymal hemorrhages.

Similar hemorrhages occur, in addition to corpus callosum and brainstem, in sub-cortical white matter, fornix, tela choroidea, walls of third ventricle, basal ganglia and hippocampal region. In very severe cases larger streaks of hemorrhage are seen in the white matter. As the hemorrhagic lesions age, they become softened, granular and finally cystic. In the later stage there is dilatation of the ventricles because of reduced bulk of white matter.

On microscopic examination, the hallmark of DAI is axonal swelling **(retraction balls)** in the cerebral white matter, corpus callosum and upper brainstem. Axonal swelling becomes apparent within hours of the injury and may persist for a year or more. In patients who survive, **microglial stars** (clusters of microglial cells) develop at the site of injury and replace the swollen axons.

To diagnose DAI, evidence of axonal injury needs to be found independent of other lesions such as infarcts and hematoma. The histologic appearance of axonal injury depends upon the duration of survival after injury. Affected patients, have a high mortality, and if they survive, a high morbidity, often improving into only a persistent" vegetative state. Diffuse axonal injury can be diagnosed by diffusion-weighted MRI.[23] If the survival is from hours to a few days, many irregular swellings of the axons and oval or rounded bulbs at the end of the axon are seen which appear bright pink (eosinophilic) on H and E staining. Axons may appear tortuous or varicosed and show irregular thickening. These findings are better broughtout in silver staining. Identification of axonal swelling can be augmented by staining for **ubiquitin** or **amyloid precursor protein (APP).** If patient survives for many months in vegetative state then Wallerian degeneration appear.

DAI appears to be a distinct clinicopathological entity which may develop after mild concussion. The findings of occasional clusters of microglia in the patients dying soon after a minor head injury suggested that axonal injury had occurred.[23] More recently axonal damage have been demonstrated in patients who died from unrelated causes after sustaining a mild injury by using **antibody against amyloid precursor proteins.**[24–26]

Adams et al[27] proposed a grading system based on the severity of injury. **In grade I DAI,** the histological evidence of axonal damage is found in the white matter of the cerebral hemispheres; corpus callosum, brainstems and less commonly in the cerebellum. **In grade II DAI**, in addition to widely distributed axonal injury there is also focal lesion in the corpus callosum. **Grade III**, represents the most severe spectrum of DAI and takes the form of diffuse damage to axons and focal lesions in both corpus callosum and dorso-lateral quadrant or quadrants of the rostral brainstem. These authors have shown correlation between the grade and level of consciousness.

Strich[28] proposed that axonal damage is produced by mechanical forces engendered at the moment of impact that physically disrupt axons. Some authors have suggested that the damage to white matter is a secondary event and is due to **hypoxic brain** damage, oedema or **herniation.**[29] Gennarelli et al[19] experimentally produced diffuse axonal injury in monkeys using only controlled angular head accelerations in the sagittal, oblique or lateral direction without the necessity of impact to the head. Experimental studies by Porlishock and Coworkers[30,31] have identified the axonal changes that produced the **axonal retraction balls**. The mechanism postulated to cause diffuse axonal injury is the shearing force regenerated by movements of the head, which physically tear the axons. Retraction balls formed from swelling of the axons, which resulted from accumulation of organelles as axoplasmic transport was impaired. The separation of proximal and distal segments did not occur until the reactive swelling was formed.

BRAIN SWELLING

Brain swelling is an increase in the size of one or both cerebral hemispheres. The extent of involvement depends on a number of features such as patient's age and nature of the injury. The term brain swelling includes both edema and cerebrovascular congestion.[33] Two closely related clinicopathologic syndromes of diffuse brain swelling were identified by CT scanning. These syndromes occur almost exclusively in children and adolescents.[34] In the first scenario, diffuse swelling is the result of edema which is of vasogenic in nature. This edema is the result of injury to the capillary endothelial junctions, the site of blood–brain barriers, leading to the passage of plasma proteins and electrolytes into the brain extracellular space. Edema fluid flows from the site of capillary injury in the white matter towards the ventricles under hydrostatic pressure of circulation. In the grey matter, the oedema fluid does not extravasate into the extracellular space and the astrocytes take in the fluid and swell. Edema fluids in the white matter move into the ventricles and enters CSF pathway. Presence of oedema contributes to increase in the intracranial pressure which further decrease the cerebral blood flow and impair auto-regulations of cerebral blood flow.

The other type of diffuse brain swelling is due to increased blood flow and severe hyperemia. The clinical importance of these two types of diffuse brains swelling lies in the fact that in first type, patients often follow relentless course to death whereas in second type recovery follows without any sequelae.

Diffuse swelling causes flattening of gyri, narrowing of sulci and symmetrical collapse of the ventricular system. In localized swelling distortion and herniation occur. Minimal swelling may not be recognized early. Cerebral edema produces pallor of the myelin, distention of perivascular and pericellular spaces, rarefaction of subpial spaces, a vacuolar appearance of the neuropil, and pools of proteins rich fluid in the spongy looking areas. However, measurement of water content is the most reliable method of diagnosing **cerebral edema.**

HEMORRHAGE

In head injury patients' hemorrhages develop in the epidural, subdural, subarachnoidal space and in the brain parenchyma.[34,35] When such bleeds form mass lesions, they often produce devastating neurophysiologic effects and cause significant mortality and morbidity.

Epidural Hematoma

Epidural hematoma follows cranial trauma complicated by temporal bone fracture and result from laceration of middle meningeal artery branches that penetrate the skull in the regions of the pterion.[35] The accumulation of blood between calvarium and endosteal surface of the dura mater is rapid and is accompanied by rapid deterioration of consciousness. If not evacuated promptly, it leads to **transtentorial herniation** and compression of brainstem. Small streak hemorrhages which occur in the midbrain and pons secondary to transtentorial herniation know as Duret hemorrhages. Chronic subdural hematomas are usually of venous origin.

Subdural Hematoma

Normally, the space between dura mater and arachnoid is closely opposed. Subdural hematomas result from the dissection of blood into this potential space. Most common location is over the cerebral convexities and supposed to be because of rupture of delicate bridging veins that traverse the arachnoid dura interface enroute to the superior sagittal sinus. These vessels are susceptible to shearing forces generated by sudden angular acceleration of the head. Patients on anticoagulants are more prone to subdural hematoma. Subdural hematomas may be acute, subacute or chronic depending upon the interval of injury and onset of symptoms. Acute hematoma becomes symptomatic within 3 days and if the symptoms develop between 3 and 21 days then subacute. If they become symptomatic after 21 days,

they are chronic. However, these distinctions are arbitrary and some authors prefer to identify age of the lesion from its **pathologic appearance.**[36]

The pathology of subdural hematoma depends upon the age. If evacuated early it consist of clotted blood. In later stages organization start and hematoma gets surrounded by collagenous membranes leading to see formation. The membrane may attain thickness of several millimeters and are composed of proliferating spindle cells, loose connective tissue budding capillaries, **siderophages** and lymphocytes. In some cases a significant number of eosinophils are also seen[9] (Fig. 5.1) and these eosinophils are more common in chronic subdural hematomas/membranes.[37]

Subdural Hygroma

A subdural hygroma is the accumulation of watery serious fluid in the subdural space. The other terminologies used for this condition are **meningitis** serosa traumatica and traumatic subdural effusion. **Hygroma** may develop immediately after head injury or after sometime. **Hygroma** occurs alone or concomitantly with other head and brain injuries. Symptoms depend upon the rate at which fluid collects. Tears of the arachnoid or impaired CSF absorption are likely to be etiological factors.

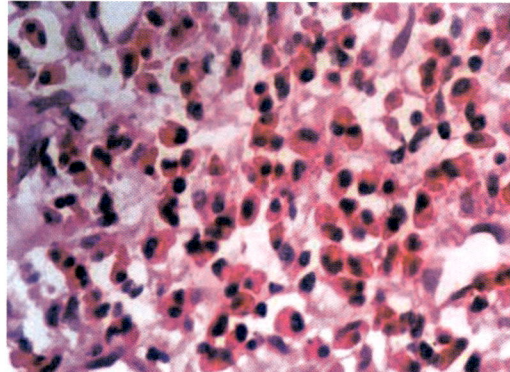

Fig. 5.1: Photomicrograph showing numerous eosinophils in a subdural hematoma

Subarachnoid Hemorrhage (SAH)

Trauma is the most frequent cause of subarachnoid hemorrhage besides other non-traumatic causes. Injury of any magnitude can cause subarachnoid hemorrhage. Subarachnoid hemorrhage is found overlying contusions, spreading outwards from lacerations and around gunshot wounds. In subdural hemorrhage if veins are teared in the subarachnoid space then hemorrhage lies under the subdural hematoma also. Traumatic basilar subarachnoid hemorrhage is a massive hemorrhage over the ventral surface of the brainstem.

Within a few hours of bleeding into the CSF, fever and meningisms develop. There is polymorphonuclear response within 24 hours and becomes prominent by 48 hours. After 48 hours, lymphocytes and macrophages start replacing them. Macrophages phagocytose RBCs and such lipid laden phagocytes may persist for years in the arachnoid meninges and Virchow-Robin spaces. Repeated episodes of CSF hemorrhage may impair the absorption of CSF and may produce hydrocephalus.[38]

Intracerebral Hemorrhage (ICH)

Intracerebral hemorrhages vary in size from a small petechial hemorrhage of less than 0.5 cm to a large hematoma and may be single or multiple in number. An intracerebral hematoma may also be accompanied with epidural hematoma alone or combined with subdural hematoma.

The large intracerebral hematomas are most commonly located in the frontal and temporal lobes and are associated with adjacent contusions and lacerations.[39] The large parenchymal hemorrhages can extend into the ventricles.

The other subgroup of intracerebral hemorrhages is associated with diffuse axonal injury. Small hemorrhage appears in the white matter and basal ganglia and probably due to tearing of small vessels by the same shearing force which damage axons. These small hemorrhages may enlarge over several days.

Delayed Traumatic Intracerebral Hematoma

A delayed traumatic intracerebral hematoma is one that arises in an area of brain that has been previously injured by impact usually in a contusion. Due to injury, vessels are weakened within the contused area and if autoregulation fails or systemic hypertension develops then bleeding occurs.

Burst Lobe

A burst lobe is severely combined frontal or temporal pole whose cortical surface is pulled out and lacerated with extension of hemorrhage through the arachnoid into subdural space. Burst lobe occurs most commonly in association with contrecoup contusions.

Intraventricular Hemorrhage (IVH)

Intraventricular hemorrhage is bleeding within the lateral ventricles that may extend into subarachnoid space. Traumatic intraventricular hemorrhage occurs commonly in association with other intracranial injury. The volume of blood varies from a few milliliter to large hemorrhage of 40 to 60 ml.

Brain Damage Related to Trauma

Immediate impact injuries are traumatically caused lesions that are generated at the time of impact and are produced by the direct damage of the impact itself rather than as a complication of the traumatizing force.

Concussion

A cerebral concussion (**commotio cerebri**) is a temporary, reversible neurologic deficiency caused by trauma, which results in immediate loss of consciousness which is temporary. Concussion is accompanied by **retrograde** and **post-traumatic amnesia** and duration of which depends upon the severity of concussion. When concussion lasts more than 24 hours or longer, diffuse brain injury is usually present. Experimental studies of concussion have shown minimal non-specific neuronal changes.[9,10] Neuropathology studies of classical cerebral concussion in humans have rarely been available to study. Concussion is usually accompanied by other injuries like contusions, skull fractures and multiple brain injuries. The morbidity and mortality of cerebral concussion depends on the severity of the associated brain injuries.

Contusions

A contusion is a bruise of the cortical surface of the brain which results as a hemorrhage around the blood vessel secondary to the injury to small vessels (Fig. 5.2). The overlying pia mater always remains intact. Contusions are usually result of mechanical injury and extent depends upon the forcefulness of the impact which results in contusions. They may occupy part or all of the cortical layers. Contusions tend to be wedge-shaped with base towards the surface and apex towards the white matter. They can cause full thickness necrosis of the cortex. Continuous bleeding within a contusion results in contusion bleeding which may extend into the white matter or cortical surface and CSF. Contusions are focal damage and even in severe cases, there may be complete recovery, clinically if there is no accompanying diffuse axonal injury.

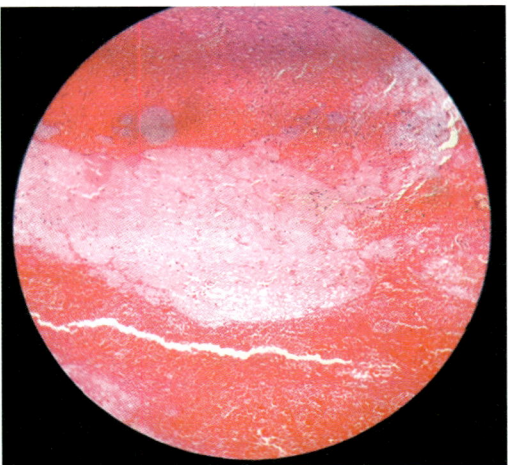

Fig. 5.2: Photomicrograph showing contused brain, i.e. petechial hemorrhages around the small vessels in the cerebral cortex

Contusions tend to be large and more hemorrhagic in hypertensive, alcoholic or who have **bleeding diathesis.** Adams et al[11] developed a contusion index in which the depth and extent of the contusions were graded in frontal, temporal, parietal and occipital lobes and in the cortex above and below the Sylvian fissures and the cerebellum. The indices that reflected the severity of contusion at each site and their mean were used to assess other types of head injury such as skull fractures or diffuse axonal injury.

Contusions formed at the site of cranial impact are **coup contusions;** those opposite the cranial impact, **contrecoup contusions;** and those at the margins of brain herniation, herniation contusions. Herniation contusions are most frequently located along the margin of the falx cerebri, tentorium or foramen magnum. Bruises found along the edges of skull fractures are **fracture contusions.** **Gliding contusions** are deep parenchymal injuries that may or may not be comparable to surface contusions.

Contusions form in certain locations depending upon the position and motion of the body at the time of impact which has been supported by experimental studies. A number of theories have been proposed to explain the phenomenon of contusion.

Houlbourn's **rotational shear force theory** to some extent explains the contrecoup contusions.[12,13] This theory suggests that rotational movements of the brain generate shearing forces that produce contusions in a distribution referred to as contrecoup.

As the contusion ages, the necrotic cortical tissue is removed, leaving behind a shrunken orange brown scar. Some contusions are large enough to produce subcortical hematoma. Spinal cord may be contused over an extended area or may show hemorrhagic necrosis. Evolution of damage to the cord includes gliosis and cavitation of the spinal cord adjacent to a transection. Ascending and descending Wallerian degeneration of injured fibers tracts evolve. Traumatic neuromata and post-traumatic syringomyelia may develop.

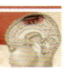
Secondary Complications

Increased intracranial pressure: Increased intracranial pressure is the most common cause of death in head injury. Pressure necrosis in one or both parahippocampal gyri at autopsy may be used as a criterion of whether intracranial pressure had been raised to a significant level. The common causes of increased intracranial pressure are intracranial hematomas and brain swelling.

Hypoxic brain damage: In patients who die from head injury, the ischemic change is a frequent finding (Fig. 5.3). Ischemic damage is more common in patients who have had a clinical episode of **hypoxia**, either as hypotension or **hypoxemia**, or in patients who have had elevated intracranial pressure. In addition, vascular spasm contributes to the etiology of ischemia. Ischemic damage is more common in the **watershed zones** or throughout the cerebral cortex, basal ganglia and cerebellum.

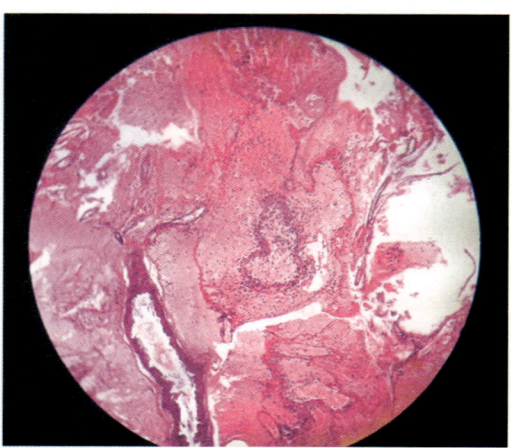

Fig. 5.3: Photomicrograph contused hemorrhages in the grey matter along with ischemic charges in the neurons. Some of the neurons show more eosinophilic cytoplasm

REFERENCES

1. Faul M, Xu L, Wald MM, Coronado VG. Traumatic brain injury in the United States: emergency department visits, hospitalizations, and deaths. Atlanta (GA): Centers for Disease Control and Prevention, National Center for Injury Prevention and Control; 2010.
2. Kraus JF, et al. Incidence, severity and external causes of pediatric head injury Am J Dis Child 1986;140:687.
3. Povilshock JT, Jenkins LW: Are the pathobiological changes evoked by traumatic brain injury immediate and irreversible? Brain Pathology 1995;5:415.
4. Adams JH: The neuropathology of head injuries. In: Vinken PJ, Bruyn GW, ed. Handbook of clinical neurology. Vol. 23, Amsterdam : North-Holland 1975;35.
5. Servadei F, Giucci G, Morchetti A. et al. Skull fracture as a factor of increased risk in minor head injuries. Indication for a broader use of cerebral computed tomography scanning. Surg Neurol 1988;30:364.
6. Ehler E, Ivankievicz D, Schomachar GH: Diagnosis of skull fractures by autopsy and radiology. Acta Morphol 1980;28:291.
7. Hobbs CJ: Skull fracture and the diagnosis of abuse. Arch Dis Child 1984;56:246.
8. Taveres J, Ransokoff J: Leptomeningeal cysis of the brain following trauma with erosion of the skull. A study of seven casestreated by injury. J Neurosurg 1953;10:233.
9. Adams JH, Graham DI, Gennarelli TA. Acceleration induced head injury in the monkey. Acta Neuropathol 1991;7(Suppl),26.
10. Groat RA, Windle WF, Magoun HW. Functional and structural changes in the monkey's brain during and after concussion. J Neurosurg 1994;2:26.
11. Adams JH, Doyle D, Graham DI, et al. The contusion index: a reappraisal in man and experimental non-missile head injury. Neuropathol Appl Neurobiol 1985;11:299.
12. Holbourn AHS. Mechanics of head injuries. Lancet 1943;2:438.
13. Holbourn AHS. Mechanics of head injuries. Brit Med Bull 1945;3:147.
14. Lindenberg R, Freytag E. Brainstem lesions characteristics of traumatic hyperextension of the head. Arch Pathol 1970;90:509.
15. Strich SJ. Diffuse degeneration of the cerebral white matter in severe dementia following head injury. J Neurol Neurosurg Psychiat 1956;19:163.
16. Greevic N. Topography and pathogenic mechanisms of lesion in "inner cerebral trauma". Rad Acad Sci 1982;402:265.
17. Peerless SJ, Rewcastle NB. Shear injuries of the brain. Can Med Assoc J 1967;96:577.

18. Adam JH, Graham DI, Murray LS, Scott G. Diffuse axonal injury due to non-missile head injury in human. An analysis of 45 cases. Ann Neurol 1982;12:557.

19. Gennarelli TA, Jhibault LE, Adams JH, Graham DI, Thompson CJ, Marcincin RP. Diffuse axonal injury and traumatic coma in the primate. Ann Neurol 1982;12:567.

20. Adams JH: Head injury. In : Adams JH, Duchen W.Ed. Greenfield's Neuropathology, 5th Ed. London. Arnold 1992;106.

21. Blumbergs PC, Jones NR, North JB: Diffuse axonal injury in head trauma. J Neurol Neurosurg Psychiatr 1989;52:838.

22. Clerk JM: Distribution of microglial clusters in the brain after head injury. J Neurol Neurosurg Psychiatr 1974;37:467.

23. Liu AY, Maldjian JA, Bagley LJ, et al. Traumatic brain injury diffusion: weighted MR imaging findings. AINR 1999;20:1636–41.

24. Blumbergs PC, Scott G, Manavis J, Wainwright H, Simpson DA, Mclean AJ. Staining of amyloid precursor protein to study axonal damage in mild head injury. Lancet 1994;344:1055.

25. Grady MS, McLaughlin MR, Christman CW, Valadka AB, Flinger CL, Povlishock JT. The use of antibodies targeted against the neurofilament submits for the detection of diffuse axonal injury in humans. J Neuropathol Exp Neurol 1993;52:143.

26. Gultekin SH, Smith TW. Diffuse axonal injury in craniocerebral trauma: A comparative histologic and immunohisto chemical study. Arch Pathol Lab Med 1994;118:168.

27. Adams JH, Doyle D, Ford 1, Gennarelli TA, Grahm DI, McLellan DR. Diffuse axonal injury in head injury: definition, diagnosis and grading. Histopathology 1989;15:49.

28. Strich SJ. Shearing of nerve fibres as a cause of brain damage due to head injury. Lancet 1961; 2:443–48.

29. Jellinger K, Seiterberger F. Protracted post-traumatic encephalopathy: Pathology, patho-genesis and clinical implications. J Neurol Sci 1970;10:51.

30. Povlishock JT, et al. Axonal change in minor head injury. J Neuropathol Exp Neurol 1983; 42:225.

31. Buki A, Povlishock JT. Evidence for Calpain — Mediated spectin protrolysis in the pathoguries of traumatically induced axoval injury. J Neuropath Exp. Neurol 1999;58:365–375.

32. Povlishock JT, Erb DE, Astrue J. Reactive axonal change, deafferentation and Neuropathology. J of Neurotrauma 1992;9:S189–5200.

33. Klagzo I. Neuropathological aspects of brain oedema. Neuropath Exp Neurol 1967;26:1.

34. Graham DI, Ford I, Adams JH, Doyle D. Lawrence AE, Me Clellan DR: Fatal head injury in children. J Clin Pathol 1989;42:18.

35. Hardman JM. Cerebrospinal trauma. In Davis RL, Robertson DM, ed. Textbook of neuropatho-logy, ed. 2. Baltimore. Williams and Wilkins 1991;973–74.

36. Fogetholm R, Heiskanen O, Waltimo O. Chronic subdural hematoma in adults. Influence of patient's age on symptoms, signs and thickness of hematoma. J Neurosurg 1975;42:43.

37. Sarkar C, Lakhtakia R, Gill SS, Sharma MC, Mahapatra AK, Mehta VS. Chronic subdural hematoma and the enigmatic eosinophilActa Neurochir (Wien) 2000;144:983–8.

38. Gilles FH, Shilliot J Jr. Infantile hydrocephalus Retrocerebellar subdural hematoma. J Pediatr 1970;76:529.

39. Gurdigian ES. Cerebral contusions: Re-evaluation of the mechanism of their development. J Trauma 1976;16:35.

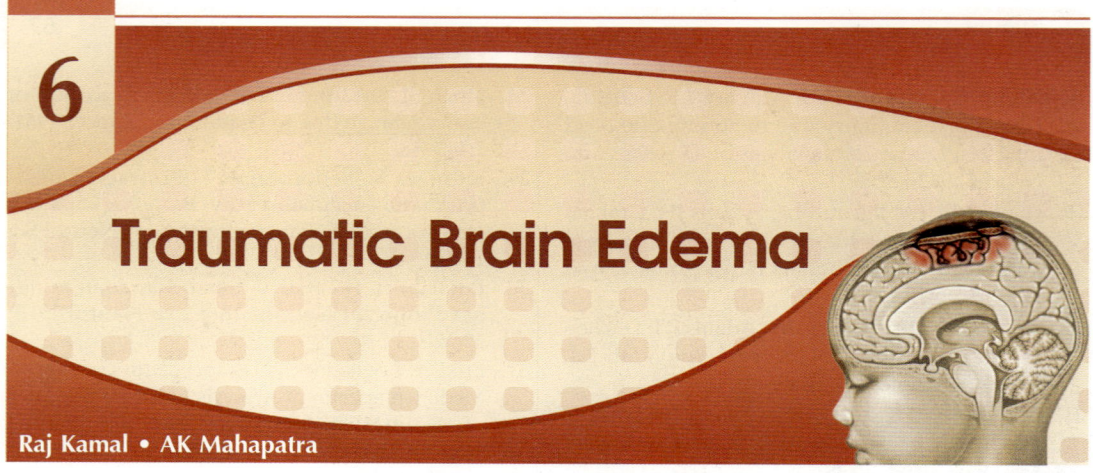

6

Traumatic Brain Edema

Raj Kamal • AK Mahapatra

INTRODUCTION

Brain edema is defined as a net increase in the water content of cerebral tissue that leads to an increase in overall brain mass. Brain swelling refers to increase in brain volume caused by increase in intracranial blood volume and brain edema.[1-4] Traumatic brain edema is a distinct condition[1-4] which can be present alone or in association with other focal pathological processes like contusion, laceration or intracerebral hematoma. The traumatic brain edema is one of the most undesirable pathology, associated frequently, and difficult to treat. Classically, two major types of traumatic brain edema exist: **"vasogenic"** due to blood–brain barrier (BBB) disruption resulting in extracellular water accumulation and "cytotoxic" due to sustained intracellular water collection.[1-4] **Vasogenic edema** refers to the influx of fluid and solutes into the brain through incompetent blood–brain barrier (BBB). **Cytotoxic edema** is due to breakdown of cell membrane following traumatic brain injury.[4,5] Cell membrane breakdown results from ischemia which causes failure of Na^+-K^+ pump and Ca^{2+} pump, release of free fatty acids (FFA) and free radicals. The formation of post-traumatic brain edema can raise intracranial pressure inside the unyielding cranial cavity, and this can reduce cerebral perfusion pressure and cause ischemia. Unfortunately, edema is the cause of death in large number of head injury patients, in whom intracranial pressure persistently remains high leading to widespread damage. In young children, edema behave very differently and may lead to death more often, hence, recently termed as malignant brain edema.[6] This chapter deals with some aspects of traumatic brain edema.

PATHOPHYSIOLOGY OF BRAIN EDEMA

Brain edema (Figs 6.1a, 6.1b and 6.2) is a dynamic process in which a series of changes occur in endothelial cells in blood vessel, blood–brain barrier and cell membrane, leading to biochemical changes which ultimately result in fluid extravasation. However, the process is very complex and involves a large number of neurotransmitters.[7-10] Generally, edema is a secondary pathology in the brain following head injury, and may be of vasogenic or cytotoxic in origin. Due to injury, there is breakdown in **blood–brain** barrier (BBB), and **exudation** of fluid (Figs 6.3 to 6.5). This process sets in around the focal brain lesions like contusion, intracerebral hematoma and give rise to focal brain edema.[9] Rarely after TBI do we encounter a "interstitial" brain edema (third type of edema) related to an obstruction of cerebrospinal fluid outflow. Following TBI, various mediators are released which enhance vasogenic and/or cytotoxic brain edema. These include glutamate, lactate,

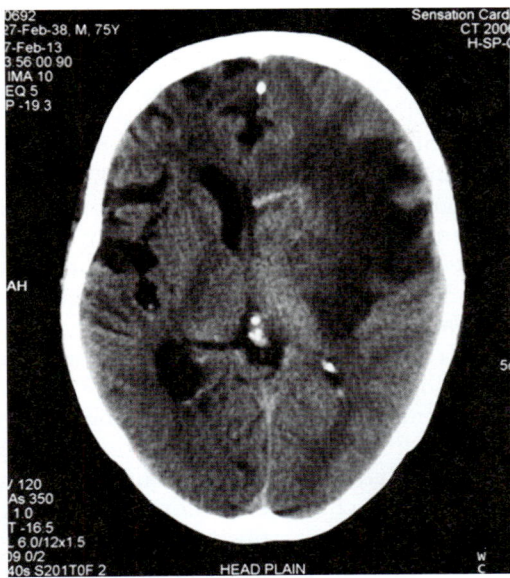

Fig. 6.1a: NCCT head of a patient with severe head injury showing left frontal lobe extensive edema

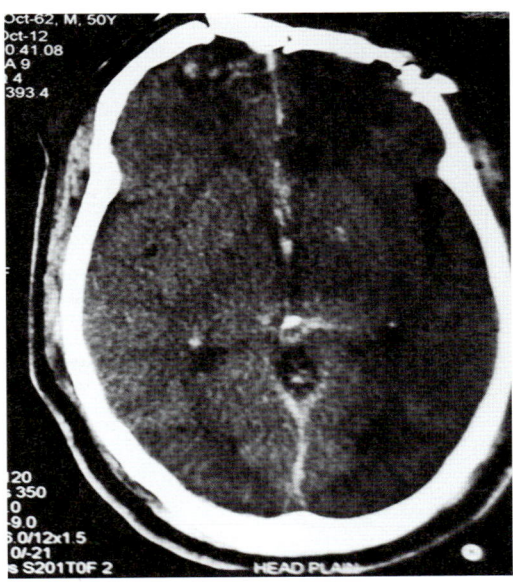

Fig. 6.2: NCCT head of a patient with severe head injury showing almost hemispheric edema on left side

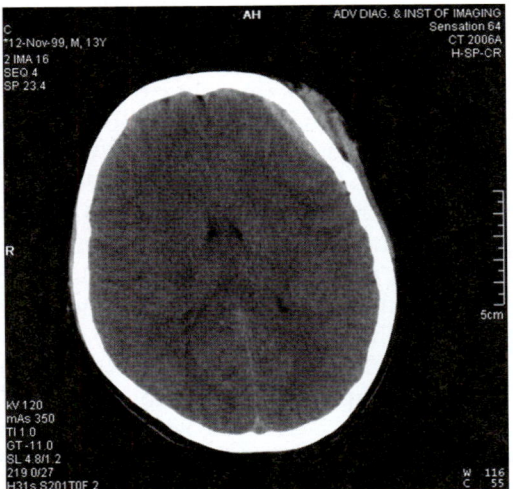

Fig. 6.1b: NCCT head of a patient with severe head injury showing generalized edema

H^+, K^+, Ca^{2+}, nitric oxide, arachidonic acid and its metabolites, free oxygen radicals, histamine, and kinins.[1] Vasogenic edema refers to the influx of fluid and solutes into the brain through incompetent blood–brain barrier (BBB). Thus, vasogenic edema, is the result of a vascular insult leading to increased permeability of endothelial cells to macromolecules, which includes protein and other molecules (Fig. 6.3).

The fluid resultant from BBB disruption is usually protein rich, having more characteristics of blood ultrafilterate. Vasogenic edema extends preferentially through white matter. The spread of vasogenic edema compromises local micro circulation, adding further ischemic insult to edematous area. Clinically, vasogenic edema is demonstrated by hypodensity of the white matter on computed tomography (CT) (Figs 6.1a, 6.1b and 6.2). In cytotoxic edema cellular swelling occurs. BBB remains intact. Following severe head injuries astrocytic swelling was seen three hours to three days after injury. Breakdown of cell membrane following traumatic brain injury is the cause of cytotoxic edema. As discussed above, cell membrane breakdown results from ischemia which causes failure of Na^+-K^+ pump and Ca^{2+} pump, release of free fatty acids (FFA) and free radicals.[11] Cellular swelling can produce

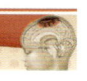
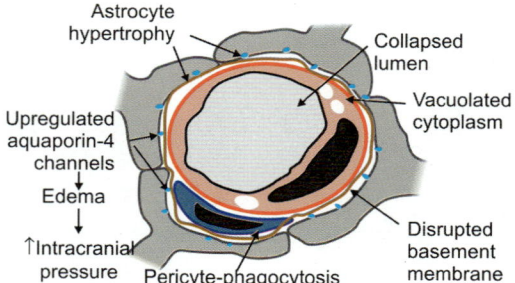

Blood–brain barrier changes

Fig. 6.3: Blood–brain barrier changes following head injury

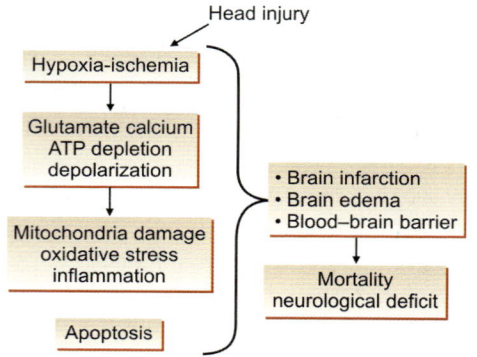

Fig. 6.4: Cascade of events in the formation of brain edema following head injury

numerous deleterious secondary effects in the cell, including membrane depolarization secondary to loss of intracellular K^+ release and decreased uptake of excitatory amino acids, as seen in astrocytes. The traumatic brain edema is a combination of vasogenic and cellular with the cellular component predominating.[12]

According to Marmarou,[13] the type of edema in traumatic brain injury with or without associated mass lesion is predominantly a cellular edema, although a vasogenic component may be present. He suggested that closed head injury is associated with a rapid and transient BBB opening that begins at the time of the trauma and lasts no more than 30 minutes. It has also been shown that addition of post-traumatic secondary insult-hypoxia

and hypotension-prolongs the time of BBB breakdown after closed head injury.[13,14] A lack of BBB opening in the presence of continued swelling has been noted in clinical studies of head-injured patients in whom magnetic resonance "water maps" were obtained with gadolinium challenge. The net balance of ionic movement that accompanies brain injury results in the movement of cations out of the extracellular space into cells. Membrane depolarization resulting from ionic flux and trauma triggers voltage-sensitive ion channels, providing further routes for ionic movement. These ionic disturbances are identified by an increase in extracellular potassium with a concomitant decrease in extracellular sodium, calcium, and chloride. Restoration of ionic homeostasis is accomplished via cotransport and countertransport processes such as the Na^+-K^+ ATPase, $Na^+/K^+/2Cl^-$ cotransporter, Na^+-H^+ transporter, and Na^+ - Ca^{2+} exchanger. However, if the injury is severe, or if secondary insults occur, disruption of ionic homeostasis persists as the cotransport and countertransport processes are impaired and become incapable of returning ion concentrations to their normal levels.[13] Moreover, in the absence of adequate levels of ATP resulting from either an ischemic reduction in cerebral blood flow or insufficient production of ATP due to mitochondrial dysfunction, energy-dependent ion pumps and cotransport and countertransport processes are inefficient in counteracting the normal dissipative flux of ions down their electrochemical gradients. Marmarou hypothesized that the movement of sodium and calcium is passively followed by chloride to maintain electroneutrality, and is followed isosmotically by water.[13–15]

Astrocytes express **aquaporin 4 (AQP4)**, the water channel protein, involved in water homeostasis and edema formation (Fig. 6.3). Aside from its function in water homeostasis, recent studies started to show possible interrelations between aquaporin 4 and neuroinflammation in recent years, AQP4 has been associated with brain edema and neuroinflammation in chronic and acute brain

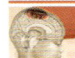

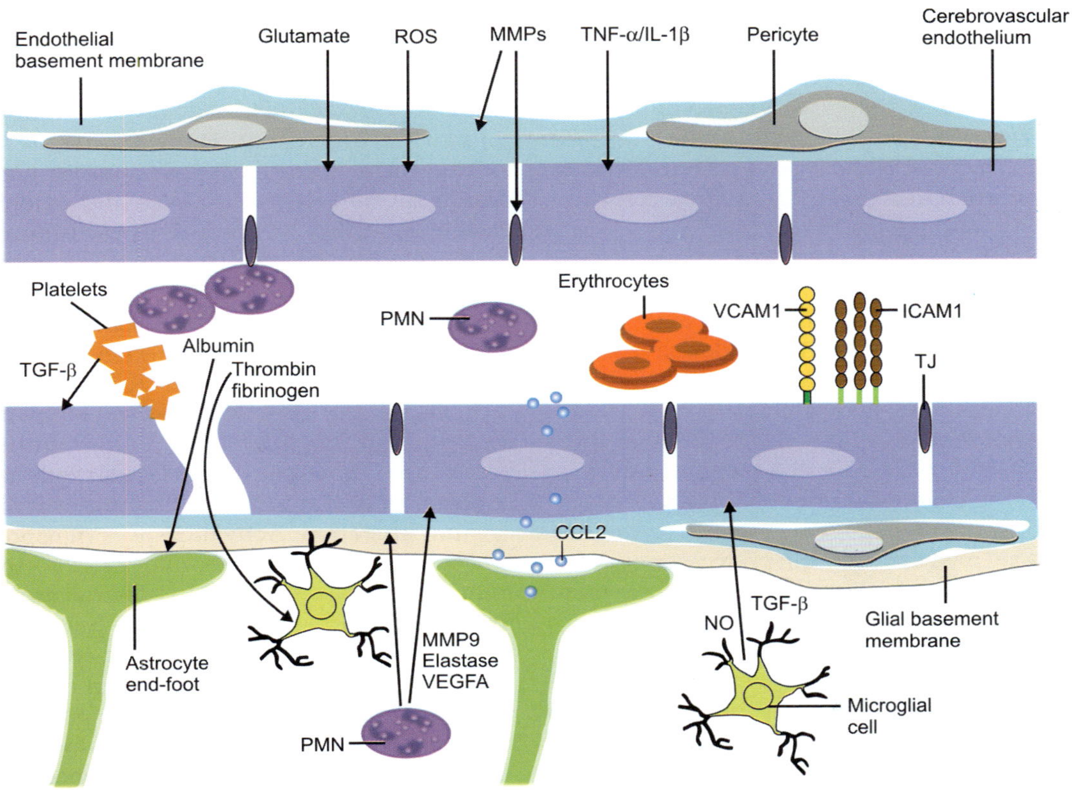

Fig. 6.5: Disruption of vascular integrity following head injury allows albumin, fibrinogen and thrombin to enter brain. In presence of thrombin and albumin microglia produces TNF-α, NO, IL-6 and IL-12. Following injury glutamate, ROS, MMPs, pro-inflammatory cytokines, TNF-α, IL-1β, VEGFA are released by parenchymal cell. PMN (polymorphoneutrophils) causes increased permeability of BBB. These cytokines stimulates expression of (1) adhesion molecules (AMs) like ICAM 1 (intercellular adhesion molecule), VCAM 1 (vascular cell adhesion molecule), (2) chemokines CKCL1 and CCL 2. End result of above processes is increased permeability of BBB and neuroinflammation. A major factor for neuroinflammation is TGF-β which is produced by platelets and microglia. TNFα: tumor necrosis factor-α, NO; nitric oxide, IL: interleukin, ROS: reactive oxygen species, MMP: matrix metalloproteinases, VEGFA: vascular endothelial growth factor A

diseases.[15–19] AQP4 is one of the key players in edema formation and resolution[20–25] and increase in its expression is observed in reactive astrocytes after brain injury. Edema is frequently observed in brain injuries and is associated with BBB disruption. Compromised BBB integrity leads to plasma protein leakage and extravascular fluid accumulation.[20–25] The breakdown of the BBB is a complex process partially caused by the activation of matrix metalloproteinases (MMPs), which is part of the neuroinflammatory response.[24, 25] MMPs are released by parenchymal cells and invading leukocytes.

Pro-inflammatory cytokines such as IL-1β and TNF-α has been shown to produce MMP-9 and MMP-3 in cultured astrocytes and microglia. (Fig. 6.5) MMP-9 aggravates vasogenic edema development by degrading the basal lamina located between the astrocytic end-feet and endothelia.[25] Of particular interest is the link of MMP with AQP4; MMP-2 and MMP-9 are known to degrade agrin and MMP-3 degrades dystroglycan,[25] two proteins that have a critical role in the maintenance of the OAP (orthogonal array of particles). So, when MMP are upregulated after a neuroinflammatory response, more AQP4-OAPs

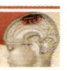

will be disorganized, leading to a possible disruption of the BBB and edema. Vasogenic edema development can further damage the endothelia by increased water volume, and therefore, increased hydrostatic pressure. Thus, if there is decreased BBB disruption, there will be less pro-inflammatory cytokines, MMPs, and edema.

Penfield and Cone 1938[26] proposed involvement of oligodendroglia in the process of acute brain swelling. However, recent clinical and experimental studies have shown wide range of chemical neurotransmitter changes following head injury which leads to brain edema (Table 6.1).[26–29] Some authors have shown the role of vasogenic amine in increase permeability of endothelial cells[30,31] giving rise to vasogenic edema. Cytokines, capsain mediated spectrin proteolytic enzymes capase activation also induces post-traumatic edema.[32–34]

Most important in production in brain edema is ischemia which alters the membrane permeability, which on the other hand leads to (a) vasogenic edema because of opening of tight junction in endothelial cells and (b) cytotoxic edema due to cellular membrane damage leading to abnormal fluid accumulation in cells.[29] The combination of cytotoxic and vasogenic edema increases the brain volume and decreases perfusion to brain tissue causing more damage.

Cell membrane damage plays an important role in pathological manifestation in head injury. Neuronal membrane damage causes efflux of K^+ into extracellular space and intracellular Ca^{++} increases. There is increase in extracellular glutamate. **Glutamate** also damages the cell membranes and causes further K^+ efflux,[9,18] leading to the disturb feedback between K^+ and glutamate liberation. This also leads to damages of calcium homeostasis. Large number of membrane receptor such as N-Methyl-D-Aspartate (NMDA) and Alpha-amino-3-hydroxy-3-methyl-4 isoxasol (AMPA) and **kinate receptors** also play an important role in membrane breakdown. **Phospholipase C,** and inositol triphosphate (IP_3) enhance the intracellular calcium liberation. Activation of AMPA and kinate receptor helps in sodium and chloride influx leading to cellular edema and cell death. Sodium influx depolarize the neuronal membrane rapidly by operating through voltage operated channel (VOC). While sodium influx is rapid, calcium influx is mediated through NMDA receptor and relatively slow process (Table 6.2).[9] Recently, cytokine and calpain-mediated spectrin proteolysis is postulated in the pathogenesis of traumatically induced axonal injury.[32–34]

Recently, calcium bind **Calmodulin** (Cam) and **Nitric oxide** synthetase (NOS) are reported to be important in formation of

---

Tabel 6.1: Potential cellular mechanism of damage

a. Phospholipid metabolism abnormality
  • Lipid peroxidation
  • Prostaglandin, leukotrienes
  • Platelet activating factors (PAF)
b. Liberation of oxygen free radicals (OFR)
  Free iron catalysis
c. Excitatory mechanism
  Glutamate increased
d. Neuropeptides raised
  • Endorphin
  • Thyrotropin releasing hormone
e. Calcium and magnesium metabolism abnormality
f. CNS lactic acidosis

Table 6.2 : Mechanism of edema

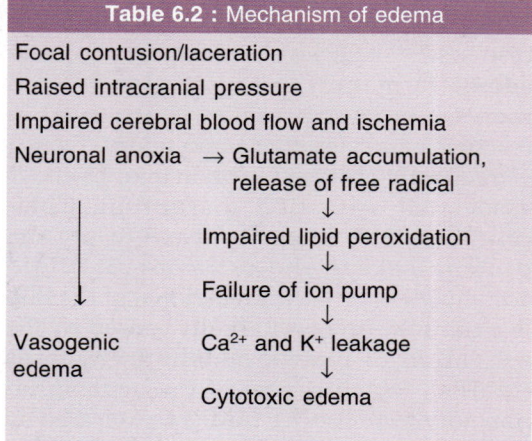

Focal contusion/laceration

Raised intracranial pressure

Impaired cerebral blood flow and ischemia

Neuronal anoxia → Glutamate accumulation, release of free radical
↓
Impaired lipid peroxidation
↓
Failure of ion pump
↓
Vasogenic edema Ca^{2+} and K^+ leakage
↓
Cytotoxic edema

edema. NOS is a very important factor giving rise to edema in not only head injury but also in brain tumours.[11,35,36] These chemicals, damage DNA and inhibit **mitochondrial** function leading to more free radical release. Nitric oxide, a water- and lipid-soluble free radical, is generated by the action of nitric oxide synthases. Ischemia causes a surge in nitric oxide synthase 1 (NOS 1) activity in neurons and, possibly, glia, increased NOS 3 activity in vascular endothelium, and later an increase in NOS 2 activity in a range of cells including infiltrating neutrophils and macrophages, activated microglia and astrocytes. The effects of ischemia on the activity of NOS 1, a Ca^{2+}-dependent enzyme, are thought to be secondary to reversal of glutamate reuptake at synapses, activation of NMDA receptors, and resulting elevation of intracellular Ca^{2+}. The up-regulation of NOS 2 activity is mediated by transcriptional inducers. In the context of brain ischemia, the activity of NOS 1 and NOS 2 is broadly deleterious, and their inhibition or inactivation is neuroprotective.[11] In head injury, lipid peroxidation can also be directly activated by the presence of ferrous ion. **Intracellular calcium influx activates Phospholipase A_2, lipoxygenase and Cyclo-oxygenase. The above substances degrade arachidonic acid into large number of metabolites like thromboxane A_2, prostaglandins and leukotrienes, oxygen and hydroxyl free radical.[37] Superoxide radicals are also increased in extracellular space and also involved in membrane damage and enhances the edema** (Table 6.3).

Overall cerebral function is dependent on adequate and continuous supply of blood and oxygen. The regulated blood flow and intact blood–brain barriers are general requirements for maintenance of **microenvironment** of the brain. Damage in the mechanism of maintenance of **microenvironment** leads to chemical changes, cell death and edema (Table 6.4).

Pathology and Natural Course of Brain Edema

Microscopically, astrocytes are specially vulnerable for damage in brain edema. Astrocytes look swollen and pale. In the initial phase, neurons look normal. Subsequently, because of cytotoxic effect neuron may get swollen. Most remarkable changes do occur in white matter. However, **oligodendroglia** and myelin do not get affected. Maximum damage is seen in pericapillary area. Vascular damage and ischemic changes are invariably observed histologically. Few days later, **macrophages** appear and try to engulf the debris. Subsequently, gliosis sets in 3–4 weeks time.

Resolution of edema is well studied in human and experimental animals. Edema increases over a period of 3–4 days then reach the peak. Within a period of 7–10 days, edema

Table 6.3: Superoxide radicals enhancing the edema

Head injury → Raised ICP → ↓ Damage to BBB ↓ Edema ← Impaired ← Membrane function	Fall of cerebral Perfusion + platelet aggregation ↓ Hypoxia, release of vasoactive substances and free radicals

Table 6.4: Chemical changes leading to brain damage

a. Ischemia hypoxia (basic cause)

b. Lactic acidosis vasospasm

c. Ca^{2+} and Na^+ into cells, K^+ comes out of the cells

d. Activation of phospholipase A_2

e. Liberation of arachidonic acid

f. Membrane damage leading edema formation

g. Further compromise in glucose and oxygen supply:

Vascular damage	Reoxidation
Prostaglandins and other free radicals	Neurotransmitter dysfunction
	Oxidation of arachidonic acid by cyclo-oxygenase and lipo- xygenase
	↓
	Brain damage

subsides.[6] However, with stimulating factor for edema, such as low perfusion, hypoxia, metabolic or electrolyte disturbances and hyperpyrexia can prolong the resolution of edema. By and large the time period for resolution of edema is unpredictable.[6] With the advent of CT scan the onset, progress and the resolution of edema are easily evaluated.[5,38,39] Bruce et al[38] had shown malignant brain swelling in children. CT scan has proved that the edema is a dynamic process and is influenced by large number of factors. CT scan also differentiate edema from brain swelling.[5,37]

Treatment of Brain Edema

Large number of substances like 20% mannitol, **hypertonic saline, furosemide** and glycerol are used routinely in brain edema with success. Use of **corticosteroids** has been proved ineffective in patients with severe head injury. It is surprising, that the steroid which works like magic in brain edema of non-traumatic origin does not work in edema due to head injury. **Barbiturate** has a limited role in head injury. While hyperventilation is not only useless but also can prove hazardous as it may wash out CO_2 and induce cerebral vasospasm, which can lead to further ischemia and edema.

Despite the predominance of cytotoxic (or cellular) edema in the first week after traumatic brain injury, brain swelling can only occur with addition of water to the cranial vault from the vasculature. As such, regulation of blood–brain barrier permeability has become a focus of recent research seeking to manage brain edema. Aquaporins, matrix metalloproteinases and vasoactive inflammatory agents have emerged as potential mediators of cerebral edema following traumatic brain injury. In particular, kinins (bradykinins) and tachykinins (substance P) seem to play an active physiological role in modulating blood–brain barrier permeability after trauma. Substance P neurokinin-1 receptor antagonists show particular promise as novel therapeutic agents.[15] Recently, free radical scavengers like

vitamin E are widely used. **Glutamate** is one of the most important factor in ischemia and production of brain edema. NMDA receptor antagonist like **phencyclidine, MK-801 and dextromethorphan** have been tried in animal models[28] of traumatic brain injury. MK-801, **phencyclidine and ketamine** have a lot of side effects in man. However, **dextromethorphan** may be useful in future, vitamin E, **selenium** and **superoxide dismutase** can reduce the free radicals and reverse or stop lipid peroxidation.[40–42]

Calcium influx into the cells can be prevented by calcium channel blockers. Few years back, expectation was raised regarding the role of **Nimodipine** in reducing ischemic, hypoxic damage and brain edema in head injury. Surprisingly, however, multicentric European trial with Nimodipine was not encouraging.[42]

Hypothermia, has long been known to reduce cerebral metabolism and protect brain.

Experimental studies; Higashida et al[16] investigated the role of hypoxia-inducible factor-1α (HIF-1α), aquaporin-4 (AQP-4), and matrix metalloproteinase-9 (MMP-9) in blood–brain barrier (BBB) permeability alterations and brain edema formation in a rodent traumatic brain injury (TBI) model (Fig. 6.5). Expression of HIF-1α, AQP-4, and MMP-9 as well as expression of the vascular basal lamina protein (laminin) and tight junction proteins (zona occludens-1 and occludin) was determined by Western blotting. Blood–brain barrier disruption was assessed by FITC-dextran extravasation, and brain edema was measured by the brain water content. The injured animals were found to have significantly ($p < 0.05$) enhanced expression of HIF-1α, AQP-4, and MMP-9, in addition to reduced amounts ($p < 0.05$) of laminin and tight junction proteins. Edema was significantly ($p < 0.01$) decreased after inhibition of AQP-4, MMP-9, or HIF-1α. While BBB permeability was significantly ($p < 0.01$) ameliorated after inhibition of either HIF-1α or MMP-9, it was not affected following

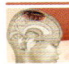

inhibition of AQP-4. Inhibition of MMP reversed the loss of laminin (p < 0.01). They concluded that HIF-1α plays a role in brain edema formation and BBB disruption via a molecular pathway cascade involving AQP-4 and MMP-9. Pharmaco-logical blockade of this pathway in patients with TBI may provide a novel therapeutic strategy.

Recently, mild hypothermia is proved to be helpful in head injury. In a randomised trial, Marion[43] had shown lowering of brain temperature and reduction of CBF with a 40% drop of ICP by using **cooling blankets** and cold saline gastric perfusion. Thus, it may be possible to get a beneficial effect by mild **hypothermia** of 33–34°C.

CONCLUSIONS

Brain edema is an important secondary pathology in brain following head injury. Edema is a complex and dynamic process mediated through large number of chemicals and **neurotransmitters.** Basic trigger points are ischemia and hypoxia. Liberation of free radicals and damage to all membranes are probably two important steps in formation of edema. Availability of CT scan has helped us in studying brain edema in patients. **Corticosteroids** are of no value in traumatic brain edema. Mild hypothermia, adequate oxygenation, perfusion and free radical scavengers can reduce brain edema and change the out-look of head injury patients.

REFERENCES

1. Shlosberg D, et al. Blood-brain barrier breakdown as a therapeutic target in traumatic brain injury. Nat Rev Neurol 2010;6,(7):393–403.

2. Brock M. Basic concept of brain edema. In: Traumatic brain edema. F Cohadon, A Bethman and J D Miller (Eds) Liviana Press, Padova 1987;123–7.

3. Clasen RA, Penn RD. Traumatic brain swelling and edema. In: Head injury. PR Cooper (Eds) William and Wilkins, Baltimore 1987;285–312.

4. Long DM. Traumatic brain edema. Clinical Neurosurgery 1982;29:174–202.

5. Ito U, Tometa SH, Yamazaki V, Takada Y, et al. Brain swelling and brain edema in acute head injury. ActaNeurochir (Wien) 1986;79:120–4.

6. Bruce DA, TerWeeme C, Kaiser G, et al. Mechanism and time course for clearance of vasogenic cerebral edema. In: Neuronal Trauma. AJ Popp, et al. (Eds). Raven Press, New York, 1979.

7. Long DM, Maxwell RE, French LA. (i) The effect of glucosteroids upon cold induced edema, (ii) Ultrastructure evaluation. J Neuropath ExpNeurol 1971;30:680–97.

8. Astrop J. Energy-requiring cell function in the ischemic brain. J Neurosurg 1982;56:482–97.

9. Choic DW. Ionic dependance of glutamate neurotoxicity. Neurosciences 1987;7:379–83.

10. Klatzo I, Piraux A and Laskowski E. The relationship between edema, blood-brain barrier and tissue element in local brain injury. J Neuropath 1958;17:548–63.

11. Chodobski A, Zink BJ, and Szmydynger-Chodobska J; Blood–brain barrier pathophysiology in traumatic brain injury Transl Stroke Res 2011;2(4):492–516.

12. Love S, Oxidative Stress in Brain Ischemia. Brain Pathology 1999;9:119–131.

13. Marmarou A. Pathophysiology of traumatic brain edema: current concepts. Acta Neurochir Suppl 2003;86:7–10.

14. Barzó P, Marmarou A, Fatouros P, Corwin F, Dunbar J. Magnetic resonance imaging-monitored acute blood–brain barrier changes in experimental traumatic brain injury. J Neurosurg. 1996;85(6):1113–21.

15. Donkin JJ, Vink R. Mechanisms of cerebral edema in traumatic brain injury: therapeutic developments. Curr Opin Neurol 2010;23(3):293–9.

16. Higashida T, Kreipke CW, Rafols JA, Peng C, Schafer S, Schafer P, Ding JY, Dornbos D 3rd, Li X, Guthikonda M, Rossi NF, Ding Y, The role of hypoxia-inducible factor-1α, aquaporin-4, and matrix metalloproteinase-9 in blood–brain barrier disruption and brain edema after traumatic brain injury. J Neurosurg 2011; 114(1):92–101.

17. Li L, Zhang H, Varrin-Doyer M, Zamvil SS, Verkman AS. Proinflammatory role of aquaporin-4 in autoimmune neuroinflammation. FASEB J 2011;25:1556–66.

18. Tourdias T, Mori N, Dragonu I, Cassagno N, Boiziau C, Aussudre J, Brochet B, Moonen C, Petry KG, Dousset V. Differential aquaporin 4

expression during edema build-up and resolution phases of brain inflammation. J Neuroinflammation 2011;8:143.

19. Verkman AS. Aquaporins in clinical medicine. Annu Rev Med 2012;63:303–16.

20. Badaut J, Ashwal S, Obenaus A. Aquaporins in cerebrovascular disease: a target for treatment of brain edema? Cerebrovasc Dis 2011;31:521–31.

21. Badaut J, Ashwal S, Adami A, Tone B, Recker R, Spagnoli D, Ternon B, Obenaus A. Brain water mobility decreases after astrocytic aquaporin-4 inhibition using RNA interference. J Cereb Blood Flow Metab 2011;31:819–31.

22. Berezowski V, Fukuda AM, Cecchelli R, Badaut J. Endothelial cells and astrocytes: a concerto en duo in ischemic pathophysiology. Int J Cell Biol 2012;176–287.

23. Rosell A, Ortega-Aznar A, Alvarez-Sabin J, Fernandez-Cadenas I, Ribo M, Molina CA, Lo EH, Montaner J. Increased brain expression of matrix metalloproteinase-9 after ischemic and hemorrhagic human stroke. Stroke 2006; 37:1399–406.

24. Rosenberg GA, Estrada EY, Dencoff JE. Matrix metalloproteinases and TIMPs are associated with blood–brain barrier opening after reperfusion in rat brain. Stroke 1998;29:2189–95.

25. Candelario-Jalil E, Yang Y, Rosenberg GA. Diverse roles of matrix metalloproteinases and tissue inhibitors of metalloproteinases in neuroinflammation and cerebral ischemia. Neuroscience 2009;158:983–94. doi: 10.1016/ j.neuroscience.

26. Penfield W, Cone W. Acute Swelling of the oligodendroglia. Arch Neurol Psychiat 1938;20:1.

27. Kontos HA, Wei EP. Superoxide production in experimental brain injury. J Neurosurg 1986; 64:803.

28. Faden A, Demediuk P, Panter S, Vink R. The role of excitatory amino acids and NMDA receptors in traumatic brain injury. Science 1989;244:298.

29. Suguru I, Marmarou A, Clarke GD, Andersor BJ, et al. Production and clearance of lactate from brain injury. J Neurosurg 1988;69:736.

30. Fishman R, Chan PH. Metabolic basis of brain edema. In: Advances in Neurol. 28: Cervos-Navarroj, Ferszt XR (eds) Brain edema, Raven Press, New York; 1980.

31. Mohanty S, Dey PK, Ray AK. Role of serotonin in cerebral edema. Ind J Med Res 1979;69:1001.

32. Mohanty S, Dey PK, et al. Role of histamine in traumatic brain edema. An experimental study in rat. J Neurolsci 1989;90:87–97.

33. Shohami E, Gallily R, Mechoulam R, et al. Cytokine production in brain following closed head injury: Dexanabinol is a novel TNF (Alpha) inhibitor and effective neuroprotectant. J. Neuroimmunol 1997;72:169–77.

34. Buki A, Povlishock JI. Evidence for calpin-mediated spectrinproteclysis in pathogenesis of traumatically induced axonal injury. J. Neuropathol Exp Neurol 1999;58:365–75.

35. Nicholls D, AHwell D. The release and uptake of excitatory amino acids. Trends in Pharmacological Sci, 1998;11:462–68.

36. Bakshi A, Nagi C. Wadhwa S, Mahapatra AK, Sarkar C. The expression of nitric oxide synthetase in human brain tumour and peritumoural areas. J Neurological Sci 1998;155:196–203.

37. Wolfe L. Eicosanoids, Prostaglandins, thromboxane leukotrienes and other derivatives of carbon-20, unsaturated fatty acids. Neurochem, 1982;38:74.

38. Bruce DA, Alavi BK, Dolinskas L, et al. Diffuse cerebral swelling following head injuries in children. The syndrome of malignant brain edema. J Neurosurg 1981;54:170–8.

39. Lobato RD, Sarabia R, Cordabe F, Riivas JJ.Posttraumatic cerebral hemispheric swelling. Analysis of 55 cases studied with CT. J Neurosurg 1988;68:417–23.

40. Muizelaar JP, Marmarou A, Young HF, et al. Improving the outcome of severe head injury with oxygen radical scavenger polyethylene glycol conjugated superoxide desmutase. A phase II trial. J Neurosurg 1993;78:375–82.

41. Anderson D, Saunders Ra, Deme dink P, et al. Lipid hydrolysis and peroxidation in injured spinal cord. Partial protection with methyle prednisolone, Yit.E and Selenium. CNS Trauma 1985;2:257–67.

42. Cohadon F. Brain protection. In: Advances in technical standard in Neurosurgery. L. Symon (Eds). Springer Verlag (Wien) 1994;21.

43. Marion DW, Obrist WD, Carlier PM, et al. The use of moderate therapeutic hypothermia for patients with severe head injuries. A preliminary report. J Neurosurg 1993;79:354–62.

7

Abnormal Calcium Homeostasis in Head Injury

P Sarat Chandra • Raj Kamal

INTRODUCTION

The following chapter will review the normal and pathological Ca^{2+} homeostasis in neurons that relate to traumatic brain injury and the possible role of neuroprotective strategies. Of interest particularly is the contribution of Ca^{2+} permeable ionic channels, Ca^{2+} pumps, intracellular Ca^{2+} stores, intracellular Ca^{2+} buffering systems and the roles of secondary, Ca^{2+} dependent processes in neurodegeneration. A number of hypotheses linking Ca^{2+} ions and Ca^{2+} permeable channels to neurotoxicity are discussed with an emphasis on strategies for lessening Ca^{2+} related damage. A number of these strategies may have a future role in the treatment of traumatic brain injury. Clinical recovery after central nervous system (CNS) trauma, to a great extent affected by a neural injury process that is triggered and perpetuated at the cellular level and is more than a surgically curable operable lesion. It is widely thought that one such process (a fundamental pathological mechanism initiated by CNS injury), is the disruption of cellular Ca^{2+} homeostasis. Because of the critical role of Ca^{2+} ions in regulating innumerable cellular functions, this major homeostatic disturbance is thought to trigger neuronal and axonal degeneration and produce clinical disability.

Although, there exist multiple mechanisms by which the central nervous system (CNS) tissue may be damaged, it is now widely accepted that one of the important underlying common factors in the abovementioned cellular disturbances is the disruption of intracellular calcium ion homeostasis. A lot of recent cellular and molecular research has focussed on the study of normal and abnormal Ca^{2+} signaling in neurons. The knowledge gained forms the basis for rational design of the therapeutic interventions aimed. At reducing the Ca^{2+} induced **neurotoxicity** in CNS injury. In addition, the new informations may explain why past attempts at lessening neuronal injury by pharmacological means have failed in clinical settings. Unfortunately, it is impossible in this chapter to cover comprehensively all the potentially relevant aspects of neuronal Ca^{2+} **homeostasis**. The purpose of this article, therefore, is to review some of the issues that may have relevance to the pharmacotherapy of neurosurgical patients presently and in the future. It is highly likely that, some of the newer therapeutic strategies that are now in process of evaluation and development will be added to the existing clinical armamentarium.

A Brief Review of Normal Calcium Homeostasis

All mammalian cells use calcium ions as signals to perform innumerable vital functions such as, the control of cell-growth and differentiation,[1] the maintenance of cytoskeletal structure,[2] membrane excitability,[3] exocytosis and synaptic activity.[4, 5] Because of the pivotal role of Ca^{2+} ions as regulators of normal neuronal function, neurons have evolved homeostatic mechanisms to tightly bind this crucial ion within the intracellular organelles and thus strictly monitor the free cytoplasmic concentration of Ca^{2+} ions. These mechanisms consist of a complex interaction between four general categories of events: Ca^{2+} influx, Ca^{2+} buffering, internal Ca^{2+} storage and Ca^{2+} efflux. A fifth process, intracellular Ca^{2+} diffusion, links the aforementioned events and is also crucial to Ca^{2+} homeostasis. Together, these mechanisms maintain Ca^{2+} at extremely low levels intracellularly (100 nmol/L or 105 times lower than extracellular Ca^{2+}), so that relatively small or localized increases in Ca^{2+} can be used by the cell as a signal to trigger a physiological effect, such as the activation of an enzyme or an ion channel. From a physiological standpoint, the delicate interplay between these five processes allows multiple Ca^{2+} dependent processes to be regulated smoothly independently within the same cell. Maintaining this balance is the goal of all clinically relevant pharmacotherapeutic strategies aimed at lessening Ca^{2+} related neurotoxicity in brain injury.

Calcium Influx

This is chiefly governed by ionic channels. Ion channels are the gates on the cell membrane by which ions gain access into the intracellular space. These specialized pores in the cell membranes are classified physiologically by their specific selectivities for certain ions (Ca^{2+}, K^+, Na^+, or Cl^-) and by their gating mechanism. Some ion channels are sensitive to membrane voltage and change their conformation between a number of open and closed states, depending on whether the cell membrane is depolarized or repolarized (voltage-gated channels). Voltage-gated calcium channels are important mediators of calcium influx into electrically excitable cells. The amount of calcium entering through this family of channel proteins is not only determined by the functional

properties of channels embedded in the plasma membrane but also by the numbers of channels that are expressed at the cell surface. The trafficking of channels is controlled by numerous processes, including co-assembly with ancillary calcium channel subunits, ubiquitin ligases and interactions with other membrane proteins such as G protein coupled receptors.[6] Other ion channels are associated with receptors that when activated by a specific ligand, induce conformational changes in the ion channel pores, which cause the pore to open. These ionic channels are frequently named according to their specific ligands (for example, "nicotinic" acetylcholine receptor channels). Voltage-gated ionic channels frequently contain binding sites for certain ligands and ligandgated channels may exhibit certain forms of voltage dependence. There exist many types of voltage and ligand-gated ion channels that are either Ca^{2+} permeable or that cause Ca^{2+} to rise through a second-messenger pathway.

Calcium Buffering

Another strategy to regulate the spread of Ca^{2+} ions within neurons is by Ca^{2+} buffering. As calcium ions diffuse into the cell, they are rapidly buffered by a number of cytoplasmic proteins, such as calmodulin, calbindin, and parvalbumin.[7] Approximately 95 to 99% of Ca^{2+} ions entering the cell under physiological conditions are buffered in this fashion.[8,9] Although the precise role of Ca^{2+} buffering substances remains poorly understood, recent evidence indicates that they may act to keep Ca^{2+} at high levels in localized areas within cells, to limit those high Ca^{2+} levels to those specific areas and to rapidly dissipate the Ca^{2+} gradients and thus limit the time course of activation of Ca^{2+} dependent processes.[10, 11]

Ca^{2+} Sequestration and Storage

The Ca^{2+} buffering capacity of cytosolic Ca^{2+} binding proteins is limited. Therefore, neurons also possess mechanisms for sequestering Ca^{2+} ions into organelles, situations in which Ca^{2+} loads exceed the ability of Ca^{2+} buffers to maintain Ca^{2+} at tolerable levels. These

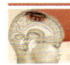
include, the smooth endoplasmic reticulum, mitochondria and synaptic vesicles. These organelles can sequester large quantities of Ca^{2+} under a variety of conditions, using active and passive Ca^{2+} transport mechanisms, similar to those found in the plasma membrane. Although, Ca^{2+} storage in the organelles is an efficient mechanism for controlling cytoplasmic Ca^{2+}, this Ca^{2+} lowering system operates at a much slower time scale than cytoplasmic Ca^{2+} binding proteins. Therefore, it is incapable of modulating rapidly changing or highly localized changes in Ca^{2+}[12].

Calcium Extrusion

All the cells must expend metabolic energy to extrude Ca^{2-}. The large extracellular-to-intracellular Ca^{2+} ion concentration gradient and the electrical driving force propelling the positively charged Ca^{2+} ions toward the negatively charged inner plasma membrane necessitate the presence of efficient Ca^{2+} extrusion mechanisms. Neurons have at least two such mechanisms, **adenosine triphosphate (ATP)-driven Ca^{2+} pumps (Ca^{2+} ATPases) and a Na^+/Ca^{2+} exchange transport** mechanism.[13–15]

Both the above systems are heavily dependent of ATP, which rapidly depletes in head injuries, thus producing a state of Ca^{2+} excess. Thus, Ca^{2+} influx may easily overwhelm cytoplasmic Ca^{2+} buffering mechanisms, resulting in an uncontrolled rise in the concentration of unbound intracellular Ca^{2+} ions, that are then free to activate numerous secondary Ca^{2+} dependent cascades, which ultimately result in cell death.

Intracellular Calcium Diffusion

Ca^{2+} concentration profiles within the cytoplasm are determined by the type and the subcellular distribution of Ca^{2+} entry sites (Ca^{2+} channels) and depend on Ca^{2+} buffering and sequestration systems and by Ca^{2+} extrusion mechanisms. These modulators have marked effects on the ability of Ca^{2+} ions to diffuse into the cell. For example, Ca^{2+} ions bound to Ca^{2+} binding proteins possess markedly different diffusion characteristics from free Ca^{2+} ions.[9, 16] Also, Ca^{2+} influx sites may be coupled with Ca^{2+} binding sites within the cell (e.g. Ca^{2+} dependent enzymes).[17] These mechanisms serve to selectively couple Ca^{2+} entry with specific intracellular targets of Ca^{2+} ions. Thus, any process that modifies cytoplasmic Ca^{2+} diffusion may disrupt this coupling process and prevent Ca^{2+} ions from reaching their sites of intracellular; action. This concept has recently been extended to the use of Ca^{2+} chelating agents, to uncouple Ca^{2+} ion entry and Ca^{2+} neurotoxicity both *in vitro*[18] and in experimental.

HOW DOES CALCIUM IONS CAUSE CELL DAMAGE?

Disturbances in Ca^{2+} homeostasis as a "final common pathway" of neurodegeneration: *A* significant step towards the understanding[19] of the mechanisms that trigger cellular injury was initiated in non-neuronal tissues, when pathologists noted the calcium deposited in areas of tissue necrosis.[20] Thereafter, Schanne, et al[21] observed that the cultured hepatocytes could be killed when exposed to various toxins in the presence, but not in the absence, of extracellular Ca^{2+}. They inferred that Ca^{2+} entry into cells was an absolute requirement for the expression of toxicity and termed this process the "final common pathway of cell death" (Figs 7.1 and 7.2). In neurons, early studies in tissue cultures showed that amputated axons degenerated only if Ca^{2+} ions were present in the culture medium.[22] More recently, neurodegeneration induced by neurotoxins such as, capsaicin and the excitatory amino acid (EAA) glutamate was shown to be associated with increases in tissue Ca^{2+}.[23] Further investigations on the toxicity of EAAs in cultured neurons and in brain slice preparations also confirmed an association between the observed toxicity and the presence of Ca^{2+} in the extracellular medium.[24, 25]

Currently, studies both *in vitro* and *in vivo* support the association between Ca^{2+} influx and damage to neural tissues. For example, experimental spinal cord injury may produce

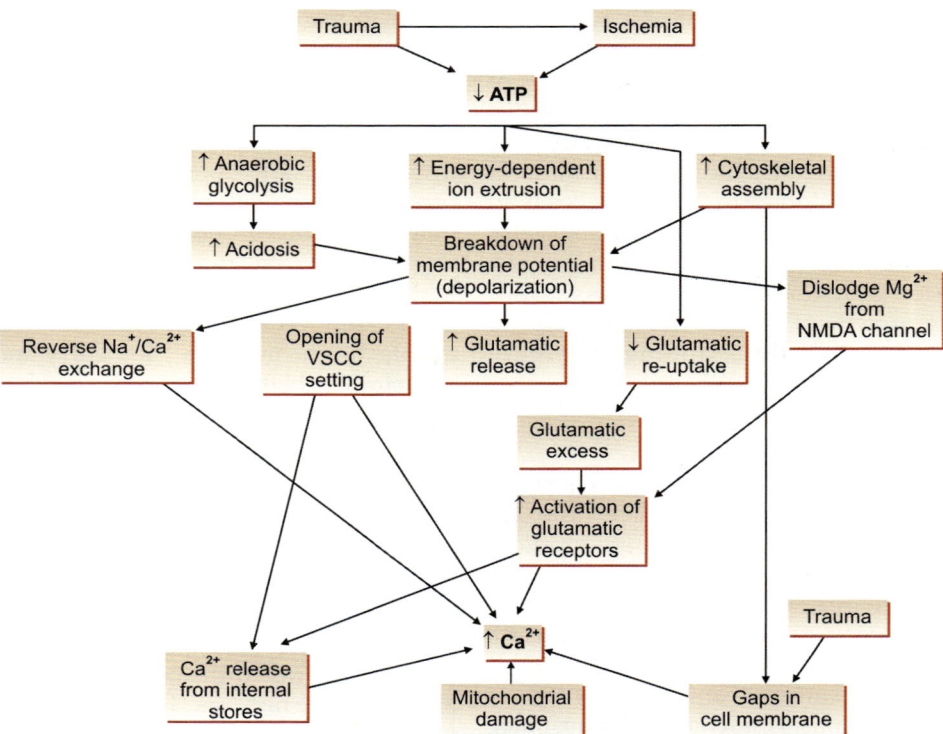

Fig. 7.1: Flow chart depicting mechanisms by which trauma and ischemia produce intracellular Ca^{2+} elevations. Voltage sensitive calcium channel (VSCC) settings, thus producing a potentially useful future clinical therapeutic strategy[18]

significant Ca^{2+} accumulation in white matter axons,[26, 27] possibly as a consequence of white matter anoxia/ischemia. Thus, although the idea that Ca^{2+} is a final common pathway of cell death has not gone unchallenged.[28] Ca^{2+} triggered injury seems to play a major role in the mammalian nervous system.

Calcium Ions, Glutamate Receptors and "Excitotoxicity"

A mechanistic link between cell destruction Ca^{2+} excess was made by physiologists studying the actions of glutamate, the major excitatory neurotransmitter in the CNS.[29] Glutamate acts on neurons and glia via a number of cell membrane receptors. These are classified into two groups, ionotropic and metabotropic receptors, based on pharmacological, electrophysiological and biochemical studies.[29] The ionotropic receptors are subdivided into the **N-methyl-D-aspartate (NMDA)** receptors and **alpha-amino-3-hydroxy-5-methyl-4-isoxazolepropionatekainate receptors,** identified according to their selective agonists. Activation of these receptors leads to the opening of their associated ion channels, which are typified by their permeabilities to Na^+, K^+ and Ca^{2+}. After the channel open, these receptors may desensitize, causing the ion channel to close again. Thus, the actions of glutamate, via a variety of membrane receptors, affects intracellular Ca^{2+} through several distinct mechanisms. Recently, recombinant deoxyribonucleic acid (DNA) techniques have revealed that many glutamate receptor subtypes exist within each receptor family.[30] The functional consequences of this diversity are incompletely understood and remain under intense investigation.

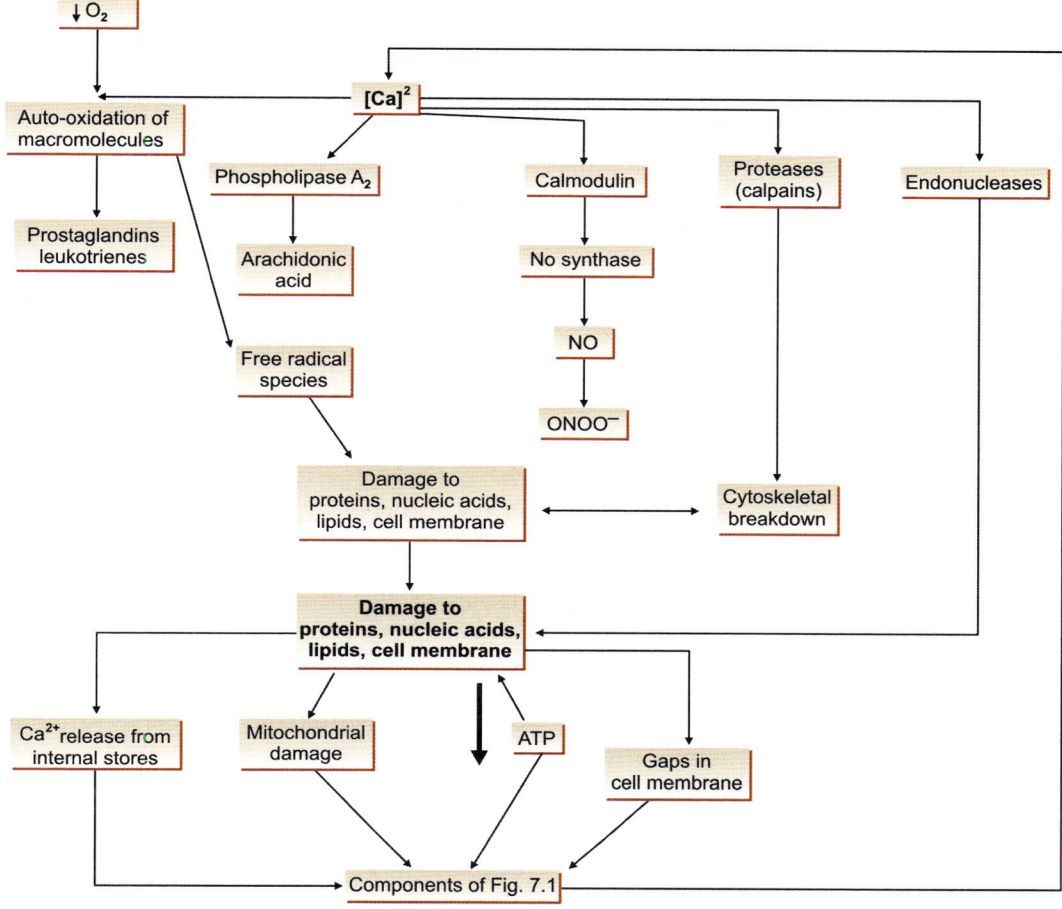

Fig. 7.2: Flow chart depicting mechanisms by which intracellular Ca^{2+} trigger the secondary Ca^{2+} dependent phenomena which result in neurotoxicity

Under physiological conditions, the synaptic release of glutamate is thought to mediate rapid neuronal excitation, plasticity, and possibly processes involved in learning and memory.[29, 31] However, glutamate excess can be toxic (Fig. 7.1). This was noted even before the realization that cellular Ca^{2+} accumulation may be critical in neurotoxicity. This notion was strengthened when glutamate receptor antagonists, such as 2-amino-7-phosphonoheptanoic acid and MK-801, were found to attenuate ischemic neuronal injury *in vivo*.[32] Thereafter, the term "excitotoxicity", initially coined by Olney,[33] came to indicate the process by which excessive synaptic release of excitotoxic amino acids (EAAs) resulted in neurotoxicity.

Several key experiments have shown mechanisms by which glutamate excess triggers toxicity. In brief, the activation of every glutamate receptor subtype has, at some point, been implicated in mediating hypoxic/ischemic neuronal death.[34, 35] Current views suggest that the activation of distinct glutamate receptor subtypes may produce distinct types of neurodegeneration. However, there is general agreement that the NMDA glutamate receptor plays a key role in mediating many aspects of glutamate neurotoxicity because of its high Ca^{2+} permeability, as compared with non-NMDA ionotropic glutamate receptors.[36, 37]

Consequently, ever since NMDA and other EAAs were found to produce calcium influx into neurons,[38] the link between synaptic over-activity, extracellular glutamate excess, and Ca^{2+} overload has been considered as the fundamental phenomenon in triggering traumatic neurodegeneration.[35, 39, 41] Recently, increased levels of EAAs have been shown to occur after traumatic head injury,[42] lending further credence to the clinical relevance of the excitotoxicity hypothesis.[43]

Mechanism of Ca^{2+} Neurotoxicity

Mechanisms leading to Ca^{2+} neurotoxicity can be classified into two stages. The first consists of the pathological mechanisms that trigger and sustain intracellular Ca^{2+} excess (Fig. 7.1), whereas the second consists of the secondary phenomena thought to be precipitated by intracellular Ca^{2+} excess (Fig. 7.2). This two-stage concept is relevant therapeutically, because most pharmacotherapeutic strategies for trauma may be classified under one of these categories. Thus, certain drugs are aimed at blocking Ca^{2+} influx into cells (e.g. Ca^{2+} channel blockers), whereas others are targeted at the consequences of this Ca^{2+} excess (e.g. free radical scavengers).

Mechanism Triggering and Sustaining Intracellular Ca^{2+} Excess

Central to the process traumatic neurodegeneration is the concept of cellular in neurons and axons after the interruption of blood flow, nutrients and oxygen (Fig. 7.1).[44, 45] Inadequate synthesis of ATP has several consequences, in addition to causing a loss of Ca^{2+} homeostasis. It is thought to produce cellular acidosis through the stimulation of anerobic glycolysis, a disruption of ion homeostasis caused by the loss of energy-dependent ion transport mechanisms and a loss of cytoskeletal integrity as a consequence of decreased synthesis of

macromolecular assemblies required for maintaining cell structure. Cellular energy failure is also hypothesized to result in Ca^{2+} overload through a number of mechanisms, including increased Ca^{2+} influx, decreased Ca^{2+} efflux and altered internal Ca^{2+} buffering and sequestration.

The increase in Ca^{2+} influx, during the energy failure, occurs by several mechanisms. First, as transmembrane ionic gates break-down; because of the failure of energy-dependent ionic/pumps (e.g. Na^+–K^+ ATPase), the plasma membrane depolarizes, causing the opening of voltage-operated Ca^{2+} channels. In traumatic injuries, the disruption of cell membranes causes an efflux of potassium ions, contributing further to ionic gradient collapse and membrane depolarization in the remaining cells. Depolarization also dislodges positively charged magnesium cations from the NMDA channel oores, where they normally prevent ion fluxes. This facilitates the activation of NMDA currents and Ca^{2+} influx by EAAs.[46, 47] Depolarization also increases glutamate release from synaptic terminals, this being coupled with a decline in energy-dependent glutamate reuptake in neurons and glia.[48–50] The resulting rise in the extracellular concentrations of glutamate and other *EAAs* is thought to trigger neuro-degeneration both *in vitro* and *in vivo*, by activating both the NMDA and non-NMDA glutamate receptors.[51, 52] Finally, an additional mechanism of Ca^{2+} influx during energy failure is through the Na^+/Ca^{2+} exchanger. The normal operation of this exchanger depends on the maintenance of a normal extracellular-to-intracellular Na^+ concentration. When the transmembrane Na^+ gradients collapse, during the energy failure, the exchanger operates in reverse, i.e. pumping Ca^{2+} in and Na^+ out instead of pumping Ca^{2+} out and Na^+ into the cells.[13, 53]

Another important process is mitochon-drial Ca^{2+} sequestration, which begins when Ca^{2+} rises to micromolar levels.[13, 54] Although this temporarily aids in keeping Ca^{2+} low, the process of Ca^{2+} transport across the mitochon-

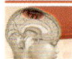

drial membrane is ATP dependent and occurs at the expense of energy production, which is already hindered by anoxia. Excessive Ca^{2+} sequestration in mitochondria may render them permanently inactive. Ca^{2+} sequestration by mitochondria during excitotoxicity also adds to cytoplasmic acidosis.[57] A further mechanism contributing to Ca^{2+} homeostatic failure and neurodegeneration may be Ca^{2+} release from intracellular stores. This is presumably because of a failure of Ca^{2+} sequestration mechanisms or to the activation of Ca^{2+} release either by metabotropic glutamate receptor activation or by Ca^{2+} induced Ca^{2+} release. All of the above mechanisms seriously limit the ability of neurons to extrude or buffer nonphysiological Ca^{2+} loads,[53] leading to an eventual deregulation of Ca^{2+} homeostasis and ultimately to an uncontrolled rise in both total and free Ca^{2+} ion concentrations.[41]

Additional mechanisms of Ca^{2+} influx probably exist. For example, in CNS trauma, Ca^{2+} ions may permeate into the cytoplasm through gaps in the cell membrane, produced by the mechanical insult. It is very clear that there exist multiple pathways by which excessive Ca^{2+} loading may occur in traumatized axons and neurons. Thus, from a clinical perspective, it is increasingly apparent that blocking a single pathway of Ca^{2+} influx may not suffice to protect neurons against Ca^{2+} neurotoxicity. This may explain why studies using single Ca^{2+} channel blockers in CNS trauma and ischemia have yielded conflicting and often contradictory results *in vitro* and *in vivo*.

SECONDARY PHENOMENA PRECIPITATED BY Ca^{2+} EXCESS (Fig. 7.3)

A complete discussion of all Ca^{2+} dependent cellular processes that may contribute to neuronal damage is beyond the scope of this chapter. However, a number of specific processes are thought to contribute significantly to Ca^{2+} related neuronal and axonal injury. It is expected that pharmacological

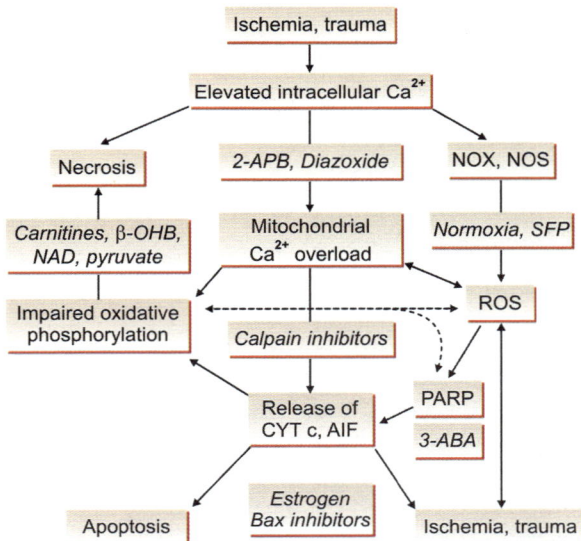

Fig. 7.3: Ca^{2+} related neuronal and axonal injury. Poly(ADP)-ribose polymerase (PARP), reactive oxygen species (ROS), **apoptosis-inducing factor** (AIF), NADPH-oxidases (NOXs), β-OHB: β-hydroxybutyrate,NOS: nitric oxide synthetase sulforaphane (SFP), calpain inhibitors, the PARP inhibitor 3-aminobenzoamide (3ABA). 2-APB: 2-Amino ethoxydiphenyl borate—it inhibits inositol 1, 4, 5-triphosphate-mediated calcium release

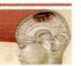

agents targeted at these processes will be useful in the clinical management of CNS trauma. These processes are thus summarized in Fig. 7.3 and are briefly reviewed here.

Formation of Free Radical Species

A free radical is any molecule, atom, or group of atoms with an unpaired electron in its outmost orbital, which accounts for its extreme reactivity. Free radical species of potential importance in cerebral trauma include superoxide (O_2^-) and hydroxyl (OH^-) radicals. Free radicals are produced in small amounts by normal cellular processes, such as the mitochondrial electron transport system, reactions catalyzed by prostaglandin hydroperoxidase and the auto-oxidation of small molecules, such as catecholamines and by the microsomal cytochrome P450 reductase system. Free radicals may play physiological roles, such as the modulation of a number of membrane receptors, including NMDA receptor function.

Free radicals are formed in excess during traumatic and hypoxic injuries, because insufficient O_2 is available to accept electrons passed along the mitochondrial electron transport chain, leading to the reduction of other components of the system, such as flavin adenine dinucleotide and coenzyme Q. These molecules then auto-oxidize to produce free radical species. Also, during reperfusion, reactive oxygen radicals may form as by-products of the reactions of arachidonic acid metabolism to produce **prostaglandins and leukotrienes.** Arachidonic acid, particularly abundant during ischemic conditions, is released from membrane phospholipids during this time. Free radicals can react with and damage proteins, nucleic acids, lipids, and other classes of molecules, such as extracellular matrix glycosaminoglycans. Sulfur-containing amino acids and polyunsaturated fatty acids are particularly vulnerable. The latter are found at very high concentrations in the CNS as components of the plasma membrane. Thus, EAA release and free radical formation may act synergistically in lipid peroxidation

and the production of ischemia-induced neuronal membrane damage.[28]

Formation of Nitric Oxide (NO)

NO, first identified as an endothelium-derived relaxing factor, is a short-lived, diffusible, highly reactive gas that has recently gained wide attention as a member of a newly discovered class of messenger molecules. NO serves a variety of functions in different tissues, including vascular endothelium, immune cells, neurons, smooth muscle and cardiac muscle. NO produced in one cell can diffuse and produce biological effects in neighbouring cells. In the brain, it is produced by both vascular endothelium and neurons. NO produced in vascular endothelium has major effects on governing cerebral blood flow and acts as a potent vasodilator. A deficiency or inhibition of NO production is postulated as one of the mechanisms of cerebral vasospasm after aneurysmal subarachnoid hemorrhage. In neurons, NO has been implicated in modulating a number of biological phenomena related to synaptic plasticity, including the NMDA receptor function and long-term potentiation.

NO production occurs at low levels during physiological function and is governed by NO synthase (Fig. 7.3). Its synthesis is regulated by the Ca^{2+} dependent regulatory enzyme, calmodulin, which is induced by the influx of Ca^{2+} ions through NMDA receptors. NO production can affect intracellular Ca^{2+} pools in neurons and adjacent cells by modulating Ca^{2+} release from intracellular stores through a cyclic guanosine monophosphate kinase-mediated mechanism. NO in itself is not highly toxic but can lead to the formation of toxic species by reacting with free oxygen radicals, particularly superoxide. NO reacts with superoxide to form the powerful oxidant peroxynitrite ($ONOO^-$), which directly oxidizes sulfhydryl groups, lipids, DNA and proteins thus leading to breakdown of the cell structure. Excessive NO production has been postulated as a causative mechanism in neurotoxicity presumably via Ca^{2+} overload leading to the ultimate overexpression of the mechanisms described above.[21, 72]

Endonucleases, Apoptosis and Necrosis

Ca^{2+} overload also activates endonucleases, a series of Ca^{2+} dependent enzymes that degrade DNA and that may play role in two well-recognized forms of cell death, necrosis and apoptosis. Apoptosis is a form of programmed cell death, which occurs during foetal development as well as during adult life. The physiological function of apoptosis in the CNS seems to be to remove those neurons of which the processes have failed to find their targets during development or regeneration. Apoptosis is pathologically distinct from necrosis, involving compaction of the cell body, nuclear fragmentation and the formation of surface blebs. Apoptosis can also be identified by a characteristic DNA fragmenta-tion resulting from the cleavage of cell chromatin into oligonucleosome-length fragments seen as a "ladder" pattern on electrophoretic gels.[22, 42, 45]

Mitochondrial Damage

Mitochondria serve as the energy generators of the cell. Considerable evidence indicates that they buffer Ca^{2+} ions during physiological and pathological states.[13, 54] Work from several laboratories suggests that mitochondrial dys-function is a common event in cell injury caused by mechanical trauma.[55] Anoxia causes the trans-mitochondrial membrane potential to collapse and then impairment of ATP production ensues. In addition to anoxia, the act of Ca^{2+} buffering by mitochondria also causes the transmembrane potential to decrease, resulting in intra-mitochondrial Ca^{2+} accumulation and a further collapse of ATP production. This process is accompanied by a concomitant release of H^+ ions from mitochondria. It is likely that extreme Ca^{2+} overload irreversibly damages mitochondria and that this event commits the cell to die.

Acidosis

CNS trauma and excitotoxicity produce acidosis. Ample evidence indicates that this occurs both at the tissue[7, 56] and at the cellular levels.[57, 58] Several mechanisms of acidosis production are in effect during neuronal injury. First, an obligatory shift from erobic to anerobic metabolism results in lactate production and the release of two H^+ atoms for every two molecules of ATP produced. However, protons are also released during many other reactions, such as phospholipid hydrolysis. Particularly, Ca^{2+} influx causes a rapid intracellular acidification[55] through a number of mechanisms, including a number of membrane exchangers ($Ca^{2+}/2H^+$ exchange at the cell and organelle membranes, Na^+/H^+ exchange to restore Na^+ gradients), the displacement of bound H^+ by Ca^{2+} at negative groups intracellularly and the release of H^+ from mitochondria during Ca^{2+} buffering as a consequence of $Ca^{2+}/2H^+$ exchange.

The mechanism by which acidosis induces cell damage is possibly due to excess accumu-lation of Ca^{2+}, enhancing free radical produc-tion,[59] or accelerating the DNA damage. At present, although experimental trials with agents such as trimethamine have been encouraging,[60] clinical trials in patients with head injuries have failed to reveal a beneficial effect of acidosis treatment.[61]

Strategies for the Treatment of Ca^{2+} Neurotoxicity

The above described cellular and molecular mechanisms of Ca^{2+} related damage constitute the foundation for the recent expansion in a number of potential pharmacological treat-ments for CNS injury. A number of these treatments have been validated *in vitro* and *in vivo* and are approaching tests in clinical trials.

Glutamate Antagonists

Antagonists of glutamate receptors are currently among the most widely investigated potential treatments of CNS injury. Studies aimed at characterizing the role of glutamate receptor-mediated mechanisms in traumatic cell death (see sections above) have produced a number of agents of potential clinical usefulness. For example, antagonists of NMDA receptors, such as **dizocilpine maleate** (MK-801), amino phosphonoheptanoic acid and its analogs and other agents (e.g. CGS 19755 and CPP), are able to markedly attenuate glutamate toxicity *in vitro*[36, 40] and hypoxic/ischemic cell death in a number of models of CNS trauma. Much of the effectiveness of these agents have been ascribed to their ability to reduce cellular Ca^{2+} loading during periods of cerebral metabolic compromise. At a concentration of 0.1 micro meter or higher, brimonidine increased survival of purified rat retinal ganglion cells (RGCs) in the presence of glutamate neurotoxicity, oxidative stress and hypoxia. The neuroprotective effect of brimonidine is mediated via α_2-adrenergic receptors at the rat retinal ganglion cells (RGCs) level.[62]

Drugs that Attenuate Excitatory Neurotransmission

Another approach has been to use agents that attenuate the excessive release of *EAAs* altogether presynaptically (Fig. 7.1), thereby attenuating the consequent neuronal damage.[63] Experimental agents, such as **nizofenone,**[64] BW1003C87,[65] phenytoin[66] and levetiracetam (LEV)[67] probably act by blocking sodium channels and preventing the propagation of action potentials to synaptic terminals, where glutamate is released. These agents have been shown to reduce hypoxic/ischemic damage *in vitro* and *in vivo* and may represent a suitable alternative strategy to glutamate antagonists.

Other Drugs that Prevent Ca^{2+} Increases

Nimodipine, an antagonist of dihydropy-ridine-sensitive (L-type) Ca^{2+} channels, reduces the incidence of ischemic sequele of vasospasm after aneurysmal subarachnoid hemorrhage. Although the precise mechanism of this action is uncertain, the action may be caused by the drug's effect on Ca^{2+} channels in cerebrovascular smooth muscle, rather than on neurons.[68] Thus, nimodipine has been successful in ameliorating outcome from ischemic CNS injury in which the primary defect is thought to lie in the cerebral vasculature rather than in the neuron.

To date, however, dihydropyridine class antagonists of voltage-gated Ca^{2+} channels have not been highly effective in reducing other forms of traumatic/ischemic CNS injury.

Agents that Act Directly on Intracellular Ca^{2+} Ions

A recent approach to protect neurons against Ca^{2+} neurotoxicity *in vitro* and *in vivo* has been the use of cell-permeant Ca^{2+} chelating agents, such as l, 2-bis-(2-aminophenoxy) ethane-N, N, N', N'-tetra-acetic acid (BAPTA). BAPTA (1, 2-bis(o-aminophenoxy) ethane-N,N,N',N'-tetra-acetic acid) is a calcium-specific poly-aminocarboxylic acid. The presence of four carboxylic acid functional groups makes possible the binding of two calcium ions. BAPTA acetoxymethyl is a lipophilic compound capable of crossing cell membranes, but it does not bind Ca^{2+} ions and does not alter extracellular Ca^{2+} concentrations. However, once the compound has crossed the neuronal membrane, intracellular esterases cleave the acetoxymethyl ester moiety, thereby forming the ionized Ca^{2+} binding compound, BAPTA, which remains trapped within the cells.[69]

Drugs that Attenuate the Secondary Processes Triggered by Ca^{2+} Excess

A comprehensive review of the many approaches aimed at attenuating the secondary sequele of Ca^{2+} excess cannot be achieved in the present review. However, a few strategies are approaching clinical applicability and will be mentioned briefly.

Considerable efforts are being extended to develop and test clinically tolerable free radical scavenging agents. For example, glucocorticoid and nonglucocorticoid steroids

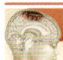

having free radical scavenging activity are currently in clinical trials for a variety of neurosurgical disorders, including stroke, head trauma, and spinal cord injury, of which **methylprednisolone** is one already in clinical use. Other free radical scavenging agents, such as polyethylene glycol-conjugated SOD[70] and vitamin E,[71] may also have a role in certain forms of Ca^{2+} dependent tissue injury.

Other strategies currently under investigation include the use of protease inhibitors to block Ca^{2+} dependent proteolysis and cytoskeletal degradation after excitotoxic or hypoxic/ischemic injuries,[68] anti-DNA fragmentation drugs to retard or abolish apoptosis,[73] and a variety of genetic and environmental manipulations of neurons to render them more resistant to hypoxic/ischemic damage.[74]

CONCLUSIONS

Central nervous system trauma produce a deregulation of cellular Ca^{2+} homeostasis by numerous mechanisms, including energy depletion, cell membrane depolarization, excessive synaptic activity and organelle dysfunction. This pathological increase in intracellular Ca^{2+} ions, which normally regulate numerous intracellular cascades, triggers further injury to neuronal and axonal elements. A key feature of Ca^{2+} neurotoxicity is that Ca^{2+} ions must rise in specific, nonrandom subcellular sites to trigger secondary cascades, which cause neurodegeneration. In some forms of injury, these sites may be located near NMDA receptors.

Considerable advances have been made in recent years in the study and understanding of neuronal Ca^{2+} homeostasis, resulting in the advent of numerous novel neuroprotective strategies. It is hoped that these strategies will find clinical applicability in the next decade. Basic research into the cellular and molecular mechanisms of CNS damage is essential and must continue for further understanding.

REFERENCES

1. Kater SB, Mattson MP, Guthrie PB. Calcium-induced neuronal degeneration: A normal growth cone regulating signal gone away. Ann NY Acad Sci 1989;568:252–61.
2. Schlepfer WW, Zimmerman UJ. Mechanisms underlying the neuronal response to ischemic injury: Calcium-activated proteolysis of neurofilaments. Prog Brain Res 1985;63:185–96.
3. Kure S, Torninaga T, Yoshimoto T, Tada K, Narisawa K. Glutamate triggers internucleosomal DNA cleavage in neuronal cells. Biochem Biophys Res Comm 1991;179:39–45.
4. Augustine GJ, Charlton MP, Smith SJ: Calcium entry into voltage-lamped presynaptic terminals of squid. J Physiol 1985;367:143–62.
5. Brose N, Petrenko AG, Sudhof TC, Jahn R. Synaptotagmin: A calcium sensor on the synaptic vesicle surface. Science 1992;256:1021–5.
6. Simms BA, Zamponi GW. Trafficking and stability of voltage-gated calcium channels. Cell Mol Life Sci 2012;69(6):843–56.
7. Baimbridge KG, Celio MR. Rogers JH. Calcium-binding proteins in the nervous system. Trends Neurosci 1992;15:303–8.
8. Neher E, Augustine GJ. Calcium gradients and buffers on bovine chromaffin cells. J Physiol 1992;450:273–301.
9. Zhou Z, Neher E. Mobile and immobile calcium buffers in bovine adrenal chromaffin cells. J Physiol 1993;469:245–73.
10. Chard PS, Bleakman D, Christakos S, Fullmer CS, Miller RJ. Calcium buffering properties of calbindin D28k and parvalbumin in rat sensory neurons. J Physiol 1993;472:341–57.
11. Kasai H. Peterson OH. Spatial dynamics of second messengers: IP3 and cAMP as long-range and associative messengers. Trends Neurosci 1994;17:95–101.
12. Balentine JD, Paris DU, Dean DL. Calcium-induced spongiform and necrotizing myelopathy. Lab Invest 1982;47:286–95.
13. Blaustein MP. Calcium transport and buffering in neurons. Trends Neuro Sci 1988;11:438–43.
14. Carafoli E. The Ca^{2+} pump of the plasma membrane. J Biol Chem 1992;267:2115–8.
15. Lwe VL, Tsien RY, Miner C. Physiological (Ca^{2+} level and pump-leak turnover in intact red cells measured using an incorporated Ca chelator. Nature 1982;298:478–81.
16. Benveniste H, Drejer J, Schousboe A, Diemer NH. Elevation of the extracellular concentrations

of glutamate and aspartate in rat hippocampus during transient cerebral ischemia monitored by intracerebral micro-dialysis. J Neurochem 1984;43:1369–74.

17. Kitamura Y, Miyazaki A, Yamanaka Y, Nomura Y. Stimulatory effects of protein kinase C and calmodulin kinase II on N-methyl-D-aspartate receptor/channels in the postsynaptic density of rat brain. J Neurochem 1993;61:100–9.

18. Tymianski M, Charlton MP, Carlen PL, Tator CH. Properties of neuroprotective cell-permeant Ca²⁺ chelators: Effects on Ca²⁺ and glutamate neurotoxicity *in vitro*. J Neurophysiol. 1994;267: 1973–92.

19. Tymianski M, Spigelman I, Zhang L, Carlen PL, Tator CH, Charlton MP, Wallace MC. Mechanism of action and persistence of neuroprotection by cell permeant Ca²⁺ chelators. J Cereb Blood Flow Metab 1994;14:911–23.

20. McLean AEM, McLean E, Judah JD. Cellular necrosis in the liver induced and modified by drugs. Int rev exp pathol 1965;4:127–57.

21. Schanne FAX, Kane AB, Young EA, Farber JL. Calcium dependence of toxic cell death: A final common pathway. Science 1979;206:700–2.

22. Schlepfer WW, Bunge RP. Effects of calcium ion concentration on the degeneration of amputated axons in tissue culture. J Cell Biol 1973;59:456–510.

23. Jancso G, Karcsu S, Kiraly E, Szebeni A, Toth L, Bacsy E, Joo F, Parducz A. Neurotoxin induced nerve cell degeneration: Possible involvement of calcium. Brain Res 1984;295:211–6.

24. Choi DW. Glutamate neurotoxicity in cortical cell culture is calcium dependent. Neurosci Lett 1985;58:293–7.

25. Garthwaite G, Garthwaite J. Neurotoxicity of excitatory amino acid receptor agonists in rat cerebellar slices: Dependence on calcium concentration. Neurosci Lett 1986;66:193–8.

26. Balentine JD: Spinal cord trauma. In search of the meaning of granular axoplasm and vesicular myelin. J Neuropathol Exp Neurol 1988;47:77–92.

27. Balentine JD, Paris DU, Dean DL. Calcium-induced spongiform and necrotizing myelopathy. Lab Invest 1982;47:286–95.

28. Cheung JY, Bonventre N, Malis CD, Leaf A. calcium and Ischemic Injury. N Engl J Med 1986;314:1670–6.

29. Dingledine R. Boland LM. Chamberlin NL, Kawasaki K, Kleckner NW, Traynelis SF, Verdoorn TA. Amino acid receptors and uptake

systems in the mammalian central nervous system. CRC Crit Rev Neurobiol 1988;4:1–97.

30. Nakanishi S. Molecular diversity of glutamate receptors and implications for brain function. Science 1992;258:597–603.

31. Collinridge GL, Singer W. Excitatory amino acid receptors and synaptic plasticity. Trends Pharmacol Sci 1990;11:290–6.

32. Ozyurt E, Graham DI, Woodruff GN, McCulloch J. Protective effect of the glutamate antagonist MK-801 in focal cerebral ischemia in the cat. J Cereb blood flow Metab 1988;8:138–43.

33. Olney JW. Brain lesion, obesity and other disturbances in mice treated with monosodium glutamate. Science 1969;164:719–21.

34. Choi DW, Maulucci-Gedde M. Kriegstein AR. Glutamate neurotoxicity in cortical cell culture. J Neurosci 1987;7:357–68.

35. Garthwaite J, Garthwaite G. The mechanism of kainic acid neurotoxicity. Nature 1983;305:138–40.

36. Gilbertson TA. Scobey R. Wilson M. Permeation of calcium ions through non-NMDA glutamate channels in retinal bipolar cells. Science 1991;251:1613–15.

37. Hollman M. Hartley M. Heinemann S. Ca2+ permeability of KA-AMPA-gated glutamate receptor channels depends on subunit composition. Science 1991;252:851–3.

38. MacDermott AB, Mayer ML, Westbrook GL, Smith SJ, Barker JL. NMDA-receptor activation increases cytoplasmic calcium concentration in cultured spinal cord neurons. Nature 1986;321:519–22.

39. Choi DW. Ionic dependence of glutamate neurotoxicity. J Neurosci 1987;7:369–79.

40. Choi DW, Maulucci-Gedde M, Kriegstein AR. Glutamate neurotoxicity in cortical cell culture. J Neurosci 1987;7:357–68.

41. Eimrel S, Schramm M. The quantity of calcium that appears to induce neuronal death. J Neurochem 1994;62:1223–6.

42. Baker AJ, Moulton RJ, MacMillan VB, Shedden PM. Excitatory amino acids in cerebrospinal fluid following traumatic brain injury in humans. J Neurosurg 1993;79:369–72.

43. Kunz A, Dirnagl U, Mergenthaler P. Acute pathophysiological processes after ischemic and traumatic brain injury.Best pract res Clin Anesthesiol 2010;24(4):495–509.

44. Astrup J, Siesjo BK. Symon L. Thresholds in cerebral ischemia: The ischemic penumbra. Stroke 1981;12:723–5.

45. Ozawa K, Seta K. Araki H. Handa H. The effect of ischemia on mitochondrial metabolism. J Biol Chem 1966;61:512–4.

46. Cox JA. Lysko PG, Henneberry RC. Excitatory amino acid neurotoxicity at the N-methyl-D-aspartate receptor in cultured neurons: Role of the voltage-dependent magnesium block. Brain Res 1989;499:267–72.

47. Nowak L, Bregestovski P. Ascher P: Magnesium gates glutamate-activated channels in mouse central neurones. Nature 1984;307:462–5.

48. Abele AE, Scholz KP, Scholz WK. Miller RJ. Excitotoxicity induced by enhanced excitatory neurotransmission in cultured hippocampal pyramidal neurons. Neuron 1990;4:413–9.

49. Rosenberg PA. Aizenman E. Hundred-fold increase in neuronal vulnerability to glutamate toxicity in astrocyte-poor culture of rat cerebral cortex. Neurosci Lett 1989;103:162–8.

50. Rosenberg PA, Amin S, Leitner M. Glutamate uptake disguises neurotoxic potency of glutamate agonists in cerebral cortex in dissociated cell culture. J Neurosci 1989;12:56–61.

51. Choi DW. Cerebral hypoxia: Some new approaches and unanswered questions. J Neurosci 1990;10:2493–2501.

52. Kiedrowski L. Brooker G, Costa E, Wroblewski JT. Glutamate impairs neuronal calcium extrusion while reducing sodium gradient. Neuron 1994;12:295–300.

53. De Erausquin GA, Manev H. Guidotti A, Costa E, Brooker G. Gangliosides normalize distorted single-cell intracellular free Ca^{2+} dynamics after toxic doses of glutamate in cerebellar granule cells. Proc Natl Acad Sci USA 1990;87:8017–21.

54. Vlessis AA, Widener LL, Bartos D. Effect of peroxide, sodium and calcium on brain mitochondrial respiration in vitro: Potential role in cerebral ischemia and reperfusion. J Neurochem; 54:1412–18.

55. Gadian DG, Frackowiak RSJ, Crockard HA, Proctor E, Alien K, Williams SR, Russell RWR: Acute cerebral ischemia. Concurrent changes in cerebral blood flow, energy metabolites, pH and lactate measured with hydrogen clearance and 31p and pH nuclear magnetic resonance spectroscopy-I: Methodology. J Cereb Blood Flow Metab 1987;7:199–206.

56. Hartley Z, Dubinsky JM. Changes in intracellular pH associated with glutamate excitotoxicity. J Neurosci 1993;13:4690–9.

57. Untenberg AW, Stover J, Kress B, Kiening KL Edema and brain trauma, Neuroscience, 2004,129(4):1021–9.

58. Siesjo BK, Katsura K, Tibor K. Acidosis related brain damage, in Siesjo BK, Wieloch T (eds): Advances in Neurology: Cellular and Molecular Mechanisms of Ischemic Brain Damage. New York, Raven Press.

59. Gaab MR, Seegers K, Smedema RJ, Heissler HE, Goetz C. A comparative analysis of THAM (Tris-buffer) in traumatic brain oedema. Acta Neurochir Suppl (Wien) 1990;51:320–3.

60. Wolf AL, Levi L, Marmarou A, Ward JD, Muizelaar JP, Choi S, Young H. Rigamonti D, Robinson WL: Effect of THAM upon outcome in severe head injury: A randomized prospective clinical trial./Neurosurg 1993;78:54–59.

61. Eimrel S, Schramm M. The quantity of calcium that appears" to induce neuronal death./ Neurochem 1994;62:1223–26.

62. Lee KY, Nakayama M, Aihara M, Chen YN, Araie M. Brimonidine is neuroprotective against glutamate-induced neurotoxicity, oxidative stress and hypoxia in purified rat retinal ganglion cells. Mol Vis 2010;17;(16):246–51.

63. Matsumoto Y, Kamata T, Goto N. The suppression by nizof enone of the release of glutamate and lactate as a mechanism of its neuroprotective effect: An in vivo brain microdialysis study./Cereb Blood Flow Metab 1993;13: S742.

64. Graham SH, Chen J, Sharp FR, Simon RP. Limiting ischemic injury by inhibition of excitatory amino acid release./Cereb Blood Flow Metab 1993;13:88–97.

65. Boxer PA, Cordon JJ, Mann ME, Rodolosi LC, Vartanian MG, Rock DM, Taylor CP, Marcoux FW. Comparison of phenytoin with noncompetitive N-methyl-D-aspartate antagonists in a model of focal brain ischemia. Stroke 21 1990 [Suppl 11]:III47–51.

66. Tymianski M, Tator CH. The direct effects of nimodipine on intracellular calcium in spinal neurons in explant culture. Drugs Dev. 1993;2: 337–47.

67. Meehan AL, Yang X, Yuan LL, Rothman SM. Levetiracetam has an activity-dependent effect on inhibitory transmission. Epilepsia 2012; 53(3):469–76.

68. Tsien RY. New calcium indicators and buffers with high selectivity against magnesium and protons: Design, synthesis and properties of prototype structures. Biochemistry 1980;19: 2396–404.

69. Tombaugh GC, Sapolsky RM. Mechanistic distinctions between excitotoxic and acidotic

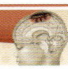

hippocampal damage in vitro model of ischemia./ Cereb Blood Flow Metab 1990;10: 527–35.

70. Fariss MW, Pascoe GA, Reed DJ. Vitamin E reversal of the effect of extracellular calcium on induced toxicity in hepatocytes. Science. 1985;227:751–4.

71. Ladecola C, Pelligrino DA, Moscowitz MA, Lassen NA. State of the art review: Nitric oxide inhibition and cerebrovascular regulation. J Cereb Blood Flow Metab 1994;14:175–92.

72. Roberts-Lewis JM, Marcy VR. Zhao Y, Vaught JL, Siman R, Lewis ME. Aurintricarboxylic acid protects hippocampal neurons from NMDA- and ischemia-induced toxicity *in vivo*. J Neurochem 1993;61:378–81.

73. Rodorf G, Koroshetz WJ, Bonventre JV. Heat shock proteins protect cultured neurons from glutamate toxicity. Neuron 1991;7:1043–51.

74. M Tymianski, Tator CH. Normal and abnormal calcium homeostasis in neurons: a basis for the pathophysiology of traumatic and ischemic central nervous system injury. Neurosurgery 1996;38:1176–95.

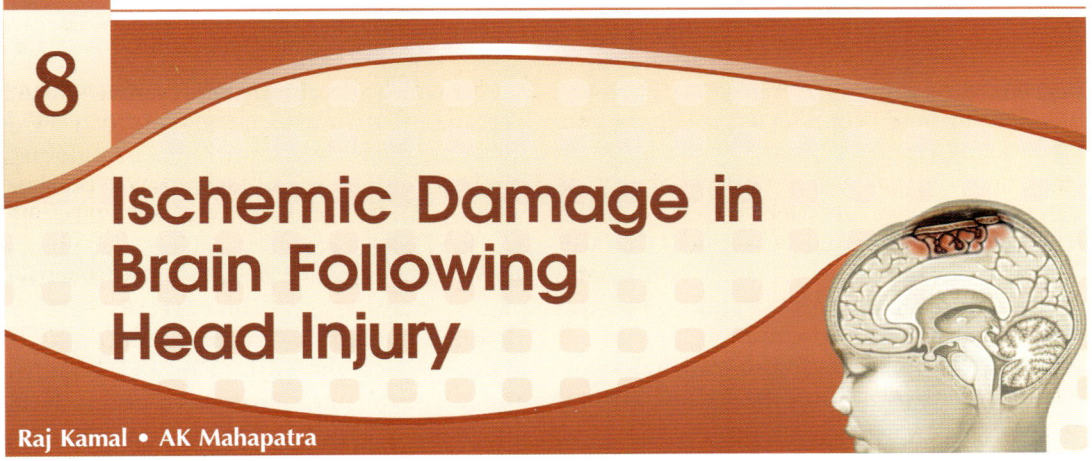

8

Ischemic Damage in Brain Following Head Injury

Raj Kamal • AK Mahapatra

INTRODUCTION

Primary brain damage occurs at the time of injury, produces its clinical detrimental effect immediately. By contrast, secondary damage occurs some time after primary head injury and is largely preventable and treatable. Severe and/or prolonged reductions in CBF lead to deprivations in oxygen and glucose delivery as well as the build-up of potentially toxic substances. Because nerve cells do not store alternative energy sources, these hemodynamic reductions can result in the reduction in metabolites such as ATP, leading to metabolic stress, energy failure, ionic perturbations, and ischemic injury. In conditions of severe TBI, reductions in CBF have been reported to reach ischemic level.[1] Secondary damage such as edema and cerebral ischemia play an important role in ultimate outcome. Graham and his colleague have demonstrated ischemic damage in fatal head injury.[2–4] However, sometimes it is possible to prevent the secondary pathological process which are almost invariably present following injury[5–10] and more harmful than primary damage. These are edema, ischemia and necrosis. Currently a controversial issue is whether ischemic events represent a primary cause of cell injury or only a secondary consequence of tissue damage.[11,12] Severe cerebral ischemic insults lead to metabolic stress, ionic perturbations, and a complex cascade of biochemical and molecular events ultimately causing neuronal death. Similarities in the pathogenesis of these cerebral injuries may indicate that therapeutic neuroprotective strategies following ischemia may also be beneficial after trauma.[13] Thus, early diagnosis, timely surgery and adequate protection of brain are probably the main objectives of modern treatment of severe head injury. The ultimate outcome of severe head injury depends on several factors. In this chapter attempt has been made to highlight the role of the ischemic brain damage following head injury.[3,5,14–17] In fatal head injury, ischemic damage is reported in 85–90% cases.[2–4] This chapter will focus on cause and effect of cerebral ischemia.

PATHOPHYSIOLOGY OF ISCHEMIC INJURY

Hypoxia is a deficiency of oxygen, which causes cell injury by reducing erobic oxidative respiration.[18] In ischemia, on the other hand, the supply of oxygen and nutrients is decreased most often because of reduced blood flow as a consequence of a mechanical obstruction in the arterial system. It can also be caused by reduced venous drainage. Hypoxia is an extremely important and common cause of cell injury and cell death. *Causes of hypoxia* include reduced blood flow (called *ischemia*), inadequate oxygenation of the blood due to cardiorespiratory failure, and decreased oxygen-carrying capacity of the blood, as in anemia or after severe blood loss. Depending on the severity of the hypoxic state, neurons may adapt, undergo injury, or die. For example, if an artery is narrowed, the tissue supplied by that vessel may initially shrink in size (atrophy), whereas more severe or sudden hypoxia induces injury and cell death. This is the most common type of cell injury in clinical medicine and has been studied extensively in humans, in experimental animals.[18]

The severity of the secondary mechanisms of head injury depends upon injury severity (mild, moderate, severe) or location of the primary insult. In conditions of severe TBI, reductions in CBF have been reported to reach ischemic levels.[1] Thus, cerebral ischemia is discussed as one secondary injury mechanism that may participate in brain trauma.[11,19] Ischemic changes are seen in autopsy specimen of fatal head injuries in most cases.[2,20,21] In severe head injury, reductions in CBF have been reported to reach ischemic levels.[1] Thus, cerebral ischemia is discussed as one secondary injury mechanism that may participate in brain trauma.[19]

Both necrotic and apoptotic cell death mechanisms have been implicated in the pathogenesis of ischemic[1,22–25] and traumatic brain injury.[22, 26–28] The brain is vulnerable to oxidative stress due to its high rate of oxidative metabolic activity. Oxidative stress leading to calcium accumulation, mitochondrial dysfunction and the production of reactive oxygen radicals is an important mechanism of cell death following both ischemic[29–37] and traumatic insults.[34–35] After cerebral ischemia and trauma, evidence for the generation of reactive oxygen species (ROS) has been demonstrated in a variety of injury models.[31,38,39] In addition, transgenic models where antioxidants including superoxide dismutase (SOD) are overexpressed have been shown to provide neuroprotection from both ischemia and traumatic insults.[29,35] Pathological changes in head injury is the widespread which affect **brainstem, cerebellum and cerebrum.** Primary pathology following injury are the various intracranial **hematomas,** cerebral **contusion and laceration.** However, with the advent of the CT scanning (Figs 8.1, 8.2a to c) it has been very well observed that a significant number of severe head injury patients may die or remain **vegetative** even in absence of demonstrated hematomas in brain.[40,41] Recently, MRI, PET, SPECT studies and **cerebral perfusion** parameters have demonstrated widespread cerebral ischemia following head injury.[5,14,42–48] SPECT studies have shown reduction of blood flow in frontal and temporal lobe even in minor head injured patients with post concussion syndrome.[49] The histopathological studies by Graham and his colleague[2–4,10] had proved beyond doubt the wide spread ischemic injury in brain, in patients with head injury. In 1977 Graham[3] described the pathological changes in brain, in patients with head injury, secondary to hypoxia and ischemic damage in 91% cases of 151 fatal non-missile head injury. Recent autopsy studies have also shown ischemic brain damage in over 85% patients with fatal closed head injury.[3,42] Low cerebral perfusion is also recorded around focal contusion, and acute SDH.[43,44]

To investigate the importance of CBF reductions in the pathogenesis of brain trauma, recent studies have utilized positron emission tomography (PET) in patients after TBI and cerebral hemorrhage (Fig. 8.2d).[12,50] In these studies, cerebral blood flow and cerebral metabolic rate of oxygen ($CMRO_2$) and oxygen extraction fraction (OEF) were evaluated to assess the O_2 availability in injured tissue. Although both CBF and $CMRO_2$ were significantly reduced in the injured hemisphere, OEF was also reduced in areas showing hemodynamic reductions. Because OEF normally increases in cerebral ischemic insults, the question of whether these hemodynamic changes are due to an ischemic insult or secondary to metabolic dysfunction and necrosis is critical.[50]

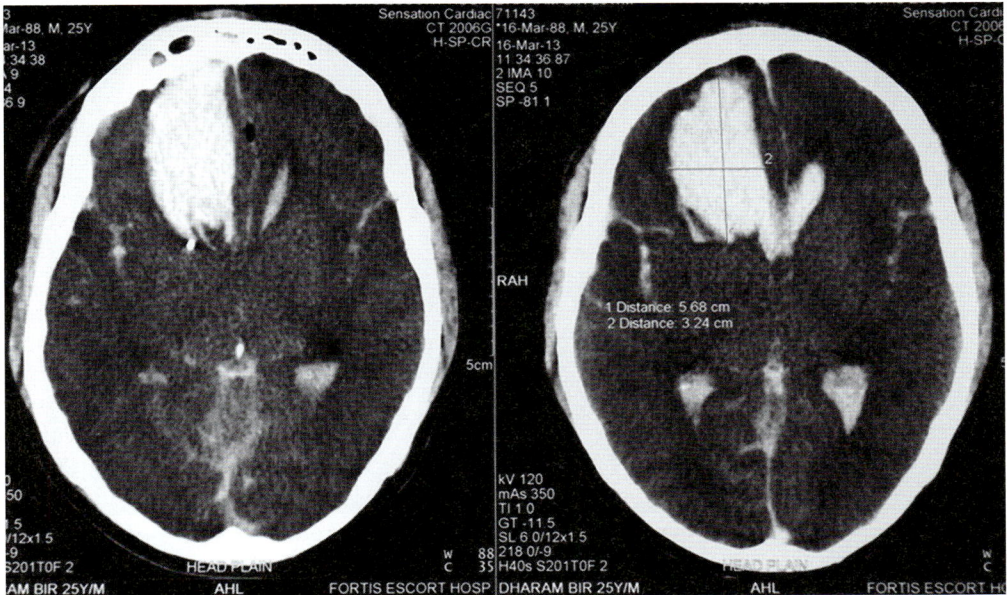

Fig. 8.1: NCCT head shows generalized diffuse ischemic changes (infarct) in a patient with severe head injury

Contusions are commonly associated with hemodynamic changes including focal reductions in local cerebral blood flow.[51,52] Focal areas of reduced CBF after brain trauma can be surrounded by regions exhibiting milder reductions in flow (Fig. 8.2b and Table 8.1).[51,52] This surrounding area may thus correspond to the penumbral region surrounding an ischemic core[53,54] This border zone area contains scattered damaged neurons within an intact neuropil.[57] Importantly, this area is sensitive to therapeutic interventions as well as at risk for secondary insults.[55–57]

Although much is known about structural changes that occur early after cerebral ischemia or trauma, less is known about the progressive nature of these acute insults to the brain. Clinically, progression of damage has been observed in stroke and TBI patients using MRI.[58] Experimentally, progressive atrophy of gray and white matter structures has been reported in models of TBI.[57,59] In one study, severe atrophy of multiple white matter tracts was described 1 year after TBI.[57,58] A greater

understanding of the pathophysiological processes in this underlying progressive injury cascade could lead to better strategies for neuroprotection and reparative processes. Head injured patients have demonstrated histopathological changes consistent with hypoxic/ischemic insults[4,60] and severe flow reductions early after TBI.[19,60] Following TBI, energy demand and tissue PO_2 in the traumatized tissue are reduced, and therefore, moderate reductions in blood flow may have severe consequences for cellular survival.[61] Experimental studies have reported reduction in ATP content in traumatized cortical regions and elevated lactate levels after severe TBI.[62]

Basic reason leading to the development of ischemic lesions in head injury is raised ICP, compromising cerebral perfusion. Systemic blood pressure remaining constant, when intracranial pressure increases the cerebral perfusion pressure (CPP) falls. However, the perfusion is maintained till the perfusion pressure is above 70 mm of Hg. When CPP reduced below 70 mm of Hg, there is likeli-

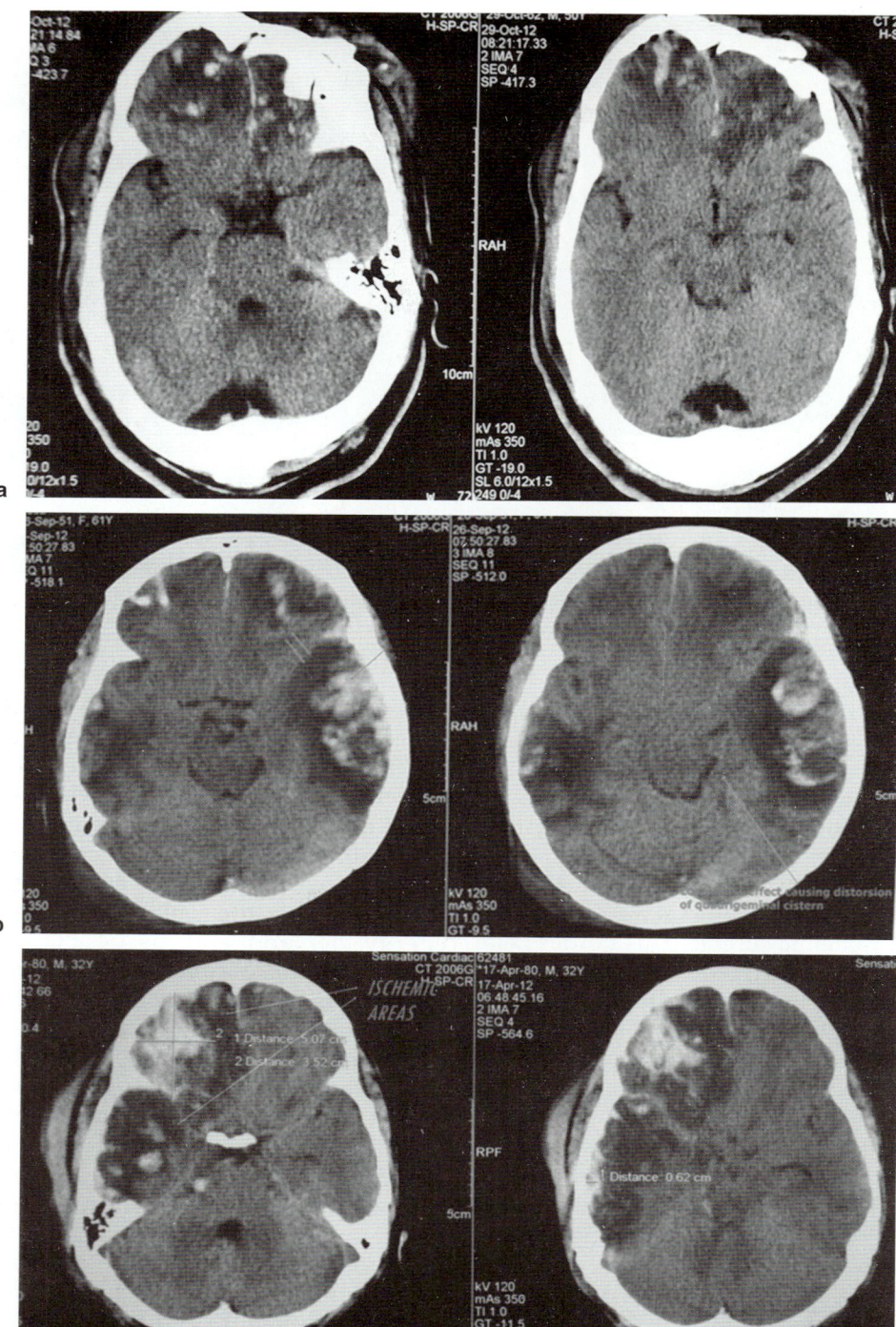

Figs 8.2a to c: NCCT head shows focal ischemic changes around contusion

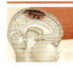

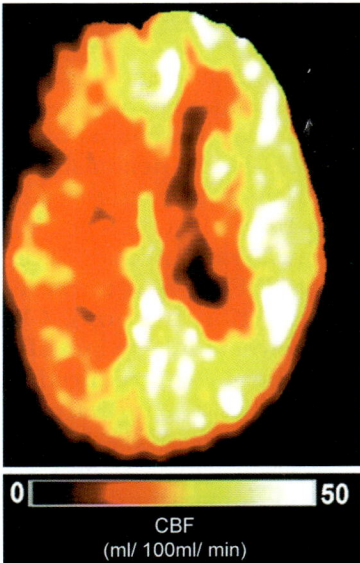

| 0 | | 50 |

CBF
(ml/ 100ml/ min)

Fig. 8.2d: PET corresponding to CT scan in Fig. 8.2c showing reduced CBF in the area of contusions

Table 8.1: Ischemic brain injury as seen in CT or autopsy		
Focal	a.	With focal lesion
	b.	Without focal lesion
Hemispheric	a.	With focal lesion
	b.	Without focal lesion
Diffuse		
Failure of microcirculation		

reported systemic insults occurring either prior to hospital admission or within hospital, during the emergency procedures. They also reported short episodes of hypotension may involve marked cerebral ischemia, which even persists after adequate systemic hemodynamic restoration. Sahuquillo et al[17] analyzed the risk factors for early post-traumatic ischemia and concluded that the ischemia is highly prevalent in the early period after severe head injury.

Arterial hypotension and intracranial hypertension are detrimental to the injured brain.[64] Although artificial elevation of cerebral perfusion pressure (CPP) has been advocated as a means to maintain an adequate cerebral blood flow (CBF), the optimal CPP for the treatment of severe traumatic brain injury (TBI) remains unclear.[64] In addition, CBF evolves significantly over time after TBI, and CBF may vary considerably in patient-to-patient. For these reasons, a more useful approach may be to consider the optimal CPP in an individual patient at any given time, rather than having an arbitrary goal applied uniformly to all patients. Important information for optimizing CBF is provided by monitoring intracranial pressure in combination with assessment of the adequacy of CBF by using global indicators (for example, jugular oximetry), supplemented when appropriate by local data, such as brain tissue oxygen tension.[64]

Botteri et al[65] systematically evaluated the evidence available on cerebral blood flow thresholds and its methodologic adequacy in adults with traumatic brain injury among the 53 diagnostic studies identified, 31 did not report any threshold value, whereas 20 studies used thresholds derived from the literature, mainly animal or clinical studies on ischemic stroke. One study measured cerebral blood flow thresholds, but did not use accepted neuroradiological criteria for the diagnosis of post-traumatic cerebral ischemia. The remaining study fulfilled all methodologic inclusion criteria, but was restricted to 14 patients with severe traumatic brain injury

hood of cerebral ischemia. There is selective vulnerability of different part of the brain to the ischemic insult, which is also of varying degree at different areas of the brain. Graham et al in 1989[3] reported almost equal incidence of ischemic injury in brain in patients between 1968–72 and 1981–82. Ischemic damage is observed more frequently in hippocampus, basal ganglia than cerebral cortex and cerebellum. As ischemic damage is related to high ICP and low perfusion pressure, this condition is reported in all the age groups.[2,4,45,63] The available evidences suggest that in majority cases ischemia occurs fairly early after injury.[2,4,9,10,17] Moeschler et al[9]

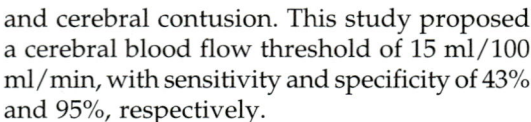

and cerebral contusion. This study proposed a cerebral blood flow threshold of 15 ml/100 ml/min, with sensitivity and specificity of 43% and 95%, respectively.

Hemodynamic Phases after the TBI

There is also a significant patient-to-patient variation in the hemodynamic response to TBI. However, a pattern of three distinct hemodynamic phases can be distinguished:

Hypoperfusion Phase (Phase 1; Day 0)

The first 24 hours after TBI are characterized by cerebral hypoperfusion. Although CBF is reduced, there is a normal velocity in the middle cerebral artery (VMCA) as assessed by transcranial Doppler and a normal cerebral arteriovenous oxygen difference (AVDO$_2$). During this hypoperfusion phase, cerebral metabolic rate for oxygen (CMRO$_2$) is about 50% of normal. It has been suggested that pathological microcirculatory resistance is responsible for the reduced blood flow. Given the normal AVDO$_2$, it is also plausible that the CBF during this stage represents physiological flow-metabolism coupling. Focal or global cerebral ischemia occurs frequently after TBI. Although the total ischemic brain volume may be less than 10% on average, the presence of cerebral ischemia is associated with poor ultimate neurological outcome.[66] The frequent association between cerebral hypoperfusion and poor outcome suggests that TBI and ischemic stroke share the same fundamental mechanisms. Regional blood flow measurements early after severe head injuriy have now demonstrated that flow levels <18 ml/100 g/min is sufficient to generate neuronal ischemic necrosis in 34% of sever TBI.[11,19,66–68] CBF below this level jeopardizes the energy dependent Na/K-ATPase pump system leading to disturbed ionic homeostasis. However, reduction in CBF does not necessarily result in ischemia. The diagnosis of cerebral ischemia requires demonstration that the CBF is insufficient for a metabolic demand. The metabolic demand is reflected by substrate (oxygen and glucose) uptake and metabolite (pyruvate and lactate) production.[66] Reductions in cerebral metabolic rates common in head injury and metabolic needs may be further reduced by sedative agents. In practice, a secure diagnosis of ischemia depends upon the the demonstration of an increased oxygen extraction fraction, an increase in tissue lactate level, or a high lactate/pyruvate ratio. Accompanying initial reduction in CBF, there is increase in OEF (oxygen extraction fraction). CMRO$_2$ is reduced somewhat initially, but falls further over a few hours. With reduced CBF and declining CMRO$_2$, the initially markedly increased OEF progressively decreases.

The relationship between CBF, CMRO$_2$ and AVDO$_2$ can be summarized by the formula **CMRO$_2$ = CBF × AVDO$_2$**. The normal values for AVDO$_2$ is approximately 6.5 ml O$_2$/100 ml blood, for CMRO$_2$ is 3.2 ml O$_2$/100 g/min and for cerebral oxygenation ranges between 50 and 75%. Ischemic brain with low CBF exhibits low SjVO$_2$ reading of less than 50%, whereas for the hyperemic brain, the reading is more than 75%. Similarly, in brain dead patient where no uptake of oxygen occurred, the SjVO$_2$ would also be higher than 75%.

Hyperemia Phase (Phase 2; Days 1 to 3)

After 24 hours (days 1 to 3) the CBF increases. This is associated by a fall in AVDO$_2$ and hence a rise in the SjO$_2$. CMRO$_2$ remains depressed. CBF is often normal in presence of low metabolism (relative hyperemia) or high CBF in relation to normal metabolism (absolute hyperemia).

There is both a relative hyperemia (relative to blood flow demand during this stage) and an absolute hyperemia (CBF above the normal CBF range). VMCA begins to rise rapidly. The pathophysiological mechanism of this hyperemia is unknown. This pathology seems as detrimental as ischemia in terms of outcome because increases in CBF beyond matching metabolic demand relate to vasoparalysis with consecutive increase in cerebral blood volume and in turn increases intracranial pressure (ICP).[11,19,68]

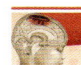

It is important to note that diagnosing *hypoperfusion* or *hyperperfusion* is only valid after assessing measurements of CBF in relation to those of cerebral oxygen consumption. Both cerebral ischemia and hyperemia refer to a mismatch between CBF and cerebral metabolism. For example, low flow with normal or high metabolic rate represents an ischemic situation whereas high CBF with normal or reduced metabolic rate represents cerebral hyperemia. In contrast, low CBF with a low metabolic rate or high CBF with high metabolic rate represents coupling between flow and metabolism, a situation that does not necessarily reflect a pathological condition.[69,70]

Vasospasm Phase (Phase 3, Days 4 to 15)

TBI may also cause spasm of large cerebral vessels similar to vasospasm induced by subarachnoid hemorrhage. VMCA rises further and CBF gradually declines. Interestingly, during the vasospasm phase the $AVDO_2$ remains low (hence the SjO_2 remains high). This is probably the result of either the persistently reduced $CMRO_2$ or cell death. Vasospasm may contribute further to cerebral ischemia.

Vasomotor paralysis by Langfitt[71,72] postulated an acute reduction in vasomotor tone that resulted in cerebral vasodilatation, increased CBV, and ICP. When arterial hypertension followed trauma, massive brain swelling occurred that was associated with both hyperemia and edema.

Of particular relevance to head injury is the related concept of "vasomotor paralysis" introduced by Langfitt and coworkers,[71,72,74] to explain brain swelling and intracranial hypertension in experimental studies of cerebral compression by Lassen,[73] who described a "luxury perfusion syndrome" in patients with acute brain disorders. This syndrome is characterized by cerebral hyperemia, defined as excessive blood flow relative to the brain's metabolic requirements. Lassen argued that the hyperemia was due to impaired CBF autoregulation secondary to ischemia or hypoxia, and speculated that it could lead to disruption of the blood–brain barrier and edema formation. Since then, hyperemia has been observed in a number of acute clinical conditions, and trauma. They postulated an acute reduction in vasomotor tone that resulted in cerebral vasodilatation, increased blood volume, and elevated intracranial pressure (ICP). When arterial hypertension followed trauma, massive brain swelling occurred that was associated with both hyperemia and edema. These findings suggested that brain trauma impairs CBF autoregulation, which was subsequently confirmed.[73]

It is apparent that the concepts of luxury perfusion and vasomotor paralysis refer to different aspects of the same phenomenon; namely, an acute derangement of the cerebral circulation manifested by hyperemia and a potential for brain swelling. Although repeatedly observed in human and animal studies, the pathophysiological significance of this syndrome remains obscure, including its relevance to the management of clinical head injury. Thus, the incidence and time course of hyperemia following head injury is not fully known, nor is its relationship to intracranial hypertension. Furthermore, it is not clear whether therapy should be aimed at reducing the hyperemia. Although hyperventilation therapy has been widely used to control ICP, its effect on acute hyperemia has not been systematically evaluated. Normal or increased CBF during coma is accompanied by a narrow $AVDO_2$ argues strongly that such flows are a luxury perfusion. High CBFs were associated with both an elevated ICP and increased jugular venous pO_2 (narrow AV difference). If blood flow is doubled, as in some patients with absolute hyperemia, CBV might be expected to increase by 30%.

Factors Responsible for Ischemia

Evidences from the clinical studies show that the ischemic brain damage is the major factor for bad outcome in severe head injury.

Laboratory studies and animal experiments indicate that the excitatory **amino acids** are important mediators causing brain damage.[6]

The mechanisms involved in ischemic brain damage is primarily due to calcium overload, **acidosis** and liberation of free radicals. In ischemia there is **anerobic metabolism,** leading to lactic acidosis. The presence of **glutamate** and increased intracellular calcium, the calcium channel opens up.

The early post-traumatic blood flow mapping and small vessel ultrastructure studies at different points reveals a zone of ischemic brain, invariably present around the contusion. Ischemic damage also occurs in acute subdural hematoma.[7]

Ischemia results due to increase in extracellular glutamate concentration.[29,30,56] Hence, the drugs which act at N-methyl-D aspartate, (NMDA)/receptor, which is a subtype of **glutamate,** have been shown to reduce ischemic brain damage. Inglis et al[7] in an experimental study in rats assessed the cerebral glucose utilization and CBF, by using double lable **autoradiography.** They found a hypermetabolic state and increase glucose utilization in the **hippocampus.**

Sahuquillo et al[17] studied severe head injured patients to detect early **ischemia.** They analyzed arteriojugular differences of oxygen (AVDO$_2$) and arteriorjugular lactate-oxygen ADDL/AVDO$_2$. They divided patients into ischemic group and non-ischemic group. They observed that the arterial hemoglobin and the ischemia score were significantly different in both groups.

Ischemia can develop due to large artery involvement.[15,16,75] Post-traumatic occlusive vascular problem is more frequent in children than adult. Occlusion may involve **internal carotid** or MCA artery. In a study of 220 pediatric head injury Walia[76] noticed 4 children with **hemispheric** infarcts. Rarely ischemia does involve the **basal ganglia** area.[20] In infants ischemia can also result due to hemoconcentration, resulting from the use of osmotic diuretics and restricted fluid intake.

Thus, the **microcirculation** gets involved leading to ischemic damage. Post-traumatic vasospasm can lead to ischemic brain damage, reported upto 20% patients.[15,16,77,78] Marshall and Gaotille[15] reported subarachnoid hemorrhage in 491 patients with head injury and reported small and large area of infarct as seen in CT scan. Marshall et al[77] 1978 reported **vasospasm** leading to clinical deterioration between 5th and 9th day. Recently, Bakshi and Mahapatra[78] have demonstrated high blood flow velocity in **basilar artery,** in 40% patients severe head injury. Rarely **venous sinus thrombosis** can lead to **venous infarction** brain following head injury.

Diagnosis of Ischemic Brain Injury

Ischemic brain damage in head injury was initially diagnosed in autopsy studies.[2,4] Even recent studies have shown the presence of ischemia in over 85% fatal cases.[3,5] With routine **ICP monitoring** and CBF study it is possible to find out the time of onset of ischemia.[7,14,45,79] With the advent of CT, MRI **SPECT and PET** (Figs 8.2a to d) the ischemia is well visualized and can be graded.[14,46,79] SPECT helps in assessing regional cerebral blood flow using **(HMPAO)** or mTC ethylene cyteine dimer (ECD). The tomographic image obtained with gamma camera provides cerebral perfusion in different cortical areas. Normally, there is bilateral symmetrical cortical uptake of HMPAO.

Use of TCD is helpful in assessing blood flow velocity (Fig. 8.3).[78,80] Czosnyka et al[79] in 1994 studied ICP, blood flow velocity (FV) and **pulsatility index** (PI). They estimated cerebrovascular resistance (CVR = CPP/FV). Their results showed CPP lower than 55 mm of Hg means failure of autoregulation and onset of cerebral ischemia. Chan et al[42] performed TCD in head injury patients, and the blood flow velocity in MCA was recorded. They concluded that TCD can provide an alternative mean to identify cerebral ischemia. Bakshi and Mahapatra[78] for the 1st time studied the basilar artery blood flow velocity in 16 severe

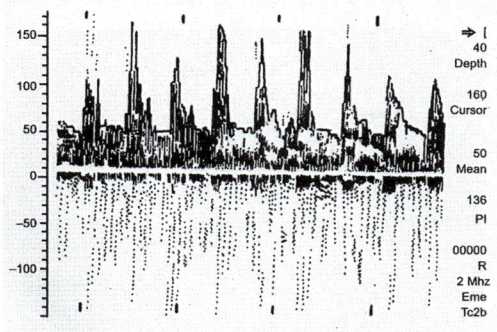

Fig. 8.3: TCD right MCA artery shows normal flow velocity and PI in a patient with severe head injury

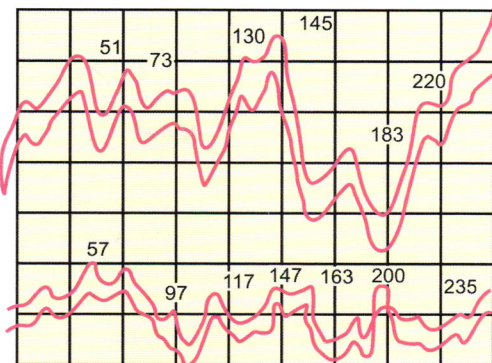

Fig. 8.4a: Brainstem auditory evoked potential

Right side median (SEP)

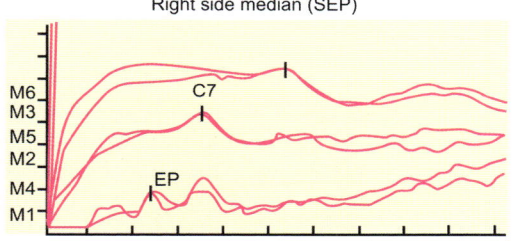

Fig. 8.4b: Sensory evoked potential (SEP) in a patient with severe head injury shows normal wave

head injury patients. They observed abnormally high flow velocity in 7 patients.

Evoked potentials (EP) are (Fig. 8.4a) helpful to assess cerebral cortical and brainstem function in head injury patients.[40,48] In absence of detectable CT pathology abnormal BEP or SEP mean impaired function most likely due to ischemia. Lesnick et al[48] reported altered sensory evoked potential (SEP) in patients with global cerebral ischemia (Fig. 8.4b).[49] Thus indicating usefulness of SEP.

Prevention and Treatment of Ischemic Injury (Tables 8.2 and 8.3)

Ischemic injury to brain is one of the most important preventable cause of death, even today.[3,6,10,17] In a study conducted by Bullock[6] it was observed that in a third of the cases, death could have been prevented and among them 88% were due to hypoxic ischemic damage.

Factors included in preventable cause of death are, failure to prevent hypoxic brain damage by timely intubation and quick resuscitation. This happens mostly prior to arrival in a specialized center. Delay in referral and inadequate control of raised ICP are the most important causes. Systemic insults can occur even before the patients reach the hospital, during intrahospital transport or at the time of emergency management. Recent studies have indicated that the short episodes

of hypotension may result in severe ischemic brain damage, that will persist even after complete **hemodynamic** restoration (Table 8.2). Hence, the treatment of the episodic hypotension should be quick and aggressive. Korosue[28] suggested **hemodilution** to increase the cerebral blood flow, which is likely to reduce ischemic damage (Table 8.3). Thus, one important key to prevent the ischemic brain damage is to maintain the oxygenation and systemic blood pressure, which can prevent perfusion defect and **anaerobic metabolism.**

Table 8.2: Protection from ischemia
Prevention of hypoxia by timely intubation
Reduction of ICP
Maintenance of systemic blood pressure and CPP
Role of steroid
Role of hypervolemia
Raising hemoglobin contain of blood

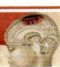

Table 8.3: Mode to increase cerebral perfusion

a. **By reducing ICP**
- Mannitol
- High dosage steroid
- Ventricular drainage

b. **By increasing systemic pressure**
- Maintaining blood pressure
- Increasing circulating volume
- Reducing viscosity of blood

c. **By preventing dehydration**
- Adequate treatment of fever, electrolyte disturbance and infection

Adequate prevention of raised ICP is important. Raised ICP reduces cerebral perfusion pressure. Hence, it is necessary to continuously monitor ICP for 2–3 days and adequately control ICP to maintain cerebral perfusion. Intravenous mannitol is one of the widely used method to reduce ICP. However, prolonged use is some time harmful and ineffective. Recently, methylprednisolone is a widely used neuroprotective drug.[81] **Glucocorticoid** and nonglucocorticoid steroids exert free radicl scavanging activity and are tried in neurosurgical disorders including head injury. **Methylprednisolone** is already in common clinical use in spinal for injury and is also used as **neuroprotective** agent in the management of subarachnoid hemorrhage and severe head injury. Chen et al[81] studied the cellular uptake and transport of methylprednisolone (MP) at the level of **blood–brain barrier,** in guineapigs. MP has a membrane effect by binding to cytoplasmic endothelial **glucocorticoid receptors.**

Recently, **calcium channel blockers** have been tried. In a multicentric study, no beneficial effect was noticed using calcium channel blocker. As the hypoxia leads to acidosis, it is most important to treat acidosis. **Tris (hydroxymethyl) aminoethane** (THAM) is widely used to raise the cellular pH and combat acidosis. Recently, NMDA antagonists are used to reduce ischemic damage.[6,7] In an experimental study Bullock[5] reported dramatic reduction of ischemic damage in cats pre-treated with NMDA antagonist, prior to MCA occlusion. Similar results were observed in rats with experimental subdural hematoma. Identical observations were made by Inglis, et al in 1990[7] in an experimental study in rats. MK 801, a potent NMDA blocker helps in reducing ischemic injury to brain. However, these agents are not widely used in clinical practice.

CONCLUSIONS

Ischemic brain damage is one of the most important secondary change that occurs following head injury. Ischemia is noticed over 85% patients with fatal head injury. Very often it is preventable. Hypoxia and hypotension are the two most important causes which lead to ischemic brain damage. Adequate prevention to hypoxia and hypotension will significantly reduce the ischemic brain lesion and increase the chance of survival and recovery in patients with severe head injury.

REFERENCES

1. Zauner A, Bullock R, Kuta AJ, Woodward J & Young HF. (1996) Glutamate release and cerebral blood flow after severe human head injury. Acta Neurochir Suppl **6740**: 6744.
2. Graham DI, Adam JH, Doyle D. Ischemic brain damage in non missile head injury. J Neurol Sciences 1978;39:213–34.
3. Graham DI, Ford I, Adam JH, Doyle D, Teasdale GM, Lawrence E, McLellan DP. Ischemic brain damage is still common in fatal non-missile head injury. J Neurol Neurosurg Psychiat 1989;52: 346–50.
4. Graham DI. In: Pathology of hypoxic brain damage in man, hypoxia and ischemia. BC Mirson (Ed). J of Clin Pathol (Suppl) Royal College of Pathology 1977;11:170–80.
5. Bennett M, O'Brien DP, Phillips JP, Farrell MA. Clinicopathological observation in 100 consecutive patients with fatal head injury admitted to a neurosurgical unit. Irs Med J. 1995;88:168–68.
6. Bullock R. Introducing NMDA antagonist into clinical practice. Why head injury trials? Br J Clin Pharmacol 1992;34:396–401.
7. Inglis EM, Bullock R. Chen MH, Graham DI, Miller JD, McCulloch J. Ischemic brain damage

associated with tissue hypermetabolism is acute subdural hematoma, reduction by a glutamate antagonist. Acta Neurochir Suppl. (Wien) 1990;51:277–79.

8. Kriger AJ, Adler RJ. Advances in the prevention and treatment of secondary brain injury. In: Modern Trend in the Management of Neurotrauma. PS Ramani and Alok Sharma (eds), 1994, Lavanya Prints, Bombay 29–32.

9. Moeschler O, Boulard G, Ravassin P. Concept of secondary cerebral injury of systemic origin. Ann Ere Anesth Reavin, 1995;14:114–21.

10. Siesjo BK. Pathophysiology and treatment of focal cerebral ischemia. Part II Mechanism of damage and treatment. J Neurosurg 1992;77: 337–53.

11. Bouma GJ, Muizelaar JP, Stringer WA, Choi C, Fatouros P, Young HF . Ultrearly evaluation of regional cerebral blood flow in severely head-injured patients using xenon-enhanced computerized tomography. J Neurosurg 1992;77:360–8.

12. Diringer MN, Videen TO, Yundt K, Zazulia AR, Aiyagari V, Dacey RG, Grubb RL & Powers WJ. Regional cerebrovascular and metabolic effects of hyperventilation after severe traumatic brain injury. J Neurosurg 2002;96:103–8.

13. Bramlett HM, Dietrich WD, Pathophysiology of cerebral ischemia and brain trauma: similarities and differences. J Cereb Blood Flow Metab. Feb; 2004;24(2):133–50.

14. Bullock R, Sakas D, Patterson J, Wyper D, Hodley D, Maxwell W, Teasdale GM. Early post-traumatic cerebral blood flow mapping. Correlation with structural damage after focal injury. Acta Neurochir Suppl. (Wien) 1992;55: 14–17.

15. Marshall LF and Gaotille TH. Large and small "Holes in the brain, reversible or irreversible change in head injury. Acta Neurochir (Suppl), 1990;51:300–1.

16. McPherson P, Graham DI. Correlation between angiographic findings and the ischemia of head injury. J Neurol Neurosurg Psychiat, 1978;41: 122–7.

17. Sahuquillo J. Pica MA, Garnacho A, Robles A, Coello F, Godot C, Triginer C, Rubio E. Early ischemia after severe head injury. Preliminary result in patient with diffuse brain injury. Acta Neurochir (Wien) 1993;122:204–14.

18. Kumar V, Abbas AK, Fausto N, Aster J, Cellular Responses to Stress and Toxic Insults: Adaptation, Injury, and DeathRobbins and Cotran Pathologic Basis of Disease 8E, 2009.

19. Bouma GJ, Muizelaar JP. Cerebral blood flow, cerebral blood volume, and cerebrovascular reactivity after severe head injury. J Neurotrauma 1992;9:S333–48.

20. Adams JH, Graham DI, Jennett B. The neuropathology of the vegetative state after an acute brain insult. brain 1999:123(7):1327–38.

21. Adams JH, Graham DI, Murray LS, Scott G. Diffuse axonal injury due to nonmissile head injury in humans: An analysis of 45 cases. Ann Neurol 1982;12:557–63.

22. Clark RS, Schiding JK, Kaczorowski SL, Marion DW, Kochanek PM. Neurotrophil accumulation after traumatic brain injury in rats: Comparison of weight drop and controlled cortical impact models. J Neurotrauma 1994;11: 499–506.

23. Kirino T. Delayed neuronal death in the gerbil hippocampus following ischemia. Brain Res 1982;239:57–69.

24. Liu PK, Hamilton WJ, Hsu CY. Apoptosis: DNA damage and repair in stroke. (In) *Stroke Therapy Basic, Preclinical, and Clinical Directions* (Miller LP, ed) John Wiley & Sons Inc. 1999;11: 299–320.

25. Snider BJ, Gottron FJ, Choi DW. Apoptosis and necrosis in cerebrovascular disease. Ann NY Acad Sci 1999;893:243–53.

26. Yakovlev AG, Knoblach SM, Fan L, Fox GB, Goodnight R, Faden AI. Activation of CPP32-like caspases contributes to neuronal apoptosis and neurological dysfunction after traumatic brain injury. J Neurosci 1997;17:7415–24.

27. Eldadah BA, Faden AI. Caspase pathways, neuronal apoptosis, and CNS injury. J Neurotrauma 2000;17:811–29.

28. Korosue K, Heros RC. Mechanism of cerebral blood flow augmentation by hemodilution in rabbits. Stroke 1992 Oct; 23(10):1487–92; discussion 1492–3.

29. Chan PH, Epstein CJ, Li Y, Huang TT, Carlson E, Kinouchi H, Yang G, Kamh H, Mikawa S, Kondo T, Copin JC, Chen SF, Chan T, Gafni CJ, Gobbel G, Reole E. Transgenic mice and knockout mutants in the study of oxidative stress in brain injury. J Neurotrauma 1995;12:815–24.

30. Chan PH, Schmidley JW, Fishman RA, Longare SM. Brain injury, edema, and vascular permeability changes induced by oxygen-derived free radicals. Neurology 1984;34: 315–20.

31. Kim GW, Kondo T, Noshita N, Chan PH. Manganese superoxide dismutase deficiency exacerbates cerebral infarction after focal

cerebral ischemia/reperfusion in mice: implications for the production and role of superoxide radicals. Stroke 2002;33:809–15.

32. Globus MY-T, Alonso O, Dietrich WD, Busto R and Ginsberg MD. Glutamate release and free radical production following brain injury: Effects of posttraumatic hypothermia. J Neurochem 1995;65:1704–11.

33. Globus MY-T, Busto R, Lin B, Schnippering H, Ginsberg MD. Detection of free radical activity during transient global ischemia and recirculation: Effects of intraischemic brain temperature modulation. J Neurochem 1995;65: 1250–56.

34. Lewen A, Fujimura M, Sugawara T, Matz P, Copin JC, Chan PH. Oxidative stress-dependent release of mitochondrial cytochrome c after traumatic brain injury. J Cereb Blood Flow Metab 2001;21:914–20.

35. Mikawa S, Kinouchi H, Kamii H, Gobbel GT, Chen SF, Carlson E, Epstein CJ, Chan PH. Attenuation of acute and chronic damage following traumatic brain injury in copper, zinc-superoxide dismutase transgenic mice. J Neurosurg 1996;85:885–91.

36. Yamamoto T, Maruyama W, Kato Y, et al. Slective nitration of mitochondrial complex I by peroxynitrite: involvement in mitochondria dysfunction and cell death of dopaminergic SH-SY5Y cells. J Neural Transm 2002;109:1–13.

37. Chan PH. Reactive oxygen radicals in signaling and damage in the ischemic brain. J Cereb Blood Flow Metab 2001;21:2–14.

38. Siesjo BK, Bengtsson F. Calcium fluxes, calcium antagonists, and calcium-related pathology in brain ischemia, hypoglycemia, and spreading depression: a unifying hypothesis. J Cereb Blood Flow Metab 1989;9:127–40.

39. Siesjo BK, Agardh C-D, Bengtsson F. Free radicals and brain damage. Cereb Brain Metab Rev 1989;1:65–211.

40. Mahapatra AK. Tandon PN. Brainstem auditory evoked response and vestibulo occular reflex in severe head injury. A prospective study of 60 cases. Acta Neurochir (Wien) 1987;87:40–43.

41. Mahapatra AK. Tandon PN. Bhatia R. Banerji AK. Bilateral decerebration in head injury patients.An analysis of 62 cases. Surg Neurol, 1985;23:36–40.

42. Chan KH. Dearden NM. Miller JD. Transcranial doppler sonography in severe head injury. Acta Neurochir Suppl (Wien) 1993;59:81–85.

43. McLaughlin MR, Marion DW.Cerebral blood flow and Vasoresponsibility within and around cerebral contusion. J Neurosurg 1996;85:871–76.

44. Salvant JB, Muizelaar JP. Changes in cerebral blood flow and Metabolism related to subdural hematoma Neurosurg 1993;33:387–93.

45. Jenkin A. The importance of cerebral perfusion pressure maintenance in severe head injury. In: Modern Trend in the management of Neuro-trauma. PS. Ramani and Alok Sharma (Eds), Lavanya Print, Bombay 1994;33–34.

46. Lele VR. Single photon emission computed tomography (SPECT) studies in head trauma. In: Modern trend in management of Neurotrauma, Lavanya Prints, Bombay 1994;27–28.

47. Agrawal D, Naveen K, Bala CS, Mahapatra AK. Post Concussion. Syndrome in the Pediatric Population. Is medial temporal damage is responsile? Correlation with Brain SPECT. A prospective controlled study. Child's Nerves Syst. IT: 2003;628 (Abstract).

48. Lennick JA. Michele JJ. Simeone FA. Defeo S. Walsh FA. Alteration of Somatosensory evoked potentials in response to global ischemia. J. Neurosurg 1984;60:490–4.

49. Cater GB, Butt W. Review of the use of Somatosensory evoked potential in the prediction of outcome after severe brain injury. Crit Care Med 2001;29:178–86.

50. Zazulia AR, Diringer MN, Videen TO, Adams RE, Yundt K, Aiyagari V, Grubb RLL, Powers WJ. Hypoperfusion without ischemia surrounding acute intracerebral hemorrhage. J Cereb Blood Flow Metab 2001;21:804–10.

51. DeWitt DS, Jenkins LW, Wei EP. The effects of fluid-percussion brain injury on regional cerebral blood flow and pial arteriolar diameter. J Neurosurg 1986;64:87–794.

52. Dietrich WD, Alonso O, Busto R, Prado R, Zhao W, Dewanjee MK, Ginsberg MD. Posttraumatic cerebral ischemia after fluid percussion brain injury: An autoradiographic and histopathological study in rats. Neuro-surgery 1998;43:585–94.

53. Back T, Ginsberg MD, Dietrich WD, Watson BD. Induction of spreading depression in the ischemic hemisphere following experimental middle cerebral artery occlusion: effect on infarct morphology. J Cereb Blood Flow Metab 1996; 16:202–213.

54. Back T. Pathophysiology of the ischemic penumbra revision of a concept. Cell Mol Neurobiol 1998;18:621–38.

55. Bramlett HM, Green EJ, Dietrich WD. Exacerbation of cortical and hippocampal CA1 damage due to posttraumatic hypoxia following moderate fluid-percussion brain injury in rats. J Neurosurg 1999;91:653–9.

56. Vespa P, Prins M, Ronne-Engstrom E, Caron M, Shalmon E, Hovda DA, Martin NA, Becker DP. Increase in extracellular glutamate caused by reduced cerebral perfusion pressure and seizures after human traumatic brain injury: a microdialysis study. J Neurosurg 1998;89:971–82.

57. Bramlett HM, Kraydieh S, Green EJ, Dietrich WD. Temporal and regional patterns of axonal damage following traumatic brain injury: A beta-amyloid precursor protein immunocytochemical study in rats. J Neuropathol Exp Neurol 1997;56:1132–41.

58. Anderson CV, Bigler ED. Ventricular dilation, cortical atrophy, and neuropsychological outcome following traumatic brain injury. J Neuropsych Clin Neurosci 1995;7:42–48.

59. Smith DH, Nakamura M, McIntosh TK, Wang J, Rodriguez A, Chen XH, Raghupathi R, Saatman KE, Clemens J, Schmidt ML, Lee VM, Trojanowski JQ. Brain trauma induces massive hippocampal neuron death linked to a surge in beta-amyloid levels in mice overexpressing mutant amyloid precursor protein. Am J Pathol 1998;153:1005–10.

60. von Oettingen G, Bergholt B, Gyldensted C, Astrup J. Blood flow and ischemia within traumatic cerebral contusions. Neurosurg 2002;50:781–90.

61. Lee SM, Wong MD, Samii A & Hovda DA. Evidence for energy failure following irreversible traumatic brain injury. Ann NY Acad Sci 1999;893:337–40.

62. Giri BK, Krishnappa IK, Bryan RM, Robertson C. Regional cerebral blood flow after cortical impact injury complicated by a secondary insult in rats. Stroke 2000;31:961–7.

63. Dharkar SR. Traumatic ischemic lesion in children. Neurology Ind (Suppl) 1995;43:61–65.

64. Hlatky R, Valadka AB, Robertson CS. Intracranial hypertension and cerebral ischemia after severe traumatic brain injury. Neurosurg Focus 2003;15:14(4).

65. Botteri M, Bandera E, Minelli C, Latronico N, Cerebral blood flow thresholds for cerebral ischemia in traumatic brain injury. A systematic review. Crit Care Med 2008;36(11):3089–92.

66. Kelly DF, Korndestani RK, Martin NA, et al. Hyperemia following traumatic brain injury: relationship to intracranial hypertension and outcome. J Neurosurg 1996;85:762–71.

67. Schroder ML, Muizelaar JP, Bullock MR, et al. Focal ischemia due to traumatic contusions documented by stable xenon-CT and ultrastructural studies. J Neurosurg 1995;82:966–71.

68. Huthinson PJ, Menon DK, Czosnyka M, Kirkpatrick PJ. Monitoring cerebral blood flow and metabolism. In; Head Injury Pathophysiology and management (eds) Reilly Pl and Bullock R). Hodder Arnold 2005;215–45.

69. Coles JP, Fryer TD, Smielewski P, et al. Defining ischemic burden after traumatic brain injury using ^{15}O PET imaging of cerebral physiology. J Cereb Blood Flow Metab 2004; 24:191–201.

70. Coles JP, Fryer TD, Smielewski P, et al. Incidence and mechanisms of cerebral ischemia in early clinical head injury. J Cereb Blood Flow Metab 2004;24:202–11.

71. Langfitt TW, Weinstein JD, Kassell NF. Cerebral vasomotor paralysis produced by intracranial-f hypertension. Neurology 1965;15:622–41.

72. Langfitt TW, Weinstem JD, Kassell NF, et al. Transmission of increased intracranial pressure within the craniospinal axis, J Neurosurg 1964;21:989–97.

73. Lassen NA, and Ingvar DH: The blood flow of the cerebral cortex determined by radioactive krypton-85. Experientia L961;L7:42–45.

74. Obrist WD, Langfitt TW, Jaggi JL, et al. Cerebral blood flow and metabolism in comatose patients with acute head injury. Relationship to intracranial hypertension. J Neurosurg 1984; 61:241–53.

75. Willkin RH, Odoms GL. Intracranial arterial spasm associated with craniocerebral trauma. J Neurosurg 1970;32:626–33.

76. Walia B. Head Injury in Pediatric age group. M. Ch. Thesis submitted AIIMS; 1996.

77. Marshall LF. Bruce DA, Bruno L, Langfit TW. Vertebrobasilar spasm, a significant cause of neuro-logical deficit in head injury. J Neurosurg 1978;48:560–4.

78. Bakshi A, Mahapatra AK. Basilar artery vasospasm in severe head injury. A preliminary transcranial Doppler study. NMJI 1998;113:220–1.

79. Czosnyka M, Guazzo E, lyre. V, Kirkpatrick P, Smielewski P, White house H, Picard JD. Testing of cerebral autoregulation in head injury by waveform. Analysis of blood flow velocity and cerebral perfusion pressure. Acta Neurochir Suppl (Wien) 1994;6:468–71.

80. Yang BO, Feng Z, Zhang Z and Sun H. A Transcranial Doppler study of drainage of CSF and intracranial hematoma. In modern trends in the management of Neurotrauma. PS Ramani and Alok Sharma (Eds), Lavanya Prints, Bombay 1994;36.

81. Chen TC, Mackic JB, Mccomb JG, et al. Cellular uptake and transport of methyleprednisolone at the blood brain barrier. Neurosurgery 1996;38:348–61.

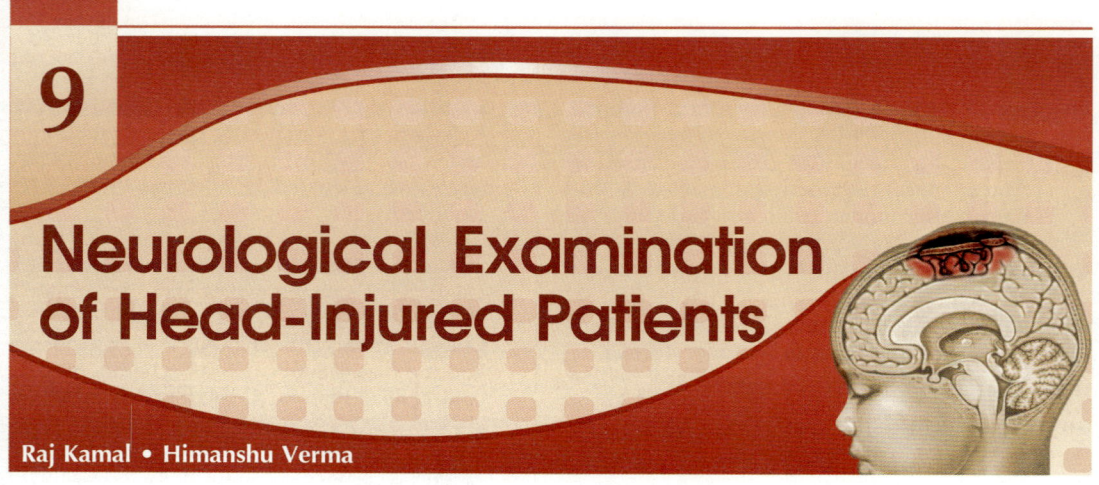

9

Neurological Examination of Head-Injured Patients

Raj Kamal • Himanshu Verma

Introduction

The neurological evaluation of the patient with head injury remains an important comprehensive process in the diagnostic evaluation and as a baseline in assessing progress. Thorough and careful examination provides an index of generalized and focal dysfunction of the nervous system which is not provided by CT scanning, ICP monitoring or any other modern technology. Repeated good, reliable thorough examination indicates the ongoing neurological state and the progress or failure of treatment rendered. The clinical value of neurological examination thus remains prominent in the initial assessment and subsequent management of head injured patients.

Also, careful general examination must define associated injuries, any source of internal bleeding or any other clinical problem requiring prompt therapy.

The major goals in the evaluation of patients with head injury are:

1. To define the presence of intracranial mass lesion requiring operative removal.
2. To determine abnormal intracranial mass lesion in order to guide and direct appropriate operative or nonoperative therapy.
3. To diagnose associated serious injuries.

In patients who are conscious, the initial examination is as thorough as possible. In patient with altered consciousness, emphasis is given to certain critical aspects that will guide immediate treatment.

History

Information regarding precise time of injury and mechanism of injury should be obtained. Acceleration injuries as a result of vehicular accidents and falls is associated with serious diffuse brain injury and polar contusion. Impact injuries such as blow to cranial vault result in underlying focal brain damage.

A history of the patient's neurological function at the scene of the accident and during transport to the hospital should be sought from police, relatives or witnesses. Any history of loss of consciousness and seizures should be obtained. A report from a referring hospital of the patient's condition should also be sought and recorded.

Information regarding drug or alcohol intake and the past medical history is also valuable.

Initial Examination

The American College of Surgeons Committee on Trauma (1997)[1] has given in its manual ATLS program for physicians, a sequence ABCDE. The airway (A), breathing (B), and circulation (C) are assessed before neurological assessment (D) and general examination (E) assessment of the consciousness is most important. The secondary survey of the

94

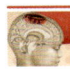

patient is done after resuscitation. Resuscitation may improve some clinical signs. Simultaneously need for intubation and elective ventilation should be assessed. Before paralyzing patients baseline clinical record is mandatory. Pulse rate, blood pressure and respiration should be assessed and given top priority in the management of traumatic brain injury.

Hypertension associated with bradycardia suggests severely increased intracranial pressure from increasing intracranial clot. Unexplained hypotension with bradycardia points towards a possibility of cervical injury. Hypotension associated with tachycardia usually indicates presence of visceral injury elsewhere such as abdominal or thoracic injury.

In our clinical practice, importance of BP is high. CPP is directly dependent on systolic BP. Marmarou et al[2] found that the proportion of hourly BP readings less than 80 mm Hg was highly significant in explaining outcome (p < 0.0001). Although critical ICP levels from 0 to 80 mm Hg in increments of 5 mm Hg were tested, the ICP level of 20 mm Hg emerged with the highest level of significance. Again, low BP critical levels from 120 to 20 mm Hg in increments of –5 mm Hg were available as candidates. Yet, the BP level of 80 mm Hg emerged with the highest level of significance. They concluded that, in addition to the factors of age, admission motor score, and admission pupillary response, the factor most indicative of outcome was the proportion of ICP measurements greater than 20 mm Hg. The next most significant factor was the proportion of BP measurements less than 80 mm Hg.

According to Stening[3] BP below 90 mm Hg persisting for more than 60 minutes in acute subdural hematoma was strong predictor of bad outcome. **Arterial hypotension seems to be preventable cause of bad outcome, and this is indisputable when hypotension is due to in adequate resuscitation or failure to treat any other source of blood loss.** Lyle et al[4] found that a systolic BP below 90 mm Hg was

significantly associated with death on univariant analysis, however, in this study hypotension correlated closely with a low Glasgow Coma Scale (GCS) score, and on multivariant analysis is the only significant variables were the GCS score and the papillary light reflexes.

Hypertension, on the other hand did not adversely affect mortality. In an interesting study, White et al[5] found that in pediatric trauma odds of survival increased 19-fold when maximum systolic blood pressure was greater or equal to 135 mm Hg (p < 0.01). In this study, predictors of outcome were abstracted, including Pediatric Trauma Score, GCS score, Pediatric Risk of Mortality, physiologic variables, computed tomography evidence of brain injury, and neuroresuscitative medications. The fatality rate was 24%. Age and gender were similar between groups (p > or = 0.1). Survival was independently predicted by 6 hr GCS score (odds ratio [OR] 4.6; 95% confidence interval [CI] 2.06–11.9; p < 0.001) and maximum systolic blood pressure (OR 1.05; 95% CI 1.01–1.09; p < 0.02). Odds of survival increased 19-fold when maximum systolic blood pressure was greater or equal to 135 mm Hg (OR 18.8; 95% CI 2.0–178.0; p < .01). They concluded that patients with higher 6-hr GCS scores were more likely to survive. Adjusting for severity of injury, survival was associated with maximum systolic blood pressure greater or equal to 135 mm Hg, suggesting that supranormal blood pressures are associated with improved outcome

Hypertension may be seen as phenomenon arising from cerebral autoregulation due to raised ICP. Hypotension following hypertension carries poor prognosis as it might indicates irreversible brainstem failure.

Zafar et al[6] (using the National Trauma Data Bank) analyzed patients older than 16 years with isolated moderate to severe blunt TBI. Scores and rates were plotted against emergency department systolic blood pressure (EDSBP). A total of 7,238 patients were included in the analysis. Plots of adverse outcomes versus EDSBP demonstrated bimodal distributions. The mortality curve had one inflection point at EDSBP 120 mm Hg, indicating higher mortality when blood pressures were lower than this threshold. Another inflection began at EDSBP 140 mm Hg. The mortality rate was 21% when EDSBP was < 120 mm Hg, 9% when it was between 120 and 140 mm Hg, and 19% when EDSBP was ≥ 140 mm Hg. Multivariate analysis demonstrated that patients presenting with an EDSBP of < 120 mm Hg and ≥ 140 mm Hg were 2.7 (95% confidence interval = 2.13,3.48) and 1.6 (95% confidence interval = 1.32,1.96) times more likely to die, respectively, than those who presented with a EDSBP of 120 to 140 mm Hg. It was concluded that mortality in moderate to severe TBI has a bimodal distribution. Like hypotension, hypertension at hospital admission seems to be associated with increased mortality in TBI.

Shallow and deep respirations in a cyclical fashion known as **Cheyne-Stokes breathing**.[7] It occurs in diffuse, bilateral cortical dysfunction, sufficient to result in drowsiness. Cheyne-Stokes breathing result in hypoventilation and hypercarbia leading to increased intracranial pressure, secondary to vascular stasis and blood pooling. Spontaneous hyperventilation with deep respiration may occur in injury at pontine level often leading to hypocarbia from hyperventilation. Ataxic or irregular respiration occurs in medullary or pontomedullary injuries resulting in hypercarbia.

General Examination

Scalp wounds include small lacerations, perforating lacerations, contused lacerations and massive avulsions. Scalp wounds may be associated with underlying skull fracture (compound injury). Wound and swelling should be recorded on diagram and also photographed for medicolegal reasons.

Bleeding from the nose and ear should be recorded. Associated CSF leak from nose (CSF rhinorrhea) and from ear (CSF otorrhea) are usually secondary to basal skull fractures.

Fractures of the orbital roofs (Figs 9.1a and b) result in bilateral periorbital hematomas (raccoon eyes). Orbital swelling points towards anterior cranial fossa. Its auscultation may detect carotid-cavernous fistula. Associated bleeding beneath the pericranium over the mastoid **(Battle's sign)** (Fig. 9.2a) is clinically apparent after 2 or 3 days. Facial paresis or paralysis can occur in patients with fracture of the petrous bone. The forehead should be palpated for signs of depressed fracture or frontal sinus injury. Asymmetry or irregularity of orbital margins and nose should be checked. Dental occlusion should be checked to rule out mandibular fracture. Cervical injury should be suspected in all severe head injuries and should be ruled out radiologically.

LEVEL OF CONSCIOUSNESS

Level of consciousness is the single most important parameter in a patient of head injury. Many pathological process may impair conscious level and numerous terms have been employed to describe the various clinical states which result, including stupor, semicoma and deep coma. These term result in ambiguity and inconsistency when used by different observers. Teasdale and Jennett[8] proposed that the degree of coma after severe head injury is the most reliable clinical indicator of the severity of brain damage and present a scale to assess the depth and duration of

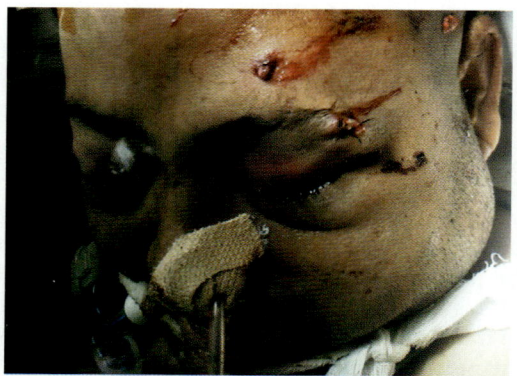

Fig. 9.1a: Bilateral black eye

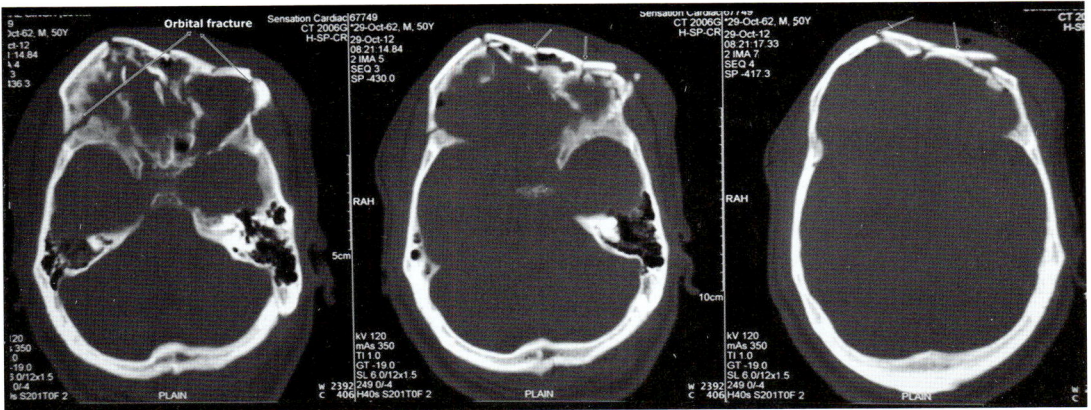

Fig. 9.1b: CT scan shows bilateral orbital fracture in th patient of Fig. 9.1a

impaired consciousness and coma. Coma was defined as the inability to obey commands, to speak, or to open the eyes, and these three behavioral aspects were incorporated into the GCS[8,9] first introduced in 1974 and then revised by the addition of another motor response level in 1977 (Table 9.1). The sum of the E + M + V value indicates the level of consciousness. Fully conscious patients will have a GCS of 15. GCS of 8 or less is found in coma. Prasad[10] confirmed that scale has good discriminative value, if used by competent observers, but urged further evaluation of interobserver reliability. GCS has found wide acceptance among trauma surgeons, residents, nurses and ambulances officers. In head injury management the chief uses of the GCS are in early evaluation of the primary effects of a

head injury in postoperative evaluation, and in routine monitoring of less severe had injury to detect changes due to complications. The ATLS manual[1] recommended a simpler non-quantitative AVPU scale, which has four levels. Alert (A): response to vocal stimuli V; response to pain (P); and unresponse (V). But GCS is generally more accepted. The GCS has greater prognostic value. According to Jennett,[10] eighty-seven percent died or because

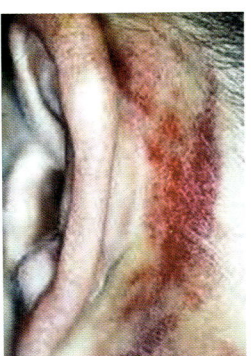

Fig. 9.2a: Battle's sign

Table 9.1: Glasgow Coma Scale	
Eye opening	
Spontaneous	E4
To Speech	3
To pain only	2
No eye opening	1
Best motor response	
Obeys command	M6
Localizes to stimulation	5
Withdraws from stimulation	4
Abnormal flexion	3
Abnormal extension	2
No motor response	1
Best verbal response	
Oriented and appropriate	V5
Confused	4
Inappropriate words	3
Incomprehensible sounds	2
No verbal response	1
Total score = 15	

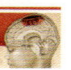

vegetative with best GCS scores of 3/4 in first 24 hours, where as bad outcomes were recorded in only 53 percent of those with GCS scores of 5/6/7. Effects of alcohol, hypoxia and other corresponding factors were excluded by including only those cases which remained comatosed for more than six hours. Deterioration or improvement can thus be made out at subsequent examinations.

Glasgow Coma Scale has been adopted by neurosurgical units throughout the world to evaluate their patients with head injuries.[11] Despite its wide acceptance GCS has numerous valid drawbacks.

GCS has been criticised on following points:
1. GCS does not take account of pupillary size and reactivity, pulse rate, respiration, BP.
2. Eye movements and other brainstem reflexes are not included in the scale.
3. Inaccurate recording in patients with bilateral ecchymosis of the eyelids (cannot open his eyes even though fully conscious), aphasia or dysphasia.

It is not easy to assess the conscious level in infants and young children, and mistakes are often made. Sometimes the severity of a head impact is overestimated, but the converse error is much commoner; because an injured infant cries or whimpers, it is thought to be fully 'conscious' and serious brain damage is overlooked. Simpson and Reilly[12,13] preferred a much simpler system, directly based on the original GCS but with age related norms for the verbal and motor responses. This scale expresses the concept that the range of responses ion head-injured infants and young children is narrower than is the case over the age of four years. This scale, which is termed

as the Pediatric Glasgow Coma Scale (PGCS), was independently compared by Yager et al[14] with five other systems of quantifying the conscious level in early life, and found to be one of the two best from the view-point of observer disagreement (< 0.10).

Severe head injuries in young children are caused by falls and abuse (inflicted head injuries). The more force that is involved in a head injury, the more likely it is that a serious injury to the brain has occurred. If there has been a high-energy injury to the head, there is a greater likelihood that a serious injury has occurred. When a high-energy injury occurs, it is even more important to assess the child for signs of a serious head injury. Responsiveness is assessed with the alert, verbal, pain, unresponsive (AVPU) system and with the GCS and its pediatric modification, the PGCS[12,13] (Table 9.2). The PGCS was developed for children younger than 5 years as a more accurate tool that would avoid the errors that occur when the GCS is applied to children and infants with limited verbal skills. A total PGCS score of 13–15 represents minor injury, a score of 8–12 represents moderate injury, and a score lower than 8 represents severe injury (Table 9.2).

Shaken baby syndrome is thought to occur when a baby is violently shaken, thrown, or slammed, causing the baby's head to move forward and backward rapidly. This movement causes the brain to hit the sides of the skull forcefully, leading to bleeding in the eyes and injury and bleeding in the brain. Brain injury and bleeding can cause increased pressure in the brain. Increased pressure in the brain can lead to serious, permanent brain damage.

Table 9.2: Pediatric Glassgow Coma Scale (Simpson & Reilly)[12,13]		
Eyes open	*Best verbal response*	*Best motor response*
	○ Orientated (5)	○ Obeys command (5)
○ Spontaneously (4)	○ Words (4)	○ Localizes pain (4)
○ To speech (3)	○ Vocal sounds (3)	○ Flexion to pain (3)
○ To pain (2)	○ Cries (2)	○ Extension to pain (2)
○ None (1)	○ None (1)	○ None (1)
Total score = 14		

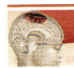
Babies who have trouble breathing or who stop breathing during an episode of being shaken, thrown, or slammed may have more brain damage.

Adjustment to Age

- During the first 6 months
  - The best verbal response is normally a cry, though some infants make vocal responses during this period. Normal verbal score expected is 2.
  - The best motor response is usually flexion. Normal motor score expected is 3.
- 6 to 12 months
  - The normal infant makes noises: Normal verbal score expected is 3.
  - The infant will usually locate pain but not obeys commands: Normal motor score expected is 4.
- 12 months to 2 years
  - Recognizable words are expected: Normal verbal score expected is 4.
  - The infant will usually locate pain but not obeys commands: Normal motor score expected is 4.
- 2 to 5 years
  - Recognizable words are expected: Normal verbal score expected is 4.
  - The infant will usually obeys commands: Normal motor score expected is 5.
- After 5 years
  - Orientation is defined as awareness of being in hospital: Normal verbal score expected is 5.

Normal aggregate score:

0–6 months	9
> 6–12 months	11
> 1–2 years	12
> 2–5 years	13
> 5 years	14

THE PERSISTENT VEGETATIVE STATE, LOCKED-IN SYNDROME, AKINETIC MUTISM

The patient who appears to be asleep and is at the same time incapable of being aroused by external stimuli and inner needs is in a state of coma.[15] There are various degrees of coma. In deep coma no reaction of any kind is obtainable: Corneal, pupillary, pharyngeal, tendon and plantar reflex are all absent. With lesser degrees of coma, pupillary reactions, reflex ocular movements and other brainstem reflexes are preserved, and there may be signs of decerebration.

"Consciousness (or awareness), in all its aspects, is a matter of degree", and "The vegetative state (is) a condition of wakefulness without awareness".[16]

A vegetative state is said permanent when one predicts that the patient will not recover. This distinction was introduced by the American Multi-Society Task Force[17] on PVS in 1994 to denote irreversibility after three months following a nontraumatic brain injury and twelve months after traumatic injury (Table 9.3).

Someone who is in a vegetative state is:

1. Not aware of their surroundings
2. Not aware of bodily sensations, such as feeling pleasure or pain
3. Not able to follow and understand speech
4. Not able to have thoughts, memories, emotions, and intentions of any kind.

As some sections of their brain are still functioning, they may perform a number of reflex actions that they are unaware of, such as:

1. Sleeping and waking at regular intervals
2. Making movements with their mouth such as smiling and grimacing
3. Gripping objects or other people's hands

A vegetative state is said permanent when one predicts that the patient will not recover. This distinction was introduced by the American Multi-Society Task Force on PVS in 1994 to denote irreversibility after three months following a nontraumatic brain injury and twelve months after traumatic injury.

Following modern treatment of severe cerebral injury more and more patients survive for indefinite periods without

Table 9.3: Criteria of vegetative state[17]
• No evidence of awareness of self or environment and an inability to interact with others.
• No evidence of sustained, reproducible, purposeful, or voluntary behavioral responses to visual, auditory, tactile, or noxious stimuli
• No evidence of language comprehension or expression
• Intermittent wakefulness manifested by the presence of sleep-wake cycles
• Sufficiently preserved hypothalamic and brainstem autonomic functions to permit survival with medical and nursing care
• Bowel and bladder incontinence
• Variably preserved cranial-nerve and spinal reflexes

From the Multi-Society Task Force on PVS (1994).[17]

regaining any meaningful mental function. For the first week or two after the cerebral injury these patients are in a state of deep coma. Then they start opening their eyes spontaneously. The patient may blink eyes spontaneously. However, the patient remains inattentive, shows no signs of awareness of the environment or the inner need; responsiveness is limited to primitive postural and reflex movements of limbs. The EEG may approach normality, even showing alpha rhythm and sleep patterns. If lasting, this syndrome referred to as the persistent vegetative state.

Neurologic conditions that produce unresponsiveness are given in Table 9.4.

The locked-in state is due most often to a lesion of the basis pontis in which there is a little or no disturbance of awareness but only an inability to respond adequately. Such a lesion interrupts corticospinal and corticobulbar pathways sparing the ascending neuronal systems and somatosensory pathways which are responsible for arousal and wakefulness.[15,18]

Akinetic mutism refers to a partially or fully awake patient who is immobile and silent. The

Table 9.4: Neurologic conditions that produce unresponsiveness					
Condition	Self-awareness	Motor function	Experiences suffering	Respiratory function	Prognosis
Presistent vegetative state	Absent	No purposeful movements, no visual tracking	No	Normal	One year outcome in traumatic cases: Died 33% Severely disabled 28% Moderately disabled 17% Good recovery 7% Persistent vegetative state 15%
Locked-in syndrome	Present	Quadriplegia, pseudobulbar palsy, preserved vertical eye movements	Yes	Normal	Recovery unlikely, remains quadriplegic prolonged survival possible
Akinetic mutism	Present	Paucity of movement	Yes	Normal	Recovery unlikely
Brain death	Absent	Absent	No	Absent	None

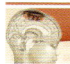

state may result from large bilateral lesion both frontal lobes or in cingulate gyrus.

MEMORY FUNCTION

Memory is usually divided into three categories: **Immediate, recent and remote.** Immediate memory has a finite capacity and information remains in the store for relatively brief period of time (seconds to minute). This type of store would hold a telephone number for a short time. Immediate recall is tested by forward and backward repetition of digit spans (seven digits forward and six back-wards). Immediate memory is mostly related to attention and consciousness.

Recent memory is assessed at the bedside by telling the patient to remember four different words or objects. After ten minutes, the patient is requested to recall from memory, the four original objects. Known anatomical substrates for recent memory are located within hippocampal fornicial mamillo-thalamic pathways. The exact pathophysio-logy accounting for loss of recent memory in head trauma is not yet correctly known.

Recent memory typically refers to memories in hours to days, in duration and remote memory refers to distant past memories of many years. These memories are thought to be retained in cerebral cortex.

Memory loss for events prior to injury is termed retrograde amnesia. With recovery, retrograde amnesia shrinks from several hours to several minutes. Hence in retrograde amnesia the problem is in retrieval not in registration. Antegrade amnesia is an inability to lay down new memories following the head injury.

In severe head injuries, antegrade amnesia may persist indefinitely. Post-traumatic amnesia (PTA) refers to the time from injury until the return of a full, ongoing memory process. It is same as antegrade amnesia. Russell and Collaborators[19] have established a direct correlation between severity of the head injury and duration of post-traumatic amnesia (PTA). They established the following scale:

PTA

0–1 hour—Mild head injury
1–24 hours—Moderate head injury
1–7 days—Severe head injury
> 7 days—Very severe head injury

Studies have shown a close correlation between neurosurgical estimation or post-traumatic amnesia and neuropsychological deficits.

EYES

Pupils: Pupillary size is determined by balance of tonic forces consisting of the pupillo-constrictor parasympathetic and pupillo-dilator sympathetic controls.

Pathway of pupillary constriction and the light reflex (parasympathetic) are demon-strated in Fig. 9.2b.

A stimulus, such as bright light shone in the left eye will send an efferent from the retinal ganglion cell through the optic nerve, chiasma, and tract, terminating medially in the pretectal nuclear area, here a second order fiber (intercalated neurons) passes to the Edinger-Westphal nucleus (a IIIrd nerve nucleus) on the same and opposite side via the posterior commissure (Fig. 9.2b). The efferent limb of the arc consists of preganglionic parasympa-thetic neurons joining the oculomotor nerve. The pupillomotor fibers are superficially located in IIIrd nerve. At the level of the superior orbital fissure of the oculomotor nerve divides and the parasympathetic fibers follow the branch to the inferior oblique muscle to synapse in the ciliary ganglion. Postganglionic short ciliary fibers penetrate the globe.

Sympathetic fibers descend from hypo-thalamus through the lateral aspect of brainstem into the spinal cord. The pupillary fibers emerge through the ventral roots of C8, and Tl, enter the sympathetic chain and, in the superior cervical ganglion (Fig. 9.2c). The postganglionic fibers, arise in the superior cervical ganglion, ascend on the wall of internal carotid artery to enter the cranium. The sympathetic plexus around the internal

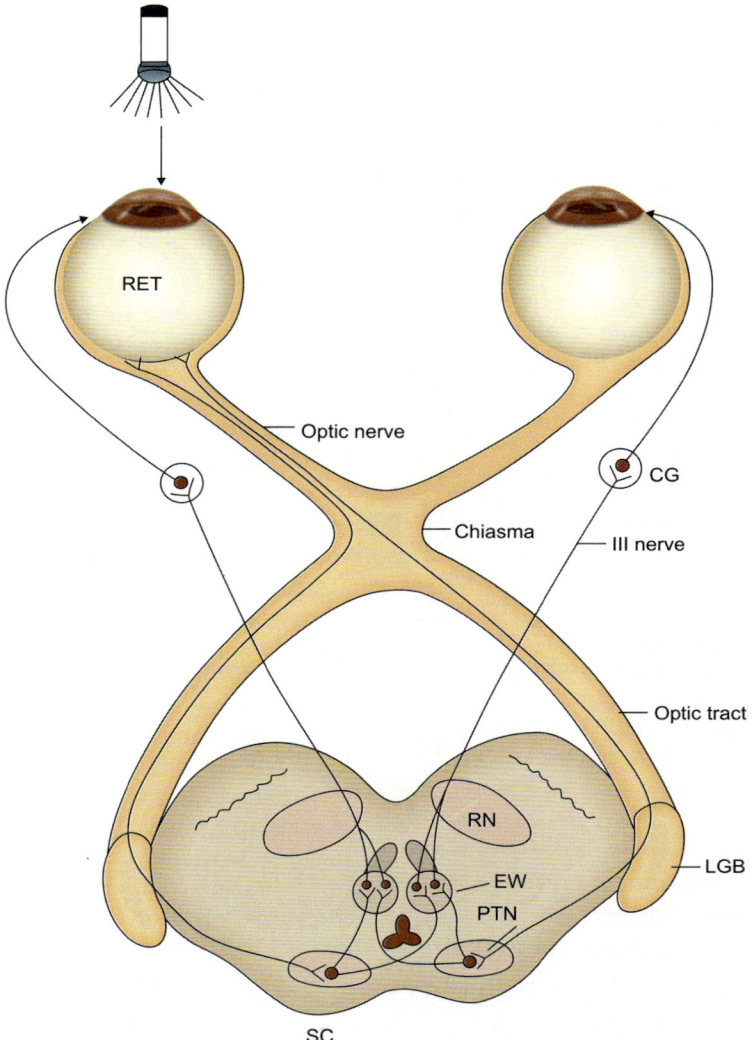

RET

Optic nerve

CG

Chiasma

III nerve

Optic tract

RN

LGB

EW

PTN

SC

Fig. 9.2b: Pupillary light reflex: Parasympathetic pathway stimulation of the retinal photoreceptors, results in excitation of ganglion cells whose axon travel within optic nerve partially decussate in the chiasma, then leave the optic tract and pass through brachium of the superior colliculus (SC) before synapsing at the pretectal nucleus. This structure connects bilaterally within oculomotor nuclear complex at Edinger-Westphal (EW) nuclei, parasympathetic fibers that travels through inferior division of third nerve and end at the ciliary ganglion (CG) in the orbit, RN: red nucleus, PTN: pretectal nucleus, LGB: lateral geniculate body

carotid artery sends a branch through the ciliary ganglion, and these postganglionic fibers reach the eyeball through the short ciliary nerves; but some sympathetic fibers may travel through the long ciliary nerves to reach the eyeball. Sudomotor fibers (concerned with sweating) passes through the external carotid artery to the dermis of the face.

Unilateral, non-reactive dilatation of pupil indicates of transtentorial herniation secondary to an expanding hematoma. Initially pupil on the side of injury contracts due to irritation of the oculomotor nerve, the opposite pupil remains normal size. In the next stage, the ipsilateral pupil dilates due to paralysis of oculomotor nerve. Finally the pupils of both sides become dilated and fixed, not reacting to light (Hutchinson's pupil) (Fig. 9.3a). The light reflex is also excellent for assessment of midbrain function, assuming that the efferent arc is intact.

Direct and Consensual Light Reflexes[20]

If a light is shone into an eye, the pupils of both eyes normally constrict. The constriction of the pupil on which the light is shone is called direct light reflex; the constriction of the opposite pupil even though no light fell on that eye is called consensual light reflex. Pupillary size, shape and reactions are routinely recorded at the initial examination, and routinely checked at specified intervals thereafter. If the pupillary light reflex is impaired on one side, the consensual light reflex is tested to exclude an optic nerve lesion.

Unilateral dilated, non-reactive pupil with absent consensual reflex will point to an optic nerve injury. When the light is directed to the unaffected eye, both pupil will react normally.

Marcus Gunn pupil:[21] During swinging flash light test, when the light is directed to the abnormal eye with relative efferent pupillary defect (say partial optic nerve injury), both pupil will dilate because of the comparatively weaker pupillary constriction. Apparently, light signals transmitted to the Edinger-Westphal nucleus in the midbrain through the injured optic nerve are insufficient to maintain the constriction induced by illumination of the unaffected or normal eye. The paradoxical pupillary dilation observed as the light is moved from the normal to the abnormal eye, is termed efferent pupillary defect.

Horner's Syndrome

Interruption of any oculosympathetic neurons may result in Horner's syndrome, characterized by unilateral miosis, facial anhidrosis, ptosis. The eyelid abnormality may give a false

impression that the eye is set back in orbit (pseudo enophthalmos).

Lesion of the third order neuron distal to the carotid bifurcation results in loss of sweating on forehead, whereas more proximal lesion, including those of first and second order neurons involve the whole one-half of face (Fig. 9.2c).

The Horner's syndrome can occur in the trauma patient from interruption of the sympathetic pupillodilator pathways anywhere between the hypothalamus and upper thoracic cord. Loss of sweating over the face occurs with disruption of the sympathetic pathways prior to the bifurcation of the common carotid artery, the point at which sweat fibers course with external carotid artery.

The diagnosis of Horner's syndrome associated with brachial plexus injury, or spinal cord trauma is important.

Brainstem hematoma following traumatic brain injuries may produce pin point pupils. In metabolic encephalopathies, the pupils may be small but remains reactive to light.

Extraocular movements in an unconscious patient may be tested by rotating head in various directions (provided cervical injury is ruled out). The eyes will be fixed at a particular point in space, regardless of head rotation, and the eyes kept passively at a certain gaze, a phenomenon like that found in some children dolls, i.e. the patient's eye tend to deviate in the opposite direction to the induced head movement. The movement depends on intact vestibular reflex mechanisms. This oculocephalic reflex is a test of the peripheral sense organs, the labyrinths and otoliths, and their central connections in brainstem, including the vestibular nuclei, the MLF (medial longitudinal fasciculi) and the efferent pathway through oculomotor, trochlear and abducent nerves and their nuclei (Fig. 9.3b).

Caloric Reflexes

Brainstem function can be assessed by oculocephalic reflex (Doll's head ocular

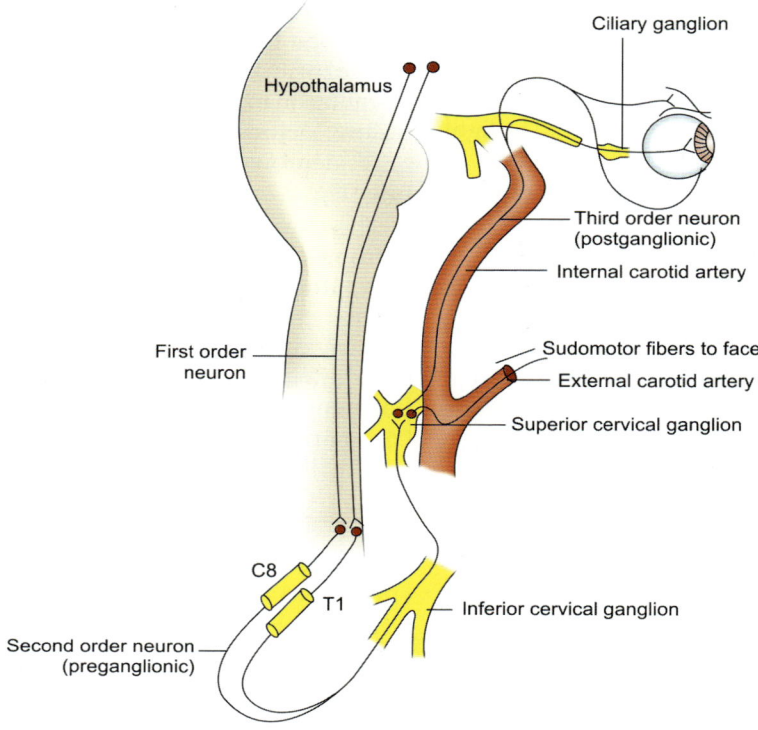

Fig. 9.2c: Sympathetic pathways to the eye

movement) and oculovestibular reflex (caloric response). The patient lies supine with head flexed 30° so that the horizontal semicircular canal lies in the vertical plane, with ampulle at the highest point. The ears are irrigated first with water at 30°C then at 44°C for 40 seconds. In the comatose patient irrigation of the external auditory meatus (after excluding perforation of tympanic membrane) on one side with atleast 20 ml of ice-cold water induces slow conjugate derivation towards the irrigated side after a few seconds delay.[22] The irrigation of cold water causes ampullofugal endolymph flow; this reduces the vestibular output from one side, creating an imbalance, resulting in conjugate deviation of eye towards irrigated side (Fig. 9.4). Rapid corrective movements result in nystagmus away from the stimulated ear. Nystagmus is absent in unconscious patient.

Disorders of Gaze of Traumatic Brain Injury

Two cortical centers of ocular control are recognized:
1. Middle gyrus of frontal lobe (area 8) for conjugate saccadic movements.
2. Occipital cortex for pursuit movements.

Frontomesencephalic and occipitomesencephalic pathways traverse the genu of internal capsule, descend and decussate in the lower midbrain and upper pons to terminate in PPRF (paramedian pontine reticular formation) which represents the brainstem center for ipsilateral conjugate gaze (Fig. 9.3b). Medial longitudinal fasciculus (MLF) interconnects oculomotor, trochlear and abducens cranial nerve nuclei (*see* legend of Fig. 9.3b) with vestibular and cerebellar complex. MLF provides the basis for normal oculocephalic and oculovestibular reflexes described above.

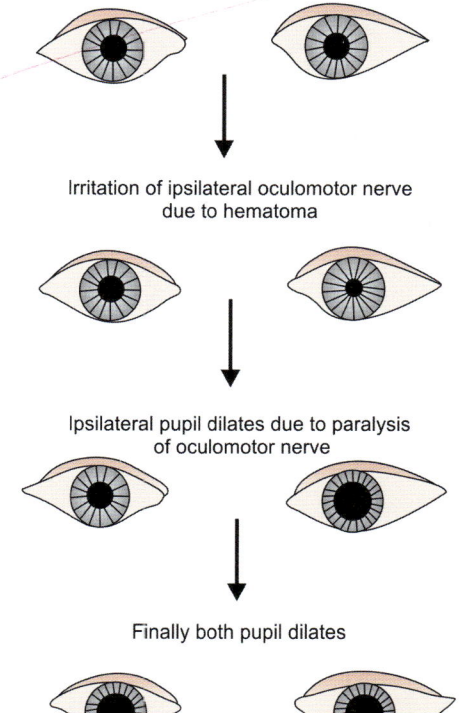

Irritation of ipsilateral oculomotor nerve
due to hematoma

Ipsilateral pupil dilates due to paralysis
of oculomotor nerve

Finally both pupil dilates

Fig. 9.3a: Hutchinson's pupil: Stages

Supranuclear Gaze Palsies

An irritative lesion in frontal area (small hematoma causing seizures) will cause contralateral gaze deviation. Large frontal contusion hematoma (destructive lesion) will cause ipsilateral conjugate gaze deviation. The patient looks towards his lesion.

If the lesion is in the pons involving pontine paramedian reticular formation (PPRF) which represents the brainstem center for ipsilateral conjugate gaze there will be conjugate deviation of the eyes to the opposite side.

Internuclear ophthalmoplegia is due to lesion in MLF in the midbrain (Fig. 9.1). It will cause impaired adduction of ipsilateral eye with nystagmus of the abducting opposite eye during attempted lateral gaze to opposite side.

In 'one and a half syndrome' a lesion involving both PPRF and MLF on the same side will cause ipsilateral gaze paresis with impairment of adduction of ipsilateral eye and nystagmus on abduction of the opposite eye.

Upward gaze paresis occurs in compressive or destructive lesions involving the pretectal area of the midbrain, posterior commissure, and dorsal midbrain tegmentum.

Skew deviation of the eyes—in which one eye is directed upwards and the other downwards reflect lesions involving the brachium pontis or dorsolateral medulla.

Intranuclear Palsies

Trochlear nerve is difficult to assess in unconscious patient. Sixth cranial nerve paresis will cause unilateral esotropia and decreased lateral excursion of that eye upon oculocephalic testing. Bilateral sixth nerve paresis will cause convergence of both eyes. Bilateral sixth nerve paresis occurs in increased ICP.

A unilateral exotropia with limited medial, superior or inferior movements associated with dilated pupil points to oculomotor nerve paresis.

CRANIAL NERVES

The Olfactory Nerve

It is impossible to examine in unconscious patient. Unilateral or bilateral anosmia may be associated with anterior cranial fossa fractures with or without CSF rhinorrhea exclusive frontal lobe contusion. CSF leak if present should be recorded.

The Optic Nerve

Anatomy: From the retina, the fibers of the optic nerve pass back to the optic chiasm. The intraorbital portion, approximately 30 to 40 mm long and 3 to 4 mm in diameter, has a sinuous course that allows for considerable excursion as the globe moves. Approximately 8 to 15 mm behind the globe, the central retinal artery penetrates and reaches the axia of the optic nerve. The intracanalicular portion, which is approximately 5 to 8 mm long, passes through the optic canal and is tightly fixed within the canal. The intracranial portion is

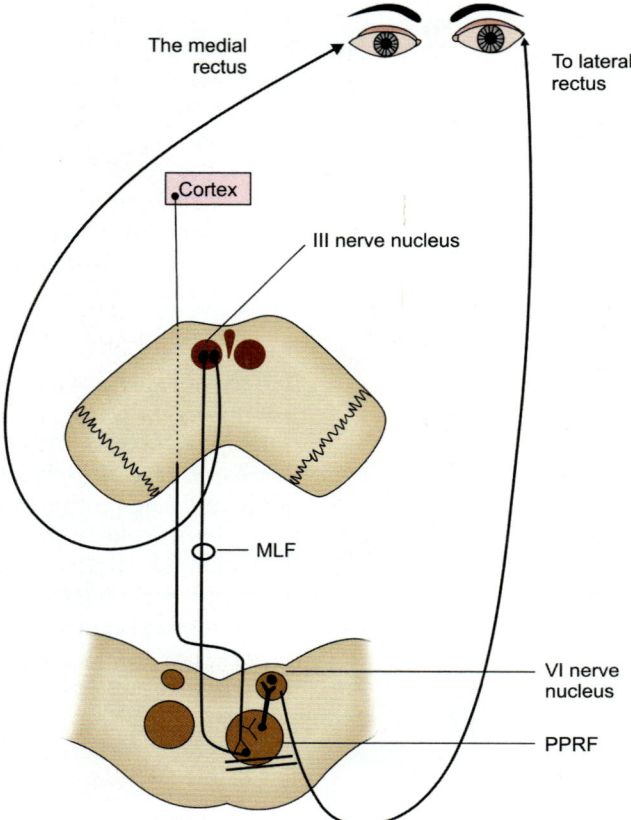

Fig. 9.3b: Pathways for horizontal eye movement involving PPRF (Paramedian Pontine Reticular Formation), MLF (Median Longitudinal Fasciculus), III and VI cranial nerves. Stimulation of PPRF causes stimulation of ipsilateral lateral rectus and contralateral medial rectus (i.e. gaze toward ipsilateral side). Right MLF lesion (A) will cause (a) Paresis of Rt. adduction (b) Nystagmus in Lt. abducting eye. Left PPRF lesion (B) will cause left lateral gaze palsy

approximately 10 mm long and joins with the contralateral nerve to form the optic chiasm. At optic chiasma, partial decussation occurs, and about 53% of the fibers cross to form the optic tracts.[23] Most of these fibers terminate in the lateral geniculate body. At the chiasm, fibers from nasal retina cross, and the most ventral axons from the inferior nasal retina bend through the contralateral optic nerve (von Willebrand knee), whereas fibers from temporal retina remain ipsilateral (Fig. 9.5). All of the CNS sheaths, including the pia mater, arachnoid, and dura mater, surround the intraorbital portion of the optic nerve.

Ipsilateral temporal fibers and contralateral nasal fibers join to form optic tracts. At the lateral geniculate body, the ganglion cell axons in optic tract synapse with neurons to become the optic radiation. Some fibers called Meyers loop course through the temporal lobe anterior to the inferior horn of lateral ventricles, subserve visual information from the lower retina and connect to the inferior bank of calcarine cortex.

The parietal portion of the optic radiation relays information from the upper retina to the superior bank of the calcarine cortex. Broadmann area 17 is the end organ of the different

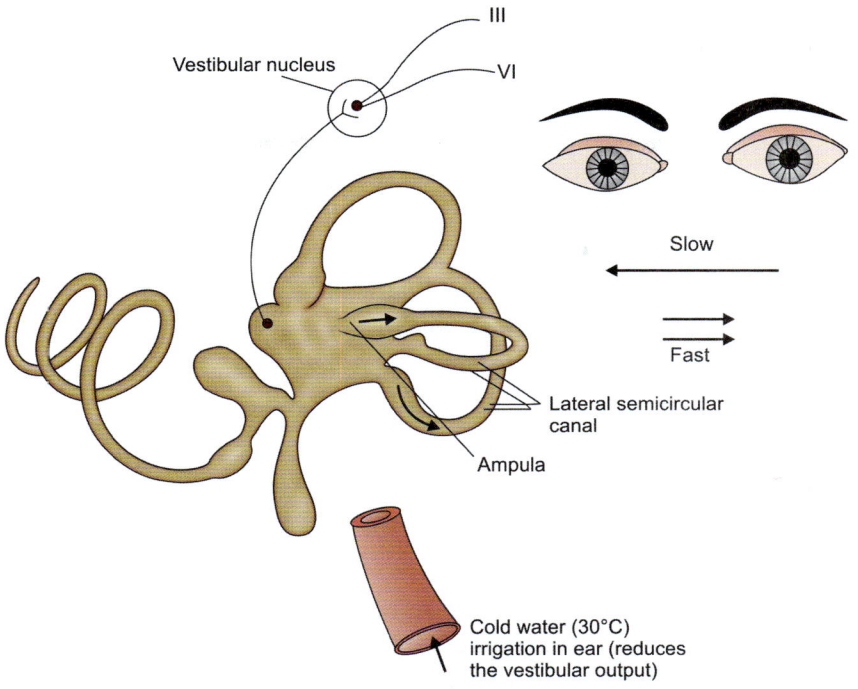

Fig. 9.4: Caloric response

visual system and is located in the calcarine cortex in the occipital lobe.

In a conscious patient visual acuity should be recorded carefully. Complete blindness is termed as no light perception (NLP).

Optic nerve injury should be suspected in a patient of head injury who has periorbital ecchymosis or complained of loss of vision.

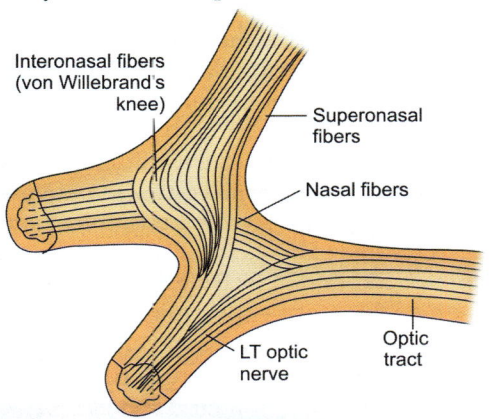

Fig. 9.5: von Willebrand's knee[23]

In unconscious patient optic nerve injury should be suspected in all patients with unilaterally dilated pupils. Optic nerve injury should be differentiated from oculomotor paresis due to transtentorial herniation. In optic nerve injury ipsilateral direct pupillary reflex and consensual reflex in the opposite eye will be absent whereas in oculomotor paresis ipsilateral direct pupillary reflex will be absent but consensual reflex in opposite eye will be present. Progressive opposite or central herniation compresses parasympathetic neurons in the upper midbrain and causes dilatation of the pupil and paralysis of light response. With full mydriasis (6 to 8 mm pupil), ptosis and paresis of the medial rectus and other ocular muscles innervated by the oculomotor nerves appear. Ophthalmoscopic examination should be done to rule out hemorrhage or distortion of the retina.

Visual field are useful in diagnosing various types of field defects involving optic tracts or geniculocalcarine pathways.

In occipital contusions, transient cortical blindness can occur. Some of these patients with acute cortical blindness are unaware of visual loss due to coincidental involvement of parietal connections (Anton's syndrome).

The trigeminal and facial nerves may be tested with corneal responses to a light cotton wisp or response to more severe facial stimuli, to assess for facial grimace and eye closure. Facial nerve injury is apparent by widened palpebral fissure and sagging facial muscles.

The seventh and eighth cranial nerves are often injured in the basal fractures involving petrous bone.

It is impossible to test auditory components of eighth nerve directly in unconscious patient (except by evoked potential using audiometric inputs). Vestibular component of eighth nerve can be tested by caloric testing.

Assessment of gag, swallowing and vocal cord function will partially evaluate the glossopharyngeal and vagus nerves. This can be observed in manipulating the endotracheal tube in a comatose patient.

Motor Response

In alert patients, muscle tone can be evaluated by passive range of movement of upper and lower limb, muscle power can be treated by voluntary movement against resistance:

The Medical Research Council Scale is used to grade muscle functions:

Grade 0	Complete paralysis
Grade 1	Flicker of contraction
Grade 2	Muscle contracts, but cannot overcome gravity
Grade 3	Muscle contraction against force of gravity only
Grade 4	Some degree of weakness, can be overcome with resistance
Grade 5	Normal power.

In an unconscious patient evaluation of the motor abilities of the uncooperative or unresponsive patient consists of observing the characteristics and strength of the skeletal muscle responses to painful stimuli. Painful stimulus is given by nibbing thumb nail in supraorbital groove thus giving painful stimuli to supraorbital nerve. In GCS, the motor responses are grouped as:

M6	Follows command
M5	Localizing to pain
M4	Withdraws from stimulation
M3	Abnormal flexion
M2	Extension
Ml	No response

Limb weakness in an unconscious patient can be determined by comparing the response in each limb to painful stimuli. The most frequently recognized combination is dilatation of pupil on one side with contralateral hemiparesis or hemiplegia (Figs 9.6a and b). The dilated and non-reactive pupil can be associated with ipsilateral hemiplegia. This is due to indentation of the contralateral cerebral peduncle by the edge of the tentorium cerebelli (Kernohan's notch).

Abnormal flexion response is characterized by adduction and internal rotation of shoulder, relatively slow flexion of the elbow, wrist, and fingers with flexion or extension of lower extrimeties. This type of response is commonly described as decorticate posture which indicates severe supratentorial damage.

Decorticate rigidity signifies lesion in cerebral white matter or internal capsules and thalamus.

In extensor motor response the head is thrown back with extension of all limbs with internal rotation of arms and opisthotonus position (decerebrate rigidity). In decerebrate rigidity the lesion is in midbrain between superior and inferior colliculus. While abnormal extensor posturing is generally assumed to occur solely in comatose patients, alert patients with decerebrate rigidity have been described. This is because of different anatomical locations which regulate consciousness and which are concerned with motor functions.

Deep tendon reflexes and superficial reflexes should be examined. Tendon reflexes include biceps jerk, supinator jerk, triceps jerk,

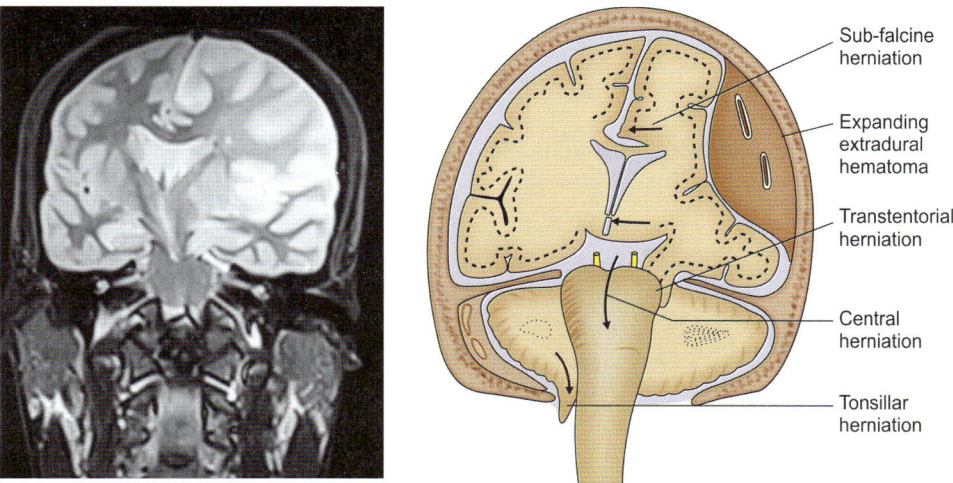

Fig. 9.6a: MRI showing transtentorial herniation and its schematic representation

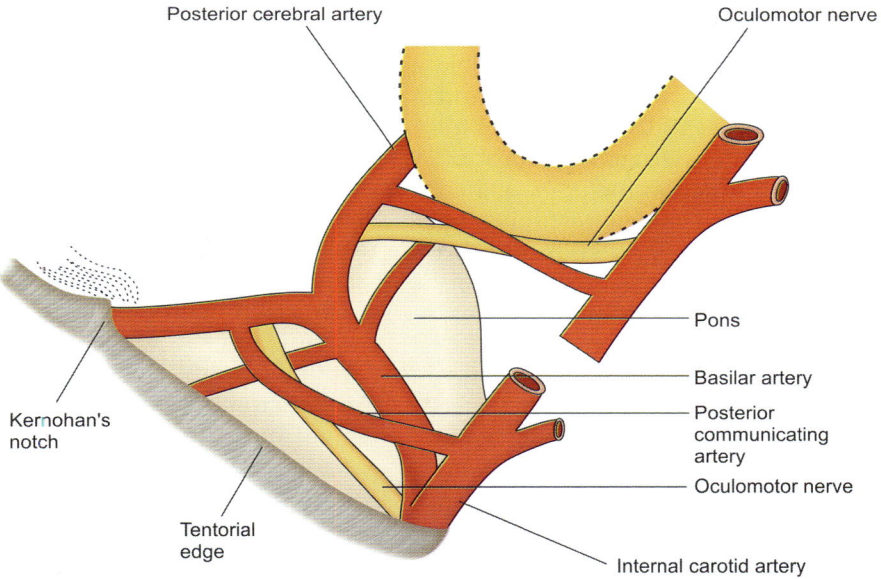

Fig. 9.6b: Kernohan's notch

knee jerk and ankle jerk. Abnormal tendon reflexes can be exaggerated, diminished or absent.

Superficial reflexes include plantar reflex, superficial abdominal reflex and corneal reflex.

Babinski's response (extensor plantar) is found in patients with corticospinal tract lesions. In conscious patients coordination, involuntary movements and gait should be included in the motor examination. Sensory examination includes examination of pain temperature touch, vibration, position sense.

Neck stiffness should be seen carefully after excluding cervical injury.

Neurological examination should conclude by detailed local examination.

Adjunct Diagnostic Modalities

Radiological investigation, X-ray films, CT scan, MRI, scanning, etc. are discussed elsewhere in this book.

BRAIN DEATH EXAMINATION

Patient with severe head injury may develop irreversible unbeatable high intracranial pressure as a result of large contusion or hematoma. The herniation may progress rapidly to an irreversible state and decompression after this time may not result in any functional improvement because of irreversible brainstem. The intracranial swelling and initial damage may lead to cessation of all valuable brain function, termed brain death.[24] The lack of brain function includes dilated unreactive pupils, no caloric response, no oculocephalic response, no spontaneous respiration and no motor or sensory response. While testing for brain function one should ensure that patient has not received any sedatives, paralytic drugs. Clinically, apnea test must be done for brain function. Apnea test is performed with 100% O_2 cannula in the endotracheal tube for oxygenation and end PCO_2 should be atleast 60 mm Hg. Patient should be re-examined at 6, 12 or 24 hours before declaring brain dead. A number of test have also been suggested, including an angiographic study showing no cerebral blood flow and silent EEG.

Brain death is defined as the irreversible loss of all function of the brain, including the brainstem. The three essential findings in brain death are coma, absence of brainstem reflexes, and apnea. The diagnosis of brain death is primarily clinical.

The Uniform Determination of Death Act indicates that "an individual who has sustained either[25] irreversible cessation of circulatory and respiratory functions, or irreversible cessation of all functions of the entire brain, including the brainstem, is dead," with brain death being determined based on "accepted medical standards." The American Academy of Neurology[26] has published practice guidelines providing medical standards for the determination of brain death. The most recent American Academy of Neurology guideline update notes that "because of the deficiencies in the evidence base, clinicians must exercise considerable judgment when applying the criteria in specific circumstances" and that ancillary tests can be used when uncertainty exists about the reliability of parts of the neurologic examination or when the apnea test cannot be performed.[22]

DIAGNOSTIC CRITERIA FOR CLINICAL DIAGNOSIS OF BRAIN DEATH (AMERICAN ACADEMY OF NEUROLOGY)[21]

A. *Prerequisites:* Brain death is the absence of clinical brain function when the proximate cause is known and demonstrably irreversible.

1. Clinical or neuroimaging evidence of an acute CNS catastrophe that is compatible with the clinical diagnosis of brain death
2. Exclusion of complicating medical conditions that may confound clinical assessment (no severe electrolyte, acid-base, or endocrine disturbance)
3. No drug intoxication or poisoning
4. Core temperature ≥ 32°C (90°F)

B. The three cardinal findings in brain death are coma or unresponsiveness, absence of brainstem reflexes, and apnea.

1. Coma or unresponsiveness—no cerebral motor response to pain in all extremities (nail-bed pressure and supraorbital pressure)
2. Absence of brainstem reflexes
   a. Pupils

i. No response to bright light

ii. Size: Midposition (4 mm) to dilated (9 mm)

b. Ocular movement

i. No oculocephalic reflex (testing only when no fracture or instability of the cervical spine is apparent)

ii. No deviation of the eyes to irrigation in each ear with 50 ml of cold water (allow 1 minute after injection and at least 5 minutes between testing on each side).

CONCLUSIONS

The clinical value of the neurological examination in the initial assessment and subsequent management of head injured patient is very important. Glasgow Coma Scale has been widely accepted for evaluation of head injured patients despite its certain drawbacks. Neurologic conditions that produce unresponsive are akinetic mutism, locked in syndrome, persistent vegetative state and brain death. Most of the cranial nerves can be examined even in unconscious patient. Direct and consensual reaction of pupil can diagnose optic nerve and third nerve injuries. Unilateral, non-reactive dilatation of pupil with deteriorating consciousness indicates of an expanding hematoma. Gaze paresis and caloric response are good parameters for evaluation of brainstem reflexes in unconscious patient. One should do all bedside tests several times before declaring brain death.

REFERENCES

1. American College of Surgeons Committee on Trauma. Chicago,IL1997: Shock in Advanced Trama Life Support, American College of Surgeons 1997;31:87–108.

2. Marmarou A, Anderson RL, Ward JD, Choi SC, Eisenberg HM, Foulkes MA, Marshall LF, Jane JA. JNS Special Supplements Impact of ICP instability and hypotension on outcome in patients with severe head trauma November 1991;75(1s):S59–66.

3. Stening WA, Berry Q, Dan NG, et al. Experience with acute subdural hematomas in New South Wales. Austral NZJ Surg 1986;56:549–56.

4. Lyle DM, Pierce JP, Freeman EA, et al. Clinical course and outcome of severe head injury in Australia. J Neurosurg 1986;65:15–18.

5. White JR, Farukhi Z, Bull C, Christensen J, Gordon T, Paidas C, Nichols DG. Predictors of outcome in severely head-injured children. Crit Care Med 2001;29(3):534–40.

6. Zafar SN, Millham FH, Chang Y, Fikry K, Alam HB, King DR, Velmahos GC, de Moya MA. Presenting blood pressure in traumatic brain injury: a bimodal distribution of death. J Trauma 2011;71(5):1179–84.

7. Levy DE: The comatose patient, Rosenberg RN (ed), Comprehensive Neurology Raven Press, 1990;817–32.

8. Teasdale G; Jennett B: Assessment and Prognosis of Coma after Head Injury. Acta Neurochir (Wien) 1976;34:45–55.

9. Teasdale G, et al, Observer variability in assessing impaired consciousness and coma. J Neurol Neurosur Psychiatry 1978;41:603–10.

10. Prasad K. The Glasgow Coma Scale; a critical appraisal of its clinometric properties. J Clin Epidemiol 1996;49:755–63.

11. Jennett B. Severe head injuries: ethical aspects of management. Br J Hosp Med 1992;47:354–7.

12. Simpson D, Reilly P. Pediatric Coma Scale. Lancet 1982;2:450.

13. Reilly P, Simpson D, et al. Assessing the conscious level in infants and young children : a pediatric version of the Glasgow Coma Scale. Child's Nerv Syst 1988;4:30–33.

14. Yager JV, Johnston B and Seshia SS. Coma scales in pediatric practice. American Journal of Diseases in Children 1990;144;1088–91.

15. Adams RD, Victor M: Coma and related disorders of consciousness. In Principles of Neurology. McGraw-Hill 1993;300–18.

16. Zeman A. Persistent vegetative state. Lancet 1997;350:795–9.

17. The Multi-Society Task Force on PVS. N Engl J Med 1994;330:1572–9.

18. Victor M: The amnestic syndrome and its anatomical basis. Can Ked J 1969;100(2):1115–25.

19. Russell WR, Smith A : Post-traumatic amnesia in closed head injury. Arch Neurol 1961;5:1–17.

20. Sambasivan, M, Ramamurti B: Assessment, Head Injuries in Textbook of Neurosurgery

Second Ed. Ed Tandon PN, Ramamurti B 1996;259–64.

21. Marcus Gunn R. Br Med J 1909;2(2554):1719–21.

22. Jadhav WR, Sinha A, Tandon PN, et al. Cold calorie test in altered state of consciousness. Laryngoscope 1971;81:391.

23. Gray H. Anatomy of the Human Body. Philadelphia: Lea & Febiger, 1918; Bartleby.com, 2000.

24. Guidelines for the determination of death. JAMA 1981;246:2184–86.

25. Webb A, Samuels O. Brain death dilemmas and the use of ancillary testing. Continuum (Minneap Minn) 2012;18(3):659–68.

26. Executive Board September 24, 1994. American Academy of Neurology, Published in Neurology 1995;45:1012–14.

10

Imaging in Head Injury

Raj Kamal • Atul Kapoor • S Chopra

INTRODUCTION

Neuroimaging methods are of considerable value for the assessment and management of acute traumatic brain injury, although their role in classifying the degree of injury and in predicting outcomes remains a topic of investigation. Currently, these assessments are made on the basis of both imaging and clinical findings, which commonly include the Glasgow Coma Scale (GCS) score.

Most commonly available imaging techniques are CT and MR imaging. CT is the preferred imaging technique for acute evaluation of traumatic brain injury and MR imaging for sub acute and chronic period if persistent and unexplained disabilities remain. Normal, fresh whole blood is hyperdense [50 to 100 Hounsfield units (HU)] relative to normal brain (20 to 35 HU).[1] This density is proportional to the protein moiety of hemoglobin. CT scan is also necessary to evaluate minor head injury. In the past, CT scan was consider unnecessary investigation. Recently, there are reports suggesting need for CT in minor head injury.[2–4] About 3–5% patients of minor head injury may have clot in brain and 33–40% them ultimately head surgery. Patients of minor head injury with severe headache, CSF leak, repeated vomiting and focal deficit need early CT scan.[2–4]

MR imaging can depict non-hemorrhagic and hemorrhagic contusions and is more sensitive for detection of diffuse axonal injury.[5,6] In many cases, the neuroimaging findings do not fully explain the clinical symptoms, and in the absence of any corroborating neuroimaging evidence, these subjects are frequently misclassified. They provide information regarding structural changes not about the functional changes. Furthermore, the correlation between early structural neuroimaging findings and long-term clinical outcomes is weak. Mild traumatic brain injury (mTBI) can induce long-term behavioral and cognitive disorders. Although the exact origin of these mTBI-related disorders is not known, they may be the consequence of diffuse axonal injury (DAI).[7] MRI at the subacute stage can detect lesions that are associated with poor functional outcome in mTBI by using anatomical images (T_1) and diffusion tensor imaging (DTI).

CT IMAGING

CT imaging is certainly the foremost investigative tool for the evaluation of a patient with traumatic head injury. The factors which establish its frontline role are its traditional use, high spatial resolution, speed due to the use of spiral techniques. A spectrum of findings are observed on CT imaging which range from presence of parenchymal injuries like hemorrhages-contusions (Figs 10.1, 10.2a to c), diffuse axonal injury, diffuse cerebral edema and brainstem hemorrhage, acute extra-axial-extradural, subdural hematomas, intraventricular and subarachnoid hemorrhage. It is needless to reconfirm its use and accuracy of detecting abnormalities of the skull vault, facial and orbital structures.

Cerebral Contusion and Hematoma
(Figs 10.1 and 10.2a to g)

Cerebral contusions are commonly seen in the frontal and temporal lobes. and usually accompany skull fractures, the so-called fracture contusion complex and appear as both hyperdense hemorrhagic contusions on CT or as non-hemorrhagic contusions which show reduced attenuation (Figs 10.1 to 10.3). The most critical feature of these contusions is their tendency to expand (Figs 10.2a and b). This usually occurs from 24 hours to as long as 7–10 days after the initial injury. For this reason, cerebral contusions are often followed with a repeat head CT scan within 24 hours after injury.

Coup injuries (contusions) are caused by direct transmission of impact energy through the skull into the underlying brain and occur directly below the site of injury. Contrecoup

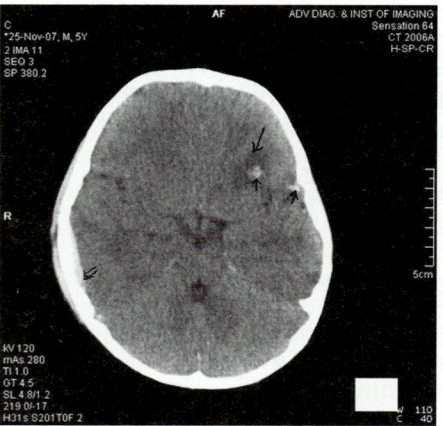

Fig. 10.1: Axial NECT scan in a patient with severe closed head injury. It shows small contusion in left frontal region. The contused brain appears as diffuse low density (large arrows) mixed with patchy hyperdense areas of petechial hemorrhages (small arrows). Thin acute subdural hematoma is present on right temporoparietal region (open arrow)

injuries are caused by rotational shear and other indirect forces that occur contralateral to the primary injury. A cerebral contusion consists of perivascular hemorrhages surrounded by necrotic brain involving crests of gyri and tend to be wedge-shaped and hence appear as having increased density on CT scan (Figs 10.2a to c). The pia-glial membrane is intact. In cerebral lacerations there is disruption of pia-glial membrane and hence results in a large area of hemorrhage. The hyperdensity mixed with hypodensity (salt pepper appearance) (Fig. 10.2b) is a mixed type of contusion while contusions which are non-hemorrhagic appear as having low attenuation. Most of the cases of post-traumatic brain injury however show all the above patterns of contusions.

Existing contusion or hematoma can increase in size between two scans (Figs 10.2a and b). This possibility is higher, if the initial CT is done very early following trauma. Studies done have shown changes in CT finding in 48% patients between initial and repeat CT. In 36% cases CT scan worsened, while in 12% cases CT scan showed resolution of hematoma (Figs 10.3a to c). MR is much more sensitive than CT scan in visualizing contusions and the demarcation is much clear and distinct (Figs 10.2d and e). Multiple superficial areas of hyperintense signal abnormalities are seen on T2WI. [8,9]

On CT scan, traumatic intracerebral hematoma is visualized as a focal, well defined rounded areas of abnormal density in the brain and is usually with other lesions (Figs 10.2e and f).

Cerebral Edema (Figs 10.4a and b)

Post-traumatic edema can be focal or generalized. Focal edema is more common and is commonly also described as non-hemorrhagic contusion.

1. Decreased gray/white matter differentiation.

In severe head injury, there can be loss of autoregulation causing high cerebral blood flow, which causes very high intracranial

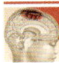

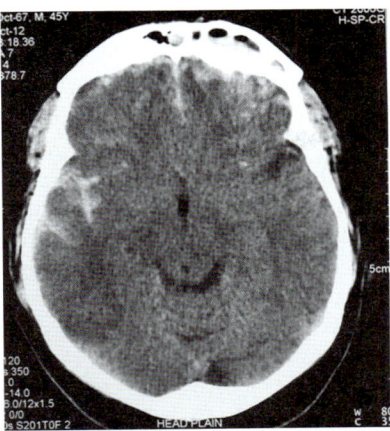

Fig. 10.2a: Axial CT scan in a patient with severe closed head injury. Immediately after head injury showing bifrontal and right temporal contusion with traumatic SAH in right Sylvian fissure

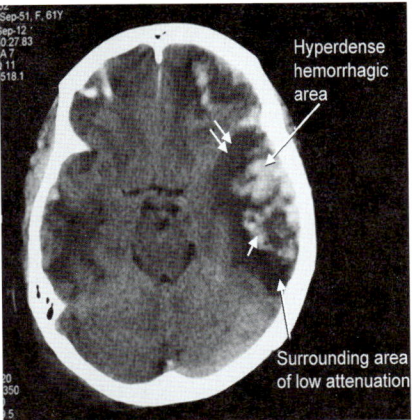

Fig. 10.2b: CT scan brain showing increase in left temporal contusion and left frontal contusion after 48 hours. Contusion appears (salt and pepper appearance) as patchy hyperdense areas of petechial hemorrhages (single arrow) mixed with low density edema (double arrows).

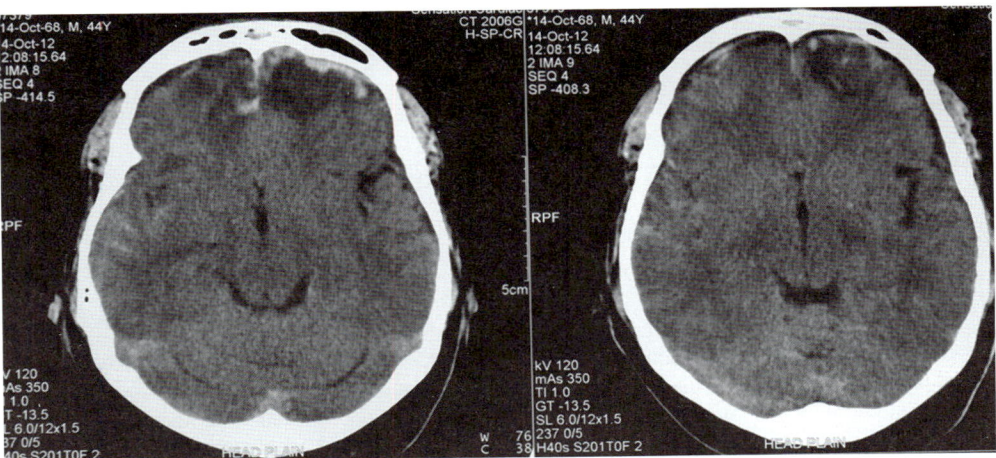

Fig. 10.2c: Resolving frontal and temporal contusions

pressure (ICP) resulting in severe cerebral, brain edema (Figs 10.4a and b). Severe cerebral ischemia produces acute cerebral edema.

Bruce et al[10] described the syndrome of diffuse cerebral edema in children and concluded that the etiology was related to increased blood volume, not oedema, since the Hounsfield values were significantly higher. On CT, focal edema is seen as uniform hypodensity. In focal injuries both edema and contusion can produce mass effect while diffuse cerebral edema appears variable effacement of sulcal spaces with compression of ventricular system and cisterns (Fig. 10.2f). It is important to observe the above changes on CT scan as patients with closed head injury may not show parenchymal or extraparenchymal hemorrhage and yet the presence and

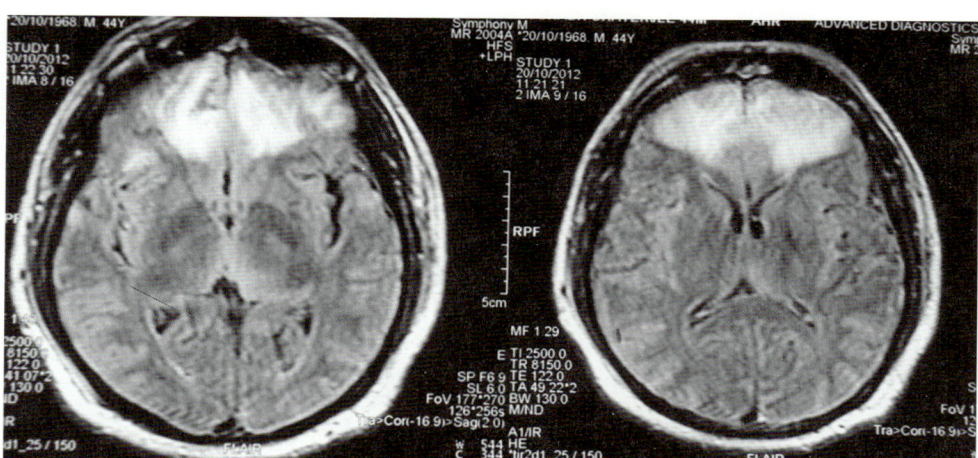

Figs10.2d and e: MRI brain of patient on 7th day after head injury. Axial T_1- and T_2-weighted images show hyperintense bifrontal contusions. Axial CT scan head is shown in Fig. 10.2a

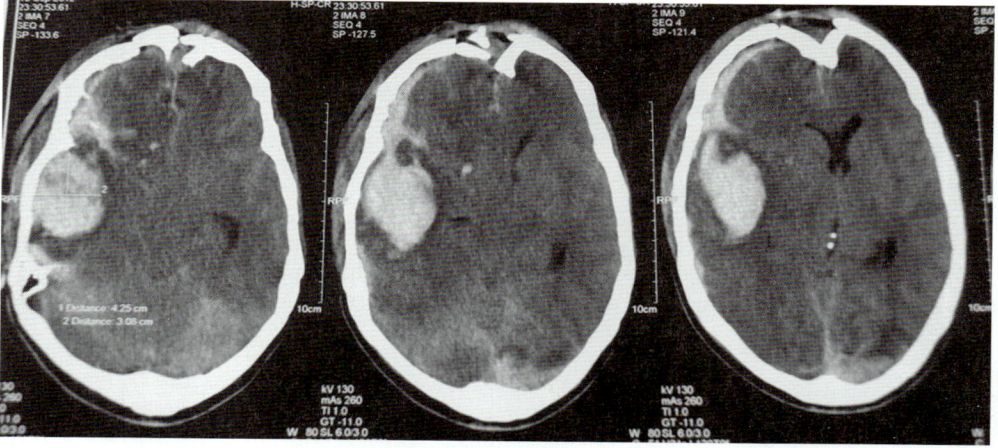

Fig. 10.2f: Axial CT scan shows right temporal contusion hematoma with acute subdural hematoma and frontal depressed fracture. There is associated right frontal contusion. This lesion is causing significant mass effect as evident by compressed-ipsilateral frontal horn, and obliterated basal cisterns. Dilated contralateral temporal horn indicates brain herniation

severity of diffuse cerebral edema can change the outcome of a brain injury patient. Cerebral edema can be primary or secondary. Primary cerebral edema is due to rotational force which causes the basal frontal and temporal cortices to impact or sweep across rigid aspects of the skull, the sphenoid wing, and petrous ridges. MR is much more sensitive than CT in visualizing contusions and the demarcation is much clear and distinct (Figs 10.2d and e). Multiple superficial areas of hyperintense signal abnormalities are seen on T2WI.[8,9]

Secondary cerebral edema appears delayed due to effects of raised intracranial pressure, mass effect of other parenchymal injuries like delayed enlargement of traumatic intra-parenchymal contusions and hematomas is hence the most common cause of clinical

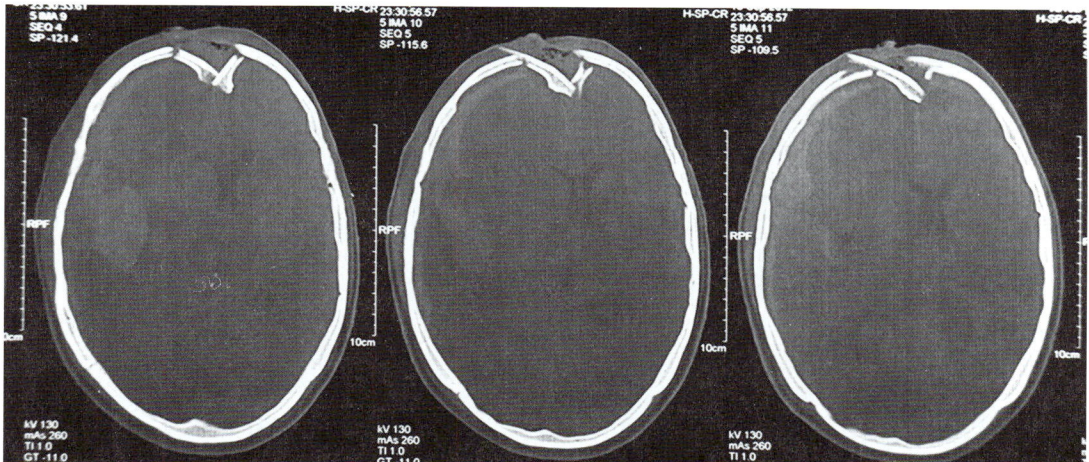

Fig. 10.2g: Depressed skull fracture. CT, bone window, large depressed fragment of frontal bone. CT, brain window of this patient (Fig. 10.2f) shows depressed fracture with underlying acute SDH and right temporal contusion hematoma

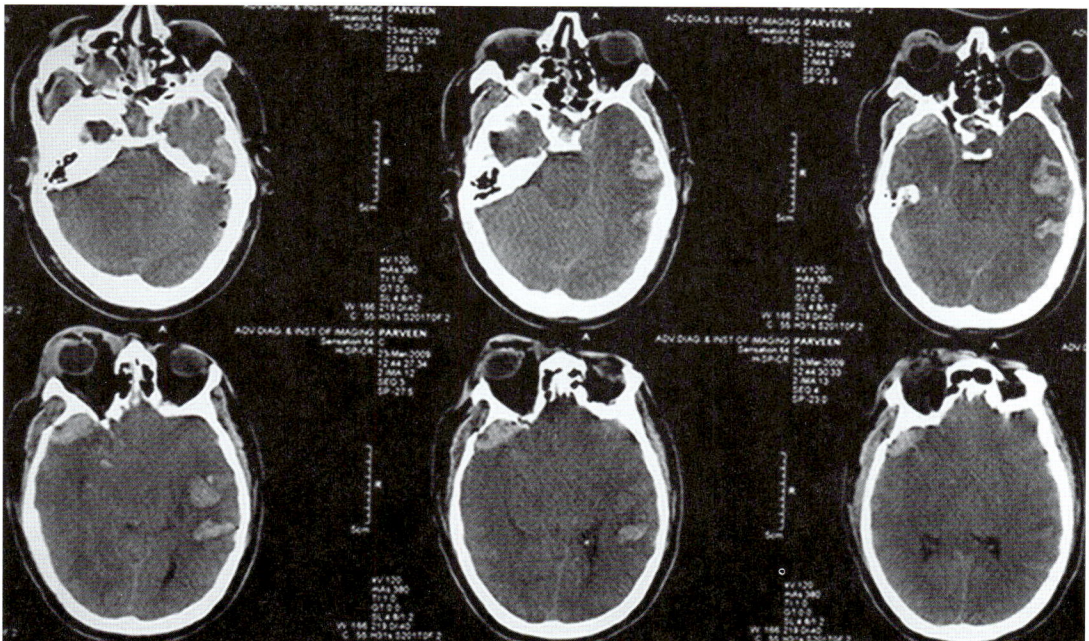

Fig. 10.3a: First day; plain CT scan (axial) in a patient with severe closed head injury. It shows large left temporal contusion, small right temporal contusion with small left temporal EDH with severe brain edema. There is significant effacement of the surface sulci and basilar subarachnoid spaces, particularly the supra-sellar and perimesencephalic cisterns. The cerebral ventricles are also severely compressed. These features are suggestive of diffuse brain edema and raised ICP (intracranial pressure)

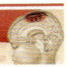

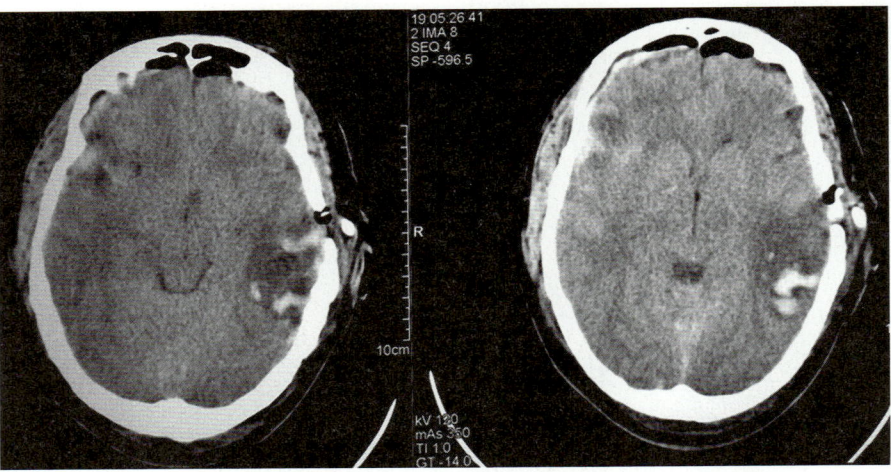

Fig. 10.3b: Fourth day after injury and surgery. Perimesencephalic cisterns have opened up and subarachnoid spaces are seen. Diffuse brain edema is also resolving

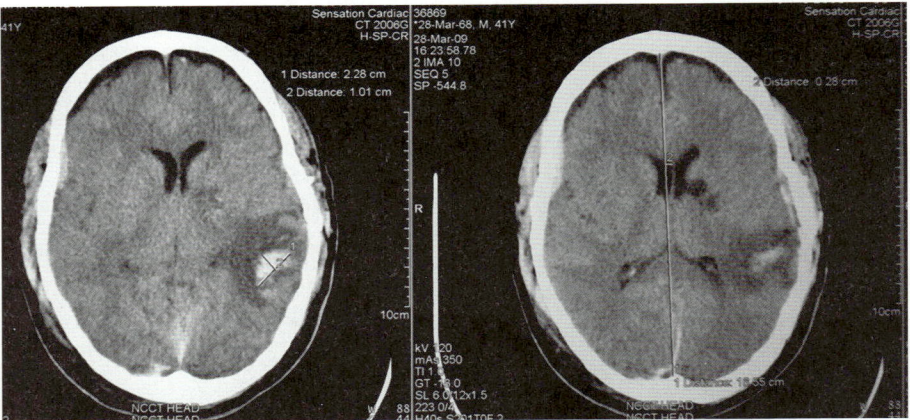

Fig. 10.3c: Sixth day following injury. Ventricles are seen well with left temporal resolving contusion. Also notice small left thalamic infarct

deterioration and death. However, progression of contusion is highly variable, and although most remain unchanged for days, a few enlarge, some quite rapidly.

Subarachnoid Hemorrhage (SAH)

The strongest prognostic factor is the presence of traumatic subarachnoid hemorrhage and appears as hyperdense areas on plain CT in the sulcal spaces and cisterns (Figs 10.5a to e). The size of the acute subarachnoid hemorrhage means that large lesions are probably in an active phase of progression at the time of the initial CT scan.

Studies have shown that while presence of acute subarachnoid hemorrhage on plain CT is a more strong predictive factor than factors such as the initial Glasgow Coma Score (GCS)

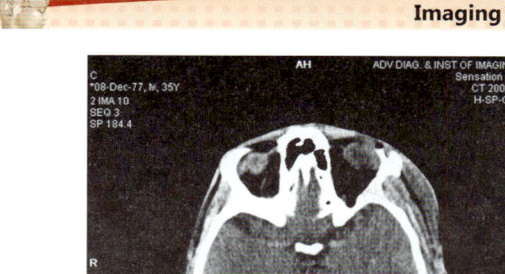
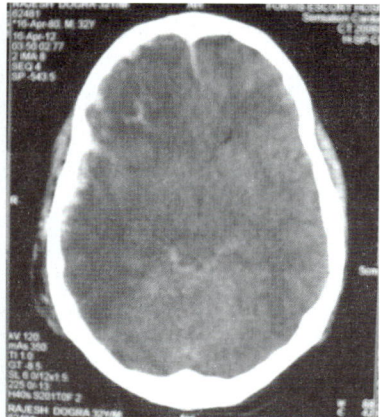

Fig 10.4a: Two examples of plain CT scan showing diffuse cerebral edema; cerebral edema is evident by decreased gray/white matter differentiation, decrease in size of ventricles, absent perimesencephalic, quadrigeminal cisterns

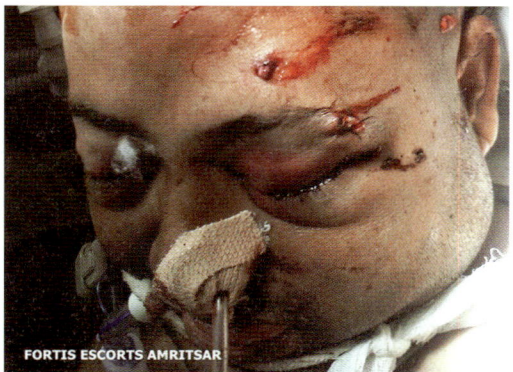

Fig. 10.4b: Anterior cranial fossa fracture. This patient had bilateral black eye, although, these can also occur with Le Fort fracture (Panda sign)

and intracranial pressure (ICP), which were not predictive of progression.

Epidural Hematomas (EDH)

The incidence of epidural hematomas is 1% of all head trauma admissions and are most commonly (85%) result from bleeding in the middle meningeal artery. Epidural hematomas, however, may occur in locations other than in the distribution of the middle meningeal artery. Such hematomas may develop from bleeding from diploic vessels injured by

overlying skull fractures.[11] Epidural hematomas appear as biconvex hyperdense extra axial areas along vault on plain CT (Figs 10.6a to d) and result because of tearing of a surface or bridging vessel (venous) which is torn because the brain parenchyma moves during violent head motion. The resulting bleeding causes a hematoma to form in the potential space between the dural and arachnoid.

Acute Subdural Hematomas (ASDH)
(Figs 10. 7a to c)

ASDH is the result of an venous or even an arterial rupture; these hematomas have the peculiar location in the temporoparietal region and differ in from those caused by the rupture of bridging veins, which typically ruptures in the frontoparietal parasagittal region. These appear as a concavo-convex hyperdense area along vault with variable mass effect (Fig. 10.7c). They differ from extradural lesions in being crescentic, i.e. concave towards brain. They may be localized to one or both lobes or may be hemispheric. Acute SDH are sometimes isodense in anemic patients or when subdural hematoma is diluted due to blood loss. The high morbidity of these lesions, particularly in the aged, is due in large part to the associated swelling,

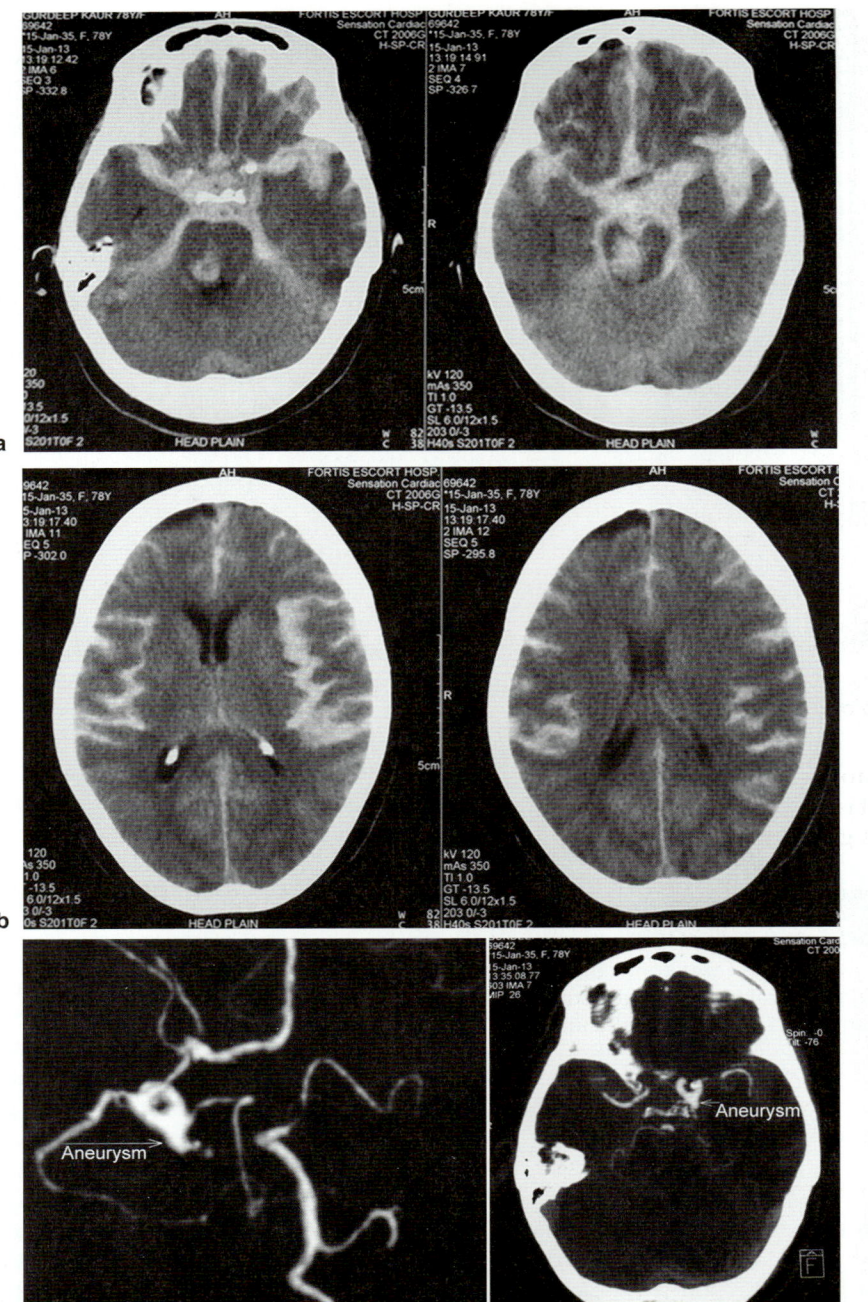

Figs 10.5a to d: CT scan showing thick severe post-traumatic SAH (Fisher's Grade 4); high attenuation within suprasellar cistern, subarachnoid spaces and throughout CSF spaces signifies severe subarachnoid bleed with guarded prognosis. Associated brainstem bleed also seen. Figures c and d CT angiogram showing left MCA aneurysm

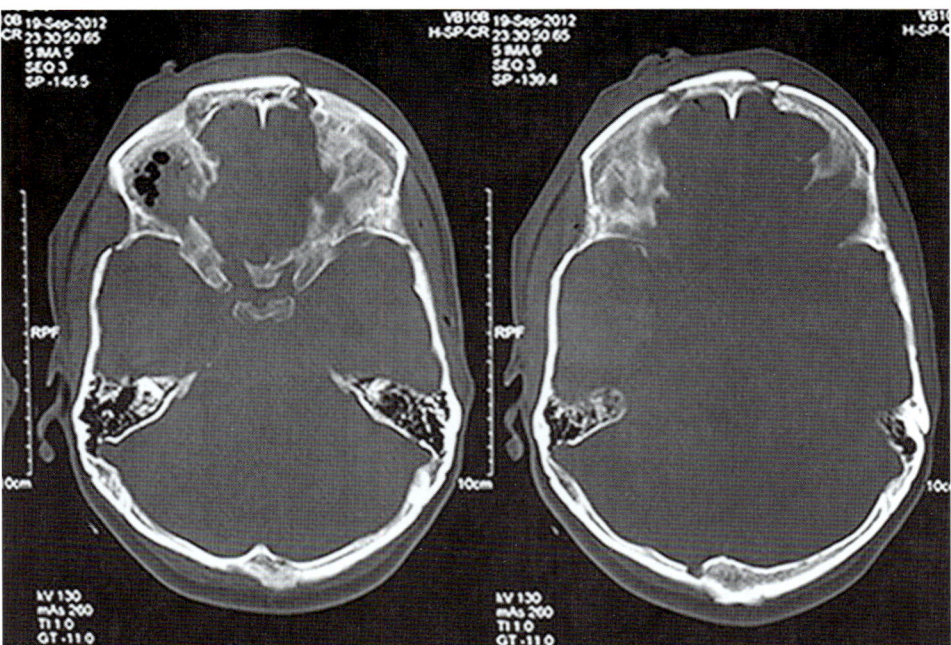

Fig. 10.5e: Anterior cranial fossa fracture. This patient had bilateral black eye (Fig. 10.4b) although, these can also occur with Le Fort fracture (Panda sign)

contusion or laceration of the underlying brain. It is often evident that mid-line displacement is greater than would be accounted for

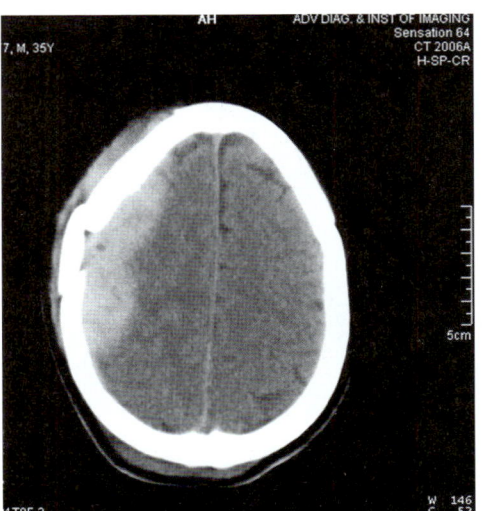

Fig. 10.6a: Plain CT scan head showing EDH with skull fracture

by the mass of the hematoma alone. The interhemispheric subdural hematoma extends along the falx cerebri and may spread onto tentorium, giving a characteristic comma shape on axial CT sections. MRI has limited role in acute SDH.

Chronic Subdural Hematoma (CSDH)

CT is the investigation of choice for evaluation of chronic SDH (Figs 10.7a to c). The density of the subdural hematoma decreases with the passage of time. A chronic subdural hematoma is hyperdense in first week after injury (Fig. 10.8a). It becomes isodense in about ten days to 2 weeks and thus could be overlooked on the CT scan examination. After 3 weeks, Chronic subdural hematoma usually appears hypodense on CT. It is often difficult to distinguish isodense chronic SDH from cerebral parenchyma. Isodense SDH displaces surface sulci of the brain away from inner table. They have been often misdiagnosed as cerebral swelling or tumor. Chances of

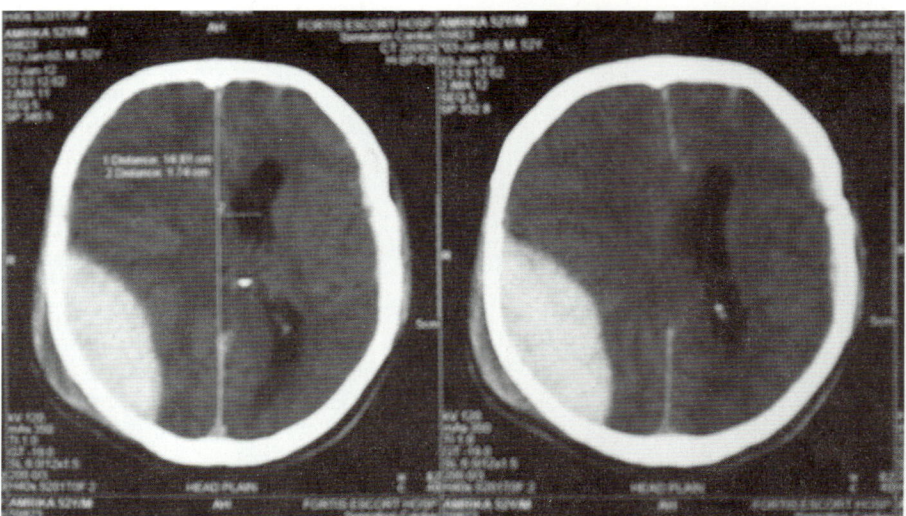

Fig. 10.6b: CT appearance of large, right temporoparietal extradural hematoma (EDH) with significant midline shift. Note the presence of biconvex extradural hematoma and compression of right lateral ventricle and midline shift towards left with dilatation of left lateral ventricle

missing bilateral isodense subdural hematoma is still higher. MRI signal intensity may vary with time, but chronic subdural hematomas are generally hyperintense on both T_1- and T_2- weighted scans. Rarely, a chronic subdural hematoma is isointense on T_1 images due to methemoglobin, which is related to the age of the extravasated blood. Often, on either CT or

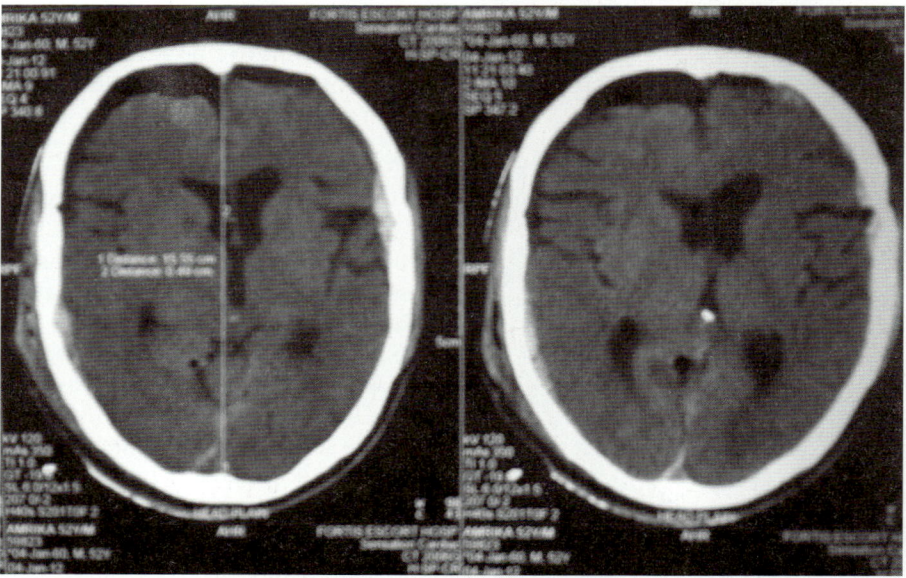

Fig. 10.6c: Postoperative CT scan shows complete removal of EDH with ventricles, cisterns and subarachnoid spaces regaining there shape

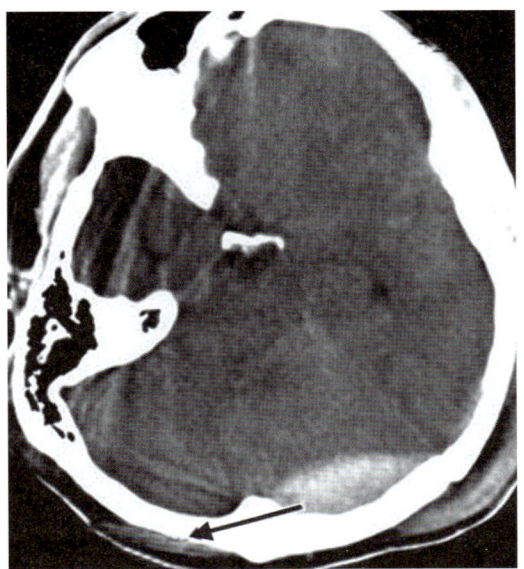

Fig. 10.6d: CT appearance of posterior fossa extradural hematoma. Mass effect is present and the fourth ventricle is compressed

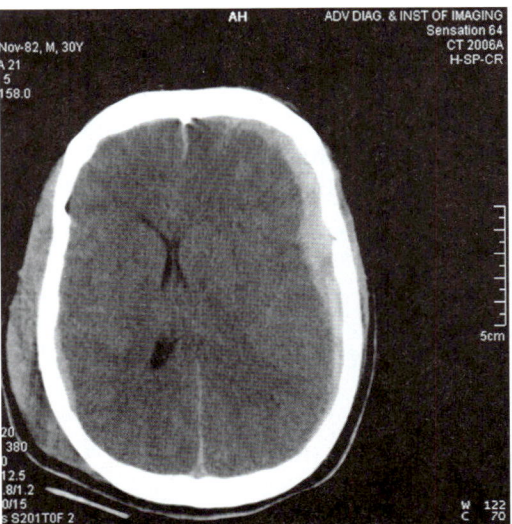

Fig.10.7a: Acute subdural hematoma. CT scan showing concavo-convex hyperdense area along vault with mass effect as evident by compressed ipsilateral ventricles. **Diffuse cerebral edema** is also present

MRI, one sees a subdural hematoma that is heterogenous or with layering of blood; these types are secondary to mixing of fresh blood (from intermittent hemorrhages from the external membrane) with the chronic subdural fluid. On T_2-weighted MRI scans, a black band is frequently observed on the inner membrane of symptomatic chronic subdural hematomas (Imaizumi et al 2003).[12]

An intraventricular hemorrhage is another intracerebral lesion that often accompanies other intracranial hemorrhages. Intraventricular blood is an indicator of more severe head trauma.

Diffuse Axonal Injury

The usual cause for persistent impairment of consciousness is the condition referred to as diffuse axonal injury, as depicted in the image below. Diffuse injuries range from concussion, with no residual damage, to diffuse axonal injury and persistent vegetative state. Diffuse injury occurs in 50–60% of patients with severe head trauma and is the commonest cause of unconsciousness, the vegetative state and subsequent disability.[13] Approximately 30–40% of individuals who die from TBI reveal postmortem evidence of DAI and ischemia. This type of injury commonly results from traumatic rotation of the head, with mechanical forces that act on the long axons, leading to axonal structural failure. DAI is caused by an acceleration injury and not by contact injury alone. The brain is relatively incompressible and does not tolerate tensile or shear strains well. Slow application of strain is better tolerated than rapid strain. The brain is most susceptible to lateral rotation and tolerates sagittal movements best. The CT findings include scattered small hemorrhages in cerebral white matter, basal ganglia, corpus callosum, or dorsal part of brainstem.[14,15] The two most common location for these hemorrhages are corpus callosum and dorsolateral quadrant of the rostral brainstem in the region of cerebral peduncle (Figs 10.9, 10.10a and b). Occasionally, hemorrhage is seen in the

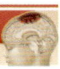

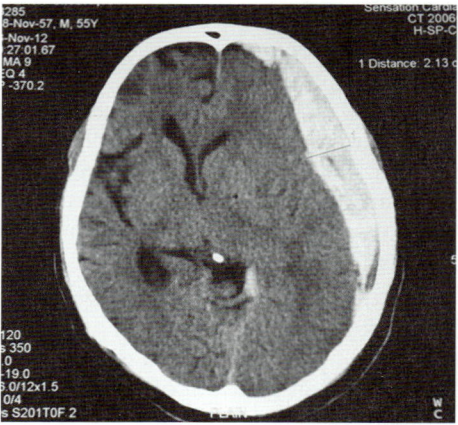
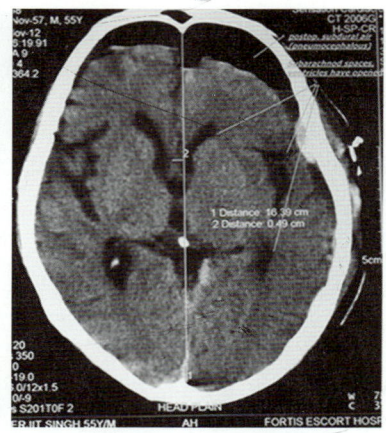

Figs 10.7b and c: Plain CT scan head showing large acute subdural hematoma. With mass effect and midline shift. Postoperative CT scan (10.7c) showing good evacuation of hematoma

structures making up the walls of the third ventricle (thalamus, column of the fornices, anterior commissure).

Role of MRI in Traumatic Brain Injury

CT is the first imaging test performed in the emergency department setting for evaluation of head trauma. The goal of emergency imaging is to depict lesions that need emergent neurosurgical treatment or in other ways alter therapy. In many institutions, MRI is reserved for showing lesions that could explain clinical symptoms and signs that are not explained by prior CT or to help better define abnormalities seen on CT. The increased sensitivity of MRI relative to CT for detection of many forms of brain injury has been well-documented.

Intracerebral Hematoma

Traumatic intracerebral hematomas may result from the coalescence of the hemorrhages within a contusion, or they may develop de novo. The margins of such hematoma tend to be more irregular and ill defined than those of hematomas due to hypertension or aneurysmal rupture.[24] A thin rim of edema usually surrounds post-traumatic hematomas. These hematomas can be multiple. Midline shift and evidence of herniation should also be looked for.

Subdural hematomas (1–2 weeks) have high signal on both T_1- and T_2-weighted images due to presence of extracellular methemoglobin (Table 10.1).

Subacute subdural hematomas are hyperintense on T_1-weighted images and hypointense (i.e. dark) relative to brain (Table 10.2) and CSF due to presence of intracellular methemoglobin (Figs 10.8a to c).

MRI can also demonstrate acute hemorrhages within chronic SDH. MRI is more sensitive than CT in identifying isodense SDH.

Table 10.1: MRI changes in hematoma on T_1- and, T_2-weighted images with time		
Hematoma	*T_1*	*T_2*
Hyper acute (< a few hours)	Hypo	Hyper (oxy Hb)
Acute	Iso to hypo	Hypo (due to deoxy Hb)
Subacute	Hyper	Hypo (intracellular-meth Hb)
Chronic	Hyper	Hyper (release of meth Hb after lysis of RBCs)

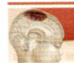

Table 10.2: Time taken for linear fractures to heal

1. Infancy and early childhood; 3 to 6 months
2. Children 5 to 12 years; ~ 1 year
3. Adolescence; months to years
4. Adult; throughout life

Use of Newer MRI Techniques

The use of diffusion-weighted imaging (DWI) and diffusion tensor imaging (DTI) in assessment of patients with traumatic brain injury is widely gaining acceptance (Fig. 10.11). DWI can detect changes in the rate of microscopic water motion, which is measured by the apparent diffusion coefficient (ADC) which is a measure of water motion limited by cellular composition. On the other hand, DTI is based on the fact that microscopic water diffusion in white matter tracts tends to occur in one direction rather than randomly, a phenomenon termed "anisotropy". The degree of anisotropy in a white matter region can be viewed as a reflection of the degree of the structural integrity of white matter.[5,6,16,17] A number of different measures of anisotropy can be used; one of the more commonly used is fractional anisotropy (FA). In an study by Jian Xu[17] the functional outcome in patients with TBI cannot be explained by focal pathology alone, and diffuse axonal injury (DAI) is considered a major contributor to the neurocognitive deficits experienced by this group. The aim of the present study was to investigate whether diffusion tensor imaging (DTI) offers additional information as to the extent of damage not visualized with standard magnetic resonance imaging (MRI) in patients with severe TBI. Nine chronic male TBI patients and 11 matched healthy controls were recruited. Results of the voxel-based analysis of fractional anisotropy (FA) maps and apparent diffusion coefficient (ADC) maps revealed significant differences in anisotropy in major white matter tracts, including the corpus callosum (CC), internal and external capsule, superior and inferior longitudinal fascicles, and the fornix in the TBI group. The FA and ADC measurements offered superior sensitivity compared to conventional MRI diagnosis of DAI. Region-of-interest (ROI) analyzes confirmed these results in the investigated regions. The findings of this study support the hypothesis that severe TBI

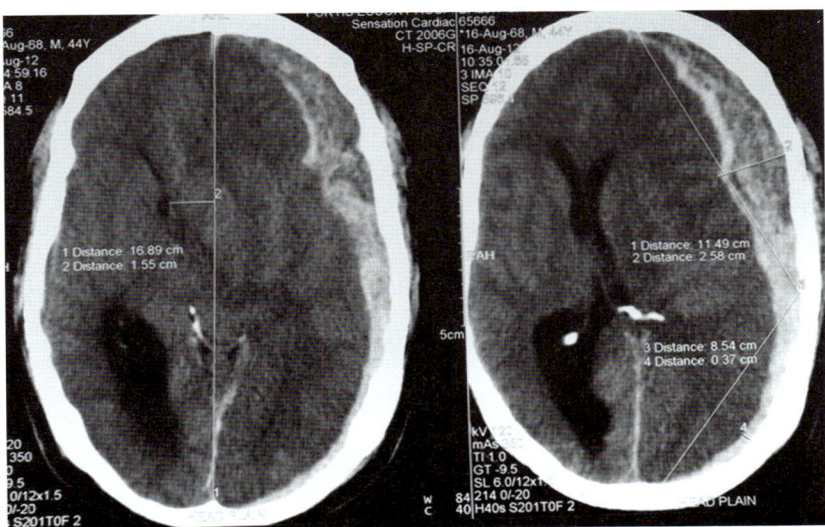

Fig. 10.8a: Chronic subdural hematoma. CT scan showing hyperdense cellular component occupying the dependent part and significant midline shift with contralateral dilated ventricles

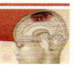

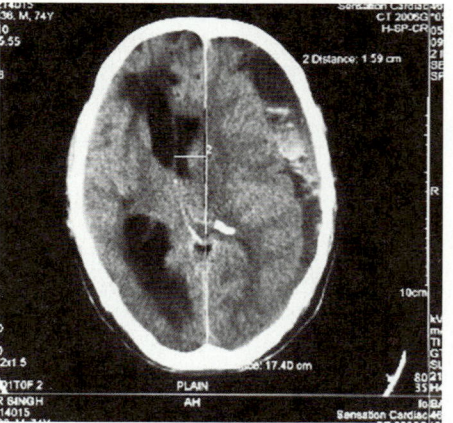

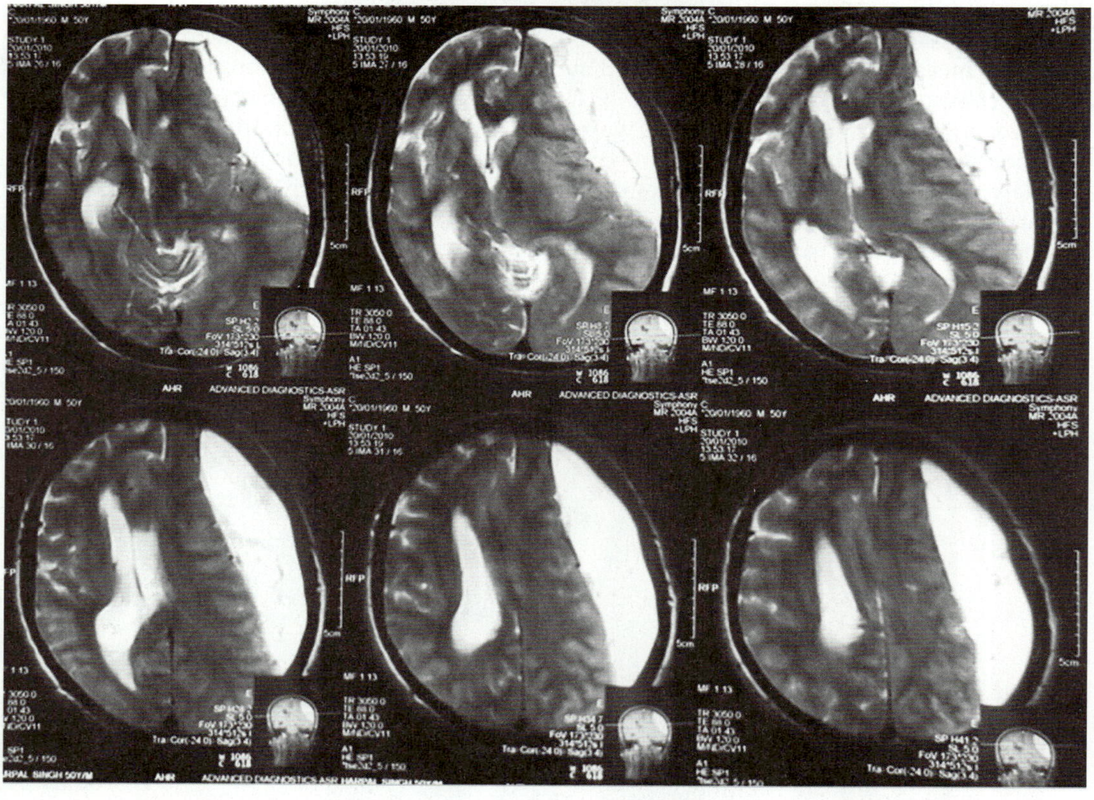

Fig. 10.8b: Chronic subdural haematoma: MRI showing bright signal on T_2-weighted images

is accompanied by DAI. The DTI changes were more prominent on the right side that contained the focal pathology in most of the patients and accurately reflected differences in both hemispheres.[16,17]

Regions of acute DAI can be depicted as bright lesions (Fig. 10. 10a). MRI is superior to CT in depicting non-hemorrhagic contusions, which appear as high intensity areas on T_2-weighted images and as iso-intense or hypo-

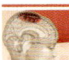

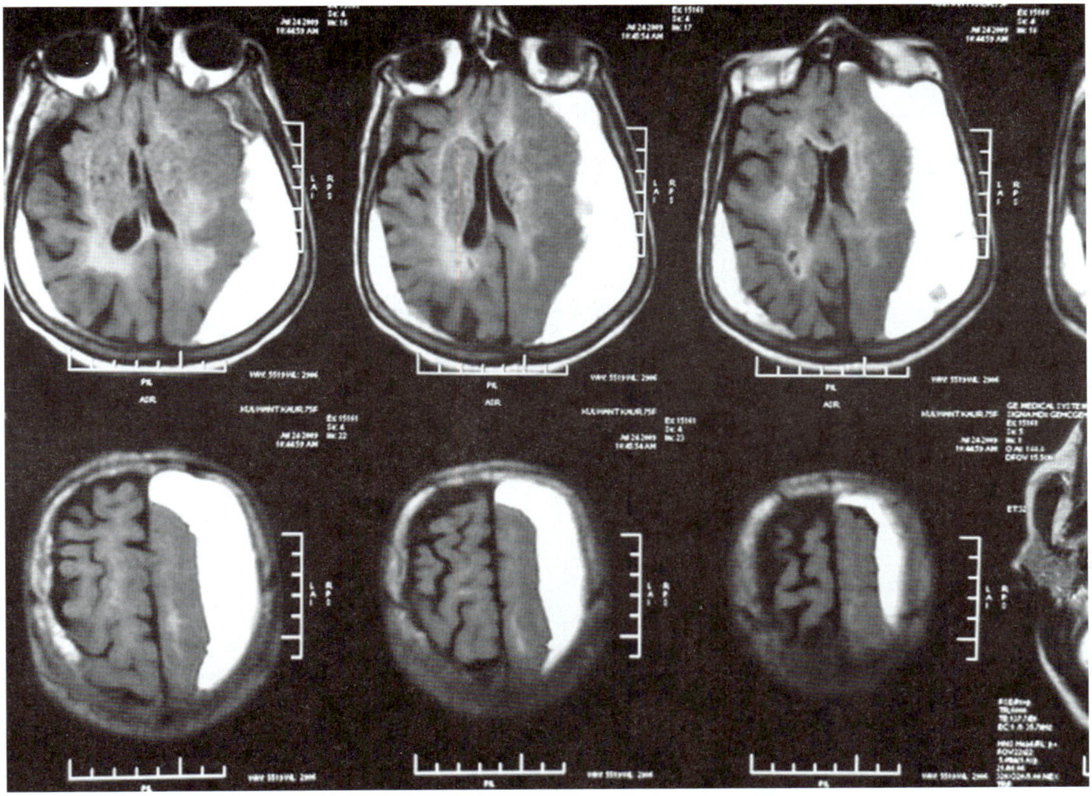

Fig. 10.8c: Chronic subdural hematoma: MRI showing bright signal on T$_1$-weighted images

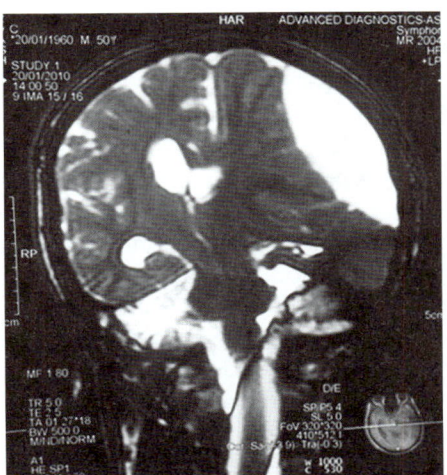

Fig.10.8d: MRI brain (coronal) T$_2$-weighted image showing large left chronic SDH with transtentorial herniation

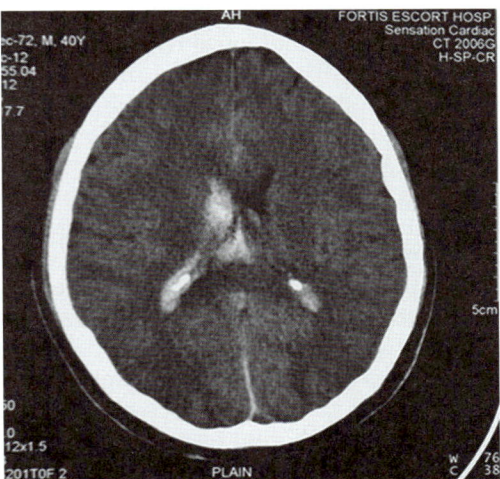

Fig. 10.9: CT scan showing corpus callosum contusion with intraventricular hemorrhage suggestive of DAI

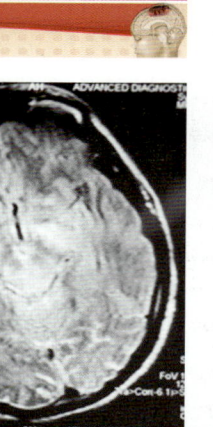

Fig. 10.10a: T_1-weighted images

intense areas on T_1-weighted images. Magnetic resonance imaging of DAI has shown hemorrhagic and non-hemorrhagic lesions in the white matter in the hemispheres, corpus callosum, and rostral brainstem, compatible with the neuropathological characteristics of this type of injury,[18] and a modified staging has been used in imaging studies. Stage 1 represents a pattern of traumatic lesions confined to lobar white matter, whereas in Stages 2 and 3, lesions are depicted in the corpus callosum and brainstem, respectively.[19,20] MRI sequences which are recommended include T_1-weighted, T_2-weighted, T_2-gradient echo, proton density-weighted, and diffusion-weighted images.[21] The degree of confidence is high, as abnormal signal in the characteristic locations, discovered in the clinical setting of recent trauma, leaves little doubt about the diagnosis of DAI. In a prospective cohort study, Skandsen et al[20] examined MRI scans from patients in the early phase of moderate to severe head injury and

determined the prognosis was better in patients with DAI whose lesions were confined to the lobar white matter or who had callosal lesions than it was in patients with DAI who had lesions in the dorsolateral brainstem.[20]

On DWI and dark regions on ADC maps because of restricted diffusion caused by acute cell death. In the past 5 years, many studies have shown that these techniques can detect regions of DAI that are subtle or undetected on T_2-weighted and FLAIR images as well as provide a quantitative assessment of DAI for large areas of the brain.[22] A large number of articles have been published on this topic, and it is possible to provide only some examples here rather than an exhaustive review.

ADC values can be measured in specific regions or in the whole brain. Galloway et al[23] measured ADC values using both methods and compared findings in 37 children with various degrees of brain injury (measured by

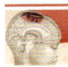
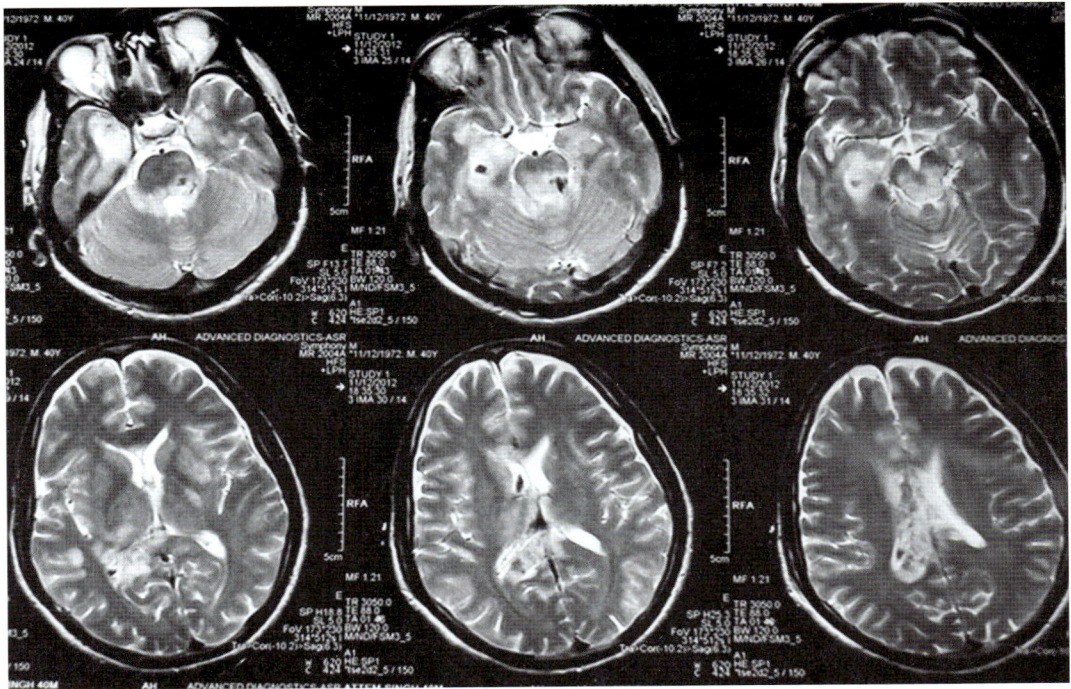

Fig. 10.10b: MRI brain of same patient (Fig. 10.9) showing the presence of multifocal areas of abnormal signal (bright on T2-weighted images) at the white matter in the temporal or parietal corticomedullary junction or in the splenium of the corpus callosum. Other areas that frequently are abnormal include the dorsolateral rostral midbrain and the corona radiata

GCS scores) and neurologic outcomes [measured by the Pediatric Cerebral Performance Category Scale (PCPCS)] and 10 normal control subjects. The authors measured ADC values in normal-appearing brain in the following regions: Deep gray matter, peripheral gray matter, deep white matter, peripheral white matter, posterior fossa, and whole brain. The major goal of the study was to determine whether ADC values in various regions or in the whole brain could predict outcome. The mean ADC value in peripheral white matter was able to predict outcome in children with severe traumatic brain injury. Overall, mean ADC in the whole brain was the best predictor of outcome among all degrees of traumatic brain injury. Susceptibility weighted imaging (SWI) is a form of MRI that utilizes the paramagnetic properties of blood products like deoxyhemoglobin, methemo-globin, and hemosiderin. Their magnetic effects increases the visibility of microscopic hemorrhages.[24] SWI is superior in detecting hemorrhagic DAI.

DTI (Fig. 10.11) and another advanced MR technique, MR spectroscopy, were recently compared for their ability to predict outcome in a group of 43 traumatic brain injury patients who were imaged, on average, approximately 3 weeks after trauma. FA values were measured at 16 sites within the supratentorial and infratentorial white matter or brainstem. The metabolite N-acetyl aspartate (NAA), a marker of neuronal integrity, was measured and compared with the stable metabolite creatine (Cr) at five locations on an axial image through the level of the lentiform nucleus and expressed as the NAA:Cr ratio. Patients were divided into either a favorable outcome group (n = 24) or an unfavorable outcome group

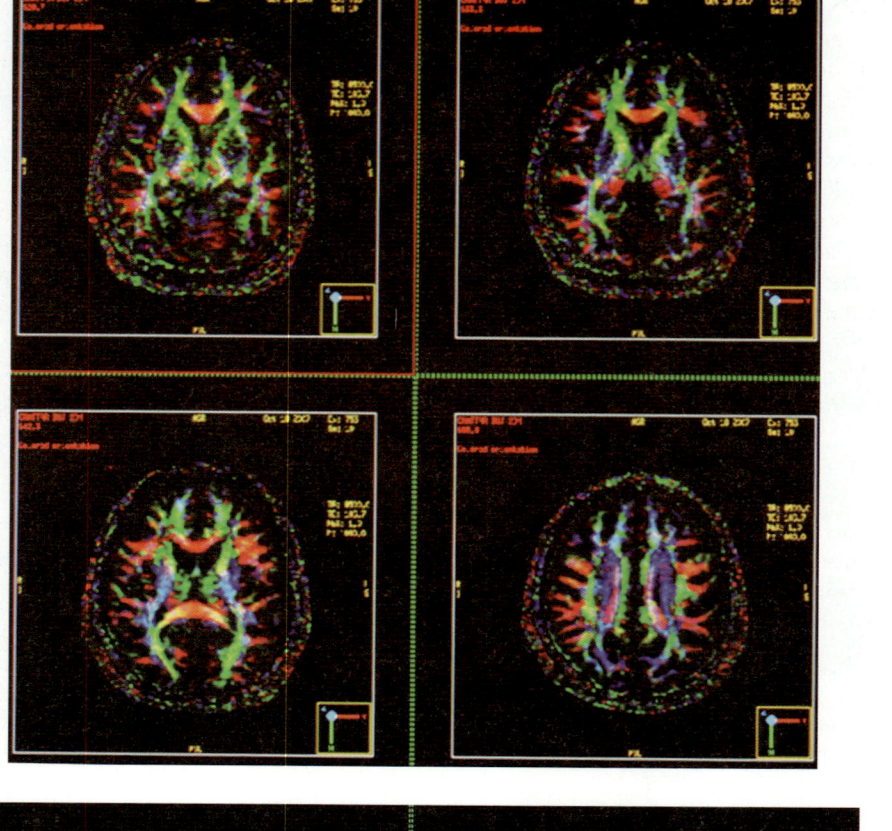

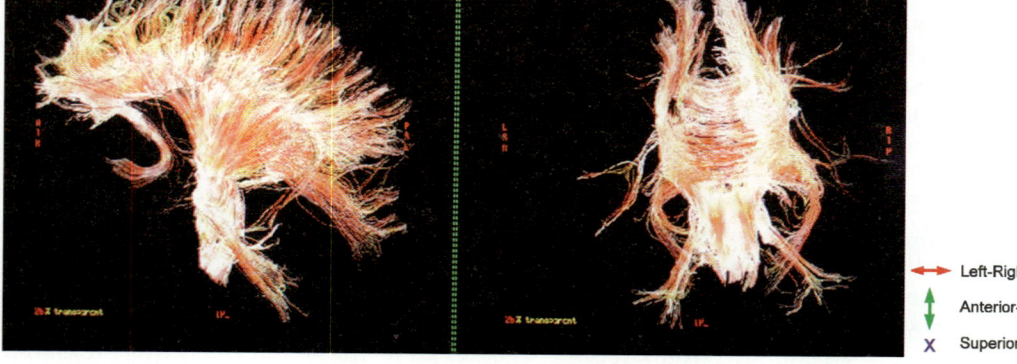

Left-Right

Anterior-Posterior

X Superior-Inferior

Fig. 10.11: Normal diffusion tensor imaging (DTI) axial tractographic image demonstrates white matter tracts in the brain in the left-right (red), anterior-posterior (green), and superior-inferior (blue) directions

(n = 19) depending on scores on the Glasgow Outcome Scale performed at 1-year follow-up after trauma. In 15 of the 16 brain regions studied, FA values were significantly reduced in the unfavorable outcome group compared with both the favorable outcome group and normal control subjects. In all of these regions, FA values were significantly decreased in the favorable outcome group compared with normal control subjects. The authors attributed decreased FA to disruption of axonal membranes and the cytoskeletal network. With regard to MR spectroscopy findings, in all five regions in which the NAA:Cr ratio was measured, statistically significant differences were found between the unfavorable outcome group and the other groups and between the favorable outcome group and normal control subjects. The authors attributed these findings to axonal loss or decreased metabolism.

CT for Prediction of Mortality in Head Trauma Patients

In 1991 Marshall classification was suggested to measure outcome of patients with traumatic bone injury as many patients on ventilation, intubation or use of sedation made it impossible to determine GCS. Hence anatomical findings on plain CT were used to predict the outcome which is as follows:

Marshall classification of predictive outcome:

Grade 1: Normal CT scan (9.6% mortality)
Grade 2: Cisterns present, shift < 5 mm (13.5% mortality)
Grade 3: Cistern compressed/absent, shift < 5 mm (34% mortality)
Grade 4: Shift > 5 mm (56.2% mortality)

Now presence of intraventricular and subarachnoid hemorrhage has also been added and the presence of acute intraventricular hemorrhage formed single important factor in short- and long-term outcome of such patients.

SPECIAL POST-TRAUMATIC BRAIN INJURY IMAGING STATES

Skull Fractures

Skull fractures often occur without significant brain injury and many patients with severe brain injury do not have skull fractures. Skull fractures can be classified as linear, com-minuted, depressed or basilar. On routine skull X-rays (Fig. 10.12d), linear fractures are typically well defined, and appear as fine lines of decreased density. They sometimes branch, and must be distinguished from the vascular markings. The fracture appears thinner and more lucent than vascular grooves. A fracture passing through a sinus or air cell is internally compound, and of great clinical significance. Fractures associated with widening (diastasis) of one or more sutures, particularly lamdoid. Linear fractures take variable time to heal (Table 10.2). In adults they can be seen throughout life. CT scan head may not detect linear fractures that lies parallel to plane of CT image. Routine CT examination of the head in axial projection, as many as 30 to 40 percent of fractures are not seen.[25]

Depressed fractures may be diagnosed by plain films but are usually diagnosed by CT (Figs 10.2f, 10.12a), which also shows any associated intracranial contusion. On plain X-rays, depressed fractures often appear as com-minuted fracture with areas of overlap in some projections and inward displacement in others.

Plain X-ray skull showing linear fracture of parietal bone.

Basilar skull fractures are often missed in routine X-rays. Basilar skull fracture (Fig. 10.4) are best demonstrated by high resolution, thin section of CT in both axial and coronal planes.[26]

Growing skull fractures (lepto meningeal cyst) usually occur after head injury in young children. The dura underlying a linear fracture is torn, sometimes intact arachnoid gets trapped in the fracture which transmits the brain pulsations. There is progressive wid-ening, eversion and smoothening of bone edges, owing to pulsation of cyst like col-lection of fluid in the partially walled off subarachnoid space. CT scan is a good investi-gation for the diagnosis of growing fractures as it shows the changes in the underlying brain, which is seen to herniate through the skull defect.

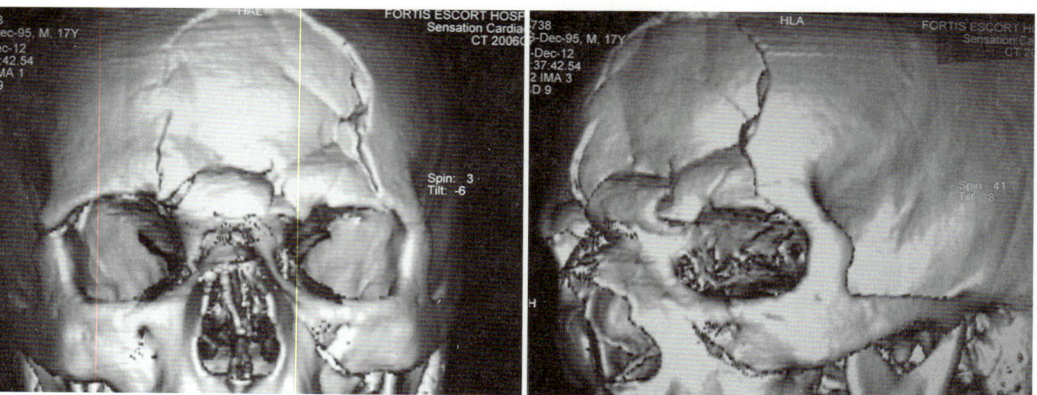

Fig. 10.12a: 3-DCT scan showing depressed fracture of frontal bone

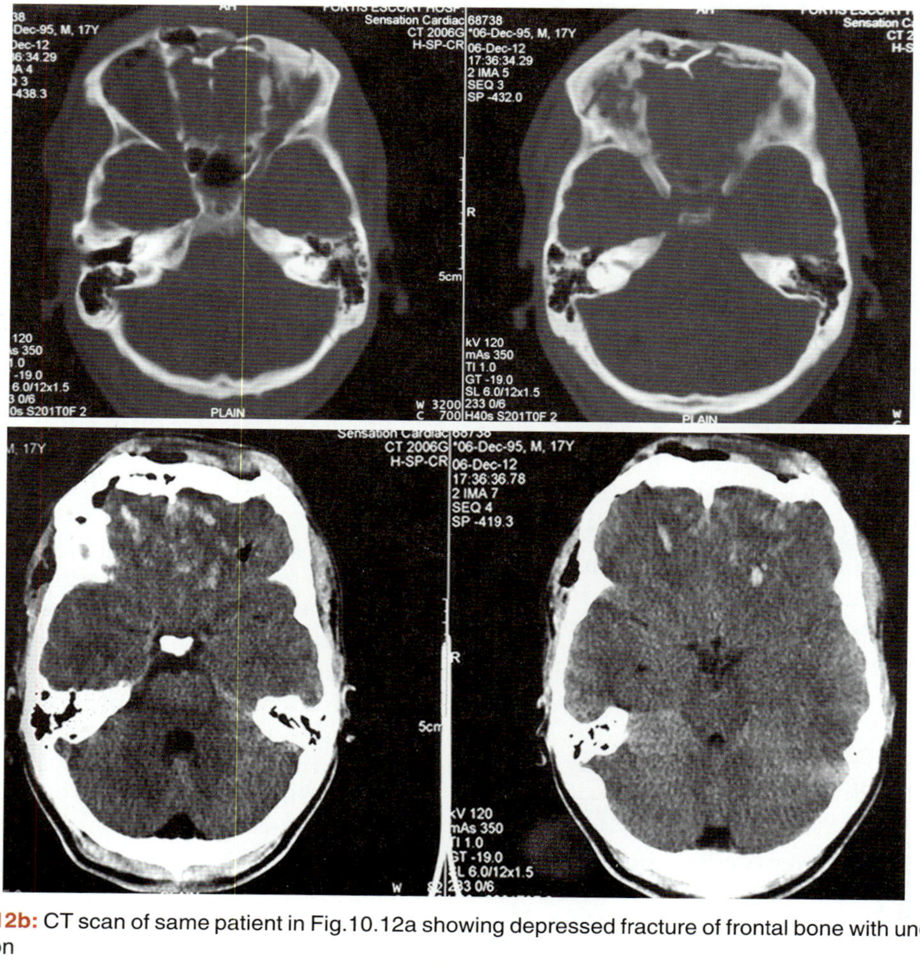

Fig. 10.12b: CT scan of same patient in Fig.10.12a showing depressed fracture of frontal bone with underlying contusion

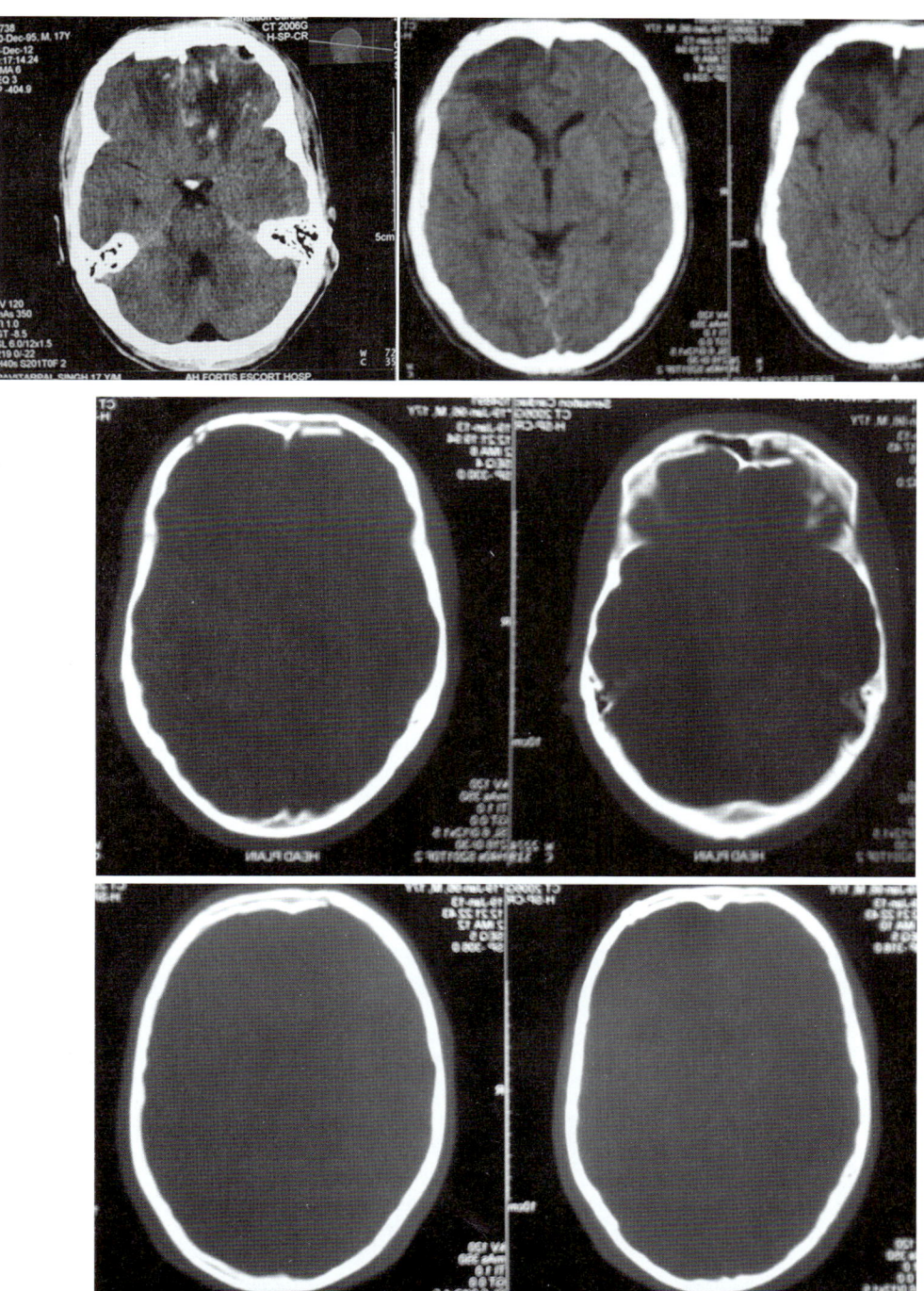

Fig. 10.12c: Postoperative CT scan showing good elevation of depressed fracture of frontal bone

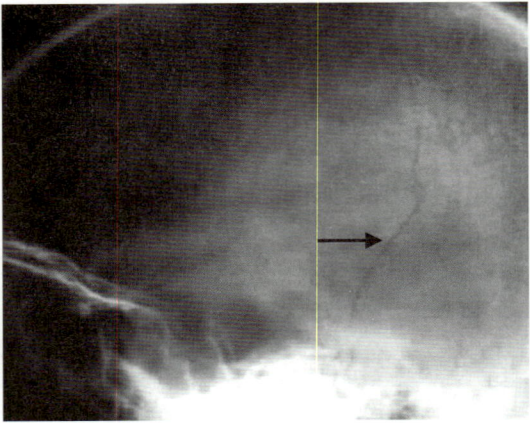

Fig. 10.12d: Skull fracture; temporoparietal fracture

CSF Rhinorrhea

It results from the rupture of basal dura and arachnoid, where it connects with the paranasal sinuses. CT is the procedure of choice.

CT scan with thin coronal cuts, occasionally augmented by cisternography using water soluble contrast such as metrizamide demonstrated defect in the anterior cranial fossa in majority of cases.[27–29] Presence of fluid levels in the ethmoid sinus or frontal sinus indicate bony defect anteriorly in cribriform plate whereas fluid level in sphenoid sinus indicates defect in sphenoid bone.

Radionuclide can be injected into the lumbar spinal canal and recovered with cotton pledgets inserted on each side of nose to detect minimal CSF leak.

MR Cisternography (Fig. 10.13)

Using fast spin echo technique has demonstrated defect in the dura at appropriate level.[28] Post-traumatic CSF rhinorrhea usually has an abrupt onset within 48 hours of the trauma with spontaneous remission in 70–80% of patients within a week. Up to 50% of those cases that do not remit develop meningitis.[17] Pneumocephalus is often present in these cases.

Posterior fossa extradural hematoma accounts for 3 to 13% of all cranial traumatic extradural hematomas. CT study is carried j low enough to adequately assess posterior fossa, j CT findings include biconvex, hyperdense collection just beneath the occipital bone, which I can extend above tentorium. Posterior fossa extradural hematoma results from injury to the transverse or sigmoid sinuses and the torcular herophili. It can be associated with occipital skull fracture invariably crossing venous sinuses.[30, 31]

Primary Brainstem Injury

Primary brainstem injury usually are nonhemorrhagic, and therefore, are better

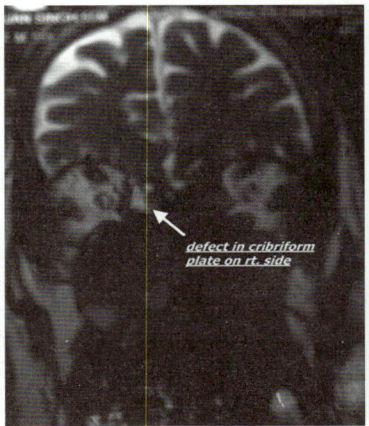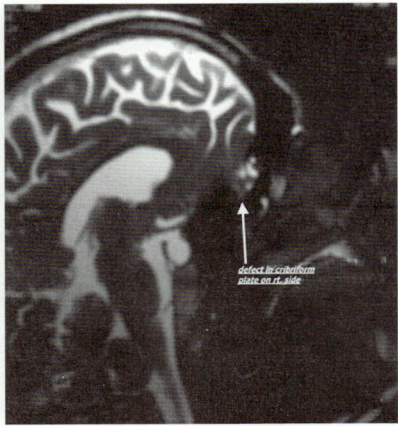

Fig.10.13: MR cisternography showing anterior cranial fossa defect

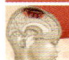

diagnosed by MR than by CT. These brainstem injuries should be differentiated from Durett hemorrhages caused by downward transtentorial herniation.[32,33] Primary brainstem lesions are usually localized to the dorsolateral midbrain and upper pons (Fig. 10.14c). Primary brainstem injuries are those that result from the initial trauma, while secondary brainstem injuries are those that develop later. The most common type of primary brainstem injury, by far, is that associated with widespread DAI. DAI lesions of the brainstem are almost invariably associated with macroscopically and microscopically similar lesions in the corpus callosum and deep cerebral white matter.

Cerebral angiography in post-traumatic contusion hematoma (a) CT scan showing left-frontal contusion hematoma (b) angiogram (lateral view) showing shift of anterior cerebral arteries posteriorly (c) angiogram (AP view) right internal carotid artery showing shift of right anterior cerebral artery (A2 and A3 segments) to right side, (d) angiogram (AP view) left internal carotid artery showing shift of left ACA (A2 and A3 segment) to opposite.

Angiography

Cerebral angiography is indicated in patients of head injury in whom there is suspicion of vascular complications. Vascular complications following head trauma are post-traumatic aneurysms, traumatic dissection of the internal carotid or vertebral arteries, arterial spasm, thrombosis, CCF (caroticocavernous fistula) and dural sinus laceration.[34]

Catheter angiography remains the definitive method of diagnosing vascular injury. However, MR angiography may be used for non-invasive evaluation.

Traumatic intracranial aneurysms are less than 1% of reported aneurysm in large series.[35,36] Traumatic aneurysms are located on the distal middle cerebral artery, distal anterior cerebral artery, basal internal carotid artery.[37,38] Basal skull fractures may be associated with cavernous internal carotid artery aneurysm.[24] Post-traumatic aneurysms can be false or true aneurysm.

False aneurysm occurs when the full thickness of vessel is lacerated and the apparent wall is actually organized hematoma. "True" aneurysm occurs following limited damage to the wall and persistence of all layers.[39] Penetrating injuries can be associated with traumatic aneurysms.

Indications for cerebral angiography after trauma include a penetrating or perforating injury, an unexplained prominent collection of subarachnoid blood.

Conventional cerebral angiography, often with digital subtraction, is the best method for detecting traumatic aneurysms. Traumatic aneurysms are usually more peripherally

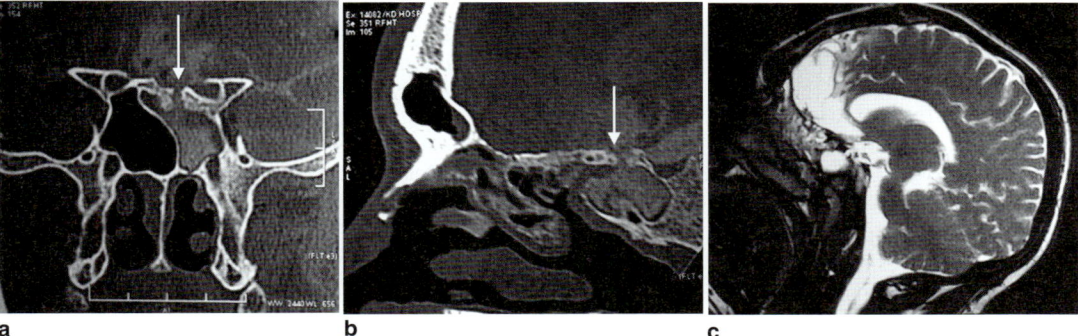

a　　　　　　　　　b　　　　　　　　　c

Figs 10.14a to c: (a and b) CT metrizamide cisternography coronal and sagittal sections showing post-traumatic bony defect in posterior part of anterior cranial fossa near sella; (c) MR cisternography of above patient showing CSF leakage in sella

situated than are berry aneurysms and typically do not occur at branching sites. A post-traumatic aneurysm is irregular in contour, may be fusiform or lobulated, often has no definable neck, and may fill and drain slowly.

Magnetic resonance angiography or three dimensional CT may eventually be able to detect traumatic aneurysms.

Traumatic dissection of internal carotid artery can occur following sudden severe sketch of the internal carotid artery over upper cervical spine when the neck is hyperextended. Other causes of traumatic dissection includes direct injury to artery, by compression between the angle of mandible and upper cervical vertebre. Dissection of internal carotid artery leads to thrombosis and embolus formation.

The angiographic abnormalities following dissection are localized narrowing of the upper cervical carotid artery or aneurysmal ourpouching between C2 and the skull base.[40,41]

CONCLUSIONS

CT scan remains the investigation of choice in head injured patients. CT scan can be repeated easily and can be done in patients on ventilator. CT scan can accurately diagnose extradural hematoma, acute and chronic subdural hematoma, contusion, post-traumatic intracerebral hematoma. However, there are some conditions, such as diffuse axonal injury, non-hemorrhagic contusion, for which MRI may be required to make the diagnosis. MRI can help by demonstrating the age of the chronic subdural hematoma. MR is a superior imaging modality, however, it is rarely used in acute head injury. MRI is more sensitive in identifying non-hemorrhagic contusion and diffuse axonal injury. MRI also demonstrate deep lesions in thalamus, brainstem and cerebellum. In chronic state MR scan demonstrate corpuscallosum degeneration following severe head injury with diffuse axonal injury. Traumatic brain injury (TBI) is the most common cause of death and disability in young people. The functional outcome in patients with TBI cannot be explained by focal pathology alone, and diffuse axonal injury (DAI) is considered a major contributor to the neurocognitive deficits experienced by this group. The Diffusion tensor imaging (DTI) offers additional information as to the extent of damage not visualized with standard magnetic resonance imaging (MRI) in patients with severe TBI.

Catheter angiography is indicated in post-traumatic aneurysms, traumatic dissection of internal carotid or vertebral arteries and caroticocavernous fistula. However, routine carotid angiography has now become investigation of the past with historical significance.

REFERENCES

1. New P, Aronow S. Attenuation measurements of whole blood and blood fractions in computed tomography. Radiology 1976;121:635–40.
2. Stein SC, Ross SE. Mild head injury: A Plea for routine early scanning. J. Trauma 1992;33:11–13.
3. Stiell IG, Well GA, Vandem heen 1C, et al. The Canadian CT head rule for patients with minor head injury. Lancet 2001;35:1391–6.
4. Jevet JS. Minor head injury and CT Scanning-Letter J. Trauma 1993;35:490–1.
5. Lei Gu, Jia Li, Dong-Fu Feng, Er-Tao Cheng, Dao-Chang Li, Xian-Qing Yang, Bo-Cheng Wang Journal of Trauma and Acute Care Surgery 2013;74(1):242–7.
6. The prognostic reliability of the Glasgow Coma Score in traumatic brain injuries: evaluation of MRI data D. Woischneck, R. Firsching, B. Schmitz, T. Kapapa European Journal of Trauma and Emergency Surgery Dec 2012.
7. Messé A, Caplain S, Paradot G, Garrigue D, Mineo JF, Ares GS, Ducreux D, Vignaud F, Rozec G, Desal H, Issac MP, Montreuil M, Benali H, Lehéricy S. Diffusion tensor imaging and white matter lesions at the subacute stage in mild traumatic brain injury with persistent neurobehavioral impairment, Human Brain Mapping 2011;32(6):999–1011.
8. Osborne AG, In diagnostic Neuroradiology, Mosby, Craniocerebral trauma 1994;199–244.
9. Lane B, Stevens JM, Moseley IF. Cranial and intracranial pathology[3]. In Grainger RG, Allison

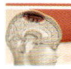

DJ (eds.), Grainger and Allison's Diagnostic Radiology, A Textbook of Medical Imaging, Churchill Livingstone 1997;2127–48.

10. Bruce DA, Alavi et al. Diffuse cerebral swelling following head injuries in children: The syndrome of "malignant brain edema/" J Neurosurg 1981;54:170–8.

11. Araujo JLV, Aguiar UP, Todeschini AB, Saade N, Veiga JCE. Epidemiological analysis of 210 cases of surgically treated traumatic extradural hematoma. Rev Col Bras Cir (periódico na Internet) 2012;39(4).

12. Imaizumi T, Horita Y, Honma T, Niwa J. Association between a black band on the inner membrane of a chronic subdural hematoma on T2*-weighted magnetic resonance images and enlargement of the hematoma. J Neurosurg 2003;99(5):824–30.

13. Graham DI, Hume Adams J, Nicoll JAR, Maxwell WL, Gennarelli TA. The nature, distribution and causes of traumatic brain injury. Brain Pathology 1995;5:397–406.

14. Kelly AB, Zimmerman RD, Snow RB, et al. Head trauma: Comparison of MR and CT - experience in 100 patients. AJNR 1988;699–708.

15. Gennarelli TA, Jhibault LE, Adam JH, et al. Diffuse axonal injury and traumatic coma in primate, Ann Neurol 1982;12:564–74.

16. Holshouser BA, Tong KA, Ashwal S. Proton MR spectroscopic imaging depicts diffuse axonal injury in children with traumatic brain injury. AJNR Am J Neuroradiol. 2005;26(5):1276–85.

17. Jian Xu, Inge-Andre Rasmussen, Jim Lagopoulos, and Asta Håberg. Journal of Neurotrauma. May 2007;24(5):753–65.
Detection of white matter lesions in the acute stage of diffuse axonal injury predicts long-term cognitive impairments.

18. Grados MA, Slomine BS, Gerring JP, Vasa R, Bryan N, Denckla MB: Depth of lesion model in children and adolescents with moderate to severe traumatic brain injury: use of SPGR MRI to predict severity and outcome. J Neurol Neurosurg Psychiatry 2001;70:350–8.

19. Gentry LR, Godersky JC, Thompson B: MR imaging of head trauma: review of the distribution and radiopathologic features of traumatic lesions. AJR Am J Roentgenol 1988;150: 663–72.

20. Skandsen T, Kvistad KA, Solheim O, et al. Prevalence and impact of diffuse axonal injury in patients with moderate and severe head injury: a cohort study of early magnetic resonance imaging findings and 1 year outcome. J Neurosurg Oct 23 2009.

21. Schrader H, Mickeviciene D, Gleizniene R, et al. Magnetic resonance imaging after most common form of concussion. BMC Med Imaging 2009; 9:11.

22. Schaefer PW, Grant PE, Gonzalez RG. Diffusion-weighted MR imaging of the brain. Radiology Nov 2000;217(2):331–45.

23. Galloway NR, Tong KA, Ashwal S, Oyoyo U, Obenaus A. Diffusion-weighted imaging improves outcome prediction in pediatric traumatic brain injury. J Neurotrauma 2008;25:1153–62.

24. Beauchamp MH, Ditchfield M, Babl FE et al. "Detecting traumatic brain lesions in children: CT versus MRI versus susceptibility weighted imaging (SWI), "Journal of Neurotrauma, 2011;28(6):915–27.

25. Taveras JM. Head Injuries and their Complications. Neuroradiology, 3rd edition, Williams & Wilkins 1996;327–64.

26. Johnson D, Hasso A, et al. Temporal bone trauma: High resolution computed tomographic evaluation. Radiology 1984;151:411–5.

27. Ozgen T, Tekkok IH, et al. CT cisternography in evaluation of cerebrospinal fluid rhinorrhoea. Neuroradiology 1989;32:481–4.

28. El Gammal T, Brooks BS: MR Cisternography: Initial experience in 41 cases. AJNR 1994;15: 1647–56.

29. Manelfe C. Cellerier P, et al. Cerebrospinal fluid rhinorrhea: Evaluation with metrizamide cisternography. AJNR 1982;3:25–30.

30. Cooper PR. Post-traumatic intracranial mass lesions. In Cooper PR, ed. Head injury. 2nd ed. Baltimore: Williams & Wilkins 1987;238–84.

31. Tsai FY, Teal JS, et al. Computed tomography of posterior fossa trauma. J Comput Assist Tomogr 1980;4:291–305.
Textbook of Diagnostic imaging 2nd edition, WB Saunders 1994;185–202.

32. Gentry LR, Godersky JC, Thompdon BH. Traumatic brainstem injury: MR imaging. Radiology 1989;171:177–87.

33. Bhatoe IH. Primary brainstem injury: Benign course and improved survival. Acta Neuro-Chirurg (Wien) 1999;141:315–9.

34. Taveras JM. Head Injuries and their complications, Neuroradiology, 3rd edn, Williams and Wilkins, Baltimore 1995;327–63.

35. Benoit BG, Wortzman G. Traumatic cerebral aneurysms: Clinical features and natural history. J Neurol Neurosurg Psychiatry 1973;36:127–38.

36. Kassell NF, Torner JC, et al. The international cooperative study on timing of aneurysm surgery. Part 1. Overall management results. J Neurosurg 1990;73:18–36.

37. Fleischer AS, Patton JM, Tindall GT. Cerebral aneurysms of traumatic origin. Surg Neurol 1975;4:233–9.

38. Kieck CF, de Villiers JC. Vascular lesions due to transcranial stab wounds. J. Neurosurg 1984; 60:42–46.

39. Crowell RM, Ogilvy CS. Traumatic Intracranial Aneurysms. In Ojemann RG, Ogilvy Cs Crowell RM, Heros RC (eds). Surgical Management of Neurovascular disease. Williams and Wilkins 1995;377–84.

40. Stringer WL, Kelly DL. Traumatic dissection of the extracranial internal carotid artery. Neurosurgery 1980;60:123–30.

41. Zelenock GB, Kazmers A, et al. Extracranial internal carotid artery dissections: Non-iatrogenic traumatic lesions. Arch Surg 1982;177:425–32.

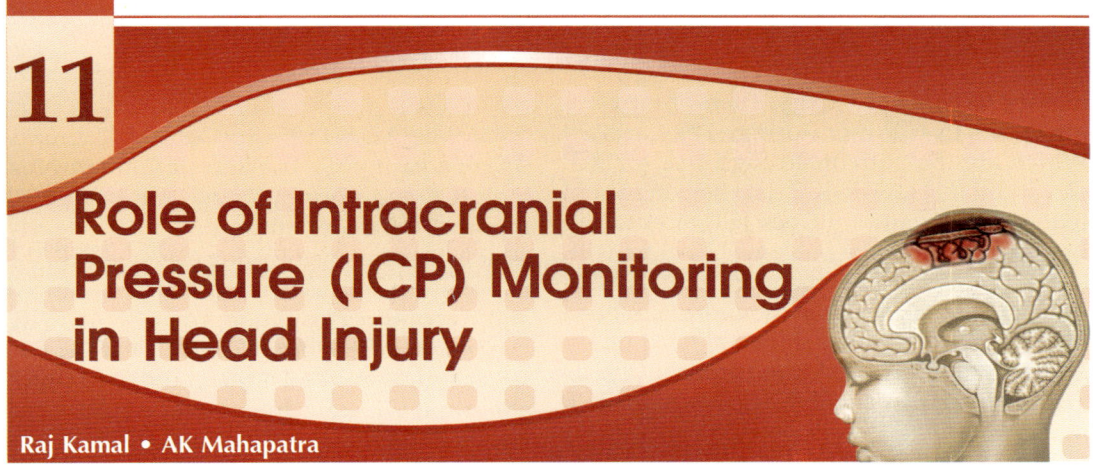

11

Role of Intracranial Pressure (ICP) Monitoring in Head Injury

Raj Kamal • AK Mahapatra

INTRODUCTION

The outcome of patients with head injury depends upon several factors, and most important among them is the raised **intracranial pressure** (ICP). Moreover, raised ICP is the most common cause of death, in patients with head injury. Uncontrolled intracranial hypertension produces secondary damage by reducing cerebral blood flow. However, surprisingly routine ICP monitoring in head injury is still continues to be a subject of controversy.[1–3] Lundberg[4,5] was the first person to introduce ICP monitoring. ICP is a reflection of the relationship between alterations in craniospinal volume and the ability of the craniospinal axis to accommodate added volume (hematoma or edema). The cranium is essentially a partially closed box which contains brain parenchyma, CSF and blood volume.[6] The properties of the container will determine what added volume can be absorbed before intracranial pressure begins to rise. So an understanding of raised ICP encompasses an analysis of both intracranial volume and craniospinal compliance and elastic elements. Today, ICP monitoring has gained a place in neurosurgical ICU management and become an integral part of ICU care. ICP monitoring is extensively studied in head injury patients in last two decades[1,7–10] either to establish its practical value for therapy or as a prognostic factor.[11–15] Surprisingly,

however, there are neither clear-cut guidelines for ICP monitoring nor there is uniform policy for duration of ICP recording. Increased ICP has been defined as pressure more than 20 mm Hg for more than 5 minutes.[14,15] Several studies linked high level of ICP with high mortality and morbidity. Persistent raised ICP has a direct effect on the brain tissue inspite of cerebral perfusion pressure being normal. ICP monitoring is recommended as per indications (Table 11.1).

Table 11.1: Indications for ICP monitoring in head injury[16]

Brain Trauma Foundation[16] recommends ICP monitoring in

1. All patients with severe TBI (GCS between 3 and 8 after resuscitation) and an abnormal CT scan that reveals hematomas, contusions, swelling, herniation or compressed cisterns (Level II recommendation)
2. Patients with severe TBI with normal CT scan if two or more features are noted at admission: age over 40 years, unilateral or bilateral motor posturing, or systolic BP < 90 mm of Hg (Level III recommendation)

INDICATIONS FOR ICP MONITORING

Indications for ICP monitoring have changed in last 15 years since routine CT scans are available worldwide. Almost all major head injury centers use ICP monitoring in the management of head injury. There are few key questions in ICP monitoring. They are: *(a)* Which are the patients at high risk for ICP elevation? *(b)* How do ICP data help in patient management? and *(c)* Does ICP monitoring improve the ultimate outcome? Dealing with above points, till 1996 there are a total of 146 published articles on ICP monitoring in head injury, forty-one publications on head injury and ICP monitoring. More importantly, 27 articles have dealt with indications for ICP monitoring.

Brain Trauma Foundation (BTF) guide-lines[16] suggest that ICP monitoring is pri-marily used when there is difficulty in clinical assessment of the patient or if there is a high risk of increased ICP. ICP monitoring is not necessary in the awake patient, in whom clinical assessment of neurological status is possible, and is contraindicated in the patient with a bleeding diathesis. In the latter case, all effort should be made to correct this if ICP monitoring is required.

Patients with head injury not requiring ICP monitoring: Patients less than 40 years without evidence of abnormal motor activity, with normal pupillary examinations, with no significant history of secondary brain insults, and with CT scans showing no pathology and open basilar cisterns.

Farahvar et al[17] studied 2134 patients with severe TBI [Glasgow Coma Scale (GCS) score < 9], 1446 patients were treated with ICP-lowering therapies. Of those, 1202 had an ICP monitor inserted and 244 were treated without monitoring. This database also contains information on known independent early prognostic indicators of mortality, including age, admission GCS score, pupillary status, CT scanning findings, and hypotension. In patients with severe TBI treated for intra-cranial hypertension, the use of an ICP monitor is associated with significantly lower mortality when compared with patients treated without an ICP monitor. Based on these findings, the authors concluded that ICP-directed therapy in patients with severe TBI should be guided by ICP monitoring.

Which Patients are at High Risk of Raised ICP?

Severe head injury: The correlation between high ICP and poor outcomes has been well reported by many authors.[18–20] It is clearly established that by lowering elevated ICP, the risk of transtentorial herniation is also reduced and cerebral perfusion improves.[9,12] In 1982, Narayan et al[12] reported 53–63% raised ICP in severe closed head injury patients with abnormal CT scan. In contrast severe head injury patients with a normal CT had 13% incidence of raised ICP. There were 3 adverse factors in normal CT scan group, those were *(a)* patients above 40 years of age, *(b)* unilateral or bilateral posturing and *(c)* patients with systolic BP lower than 90 mm of Hg. The risk of raised ICP was similar to those patients with abnormal CT.

MINOR AND MODERATE HEAD INJURY

It is an accepted belief that the patients with mild or moderate head injury, risk of raised ICP is low. The incidence of raised ICP in minor head injury is 3% and in moderate head injury 10–20%. Thus, routine ICP monitoring not indicated in mild head injury.[21–27] However, sometimes patients with minor head injury may need repeated CT scan and ICP monitoring.

Considering all above points and avail-ability of facilities one can decide his own indications. However, we feel the rational indication of ICP monitoring in head injury as follows:

a. All patients with severe head injury with mass lesion with midline shift or com-pression of the ventricles or cisterns.
b. Patients with good coma scale with hema-tomas diagnosed in CT scan.
c. Patients with multiple small intracranial hematoma and not meriting a surgical evacuation.
d. Patients with diffuse swelling, who needs aggressive management.
e. Patients with multiple hematomas of which the only largest one is being removed.

f. Postoperative ICP monitoring after evacuation of hematoma.

Pathophysiology

Normally, resting ICP is 5 to 15 mm. Transient elevations of ICP occurs normally with straining, coughing or the trendelenburg position. A sustained ICP greater than 20 mm Hg is clearly abnormal. An ICP between 20 and 40 mm Hg is considered moderate intracranial hypertension. An ICP greater than 40 mm Hg represents severe, usually life-threatening intracranial hypertension.[4,5] About 50% of the patients with severe head injury will develop increased intracranial pressure. Increased ICP occurs in 50–70% of patients even after evacuation of intracranial hematoma.

The cranium and the vertebral canal, along with the relatively inelastic dura, form a rigid container, such that the increase in any of its contents; brain, blood, or CSF, will tend to increase the ICP. In addition, any increase in one of the components must be at the expense of the other two; this relationship is known as the Monro-Kellie doctrine. Rigid bony skull offers excellent protection to brain but allows little tolerance for additional volume. The intracranial contents include brain 1400 g of which 80% is water, 75 ml of CSF mostly in ventricles, 75 ml of blood mostly in post capillary venous circulation.

Brain parenchyma account for most of the intracranial content. A 4-yr-old boy is least able to accommodate mass lesion than an elderly man. Apart from removing brain tissue or shrinking it with diuretics, the cell mass cannot be decreased.

Small increases in brain volume do not lead to immediate increase in ICP because of the ability of the CSF to be displaced into the spinal canal, as well as the slight ability to stretch the falx cerebri between the hemispheres and the tentorium between the hemispheres and the cerebellum. As the intracranial volume increases, compensation takes place and the ICP remains stable up to a point at which decompensation begins to occur, and then the ICP rises dramatically. On that part of the intracranial compliance curve where the pressure suddenly increases (Fig. 11.1), a small rise in volume will cause a dramatic increase in the ICP and will further reduce cerebral perfusion. Similarly, meticulous care of a patient who is functioning on this part of the curve can be rewarding. Any small decrease in intracranial volume that can be achieved, e.g. by sitting the patient up, keeping the head straight, using adequate sedation) can have a dramatic effect in bringing the ICP down. **Meticulous nursing care is crucial to outcomes for patients with increased ICP.**

The compliance (C) describes the volume-dependent increase of the pressure in the craniospinal space and can be used for the assessment of the cerebrospinal space reserves. The inversion is termed elastance (E) (Figs 11.1a and b).

Marmarou[28,29] demonstrated that the non-linear craniospinal volume–pressure relationship could be described as a straight line segment relating the logarithm of pressure to volume, which implies a monoexponential relationship between volume and pressure. Marmarou termed the pressure–volume index (PVI) which is the imaginary volume required to raise ICP tenfold. PVI is calculated from pressure changes by injecting or withdrawing CSF. Higher values of PVI indicates higher brain compliance. Practically, this means that withdrawing 10–15 ml of CSF through ventriculostomy could reduce ICP significantly.

For example, an increase in lesion volume (e.g. epidural hematoma) will be compensated by the downward displacement of CSF and venous blood. These compensatory mechanisms are able to maintain a normal ICP for any change in volume less than approximately 100–120 ml.

The cerebral perfusion pressure (CPP) is equivalent to the mean arterial pressure (MAP) minus the ICP.

$$CPP = MAP - ICP$$

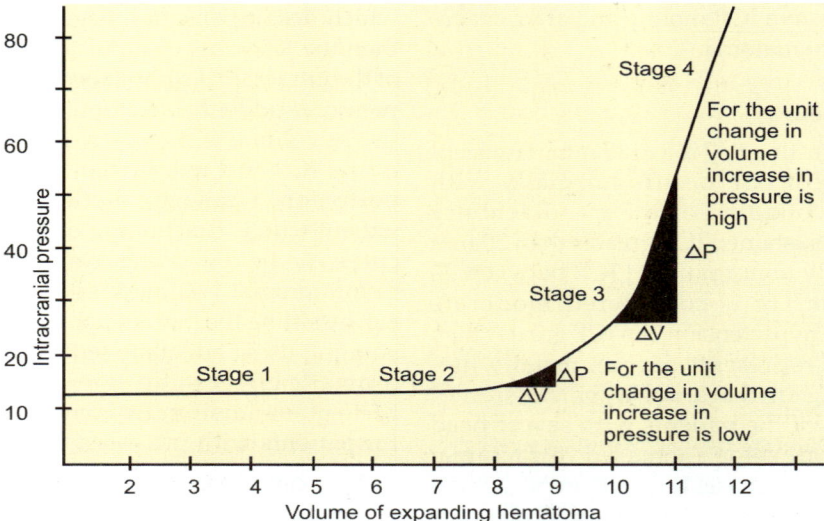

Fig. 11.1a: Graph shows the ICP-volume relationship. The change in pressure *dP* due to change in unit volume dV increases linearly with increased ICP. ICP elastance curve (change in pressure per unit change in volume; dP/dV)

Stage 1/2 = compensation phase. As one of the intracranial constituents increases in volume, the other two constituents decrease in volume in order to keep the intracranial pressure constant. Stage 3/4 = decompensated phase. When compensatory mechanisms are exhausted, small increases in the volumes of intracranial hematoma cause large increases in ICP.

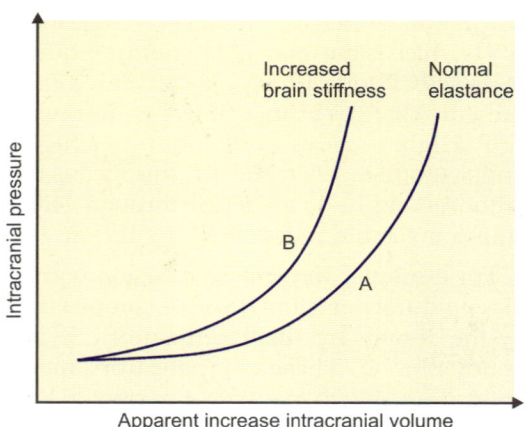

Fig. 11.1b: Two intracranial compliance or elastance curves. Curve A represents the normal situation. Curve B represents the situation with a fast increase in volume or when the compensatory mechanism is already partially exhausted by pre-existing pathology, i.e. edema or contusion hematoma

Severe head injury can cause impairment or loss of autoregulation–hence, decrease in cerebrovascular resistance, which can lead to raised ICP in both adults and children.[16,23] The principal strategy for managing head injury is to reduce the frequency and severity of secondary brain insults from intracranial pressure (ICP) and cerebral perfusion pressure (CPP), and hence improve outcome. In an experimental study of CBF by, Miller[24,27] demonstrated. In an experimental study of CBF as determined by the venous outflow technique in dogs, Miller[24,26,27] demonstrated that, when MAP and ICP rise in parallel so that CPP remains constant at about 60 mm Hg. His work also suggested that cerebral perfusion is more sensitive to arterial hypotension than to intracranial hypertension. The clinical significance of this information is that in the management of head injury it is often necessary to employ therapy to lower raised ICP. Therapeutic agents for reducing raised

ICP often do so at the expense of reduced MAP and as a consequence CPP may not improve. If autoregulation is preserved, CBF should remain unchanged despite parallel changes in MAP and ICP.

The association between the severity of intracranial hypertension and a poor outcome after severe head injury is well recognised. Miller, et al.[8,24] reported that mortality rate increased from 18 to 92% and the frequency of good outcomes decreased from 74 to 3% in patients with normal ICP compared with patients who had intracranial hypertension that could not be reduced below 20 mm Hg. Saul and Dicker[30] reported a 69% mortality rate in patients with an ICP greater than 25 mm Hg, compared with a mortality rate of 15% if ICP remained less than 25 mm Hg.[30]

Methods of ICP Monitoring (Table 11.2)

Two types of ICP monitoring devices are available:
1. Fluid coupled catheter transducer systems
2. Non-fluid coupled catheter transducer systems.

The standard intraventricular catheter connected to an external strain gauge transducer is termed a catheter-transducer system because it behaves, in many ways, like a mechanical system with a mass of fluid that acts against the spring-like elastic properties of the catheter walls and the transducer diaphragm.

The fluid coupled devices are placed in ventricles, subarachnoid space or the subdural spaces and are connected to a pressure transducer through a fluid filled line. The ventriculostomy catheter remains the **gold standard** against which all of the newer monitors are compared. This method allows the clinician to check for zero drift and the sensitivity of the measurement system *in vivo*. Ventricular catheter also allows cerebrospinal fluid drainage for therapeutic purposes. It can be placed easily and quickly in most patients with head trauma, even those with mass effect. Disadvantages of ventricular catheter include infection rate of 8 to 10% and 1 to 2% risk of intracranial hemorrhage.[4]

The Head Injury Management Guidelines published by the Brain Trauma Foundation[16,30] recommended intraventricular ICP measurement as the first-line approach to monitoring ICP: **Subdural bolt (Richmond Screws)** which is placed in subdural space is less invasive. Subdural and epidural devices are comparatively less reliable and higher rate of blockage. Richmond screw is inserted by making a twist drill hole at a site, 3 cm lateral to midline and 1 cm infront of coronal suture. Dura and arachnoid are coagulated and cut, allowing the CSF to flow, then the bolt is

Method	Advantages	Disadvantages
Table 11.2: Intracranial pressure monitoring catheters[6]		
Intraventricular	• Gold standard • Measures global values • Allows drainage of CSF • *In vivo* calibration	• Insertion may be difficult • Most invasive method • Risk of hematoma
Microtransducer system	• Intraparenchymal/ subdural placement • Low complication risk • Low infection risk	• Small zero drift over time • No *in vivo* calibration • Measures local pressure
Epidural catheter	• Easy to insert • No penetration of dura	• Limited accuracy • Rarely used

CSF: Cerebrospinal fluid

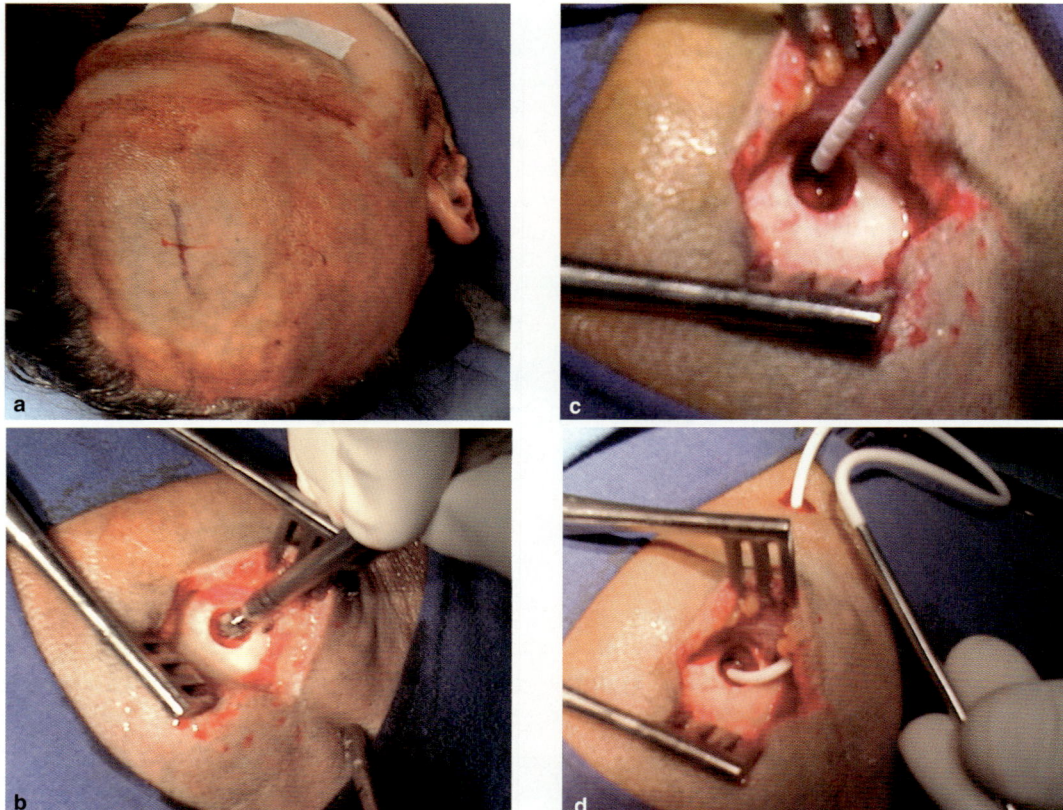

Figs 11.2a to d: Figure showing steps of placement of ventricular catheter in right frontal horn with subcutaneous tunnel. (a) Skin mark; 3 cm lateral and 1 cm anterior to coronal suture (right), (b) Right frontal burr hole, (c) Introduction of ventricular catheter, (d) Subcutaneous tunnel and connection to ICP monitor

tightened in the hole, after proper hemostasis. Intraventricular catheters are placed through a drill hole at the same site and the catheter is placed in the right frontal horn (Figs 11.2a to d). In the operated cases, a catheter can be left at the operation cavity for ICP monitoring.

Despite the existence of these guidelines, catheter tip intraparenchymal pressure monitoring remains popular, particularly in the United Kingdom, because it does not require catheter placement in the operating theater and thus requires significantly fewer resources. The two most frequently used catheter tip systems in the management of patients with head injuries are the Codman and Camino systems. Neither allows a pressure calibration to be performed *in vivo*. After these systems are zeroed relative to atmospheric pressure during a preinsertion calibration, their pressure output is dependent on zero drift of the sensor.

A ventricular catheter connected to an external strain gauge is the most accurate and low cost method for ICP monitoring. It also allows periodic re-zeroing. Presently most common method of ICP monitoring is probably intraparenchymal catheters. Both systems are accurate but they have been reported to zero-drift over 4–5 days. Most neurosurgeons use ICP only for short time, hence these shortcomings may become irrelevant. The Codman ICP Express Monitoring

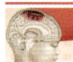
System is one such popular system readily available and gives real time accurate ICP readings, so one can make timely decisions on surgical or medical aspects, contributing to good outcome.[33] The Codman ICP Monitoring System (Fig. 11.3) provides accurate measurements of intracranial pressure at the source-subdural, parenchymal or intraventricular levels. The information is relayed electronically rather than through a hydrostatic column or fiberoptics.

Simple, Reliable Choice for Monitoring ICP

The ICP express is a digital intracranial pressure (ICP) monitor that also serves as an interface between the Codman Microsensor™ ICP transducer and patient monitors.

Non-fluid coupled system such as the Camino intraparenchymal monitor is placed within the parenchyma, and therefore, is not subjected to the discontinuities of pressure transmission afforded by the subarachnoid or dural layers and it is not prone to clogging. This system is expensive and the risks involved are similar to the fluid compiled systems.

Both intracavitary and intraventricular catheters are taken out at least 5 cm away from

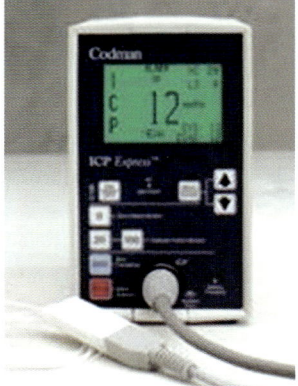

Fig. 11.3: The Codman® ICP monitoring system (the ICP express) provides accurate measurements of intracranial pressure at the source-subdural, parenchymal or intraventricular levels. The information is relayed electronically rather than through a hydrostatic column or fiberoptics

the main wound, through a subcutaneous tunnel. This is basically to prevent infection.

After placement of the catheter or a screw, all the devices are connected through a fluid filled line (containing antibiotic and saline solution) to a strain gauze transducer, zeroed at the level of external auditory meatus. The recording are made using monitor which provides waveform, as well as 24 hours trends and absolute values at an adjustable present time interval. ICP is monitored 24–48 hours. The patients are prescribed systemic antibiotics to reduce the risk of infection.

Duration of ICP Monitoring

It is difficult to decide the optimum duration of ICP monitoring in head injury. Sometimes the ICP can remain high for a long duration, as many systemic factors can give rise to brain swelling and prolong the duration of raised ICP. Thus, duration of raised ICP is unpredictable, and there is phenomenon of secondary rise of intracranial pressure. Most of the reports indicate ICP monitoring 48–72 hours[8,34,35] (Fig. 11.4). ICP monitoring for longer period increases the risk of infection. However, in patients with moderate to severe brain swelling and sustained raised ICP (Fig. 11.4), the duration of ICP monitoring may extend a longer period. The rationale of monitoring ICP for 5–6 days is due to well accepted clinical experience, that the intracranial hypertension is maximum between 48 and 72 hours following trauma. In a few patients, secondary raised ICP can occurs, between 7 and 10 days after trauma.[36]

HOW DOES ICP MONITORING INFLUENCE HEAD INJURY MANAGEMENT?

Intraventricular pressure monitoring help in assessing the level of ICP and also allow CSF drainage. However, primarily may guide the therapy.[2,3,9] It is a well known fact that one cannot ascertain level of ICP just looking at the clinical state, or pupillary size. Rise in ICP can guide to go for an early CT scan and diagnose or predict increase in contusion hematoma (Figs 11.5a to c).

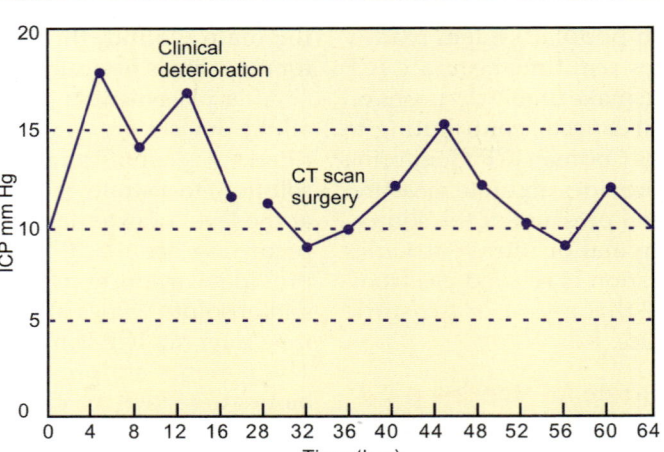

Fig. 11.4: ICP recording graph shows initially 12 hours ICP was mildly elevated then ICP remained normal

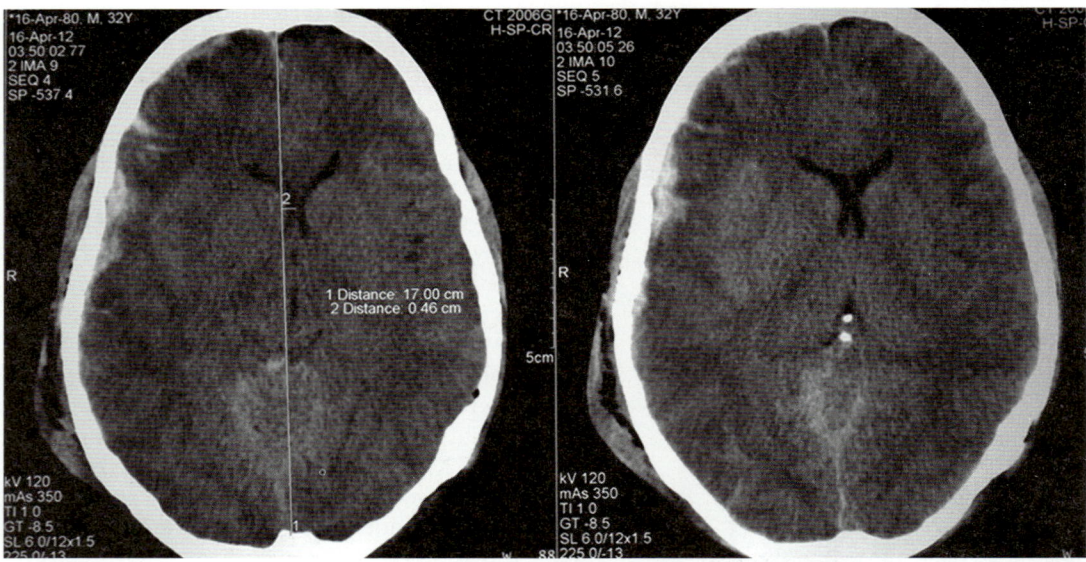

Fig. 11.5a: CT scan on admission, ICP monitoring shows increase in ICP to 30 mm Hg (initial was 18 mm Hg). Hence, immediately CT was repeated (Fig. 11.5b)

On the other hand, all the therapeutic modalities to control raised ICP are double-edged sword. For example, prolonged use of I/V mannitol create problem and prolonged **hyperventilation** has been conclusively shown to worsen the outcome in severe head injured patients. Hyperventilation reduces the PCO_2, leading to vasoconstriction and causes ischemic damage.[11,37] Surprisingly, **hyperventilation** is still liberally used in the management of head injury to reduce ICP.[38] The role of mannitol is also unpredictable, both the extent and the duration of action.[39,40] ICP recording not only helps in guiding therapy, but also helps in predicting the outcome.[1,9,14,15]

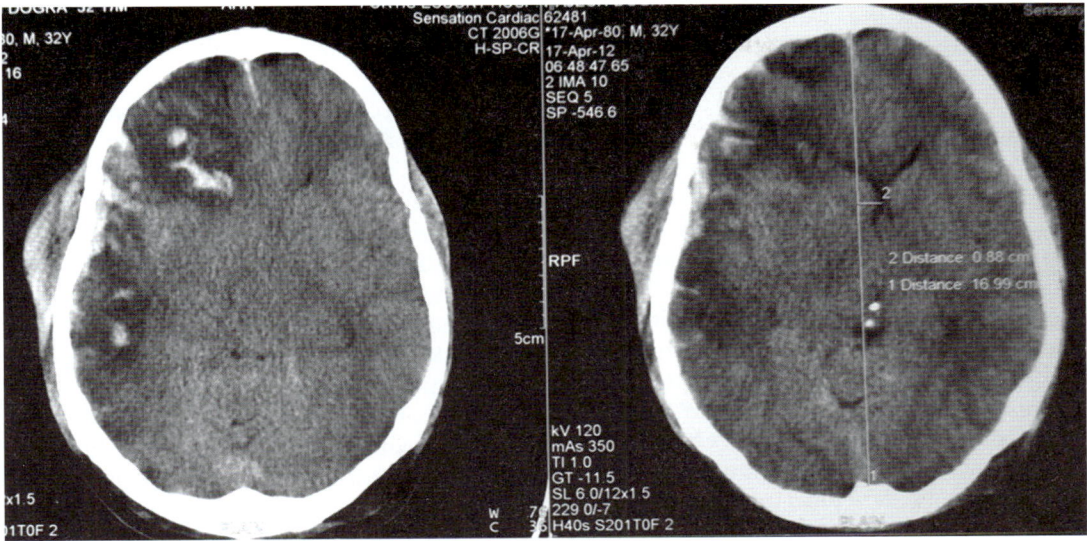

Fig. 11.5b: Repeat CT scan shows gross increase in right frontal and temporal contusion with midline shift. Immediately surgery was done (Fig. 11.5c)

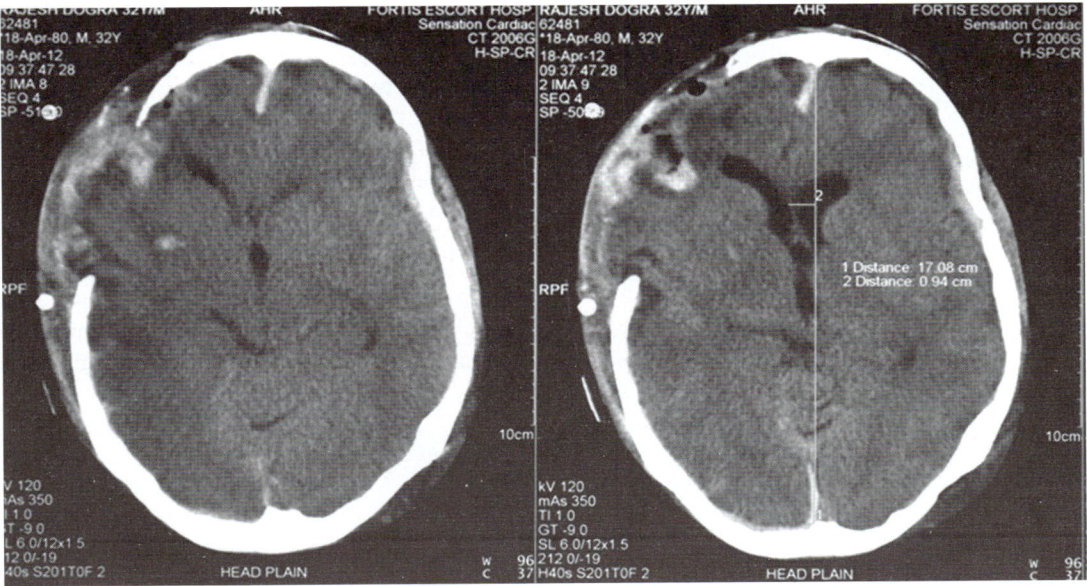

Fig. 11.5c: Postoperative CT scan showing good decompression. Midline shift was corrected. Patient survived with excellent results

Timofeev et al[36] retrospectively analysed outcomes for severe TBI patients (n = 49) treated for intractable ICH with decompressive craniectomy. Of 27 patients for whom pre- and post-surgical ICP was measured, mean ICP decreased from 25 ± 6 to 16 ± mm

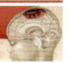
Hg (p < 0.01). Of the entire sample, 61.2% had a good recovery.

ICP and Outcome (Tables 11.3 and 11.4)

Intracranial pressure monitoring improves the mortality from head injury. Patients who respond to ICP-lowering treatment had a 64% lower risk of death at 2 weeks than those who did not respond after adjusting for factors that independently predict risk of death.[18] In 1977 Jennett et al[42] reported mortality in severe head injury around 50%. Subsequently other authors reported lower mortality with aggressive treatment.[1,8,9,14,43,44] The aggressive management means ICU care, ventilation and ICP monitoring. Saul and Ducker[30] treated two groups of severe head injury patients with mannitol and CSF drainage. In the patients in whom ICP was between 20 and 25 mm Hg had a 46% mortality as compared to 28% mortality in patients in whom ICP was 15 mm of Hg. In our study,[11] 65% patients had raised ICP. Only 26% patients with mass lesion had a normal ICP as compared to 67% normal ICP when CT scan did not reveal mass lesion. In 12 patients ICP was more than 30 mm of Hg. Overall 52%

patients with raised ICP had poor outcome and only 15% had a good outcome (Table 11.4).

The improved outcome of patients with severe head injuries in US has been ascribed to aggressive management protocol, which includes ICP monitoring and drainage of CSF to control ICP.[15,45,52]

Raised ICP has in the past been found to be associated with a poorer outcome from injury with the higher the level of ICP, particularly the peak ICP level, correlating with the expected prognosis for mortality and morbidity.[44,46] There has, however, been controversy over the usefulness of monitoring raised ICP with some groups, with a 'no ICP monitoring' policy, finding in their studies of head injury mortality and morbidity that outcome is similar to other groups that do monitor ICP. Narayan et al[47] in a prospective study in 133 severely head injured patients, demonstrated that the outcome prediction rate was increased when the standard clinical data, such as age, Glasgow Coma Score (GCS) on admission and pupillary response with extraocular and motor activity, was combined with ICP monitoring data. Recently, Chestnut et al[46] conducted a multicenter, controlled trial in which 324 patients 13 years of age or older who had severe traumatic brain injury and were being treated in intensive care units (ICUs). In the first group protocol for monitoring intraparenchymal intracranial pressure was used (pressure-monitoring group) and in

---

Table 11.3: Key prognostic factors

Key prognostic factors in outcome

1. ICP > 20 mm Hg
2. Arterial pressure < 80 mm Hg
3. CPP < 50 mm Hg
4. No response to ICP-lowering treatment[18]

Table 11.4: Outcome of head injury correlated to ICP

Authors	No. of patients	ICP (mm Hg)	Good / moderate%	Dead/ disabled%
1. Becker et al[9] 1977	160	> 20/40	60	30
2. Miller et al[8] 1977	225	> 25	56	34
3. Narayan et al[47] 1982	207	> 25	57	34
4. Smith et al[35] 1986	37	> 25	54	35
5. Saul & Ducker[30] 1982	127	> 25	–	46
6. Ghajar, et al[38] 1995	34	> 15	59	12
7. Timofeev, et al[36] 2006	27	> 16	61	18.4

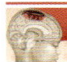

second group, a protocol in which treatment was based on imaging and clinical examination (imaging–clinical examination group) was used. They concluded that care focused on maintaining monitored intracranial pressure at 20 mm Hg or less was not shown to be superior to care based on imaging and clinical examination.[45]

Marmarou et al[28] reporting on 428 patients' data from the National Institute of Health's Traumatic Coma Data Bank, showed that, following the usual clinical signs of age, admission motor score and abnormal pupils, the proportion of hourly ICP recordings greater than 20 mm Hg was the next most significant predictor of outcome. They also found, using stepwise logistic regression, that, following ICP, arterial pressure below 80 mm Hg was also a significant predictor of outcome. Jones et al studied prospectively 124 adult head-injured patients during intensive care using a computerized data collection system capable of minute-by-minute monitoring of up to 14 clinically indicated physiological variables. They found that ICP above 30 mm Hg, arterial pressure below 90 mm Hg and cerebral perfusion pressure below 50 mm Hg significantly affected patient morbidity.

LIMITATIONS OF ICP MONITORING

The **Brain Trauma Foundation (BTF)** guidelines[16] have been endorsed by the American Association of Neurological Surgeons, the World Health Organization (WHO) Neurotrauma Committee. The guidelines provide medical personnel a protocol which has been proven to improve the survival and outcomes of TBI patients and has been shown to reduce rates of mortality.[49-51] There is a little doubt about the beneficial role of ICP monitoring in head injury. However, the routine ICP monitoring use has not been widely used in India. The basic problem is that the ICP monitoring is an invasive method and require a good ICU care. The complication of ICP monitoring is not infrequent. The frequent problem is the blocking of the device or dampened tracings.

Infections and hematoma formation are two other complications. Narayan et al[47] in 1982 reported 6.3% infection and 1.4% intracranial hemorrhage in patients undergoing ICP monitoring. In a study at AIIMS, 6% infection rate was observed in patients who had an ICP monitoring. Fortunately, there was no incident of intracranial hematoma in patients, in whom ICP monitoring was carried out.

CONCLUSIONS

ICP monitoring helps in early detection of intracranial mass, limits the indiscriminate use of therapeutic modalities to reduce raised ICP, can reduce ICP by allowing the CSF drainage, and helps in prognosticating the outcome. Routine ICP monitoring is not indicated in minor or moderate head injury, except in patients with large intracranial hematoma, when the treating neurosurgeon feels the possibility of raised ICP. Blockage is the most frequent cause for discontinuing ICP monitoring, while infection such as meningitis is the most dangerous complication. Even with all above, ICP monitoring deserve a special place in the management of head injury.

REFERENCES

1. Marshall LF, Smith RW, Shapiro, HM. The outcome with aggressive treatment in severe head injury. Part I. The significance of intracranial pressure monitoring. J Neurosurg 1979;80:20–25.
2. Chesnut RM, Crisp CB, Klauber MR, et al. Early routine paralysis for intracranial pressure control in severe head injury: Is it necessary? Crit Care Med 1994;22:1471–76.
3. Feldman Z, Narayan RK. Intracranial pressure monitoring. Techniques and pitfalls. In: Cooper PR (eds) Head injury 3rd Ed of Williams and Wilkins, Baltimore 1993.
4. Lundberg N. Continuous recording and control of ventricular fluid pressure in neurosurgical practice. Acta Psychiatr Neurol Scand (Suppl) 1960;36:1–193.
5. Lundberg N, Troupp H and Lorin H. Continuous recording of the ventricular fluid pressure in patients with severe acute traumatic brain injury. Journal of Neurosurgery 1965;22, 581–90.

6. Flavio MB. Maciel, Central Nervous System Monitoring, In AntoninoGullo, José Besso, Philip D. Lumb, Ged F. Williams (Eds.) Intensive and Critical Care Medicine, WFSICCM World Federation of Societies of Intensive and Critical Care Medicine 2009;135–43.

7. Johnston IH, Johnston JA, Jennett WB. Intracranial pressure following head injury. Lancet 1970;2:433–6.

8. Miller JD, Decker CD, Ward JD, et al. Significance of intracranial hypertension in severe head injury. J Neurosurg 1977;47:563–76.

9. Becker DP, Miller JD, Ward JD, et al. The outcome from severe head injury with early diagnosis and intensive management. J Neurosurg 1977;47:491–502.

10. Badri S, Chen J, Barber J, Tempin NR, Dikmen SS, Chestnut RM, Deem S, Yanez ND, Treggiari MM. Mortality and long term functional outcome associated with intracranial pressure after traumatic brain injury. Intensive Care Medicine 2012;38:1800–9.

11. Mahapatra AK, Bansal S. Role of ICP monitoring in head injury. A prospective study. Neurology India 1998;46:109–14.

12. Narayan RK, Kishore PR, Becker DP, et al. Intracranial pressure to monitor or not to monitor ?A review of our experience with severe head injury. I Neurosurg 1982;56:650–9.

13. Miller JD. ICP monitoring-current states and future direction.ActaNeurochir 1987;85:80–86.

14. Miller JD, Butterworth JF, Gudeman SK, et al. Further experience in management of severe head injury. J Neurosurg 1981;54:289–99.

15. Bullock MR, Chestnut RM, Clifton GL, et al. Intracranial pressure treatment threshold J. Neurotrauma 2000;17:493–5.

16. Brain Trauma Foundation; American Association of Neurological Surgeons; Congress of Neurological Surgeons; Joint Section on Neurotrauma and Critical Care, AANS/CNS, Bratton SL, Chestnut RM, Ghajar J, McConnell Hammond FF, Harris OA, Hartl R, Manley GT, Nemecek A, Newell DW, Rosenthal G, Schouten J, Shutter L, Timmons SD, Ullman JS, Videtta W, Wilberger JE, Wright DW . Guidelines for the management of severe traumatic brain injury. VIII. Intracranial pressure thresholds. J Neurotrauma 2008;24:S55–8.

17. Farahvar A, Gerber LM, Chiu YL, Carney N, Härtl R, Ghajar J. Increased mortality in patients with severe traumatic brain injury treated without intracranial pressure monitoring. J Neurosurg 2012;117:729–34.

18. Farahvar A, Gerber LM, Chiu YL, Härtl R, Froelich M, Carney N, Ghajar J. Response to intracranial hypertension treatment as a predictor of death in patients with severe traumatic braininjury. J Neurosurg 2011;114: 1471–8.

19. Marmarou A, Anderson RL, Ward JD, et al. Impact of ICP instability and hypotension on outcome in patients with severe head trauma. J Neurosurg 1991;75:S59–66.

20. Marshall LF, Gautille T, Klauber MR, et al. The outcome of severe closed head injury. J Neurosurg 1991;75:528–36.

21. Eisenber HM, Gary HE Jr, Aldrich EF, et al. Initial CT findings in 753 patients with severe head injury. A report from the NIH Traumatic coma data Bank. J Neurosurg 1990;73;688–98.

22. Stein SC, Ross SE. Mild Head injury: a Plea for routine early CT scanning J. Trauma 1992;33:11–13.14b. Jevet JS.Minor head injury and CT Scanning. Letter J. Trauma 1993;35:490–1.

23. Muizelaar JP, Marmarou A, Ward JD, et al. Adverse effects of prolonged hyperventilation in patients with severe head injury. A randomized clinical trial. J Neurosurg 1991;5:731–9.

24. Miller JD. Volume and pressure in the craniospinal axis. Clinical Neurosurgery, 1975;22:76–105. Miller JD and Adams JH. The pathophysiology of raised intracranial pressure, in Greenfield's Neuropathology, 5th edn, (eds J. H. Adams and L. W. Duchen), Edward Arnold, Sevenoaks 1992;69–105.

25. Chambers IR, Jones PA, Lo, TYM, Forsyth RJ, Fulton B, Andrews PJD, Mendelow AD, Minns, RA. Critical thresholds of intracranial pressure and cerebral perfusion pressure related to age in pediatric head injury. Journal of Neurology, Neurosurgery, and Psychiatry 2005;77:234–40.

26. Miller JD, Becker DP, Ward JD, et al. Significance of intracranial hypertension in severe head injury. Journal of Neurosurgery 1977;47:503–16.

27. Miller JD, Garibi J, Pickard JD. Induced changes of cerebrospinal fluid volume: effects during continuous monitoring of ventricular fluid pressure. Archives of Neurology 1973;28: 265–9.

28. Marmarou A, Maset AL, Ward JD, et al. Contribution of CSF and vascular factors to elevation of ICP in severely head-injured patients. Journal of Neurosurgery 1987;66:883–90.

29. Marmarou A, Foda MA, Bandoh K, et al. Elevated venous outflow pressure in head injured patients, in Intracranial Pressure VIII,

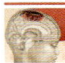

(eds CJJ Avezaat, JHM van Eindhoven, AIR Maas and JTJ Tans), Springer-Verlag, Berlin 1993;712–5.

30. Saul TG, Ducker TB; Effect of intracranial pressure monitoring and aggressive treatment on mortality in severe head injury. J Neurosurg 1982;56:498–503.

31. Piper IR, Chan KH, Whittle IR and Miller JD. An experimental study of cerebrovascular resistance, pressure transmission and craniospinal compliance. Neurosurgery 1936;32:805–16.

32. Unterberg A, Kiening K, Schmiedek P, Lanksch W. Long-term observation of intracranial pressure after severe head injury. The phenomenon of secondary rise of intracranial pressure. Neurosurg 1993;32:17–24.

33. Gupta DK, Mahapatra AK, Kumar H, Monitoring in Patients with Traumatic Brain Injury: an Experience of 98 cases. Indian Journal of Neurotrauma 2006;3:31–36.

34. Jane JA, Luerssen TG, Marmarou A, Foulkes MA. The outcome of severe closed head injury. J Neurosurg, 75 (Suppl) 1991;S28–36.

35. Smith HP, Kelly DL Jr., Me Whorter JM. et al. Comparison of mannitol regimens in patients with severe head injury undergoing intracranial pressure monitoring. J Neurosurg, 1986;65: 820–24.

36. Timofeev I, Kirkpatrick PJ, Corteen E, Hiler M, Czosnyka M, Menon DK, Pickard JD, Hutchinson PJ. Decompressive craniectomy in traumatic brain injury: outcome following protocol-driven therapy. Acta Neurochir (Suppl) 2006;96:11–6.

37. Gopinath SP, Robertson CS, Contant CF. et al. Jugular venous desaturation and outcome after head injury. J Neurol Neurosurg and Psychiat, 1994;57:717–23.

38. Ghajar JB, Ha, R, Narayan RK, et al. Survey of critical care management of comatose head injured patients in the United States: Crit Care Med 1995;23:560–67.

39. Marshall, LF, Smith RW, Ranscher IA, et al. Mannitol dose requirements in brain injured patients. J Neurosurg 1978;48:169–72.

40. Mendelow AD, Teasdale GM, Russell T et al. Effect of mannitol on cerebral blood flow and cerebral perfusion pressure in human head injury. J Neurosurg 1985;63:43–48.

41. Narayan RK, Greenberg RP, Miller JD, et al. Improved confidence of outcome prediction in severe head injury: A comparative analysis of

clinical examination, multimodal evoked potentials, CT scanning and intracranial pressure. J Neurosurg 1981;54:751–62.

42. Jennett B, Teasdale G, Galbraith S *et al.* Severe head injury in three countries. J Neurol Neurosurg Psychiat 1977;40:291–5.

43. Lane, PL, Storetz TG, Doig G, et al. Intracranial pressure monitoring and outcome after traumatic brain injury. Can J. Surg 2000;43:442–8.

44. Goldstein B, Powers ICS Head trauma in children. Peditr. Rev 1994;15:213–9.

45. Bullock MR, Chernut RM, Clifton GL, et al. Critical pathways for treatment of established intracranial hypertension. J Neurotrauma 2000;17:537–47.

46. Chesnut RM, Temkin N, Carney N, Dikmen S, Rondina C, Videtta W, Petroni G, Pridgeon SLJ, Barber J, Machamer J, Chaddock K, Celix JM, Cherner M, and Hendrix T, A Trial of Intracranial-Pressure Monitoring in Traumatic Brain Injury. N Engl J Med 2012; 367:2471–81.

47. Narayan RK, Kishore PRS, Becker DP, et al. Intracranial pressure: to monitor or not to monitor: a review of our experience with severe head injury. Journal of Neurosurgery 1982;56: 650–9.

48. Jones PA, Andrews PJD, Midgley S, et al. Measuring the burden of secondary insults in head-injured patients during intensive care. Journal of Neurosurgery and Anesthetics 1994;6, 4–14.

49. Fakry SM; Trask AL; Waller MA; Watts, Dorraine D. "Management of Brain-injured patients by an evidence-based medicine protocol improves outcomes and decreases hospital charges", J Trauma 2004;56:492–9; discussion 499–500.

50. Palmer, S; Qureshi, A; Qureshi, Azhar; Palmer, Jacques; Shaver, Thomas; Borzatta, Marcello; Stalcup, Connie, "The impact on outcomes in a community hospital setting of using the AANS traumatic brain injury guidelines Americans Associations for Neurologic Surgeons", J Trauma 2001;50:657–64.

51. Patel HC; Menon DK; Tebbs S; Hawker R; Hutchinson PJ; Kirkpatrick PJ, "Specialist neurocritical care and outcome from head injury.", Intensive Care Med 2002;28:547–53.

52. Bullock MR, Chestnut RM, Clifton GL. Indications for ICP monitoring. J. Neurotraum 2000;17:474–91.

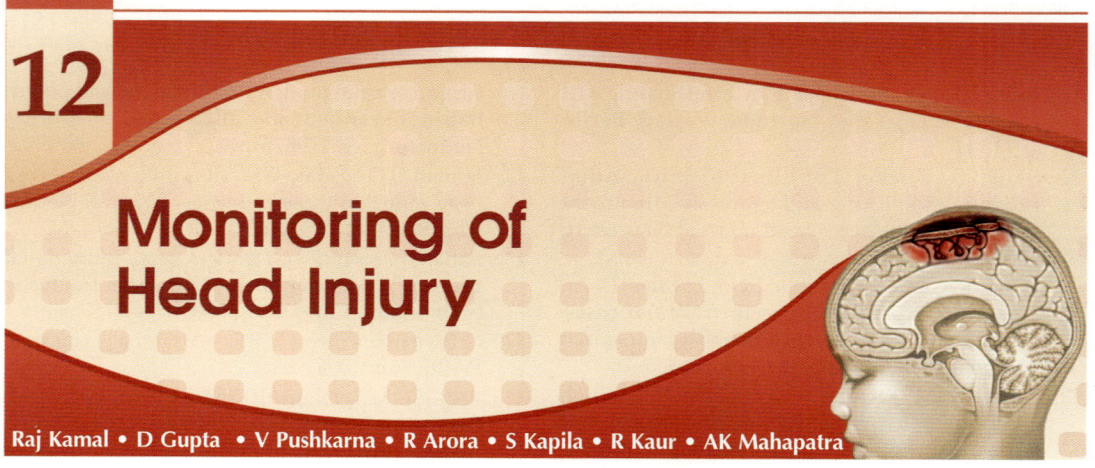

12

Monitoring of Head Injury

Raj Kamal • D Gupta • V Pushkarna • R Arora • S Kapila • R Kaur • AK Mahapatra

INTRODUCTION

The outcome of head injury is multifactorial hence; the factors influencing the outcome have to be carefully assessed from time to time to assess the progress of the patients. The goal of monitoring the injured brain is to enable the detection of harmful physiological events before they cause irreversible damage to the brain, thereby allowing diagnosis and effective management.[1] Intensive multimodal neuromonitoring, is therefore, critical in improving the neurological outcome of the patients with traumatic brain injury.

Changes in intracranial pressure (ICP), cerebral perfusion pressure (CPP), brain tissue partial pressure of oxygen ($PbtO_2$), blood pressure, brain temperature and recently cerebral blood flow (CBF) are monitored in ICU.[2] Cerebral microdialysis is a technique increasingly used as a bedside method glucose, lactate, pyruvate and glycerol levels in the brain of the patients with severe head trauma.[3] Aberrations in cerebral metabolites may indicate occult cerebral ischemia. Minimizing secondary ischemic injury common in TBI may be possible by manipulating ICP, CPP, CBF, $PbtO_2$ in brain parenchyma after acute brain injury.[1-4] The information provided by brain monitoring can supplement the clinical examinations and parameters currently measured such as intracranial pressure (ICP) and cerebral perfusion pressure

(CPP) to improve "goal-directed therapy" of patients after a wide range of neurological injuries, including SAH. Goal-directed therapy is a term borrowed from the sepsis literature in which studies have shown that rigorous attention to correcting alterations in physiological parameters early in a sepsis episode improves outcome.[3,5]

Goal-directed therapy is a term borrowed from the sepsis literature in which studies have shown that rigorous attention to correcting alterations in physiological parameters early in a sepsis episode improves outcome. Spiotta et al[5] used goal directed therapy in a similar way to correct brain physiological parameters in an attempt to improve the outcome of patients with SAH. This approach is highly recommended for patients with severe brain trauma. The information that can be gathered by multi-modal brain monitoring can be used to understand pathophysiology of the disease by studying the response of the various brain parameters being measured to medical and interventional therapies.

Various multimodal neuromonitoring techniques may be classified as follows:

1. *Clinical monitoring*
    a. Glasgow Coma Scale
    b. Focal deficits
    c. Vitals monitoring

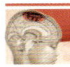

d. Pupillometry

e. Cold caloric response

2. *Non-invasive cerebral monitoring*

   a. Cerebral imaging

   b. Transcranial Doppler ultrasonography

   c. Evoked potential monitoring

   d. Continuous electroencephalography

   e. Near infrared spectroscopy

3. *Invasive cerebral monitoring*

   a. Intracranial pressure monitoring

   b. Jugular venous oxygen saturation

   c. CBF monitoring systems (intraparenchymal brain monitors)

   d. Cerebral microdialysis

   e. Brain temperature monitoring.

CLINICAL MONITORING

Head injury is a dynamic process and the changes occurring at cellular, biochemical and molecular level are continuous. However, the starting point of these changes is the point of trauma. As the changes keep on progressing or regressing patients may show deterioration or improvement. Hence, the importance of clinical monitoring cannot be over emphasized. The clinical parameters which need to be monitored are:

a. Level of consciousness

b. Cranial nerve function

c. Doll's eye movement

d. Vestibulo-ocular response.

These parameters are vital and have tremendous prognostic value. Level of consciousness must be analyzed on the Glasgow Coma Scale which is easy to follow. Even, the nurses must be trained in monitoring patients' neurological state and respiration. GCS provides an idea of patients' improvement or deterioration. If carefully evaluated, clinical monitoring will indicate in what stage patient need surgery and further observation and waiting may risk the patients' life or may lead to irreversible brain damage. Hence, clinical monitoring is vital in head injury management.

Among the clinical monitoring, most important is the close observation of GCS. GCS is internationally accepted as a standard method of assessing the conscious state, which includes:

a. Eye opening

b. Best motor response

c. Best verbal response.

The details of GCS are decribed in Chapter 9 (Table 9.1). However, over the years the limitations of GCS are well recognized. In children under 5 years of age where assessing the verbal response is difficult, GCS is of limited value, this is particularly so in infants where assessment of best motor and best verbal response is also difficult.

Monitoring of Vestibulo-ocular Reflex (Cold Caloric Response)

Vestibulo-ocular reflex (VOR) is a reliable test of assessing brainstem function.[6,8] Medial longitudinal fasciculus (MLF) in the brainstem is connected to the vestibular apparatus in the inner ear, vestibular nuclei of 3rd, 4th and 6th cranial nerves on the both sides. Thus, VOR provides a very good physiological substrate for studying brainstem function. In a normal situation, by stimulating the external ear, one can stimulate vestibular apparatus and induce a conjugate eye movement, which is otherwise called VOR. VOR is also utilized to establish the brain death, when it is absent in association with other parameters.

Over last a few decades, VOR is utilized as a reliable bedside test to establish the integrity of the brainstem function, in various neurological disorders, and more importantly, in head injury, to prognosticate the outcome. As early as 1969, Jadav et al[6] analyzed the role of VOR in patients with altered conscious state. Bruce et al[7] in 1982 reported VOR as a good predictor of outcome in pediatric head injury. Mahapatra et al[8] reported good outcome in decerebrating head injury patients with normal outcome. In another study, Mahapatra and Tandon[9] compared VOR with brainstem auditory evoked potential (BAEP) and found that VOR was as good or even better that BAEP in predicting outcome in severe head injury patients. BAEP is more difficult to perform than VOR, which is simple bedside test. It can be repeated as and when necessary, without much problem.

Normal VOR indicates a very good outcome.[6,9,10] In a study Mahapatra[10] reported good outcome in 85% patients when VOR was normal, while 100% patients with an absent VOR had a poor outcome.

Pupillometry

The pupil check with a flash light is an extremely important standard measurement of pupil reactivity and status of the nervous system and brain. Recently, devices have been invented that can quantitatively assess the changes in constriction and dilatation of pupils to light. The NeurOptics ForSite Pupillometer (Fig. 12.1) is one such non-invasive, battery operated hand-held device that uses light stimulus and rapid live photography to measure maximum and minimum aperture and constriction velocity of the pupils. Constriction velocities less than 0.8 mm/sec indicate increased brain volume and velocities less than 0.6 mm/sec suggest elevated and problematic ICP. Similarly, pupil reactivity less than 10% after light stimulus suggests elevated ICP and should be considered in conjunction with results of other monitoring systems.[11]

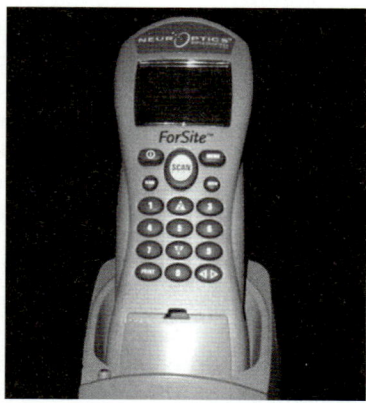

Fig. 12.1: NeurOptics® pupillometer

The NeurOptics® NPi™-100 pupillometer is a hand-held, cordless, and simple to use device which removes subjectivity in the measurement of pupil size and the pupillary light reflex (PLR). Now, even the smallest changes in pupillary function which are not discernable to the naked eye are detectable by clinicians and can be measured and quantified.

Cerebral Imaging

CT imaging is the gold standard in diagnosis of intracranial pathology in head injury. The importance of monitoring through radio-logical modality is given in Chapter 10.

Continuous Electroencephalography

Continuous EEG (cEEG) is increasingly used to monitor brain function in neuro ICU patients. It provides important information regarding brain function, particularly in comatose patients. Seizures are a source of secondary insult to the injured brain. They tend to occur in first a few days after TBI and are associated with a higher injury severity and worse outcomes. cEEG studies have demonstrated that seizures occur in around 20% of TBI patients.

Evoked potential monitoring provides the functional assessment of neuronal structures in a tested pathways.[12–17] Functional or physiological monitoring can be performed through EEG, sensory evoked potential (SEP) and auditory brainstem evoked potential (ABEP). Over last 3 decades, considerable interest has been shown in studying evoked potential in head injury patients, to predict the outcome. Greenberg and his colleagues[12,13] were the first to perform multimodal evoked potential studies in severe head injury and established the predictive value. They graded, evoked potentials into 4 different grades. Grade I was normal, Grade II mild abnor-mality, Grade III severe abnormality and Grade IV was absent response. Mahapatra and Tandon[9] and Mahapatra[15] classified EP into normal, abnormal and absent.

ICP Monitoring

ICP monitoring has become the standard of care in management of patients with TBI. Intervention is indicated when ICP rises to 20–25 mm Hg from normal levels of 0–10 mm Hg. A ventriculostomy catheter provides a method for monitoring ICP while simultaneously reducing ICP through therapeutic CSF drainage. Ventricular pressure is the reference standard in ICP monitoring and should be considered gold standard. A transducer system is required to monitor ICP through this catheter. The transducers are levelled at the tragus. The details of ICP monitoring are described in the previous chapter (Chapter 11). ICP monitoring has gained a place in neurosurgical ICU management and become an integral part of ICU care. ICP monitoring is extensively studied in head injury patients in last two decades.[18,21–23,28] Persistent raised ICP has a direct effect on the brain tissue inspite of cerebral perfusion pressure being normal. ICP monitoring is recommended as per indications (*see* Table 11.1).

Brain Trauma Foundation (BTF) guidelines[17] suggest that ICP monitoring is primarily used when there is difficulty in clinical assessment of the patient or if there is a high risk of increased ICP. ICP monitoring is not necessary in the awake patient, in whom clinical assessment of neurological status is possible, and is contraindicated in the patient with a bleeding diathesis. The correlation between high ICP and poor outcomes has been well reported by many authors.[21–26] Normally, resting ICP is 5 to 15 mm. Transient elevations of ICP occurs normally with straining, coughing or the trendelenburg position. A sustained ICP greater than 20 mm Hg is clearly abnormal. An ICP between 20 and 40 mm Hg is considered moderate intracranial hypertension. An ICP greater than 40 mm Hg represents severe, usually life-threatening intracranial hypertension.[25, 26] About 50% of the patients with severe head injury will develop increased intracranial pressure.

Increased ICP occurs in 50–70% of patients even after evacuation of intracranial hematoma.

The cerebral perfusion pressure (CPP) is equivalent to the mean arterial pressure (MAP) minus the ICP.

$$CPP = MAP - ICP$$

The principal strategy for managing head injury is to reduce the frequency and severity of secondary brain insults from intracranial pressure (ICP) and cerebral perfusion pressure (CPP), and hence improve outcome. In an experimental study of CBF by, Miller[26,27] demonstrated that, when MAP and ICP rise in parallel so that CPP remains constant at about 60 mm Hg. His work also suggested that cerebral perfusion is more sensitive to arterial hypotension than to intracranial hypertension. The clinical significance of this information is that in the management of head injury it is often necessary to employ therapy to lower raised ICP. Therapeutic agents for reducing raised ICP often do so at the expense of reduced MAP and as a consequence CPP may not improve. If autoregulation is preserved, CBF should remain unchanged despite parallel changes in MAP and ICP.

The venticulostomy catheter and intraparenchymal catheter are two most common methods for ICP monitoring. The intraparenchymal pressure monitoring remains popular, particularly in the United Kingdom, because it does not require catheter placement in the operating theater and thus requires significantly fewer resources. The two most frequently used catheter tip systems in the management of patients with head injuries are the Codman and Camino systems. The ventriculostomy catheter remains the gold standard against which all of the newer monitors are compared. This method allows the clinician to check for zero drift and the sensitivity of the measurement system *in vivo*. Ventricular catheter also allows cerebrospinal fluid drainage for therapeutic purposes. It can be placed easily and quickly in most patients with head trauma, even those with mass effect. Disadvantages of ventricular catheter include infection rate of 8 to 10% and 1 to 2% risk of intracranial hemorrhage.[19]

CBF MONITORING

Cerebral blood flow (CBF) can be estimated by various techniques, including transcranial Doppler (TCD), xenon-CT, single photon emission CT (SPECT), oxygen-15 PET, perfusion CT, and perfusion weighted MRI. Except for TCD, these methods do not offer the possibility of continuous monitoring. Placement of intraparenchymal probe offers the possibility for continuously assessing regional cerebral blood flow (rCBF). Direct measurement of CBF is relatively new in neurointensive care. Monitoring CBF could play an important role in neurological care, because the outcome depends on continuous blood flow to the injured brain. For the past two decades, two types of bedside CBF monitoring have been popular; direct method like intraparenchymal probe and indirect methods like TCD, $SjvO_2$ measurement.[29]

Two types of intraparenchymal probes are available based on different principles:

1. rCBF measurement probe using thermal dilution method (Hemedex) (Fig. 12.2)
2. rCBF measurement probe using laser Doppler flowmetry (LDF) technology (Integra).

The intraparenchymal probe (using thermal dilution method) incorporating thermistors has been evaluated in brain-injured patients.[30] It provides continuous quantitative real-time data that are in good agreement with values obtained by Xenon-CT for a volume of approximately 5 cm³ around the tip of the probe. The intraparenchymal probe is a thermodilution probe with two thermistor sensors located 5 mm apart near the tip of the catheter.[30] Local cortical blood flow is calculated from temperature difference between two thermistor plates, which decreases with rising blood flow.

Once implanted into the brain and connected to the machine, the proximal

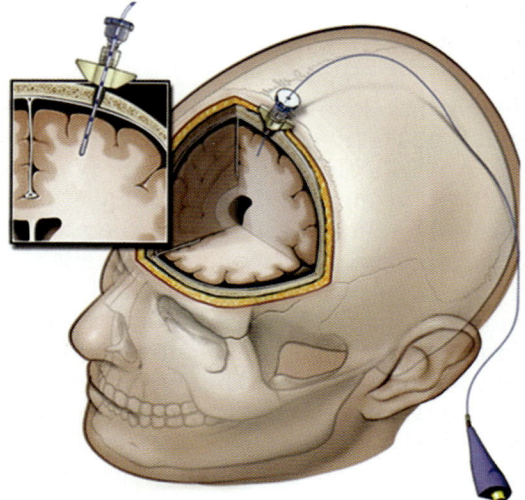

Fig. 12.2: Hemedex catheter provides constant, updated and accurate measurement of blood flow at the capillary level

thermistor measures the temperature in the brain. The distal thermistor is heated up to 2°C higher than the patient's measured temperature.[30] The monitoring system uses a series of data-reduction algorithms that factor in quantification of tissue perfusion using conductive properties of the tissue.[30] The result is a measurement of local CBF in milliliters per 100 g of brain tissue per minute. The accuracy and reliability of this system have been challenged.[31] Another cited limitation is that the system measures CBF in only one small area of the brain, although differences in global and regional CBF often occur.[29]

Another system for measuring CBF is based on laser Doppler flowmetry (LDF) technology.[31,32] Like the previous probe it must be inserted into the brain parenchyma through an introducer. The LDF measures regional CBF (Integra Neurosciences, 2005) and is considered to have excellent dynamic resolution and to be fairly reliable for local cortical nondirectional CBF.[29,31] The CBF in high and low flow compartments, sampled by placing 5 mm circular ROIs in regions containing the highest and lowest flow values

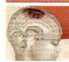

in each hemisphere, averaged, in the original paper of Yonas,[34] 84 ± 14 and 20 ± 5 ml/100 gr/min, respectively.[34] These normative values should be kept in mind and compared with traditional values of ischemia threshold for the cortex which are 18 ml/100 gr/min[33] and that for white matter, which should be at a much lower level (7 ml/100 gr/min).[35]

NON-INVASIVE NEAR-INFRARED SPECTROSCOPY (NIRS)

Continuous real-time monitoring of the adequacy of cerebral perfusion can provide important therapeutic information in a variety of clinical settings.[36] The current clinical availability of several non-invasive near-infrared spectroscopy (NIRS)-based cerebral oximetry devices represents a potentially important development for the detection of cerebral ischemia (Fig. 12.3). NIR light can be used to measure regional cerebral tissue oxygen saturation (rSO_2). This technique uses principles of optical spectrophotometry that make use of the fact that biological material, including the skull, is relatively transparent in the NIR range.[36]

Measurement of tissue oxygen saturation and tissue hemoglobin content is determined

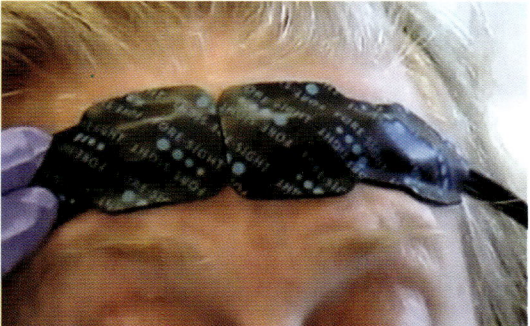

Fig. 12.3: Cerebral optically-based near infrared spectroscopic oximetry applied to patients who have suffered a stroke can help monitor regional cerebral perfusion in real time, and thus may serve as a useful, noninvasive, bedside intensive care unit monitoring tool to assess brain oxygenation in a direct manner (device is called ForeSight from Casmed of Branford)

by the difference in intensity between a transmitted and received light delivered at specific wavelengths in the 700–1300 nm range, NIR light penetrates biological tissue several centimeters.[37] Within the NIR range, the primary light-absorbing molecules in tissue are metal complex chromophores: hemoglobin, bilirubin, and cytochrome. The absorption spectra of deoxyhemoglobin (Hb) ranges from 650 to 1000 nm, oxyhemoglobin (HbO_2) shows a broad peak between 700 and 1150, and cytochrome oxidase aa3 (Caa3) has a broad peak at 820–840 nm.[37,38] The isobestic point (wavelength at which oxy- and deoxyhemoglobin species have the same molar absorptivity) for Hb/HbO_2 is 810 nm. As discussed below, the isobestic absorption spectra can be utilized to measure total tissue hemoglobin concentration. The proper management of brain oxygenation is one of the principal endpoints of all anesthesia procedures, but the brain remains one of the least monitored organs during clinical anesthesiology. There are some medical procedures where iatrogenic brain ischemia is present, including carotid endarterectomy (CEA) in patients with high-grade carotid artery stenosis, temporary clipping in brain aneurysm surgery, hypothermic circulatory arrest for aortic arch procedures, and others in which the pathology itself generates brain ischemia, such as traumatic brain injury and stroke.

It is important to recognize that confounders such as extracerebral or subdural hematoma can change the proportion of cerebral to extracerebral hemoglobin and thus offset tissue oxygen saturation values by a variable amount. Using computed tomographic assessment of skull thickness (t-skull), cerebrospinal fluid area (a-CSF), and hemoglobin concentration. In a recent study of 103 cardiac surgical and neurosurgical patients,[39] demonstrated that rSO_2 values were potentially influenced by hemoglobin concentration, t-skull, and a-CSF.

Jugular Bulb Venous Oxygen Saturation

The utilization of oxygen by the brain is critical for normal brain function. In head injury patients, this function becomes more important. Continuous monitoring of jugular venous bulb oxygen saturation ($SjvO_2$) provides valuable information regarding cerebral oxygen metabolism ($CMRO_2$). The $SjvO_2$ monitoring is carried out by fiberoptic catheter inserted into the internal jugular vein, and placed at jugular bulb. $SjvO_2$ helps in calculating arteriovenous desaturation of oxygen ($AVDO_2$) which is equal to $1.39 \times Hb \times$ arterial oxygen saturation (SaO_2) minus $SjvO_2$.[40–43] Sheinberg et al[42] reported the useful value of continuous monitoring of jugular venous oxygen saturation in head injured patients.

The jugular venous oxygen saturation ($SjvO_2$) is an indicator of both cerebral oxygenation and cerebral metabolism, reflecting the ratio between cerebral blood flow (CBF) and cerebral metabolic rate of oxygen ($CMRO_2$). $SjvO_2$ monitoring permits the early identification of patients with low CPP and high risk of cerebral ischemia.[44]

The internal jugular vein is cannulated in a retrograde direction with a catheter containing a spectrophotometric fiberoptic probe and a lumen for aspiration of blood. Infrared light at three wavelengths measures hemoglobin concentration and oxygen saturations.[44] The position of the catheter tip should be confirmed by a lateral X-ray, the ideal position is above the disc between the first and second cervical vertebre and close to skull base. This approximates with the level of the mastoid air cells.

Normal arteriojugular oxygen difference ($AJDO_2$) range[45] from 4 to 9 ml 100^{-1}. Low CBF and ischemia raise oxygen extraction fraction (OEF) and increases arteriojugular oxygen difference ($AJDO_2$), whereas hyperemia will lead to decrease in $AJDO_2$.

$$CBF = CMRO_2 / AJDO_2$$
$$CBF \sim 1 / AJDO_2$$

In the uninjured brain, reduced cerebral oxygen delivery (e.g. arterial desaturation) causes an increase in cerebral blood flow resulting in improved oxygen delivery (autoregulation). In patients with brain injury, autoregulation may be deranged and the cerebral vasculature may be unable to compensate for changing oxygen requirements. The normal jugular saturation ($SjvO_2$) ranges from 55 to 71%, a figure that is lower than mixed venous saturations, reflecting the greater cerebral oxygen extraction compared with the rest of the body. $SjvO_2$ is dependant upon arterial oxygen saturation, cerebral blood flow and cerebral metabolic rate. As long as the first two factors remain constant, the $SjvO_2$ varies with cerebral oxygen uptake. Significant increases and decreases of $SjvO_2$ are associated with poorer outcome. Studies showed that a sustained reduction of the $SjvO_2$ < 50% was associated with poor outcome, and an independent risk factor for poor prognosis.[45–48] $SjvO_2$ monitoring is mainly used in the management of severe head injury. It confirms the deleterious effects a low cerebral perfusion pressure, and reflects the effects of interventional therapies. For example, hyperventilation is used to acutely reduce ICP, but can lead to critical cerebral vasoconstriction and ischemia. $SjvO_2$ monitoring can be used to define how much hyperventilation can be safely used. $SjvO_2$ monitoring can also be used to optimize cerebral perfusion pressure: 70 mm Hg is considered optimal but it may be possible to lower this aim, minimizing the administration of vasopressors, if adequate cerebral oxygenation is confirmed.

Brain Tissue Oxygen Tension

The jugular venous oxygen saturation ($SjvO_2$) is an indicator of both cerebral oxygenation and cerebral metabolism, reflecting the ratio between cerebral blood flow (CBF) and cerebral metabolic rate of oxygen ($CMRO_2$). Both $SjvO_2$ and brain tissue oxygen tension ($PbtO_2$) monitoring measure cerebral oxygenation, however, $SjvO_2$ measures global cerebral oxygenation and $PbtO_2$ measures focal cerebral oxygenation using an invasive

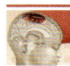

probe (Licox).[49] $PbtO_2$ is the product of CBF and the cerebral arteriovenous oxygen tension difference rather than a direct measurement of total oxygen delivery or cerebral oxygen.[50] As $PbtO_2$ provides a highly focal measurement, it is mainly used to monitor oxygenation of a critically perfused brain tissue. $PbtO_2$ is the most reliable technique to monitor focal cerebral oxygenation in order to prevent episodes of desatuartion. However, global cerebral oxygenation alterations may not be observed. The normal $PbtO_2$ ranges between 35 mm Hg and 50 mm Hg.[51] A value of a $PbtO_2$ < 15 is considered a threshold for focal cerebral ischemia and treatment. Several studies demonstrated that $PbtO_2$-based therapy may be associated with reduced patient mortality and improved patient outcome after severe TBI.[52,53] Narotam et al[53] in their study concluded that elevated ICP and a persistent low $PbtO_2$ after 2 hours represented increasing odds of death (OR 14.3 at 48 hours). Survivors and patients with good outcomes generally had significantly higher mean daily $PbtO_2$ and CPP values compared to nonsurvivors.

A few studies suggested that $PbtO_2$-based therapy, may be associated with reduced patient mortality and improved patient outcome after severe TBI.[54,55]

Oddo et al[56] suggested that combined ICP/CPP and $PbtO_2$-based therapy is associated with better outcome after severe TBI than ICP/CPP-based therapy alone.[56] Oddo et al reported that brain hypoxia or reduced $PbtO_2$ is an independent outcome predictor and is associated with poor short-term outcome after severe TBI independently of elevated ICP, low CPP, and injury severity. $PbtO_2$ may be an important therapeutic target after severe TBI.[2] $PbtO_2$ has been documented to be superior to $SjvO_2$, near infrared spectroscopy, and regional transcranial oxygen saturation[4] in detecting cerebral ischemia. $PbtO_2$ monitoring is a promising, safe and clinically applicable method in severe TBI patients; however, it is neither widely used nor available. The combinations of ICP/$PbtO_2$ intraparenchymal monitoring are important and helpful modalities in the management of severe TBI.

TRANSCRANIAL DOPPLER MONITORING

It was generally believed that the vasospasm never occurs in traumatic subarachnoid hemorrhage. Over the years it has been proved wrong, not only by carotid angiography[57] which showed focal or generalized narrowing of vessel, but also CT scan may show appearance of an infarct which may not be present in the initial scan. This finding in CT scan did confirm the focal vasospasm leading to focal infarction.

Over last 3 decades, transcranial Doppler (TCD) sonography has been routinely used (Figs 12.4a and b) to evaluate the blood flow in intracranial vessel. Intracranial blood flow velocity (BFV) can be repeatedly studied in head injury patient. It also helps in finding pulsatility index (PI) by finding out difference in systolic and diastolic flow velocity.[58] By monitoring flow velocity in ICA and MCA through TCD, post-traumatic vasospasm can be detected. In a study by Matz and Pitts, they measured BFV on consecutive days, post-traumatic vasospasm was diagnosed when MCA, flow velocity was above 120 cm/sec. In some patients increased BFC was observed 5–15 days after injury.[57]

Cerebral vasospasm was also confirmed by Lindegaard ratio[63] by comparing MCA flow velocity with extracranial ICA blood flow velocity. Bakshi and Mahapatra[59] observed basillary artery spasm in severe head injury. Thus, TCD can be used to demonstrate vasospasm and predict cerebral compliance changes in head injury, using portable TCD machine. However, the limitation of TCD is that, it only provides qualitative estimation of regional CBF.

TCD can be helpful in preventing secondary brain damage due to ischemia.[60–63] In some patients there may be unilateral increase in BFV, and these patients are likely to develop focal infraction, supplied by the vessel having vasospasm. Maneuvers to

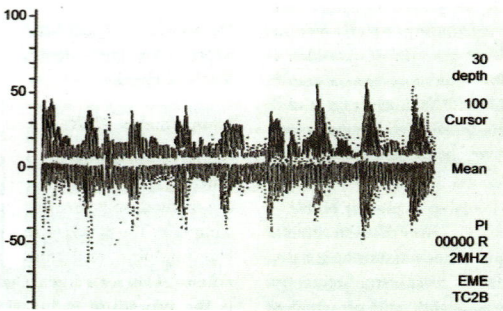

Fig. 12.4a: Transcranial Doppler (TCD) from MCA in a patient with severe head injury shows increased PI 1.75

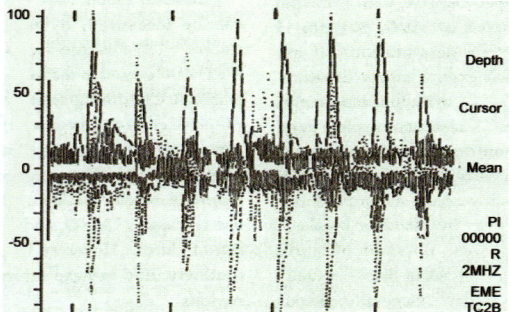

Fig. 12.4b: TCD in a severe head injury shows abnormal PI 3.[58]

Normal and threshold values of metabolic parameters used in microdialysis		
Metabolite	Normal value	Threshold value
Glucose (mg/dl)	30.6	14.4
Pyruvate (mg/dl)	1.46	0.27 (fatal)
Lactate (mg/dl)	26.1	80.2 (fatal)
Lactate to pyruvate ratio (LPR)	23	30
Glycerol (mg/dl)	184–460	21

parameter in the management of severe head injury.

CEREBRAL MICRODIALYSIS

Cerebral microdialysis (Figs 12.5 to 12.9a and b) is a minimally invasive sampling technique that is now a well-established bedside monitoring to provide online analysis of the brain tissue biochemistry in patients with TBI. Cerebral microdialysis enables measurement of the metabolic markers (glucose, pyruvate, lactate, and glycerol).[64–66] Cerebral microdialysis involves placing a catheter with a 10 mm semipermeable distal end membrane into the brain parenchyma (Fig. 12.5). The catheter is pumped with sample fluid that is isotonic to brain parenchymal interstitium. Through this catheter, molecules related to ATP generation (i.e. glucose, pyruvate, lactate and glycerol) are collected from interstitial fluid and are analyzed hourly. The metabolites analyzed represent 70% of the true interstitial fluid concentration.[67] Usually **two** micro-

increase CPP will prevent ischemic damage. Martin et al[57] reported elevated MCA, BFV (blood flow velocity) in 27% patients. In 17% patients elevated MCA velocity was associated with traumatic subarachnoid hemorrhage. Thus, a combination of traumatic SAH and vasospasm lead to a poor outcome.[57–62] Generally, raised BFV reduces in a few days time (5–15 days), the pattern is exactly similar to spontaneous SAH. Increased BFV may also be associated with cerebral hyperemia, depending on vascular resistance. Both hyperemia and vasospasm are associated with impaired autoregulations. Over the years, the role of ischemic damage is well established. The ischemia is due to traumatic SAH and vasospasm, demonstrated in TCD. Thus, TCD monitoring has become an important ICU

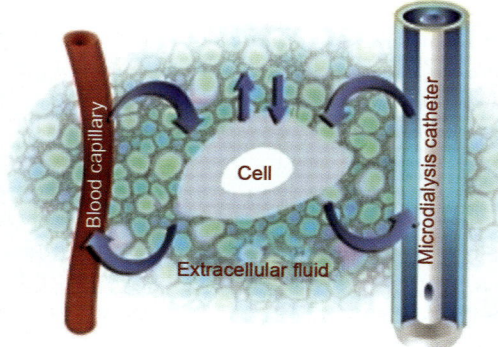

Fig. 12.5: Principles of microdialysis

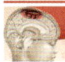

dialysis catheters are placed, one in the **pericontusional penumbra** of the injury and its position is verified by CT (Figs 12.6 to 12.8). Another catheter is placed in an area of undamaged tissue for comparison. The samples are collected and analyzed every hour, although it can be repeated every 15–20 mins, as indicated by changes in patient's condition.

Normal brain glucose levels are 30.6 mg/dl. The ischemic threshold for the same is 14.4 mg/dl. Preventing systemic hypoglycemia is extremely important in preventing metabolic crisis and ultimately secondary brain injury. It has been proved that strict adherence to tight glycemic control (blood glucose 80–110 mg/dl) often leads to dangerously low brain glucose levels that can be detected only with cerebral microdialysis.[64–66]

The normal lactate to pyruvate ratio (LPR) is 23. An LPR level near a threshold value of 30, in conjunction with low glucose levels, requires intervention to prevent cellular energy failure. Similarly, glycerol levels near 921 mg/dl indicate cellular energy failure.[64,65]

Routine interventions to lower the LPR by preventing anerobic respiration that leads to abnormally elevated glycerol levels include, increasing glucose levels to 110 to 180 mg/dl, elevating and adjusting the patients head position and augmenting CPP with vaso-pressors.

Brain microdialysis (MD) is a well-established technique to monitor the chemistry of the extracellular space in the brain during neurointensive care. MD may be useful in severe cases of traumatic brain injury (TBI) in which monitoring of intracranial pressure and cerebral perfusion pressure is required. Lactate/pyruvate (L/P) ratio, glucose, glutamate, and glycerol can be measured using a bedside device. The L/P ratio is a sensitive marker of changes in the redox state of cells caused by ischemia. Glycerol is an integral component of cell membranes. Loss of energy due to ischemia eventually leads to an influx of calcium and a decomposition of cell membranes, which liberates glycerol into the interstitial fluid. Thus the L/P ratio and glycerol have become the most important

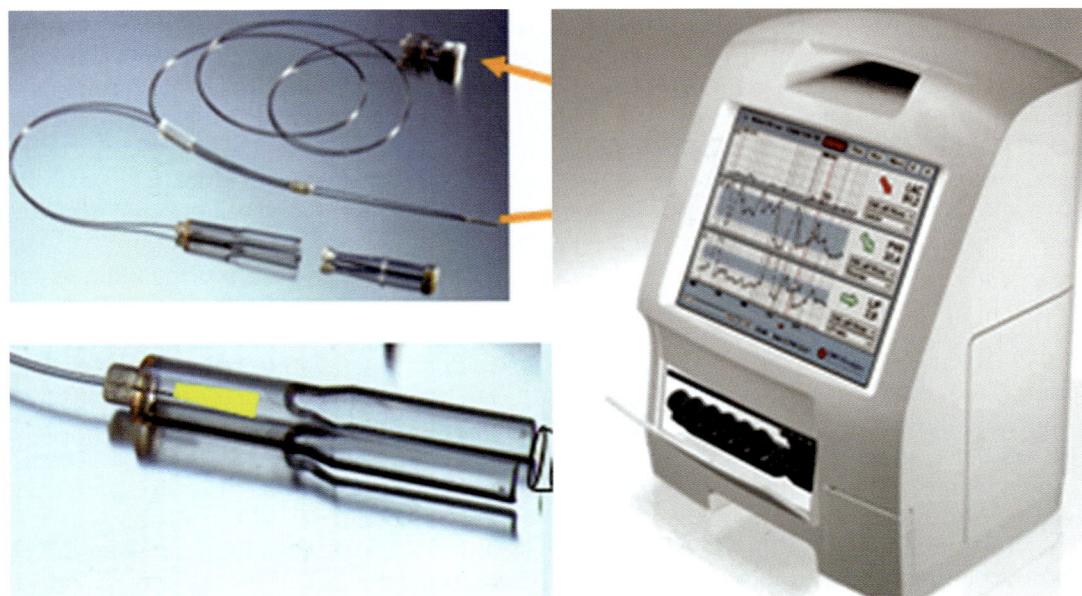

Fig. 12.6: Microdialysis instruments

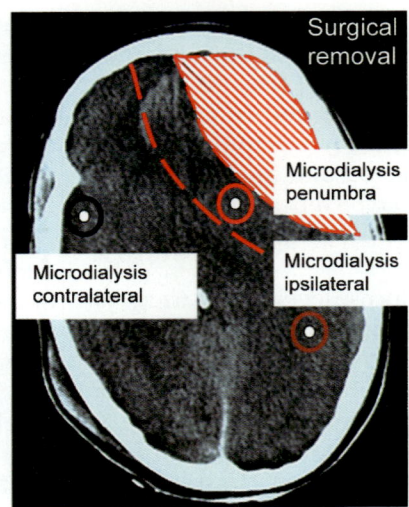

Focal hemorrhagic contusion

One microdialysis is placed in the contralateral hemisphere

One microdialysis catheter is placed in the penumbra of the contusion

One microdialysis catheter is placed outside the penumbra

Surgical removal

Microdialysis penumbra

Microdialysis contralateral

Microdialysis ipsilateral

Fig. 12.7: Microdialysis catheter is placed in the penumbra of contusion, second MD catheter is placed in contralateral hemisphere, sometimes 3rd catheter is placed in ipsilateral area outside the penumbra of contusion

markers of ischemia and cell membrane damage. As the primary source of energy, glucose is an important marker of changes in brain metabolism and the glutamate level is an indirect marker of cell damage.

The most consistent finding is the significant association of higher lactate/pyruvate ratio with increased mortality and unfavorable outcomes after TBI.[68–72] The lactate/pyruvate ratio reflects the metabolic state, and the elevation of lactate/pyruvate ratio may reflect the presence of either mitochondrial dysfunction[69] or lack of oxygen supply, due to ischemia or hypoxia. Persistent abnormalities that are refractory to clinical interventions are also common, especially in the vicinity of the injured cerebral tissue.[71,82]

Why should we monitor organ chemistry. The answer is that we get direct measure of tissue damage/ischemia directly from organ itself, continuously, bedside instead of one time study (MRI, CT, PET). There exists a window of opportunity from organ chemistry change to manifestation of clinical signs which varies between organs-to-organs. The physician

gets an early warning (for example, severe increase in lactate/pyruvate ratio) of an impending ischemic event, actually before it occurs.

In order to make effective use of microdialysis data, it is essential to relate them to other data collected bedside. This may be done by software, which allows for integrating data from the microdialysis analyzer, the ICU monitor displaying intracranial pressure (ICP) and cerebral perfusion pressure (CPP), a tissue oxygen analyzer, the ventilator, the infusion pumps, etc. (Figs 12.8, 12.9a and b).

This "multimodal monitoring" allows for the display of all data as trend curves on one computer screen. It creates the framework for individualizing therapy on the basis of clinical status, brain tissue chemistry and the effect of therapeutic interventions.

Microdialysis catheter forms a "biosensor" where samples of the tissue chemistry transported out of body for analysis c.f. traditional biosensor where analysis takes place inside body. The availability of modern analytical techniques has made microdialysis a "universal" biosensor capable of monitoring

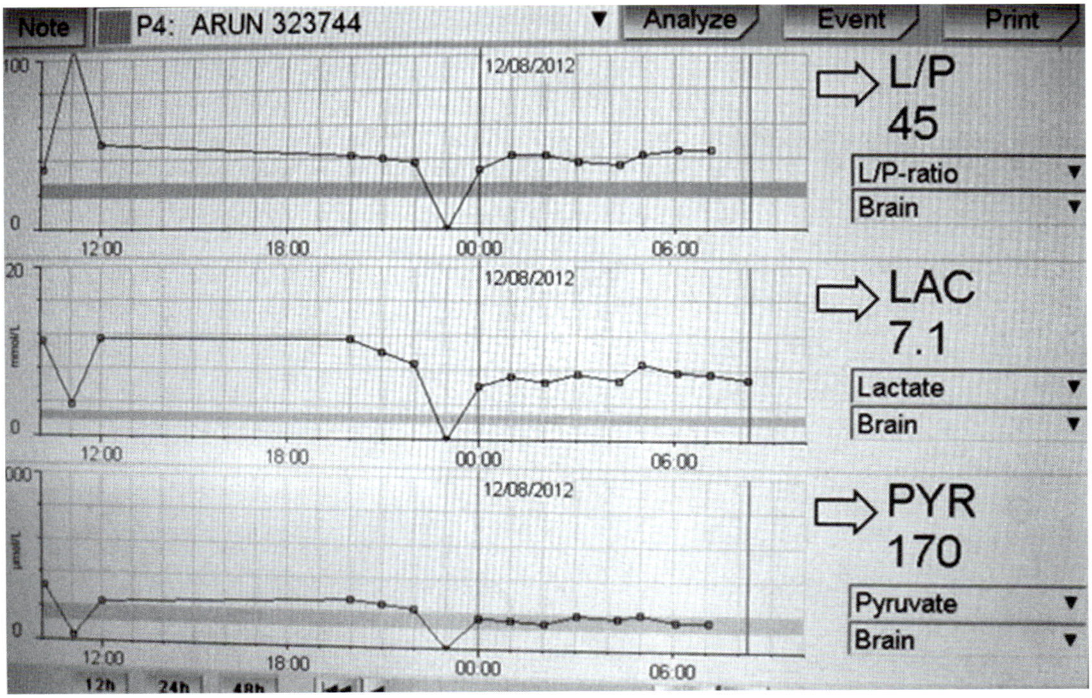

Fig. 12.8: Recording of various metabolites on monitor

essentially every small and medium sized molecular compound in the interstitial fluid of endogenous as well as exogenous origin.

Artificial CSF is slowly pumped into the microdialysis probe using a microsyringe pump capable of pumping very low volume of fluids probes wall is semipermeable to small molecules which diffuse from extracellular space of the brain into the dialysate fluid. The analyte molecule diffuses through the extracellular space and ultimately the collected analyte can be analyzed.

Principles of Microdialysis

The microdialysis catheter takes up substances delivered by the blood, e.g. glucose and drugs, but also substances released from the cells, e.g. markers of cellular metabolism.

The interstitial fluid is the "cross road" of all substances passing between cells and blood capillaries. By monitoring this compartment in the brain it is possible to get crucial informa-tion about the biochemistry of neurons and glia and how seriously brain cells are affected by for example ischemia, hyperemia, trauma, hemorrhage, vasospasm as well as various physiological, pharmacological and surgical interventions during intensive care.

Although microdialysis samples essentially all small molecular substances present in the interstitial fluid, the use of microdialysis in neurointensive care has focused on markers of ischemia, energy break down and cell damage. The reason is that they are of obvious importance for the survival of the tissue, well understood from a biochemical point of view and easy to interpret in the clinical setting of intensive care.

Microdialysis tells us how cells react to an increase or decrease in the supply of oxygen and glucose. However, while normal brain tissue may not suffer when exposed to a moderate decrease in oxygen and glucose, vulnerable cells in the pericontusional

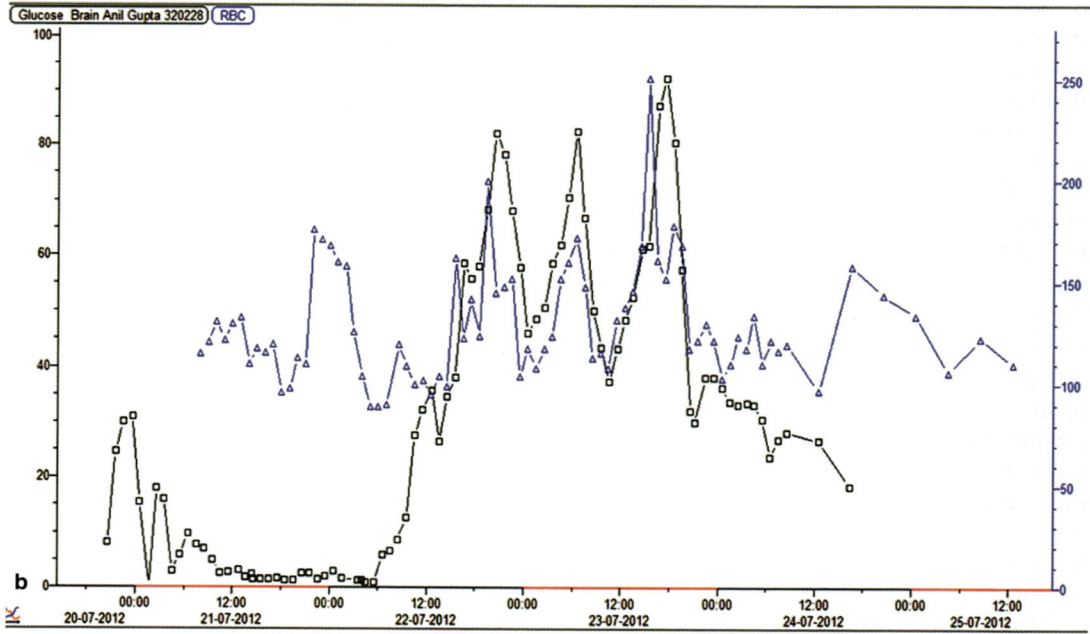

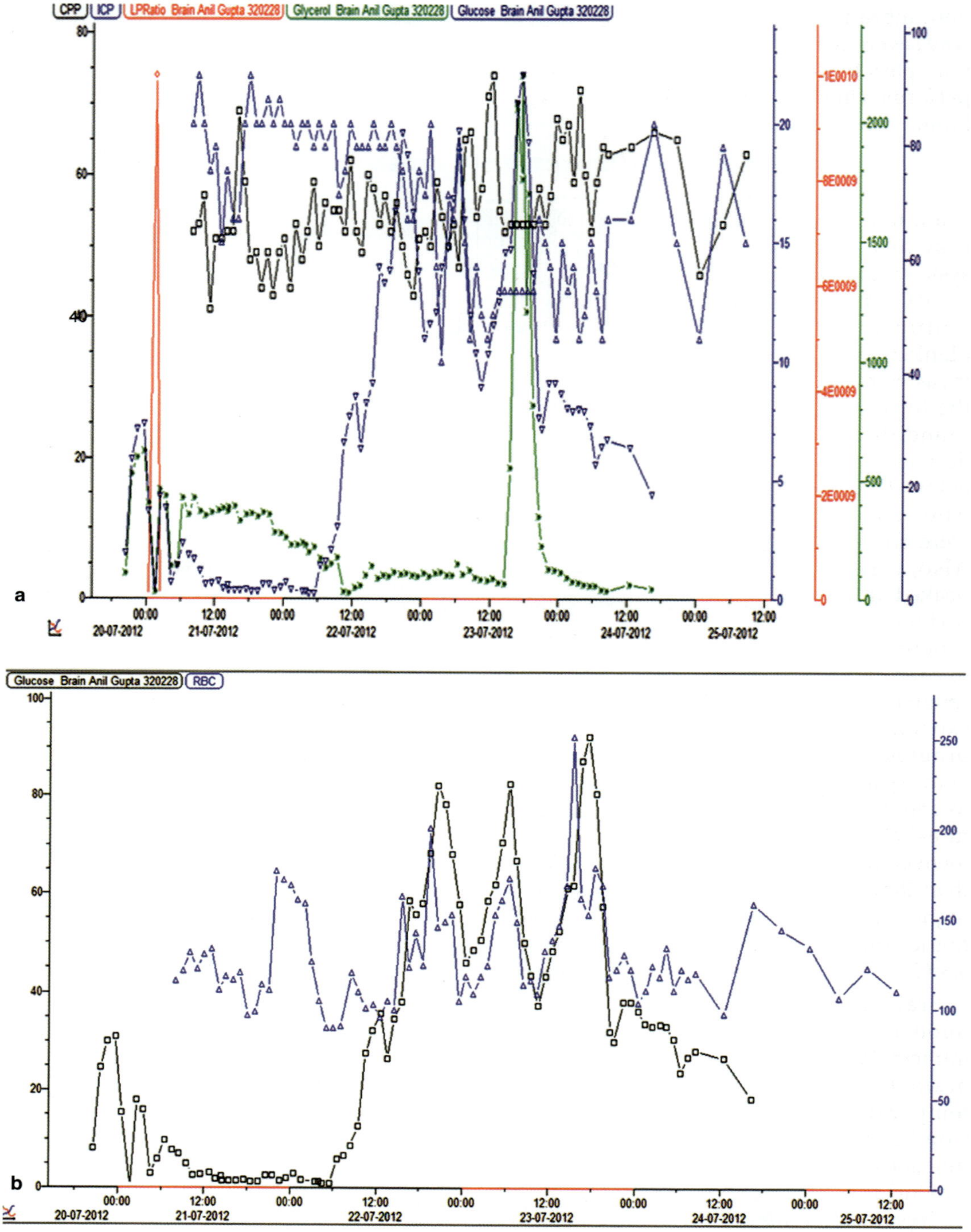

Figs 12.9a and b: A patient with severe head injury who underwent cerebral microdialysis study

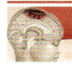

penumbra may simply not survive. In this way severe secondary damage to brain tissue may pass unnoticed if microdialysis is not performed in the most vulnerable tissue of the brain.

BRAIN TEMPERATURE MONITORING

Brain temperature monitoring is relatively easy as it is an integral part of multiple systems. Brain hyperthermia, a temperature of 38.5°C or greater, can be prevented by multiple methods. Antipyretics, cooling blankets, ice packs have all been used but invasive methods can also be used wherever the former prove futile. Tokutomi et al[73,74] found that the intracranial pressure (ICP) decreased significantly at brain temperatures below 37°C and decreased more sharply at temperatures 35 to 36°C, but no differences were observed at temperatures below 35°C. Also, cerebral perfusion pressure (CPP) peaked at 35.0 to 35.9°C and decreased with further decreases in temperature. Jugular venous oxygen saturation and mixed venous oxygen saturation remained in the normal range during hypothermia. Resting energy expenditure and cardiac output decreased progressively with hypothermia. Oxygen delivery and oxygen consumption decreased to abnormally low levels at rectal temperatures below 35°C, and the correlation between them became less significant at less than 35°C than that when temperatures were 35°C or higher. Brain temperature was consistently higher than rectal temperature by 0.5 +/− 0.3°C.

Brain temperature can be monitored through multiparameter catheters measuring intracranial pressure (ICP), partial pressure of brain tissue oxygen (PtiO$_2$), and brain temperature (TBr) (Neurovent PTO).[75,76] Combining 3 different neuromonitoring functions in 1 probe might ease monitoring by making a second (PtiO$_2$) probe unnecessary. Multipara catheters; future of brain monitoring; recording of most of essential parameters through single probes are being developed

and their reliability is still in experimental stage, but its development will be a major step towards brain monitoring in ICU.

The lab-on-a-tube system developed by Chunyan Li and colleagues[76] at the University of Cincinnati, US, comprises a film containing a microchannel sandwiched between two polymer films, one including a pressure sensor and the other containing glucose, oxygen and temperature sensors. The system is rolled into a spiral to form a tube which can be inserted into the brain (Fig. 12.10). The tube is connected to a multimodal monitor, which shows results from the four sensors, and a cerebrospinal fluid drainage bag as the tube can also be used to drain (and monitor) the fluid to lower intracranial pressure.

BIOMARKERS

A biomarker is a characteristics that is objectively measured and evaluated as an indicator of normal biological processes, pathological processes, or responses to therapeutic intervention. It should appear in easily accessible material such as blood or CSF.

Several proteins synthesized in astrocytes or neuron have been proposed as potential biomarkers. They can be summarised as S-100α, neuron-specific enolase, glial fibrillary acidic protein (GFAP), cleaved-tau (C-tau), and SBDP.

S-100α is considered a marker of astrocyte injury or death. Its level in serum has correlated well with both GCS scores and neuroradiologic findings.[77–80] This protein has been implicated in the Ca^{++} dependent

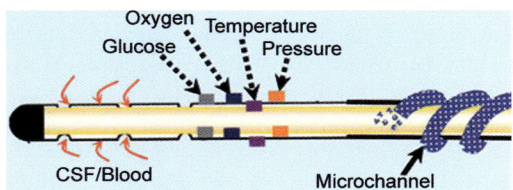

Fig. 12.10: Multiparameter catheter; Li's device[76] can measure key parameters affected by TBI and could be used to deliver drugs to the brain through the microchannel

regulation of various intracellular functions. In a few reports, S-100α levels consistent with the outcome following head injury.[79-86] S-100α is also present in adipocytes and chondrocytes, and high serum levels have been observed in trauma patients without head injuries.[87–90] Severe head injury triggers a rapid increase in S-100α concentrations which normalize after 12 hours. There is relatively robust correlation between initial S-100α serum levels and outcome after severe head injury.[90–94] S-100α is not a useful marker in children less than 2 years of age, owing to high normative values in that age group.[93–94] Therefore, although S-100α remains promising as an adjunctive marker, its utility as a biochemical diagnostic remains controversial. Kövesdi et al [95] found that only S-100β in severe traumatic brain injury has consistently demonstrated the ability to predict injury and outcome in adults.

Neuron-specific enolase (NSE) is primarily located in the cytoplasm of neurons and is probably involved in increasing neuronal chloride levels during the onset of neural activity.[97] NSE concentration has served as a marker in other neurological disorders such as in Status epilepticus and Creutzfeldt-Jacobs disease. This marker is thought to assess damage to the functional cells of the brain (i.e., the neurons), and a rapid appearance in serum after head injury has been reported.[83,84,97] Neuron-specific enolase is also released in the blood by hemolysis, which may be a serious source of error. NSE levels do not correlate with the outcome in TBI patients.[98]

Glial fibrillary acidic protein represents the major part of the cytoskeleton of astrocytes, is found only in glial cells of the CNS[99,100] and may, therefore, be considered to be a specific marker for CNS disease, and is also involved in various neuronal processes, including maintenance of the blood–brain barrier.[101] Increased serum GFAP levels have been reported in patients suffering from severe head trauma.[102] Recently, other reports have confirmed that serum GFAP is a specific marker of brain damage after head trauma.[86,104,105] GFAP has also been demonstrated to be a potential useful biomarker to predict clinical outcome. Ongoing studies in our research group have shown that serum GFAP levels are significantly higher in patients who died 6 months postinjury than in those who are alive.

C-tau; traumatic brain injury (TBI) in humans results in proteolysis of neuronally-localized, intracellular microtubule associated protein (MAP)-tau to produce cleaved tau (C-tau). Tau protein is a highly soluble microtubule-associated protein (MAP) and are mostly found in neurons compared to non-neuronal cells. One of tau's main functions is to modulate the stability of axonal microtubules. Tau is not present in dendrites and is active primarily in the distal portions of axons where it provides microtubule stabilization but also flexibility as needed.[106.]

Following traumatic brain injury, the neuronally-localized intracellular protein MAP-tau is proteolytically cleaved (C-tau) and gains access to cerebrospinal fluid (CSF) and serum.

Tau levels in the microdialysis samples were highest early and fell over time in all patients. Initial tau levels were > 3-fold higher in patients with microdialysis catheters placed in pericontusional regions than in patients in whom catheters were placed in normal-appearing right frontal lobe tissue.[107]

SBDP (NSEII-spectrin breakdown products) proteolysis as a biochemical marker of CNS injury.[107,108] αII-spectrin is primarily found in neurons and is abundant in axons and presynaptic terminals.[108] The protein is processed to breakdown products (SBDPs) of molecular weights 150 kDa (SBDP150) and 145 kDa (SBDP145) by calpain and is also cleaved to a 120-kDa product (SBDP120) by caspase-3. Calpain and caspase-3 are major executioners of necrotic and apoptotic cell death, respectively, during ischemia or TBI.[110–111] Thus, a unique feature of this technique is the ability to concurrently detect calpain and

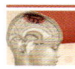

caspase-3 proteolysis of αII-spectrin, providing crucial information on the underlying cell death mechanisms.

Pineda et al[111] reported elevated levels of SBDPs in CSF from adults with severe TBI and their significant relationships with severity of injury and outcome.[111] Recently, CSF SBDP levels were found to be significantly higher in patients who died compared with those who survived.

Mondello et al[112] quantitatively assessed αII-spectrin breakdown products (SBDP145 produced by calpain, and SBDP120 produced by caspase-3) in cerebrospinal fluid (CSF) as markers of brain damage and outcome after severe traumatic brain injury (TBI). SBDP145 and SBDP120 were observed. SBDP145 provided accurate diagnoses at all time points examined, while SBDP120 release was more accurate 24 h after injury. Within 24 h after injury, SBDP145 CSF concentrations significantly correlated with GCS scores, while SBDP120 levels correlated with age. SBDP levels were significantly higher in patients who died than in those who survived. These results suggest that CSF SBDP levels can predict injury severity and mortality after severe TBI.

Ubiquitin C-terminal hydrolase-L1 was previously used as a histological marker for neurons owing to its high abundance and specific expression in neurons. A recent study reported that levels of UCH-L1 in CSF were significantly increased in severe TBI patients compared with control subjects.

REFERENCES

1. Cecil S, Chen PM, Callaway SE, Rowland SM, Adler DE, Chen JW, Advanced Multimodal Neuromonitoring; From Theory to Clinical Practice; Traumatic Brain Injury, Critical Care Nurse 2011;31:25–37.

2. Bhatia A, Gupta AK. Neuromonitoring in the intensive care unit. II. Cerebral oxygenation monitoring and microdialysis. Intensive Care Med 2007;33:1322–28.

3. Spiotta AM, Provencio JJ, Rasmussen PA, Manno E. Brain monitoring after subarachnoid hemorrhage: lessons learned. Neurosurgery 2011 Oct;69(4):755–66.

4. Leal-Noval SR, Cayuela A, Arellano-Orden V, Marín-Caballos A, Padilla V, Ferrándiz-Millón C, Corcia Y, García-Alfaro C, Amaya-Villar R, Murillo-Cabezas F. Invasive and noninvasive assessment of cerebral oxygenation in patients with severe traumatic brain injury. Intensive Care Med 2010;36(8):1309–17.

5. Rivers E, Nguyen B, Havstad S, et al; Early Goal-Directed Therapy Collaborative Group. Early goal-directed therapy in the treatment of severe sepsis and septic shock. N Engl J Med 2001; 345(19):1368–77.

6. Jadav SR, Sinha A, Tandon PN, et al. Cold caloric test in altered state of consciousness. Laryngoscope 1971;8:391–397.

7. Bruce DA, Alavi A, Balaniwk LT, et al. Diffuse cerebral swelling following head injury in children. The syndrome of malignant brain oedema. J Neurosurg 1981;54:170–8.

8. Mahapatra AK. Tandon PN, Bhatia R, Banerji AK. Bilateral decerebration in head injury patient. An analysis of 62 cases. Surg Neurol 1985;23:536–40.

9. Mahapatra AK. Tandon, PN. Brainstem auditory evoked potential and vestibulo ocular reflex in severe head injury. A prospective study of 60 cases. Acta Neurochirurgi (Wien) 1987;87:40–43.

10. Mahapatra AK. Monitoring in Pediatric Head injury patients. Neurology India (Suppl) 1995;43:64-67.

11. Taylor WR, Chen JW, Meltzer H, et al. Quantitative pupillometry, a new technology: normative data and preliminary observations of patients with acute head injury. J Neurosurg 2003;98(1):205–13.

12. Greenberg RP, Becker DP, Miller JD, et al. Evaluation of brain function in severe head trauma with multimodality evoked potential Part II. Localisation of brain dysfunction and correlation with post-traumatic neurological condition. J Neurosurg 1977;47:163–77.

13. Greenberg RP, Newlong PG, Hyatt MJ, et al. Prognostic implication of multimodal evoked potential in severe head injury patients. A prospective study. J Neurosurg 1981;55:227–36.

14. Humes AL, Cant BR. Central Somatosensory conduction time after head injury. Ann Neurol 1981;10:411–9.

15. Mahapatra AK. Evoked potentials in severe head injury. A prospective study of 40 patients. J Ind Med Asso 1990;88:217–20.

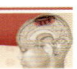

16. Seals DM, Rossiter VS, Weinstein ME. Brainstem auditory evoked responses in patients comatose as a result of blunt head trauma. J Trauma 1979;19:347–53.

17. Guerit JM. Usefulness of EEC exogenous evoked potentials, and cognitive evoked potentials in the acute stage of postanoxic and post traumatic coma. Acta Neurol Belg 2000;100:229–36.

17a. Brain Trauma Foundation; American Association of Neurological Surgeons; Congress of Neurological Surgeons; Joint Section on Neurotrauma and Critical Care, AANS/CNS, Bratton SL,Chestnut RM, Ghajar J, McConnell Hammond FF, Harris OA, Hartl R, Manley GT, Nemecek A, Newell DW, Rosenthal G, Schouten J, Shutter L, Timmons SD, Ullman JS, Videtta W, WilbergerJE, Wright DW . Guidelines for the management of severe traumatic brain injury. VIII. Intracranial pressure thresholds. J Neurotrauma 2008;24:S55–8.

18. Marshall LF, Smith RW, Shapiro, HM. The outcome with aggressive treatment in severe head injury. Part I. The significance of intracranial pressure monitoring. J Neurosurg 1979;80:20–25.

19. Lundberg N. Continuous recording and control of ventricular fluid pressure in neurosurgical practice. Acta Psychiatr Neurol Scand suppl 1960;36:1–193.

20. Lundberg N, Troupp H and Lorin, H. Continuous recording of the ventricular fluid pressure in patients with severe acute traumatic brain injury. Journal of Neurosurgery, 1965;22, 581–90.

21. Johnston IH, Johnston JA, Jennett WB. Intracranial pressure following head injury Lancet 1970;2:433–6.

22. Miller JD, Decker CD, Ward JD, et al. Significance of intracranial hypertension in severe head injury. J Neurosurg 1977;47:563–76.

23. Becker DP, Miller JD, Ward JD, et al. The outcome from severe head injury with early diagnosis and intensive management. J Neurosurg 1977;47:491–502.

24. Miller JD, Butterworth JF, Gudeman SK, et al. Further experience in management of severe head injury. J Neurosurg 1981;54:289–99.

25. Marmarou A, Anderson RL, Ward JD, et al. Impact of ICP instability and hypotension on outcome in patients with severe head trauma. J Neurosurg 1991;75:S59–66.

26. Marshall LF, Gautille T, Klauber MR, et al. The outcome of severe closed head injury. J Neurosurg 1991;75:528–36.

27. Miller JD. Volume and pressure in the craniospinal axis. Clinical Neurosurgery, 22, 76–105. Miller, JD and Adams J. H. (1992) The pathophysiology of raised intracranial pressure, in Greenfield's Neuropathology, 5th edn, (eds J. H. Adams and LW Duchen), Edward Arnold, Sevenoaks 1975;69–105.

28. Chambers IR, Jones PA , Lo, TYM, Forsyth RJ, Fulton B, Andrews PJD, Mendelow AD, Minns RA. Critical thresholds of intracranial pressure and cerebral perfusion pressure related to age in pediatric head injury; Journal of Neurology, Neurosurgery, and Psychiatry 2005;77(2):234–40.

29. Steiner LA, Czosnyka M. Should we measure cerebral blood flow in head-injured patients? Br J Neurosurg 2002 Oct;16(5):429–39.

30. Vajkoczy P, Roth H, Horn P, et al. Continuous monitoring of regional cerebral blood flow: experimental and clinical validation of a novel thermal diffusion microprobe. J Neurosurg 2000;93:265–74.

31. Springborg JB, Frederiksen HJ, Eskesen V, & Olsen, NV Trends in monitoring patients with aneurysmal subarachnoid hemorrhage. British Journal of Anesthesia 2005;94:259–70.

32. Tonnesen J, Pryds A, Larsen EH, Paulson OB, Hauerberg J, Knudsen GM. Laser Doppler flowmetry is valid for measurement of cerebral blood flow autoregulation lower limit in rats. Exp Physiol 2005;90:349–55. Epub 2005 Jan 14.

33. Jones TH, Morawetz RB, Crowell RM, et al. Thresholds of focal cerebral ischemia in awake monkeys. J Neurosurg 1981;54:773–782.

34. Yonas H, Darby JM, Marks EC, Durham SR, Maxwell C. CBF measured by Xe-CT: approach to analysis and normal values. J Cereb Blood Flow Metab 1991;11:716–25.

35. Bell BA, Symon L, Branston NM. CBF and time thresholds for the formation of ischemic cerebral edema.

36. Murkin JM and Arango M, Near-infrared spectroscopy as an index of brain and tissue oxygenationBr. J. Anesth. (2009) 103(suppl 1): i3-i13 doi:10.1093/bja/ep299.

37. Jobsis FF. Noninvasive, infrared monitoring of cerebral and myocardial oxygen sufficiency and circulatory parameters. Science 1977;198:1264–7.

38. McCormick PW, Stewart M, Goetting MG, Dujovny M, Lewis G, Ausman JI. Noninvasive cerebral optical spectroscopy for monitoring cerebral oxygen delivery and hemodynamics. Crit Care Med 1991;19:89–97.

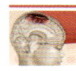

39. Yoshitani K, Kawaguchi M, Miura N, et al. Effects of hemoglobin concentration, skull thickness, and the area of the cerebrospinal fluid layer on near-infrared spectroscopy measurements. Anesthesiology 2007;106:458–62.

40. Martin NA, Dobertein C. Cerebral blood flow measurement in neurosurgical intensive care. Neurosurgia Clin North Ame 1994;5:607–18.

41. Ritter AM, Robertson CS. Cerebral metabolism. Neurosurg Clin N Ame 1994;5:633–45.

42. Sheinbergin, Kanter MJ, Robertson CS, et al. Continuous monitoring of jugular oxygen saturation in head injured patients. J. Neurosurg 1992;76:212–7.

43. Andrews PJ, Dearden NM, Miller JD. Jugular bulb cannulation. Description of a cannulation technique and validation of a new continuous monitor. Br J Anesth 1991;67:553–8.

44. White H, Baker A. Continuous jugular venous oximetry in the neurointensive care unit-a brief review. Can J Anesth 2002;49:(6);623–9.

45. Fitch W. Brain metabolism, in Cottrell j, Smith DS (eds). Anesthesia and Neurosurgery. 4th Edition, St Louis; Mosby 2001;1–17.

46. Gopinath SP, Robertson CS, Contant CF, et al. Jugular venous desaturation and outcome after head injury. J Neurol Neurosurg Psychiatry. 1994;57:717–23.

47. Robertson CS, Gopinath SP, Goodman JC, Contant CF, Valadka AB, Narayan RK. SjvO$_2$ monitoring in head-injured patients. J Neurotrauma 1995;12:891–6. [PubMed]

48. Lewis SB, Myburgh JA, Reilly PL. Detection of cerebral venous desaturation by continuous jugular bulb oximetry following acute neurotrauma. Anesth Intensive Care. 1995;23:307–14. [PubMed]

49. Haddad SH, Arabi YM. Critical care management of severe traumatic brain injury in adults. Scand J Trauma Resusc Emerg Med 2012 Feb 3; 20:12. Epub 2012 Feb 3.

50. Rosenthal G, Hemphill JC, Sorani M, Martin C, Morabito D, Obrist WD, Manley GT. Brain tissue oxygen tension is more indicative of oxygen diffusion than oxygen delivery and metabolism in patients with traumatic brain injury. Crit Care Med 2008;36(6):1917–24.[PubMed]

51. Meixensberger J, Dings J, Kuhnigk H, Roosen K. Studies of tissue pO$_2$ in normal and pathological human brain cortex. Acta Neurochir Suppl (Wien) 1993;59:58–63. [PubMed]

52. Stiefel MF, Spiotta A, Gracias VH, Garuffe AM, Guillamondegui O, Maloney-Wilensky E, Bloom S, Grady MS, LeRoux PD. Reduced mortality rate in patients with severe traumatic brain injury treated with brain tissue oxygen monitoring. J Neurosurg 2005;103:805–11. [PubMed]

53. Narotam PK, Morrison JF, Nathoo N. Brain tissue oxygen monitoring in traumatic brain injury and major trauma: outcome analysis of a brain tissue oxygen-directed therapy. J Neurosurg 2009;111(4):672–82. [PubMed]

54. Spiotta AM, Stiefel MF, Gracias VH, Garuffe AM, Kofke WA, Maloney-Wilensky E, Troxel AB, Levine JM, Le Roux PD. Brain tissue oxygen-directed management and outcome in patients with severe traumatic brain injury. J Neurosurg 2010;113(3):571–80. [PubMed]

55. Nangunoori R, Maloney-Wilensky E, Stiefel M, Park S, Andrew Kofke W, Levine JM, Yang W, Le Roux PD. Brain Tissue Oxygen-Based Therapy and Outcome After Severe Traumatic Brain Injury: A Systematic Literature Review. Neurocrit Care, 2011. in press. [PubMed]

56. Oddo M, Levine JM, Mackenzie L, Frangos S, Feihl F, Kasner SE, Katsnelson M, Pukenas B, Macmurtrie E, Maloney-Wilensky E, Kofke WA, LeRoux PD. Brain hypoxia is associated with short-term outcome after severe traumatic brain injury independently of intracranial hypertension and low cerebral perfusion pressure. Neurosurgery 2011;69(5):1037–45. discussion 1045. [PubMed]

57. Martin NA, Doberstein C, Zane C, et al. Posttraumatic cerebral arterial spasm: Transcranial Doppler ultrasound, cerebral blood flow, and angiographic findings. J Neurosurg 1992;77: 575–83.

58. Goraj B, Rifkinson-Mann S, Leslie DR, et al. Correlation of intracranial pressure and transcranial Doppler resistine index after head trauma. Am J Neuro Radio 1994;15:1333–39.

59. Bakshi A, Mahapatra AK. Basilar artery vasospasm in severe head injury. A preliminary TCD study. NMJI 1998;113:220–1.

60. Chan KH, Deardan NM, Miller JD. The significance of post-traumatic increase in cerebral blood flow velocity. A transcranial doppler ultrasound study. Neurosurg 1992;30: 697–700.

61. Shigemori M, Kikuchi N, Tokutomi T, et al. Monitoring severe head injury patients with transcranial doppler ultrasonography. Acta Neurochir Suppl (Wien) 1992;55:6–7.

62. Steiger HJ, Aaslid R, Stooss R, et al. Transcranial doppler monitoring in head injury. Relations

between injury, flovw velocity Vasor£activity, and outcome. Neurosurg 1994;34:79–85.

63. Lindegaard KF, Nornes H, Bakke SJ, et al. Cerebral vasospasm diagnosed by means of angiography and blood velocity measurements. Acta Neurochir (Wien) 1989;100:12–24.

64. Peerdeman SM, Girbes AR, Vandertop WP. Cerebral microdialysis as a new tool for neurometabolic monitoring.Intensive Care Med 2000;26:662–9.

65. Ungerstedt U, Rostami E. Microdialysis in neurointensive care. Curr Pharm Des 2004; 10(18):2145–52.

66. Peerdeman S, Tulder MW, Vandertop W. Cerebral microdialysis as a monitoring method in subarachnoid hemorrhage patients, and correlation with clinical events. J Neurol 2003;250:797–805.

67. Bellander B, Cantais E, Enblad P, et al.Consensus meeting on microdialysis in neurointensive care. Intensive Care Med 2004;30(12): 2166–2169.

68. Timofeev I, Carpenter KL, Nortje J, Al-Rawi PG, O'Connell MT, Czosnyka M, Smielewski P, Pickard JD, Menon DK, Kirkpatrick PJ, Gupta AK, Hutchinson PJ. Cerebral extracellular chemistry and outcome following traumatic brain injury: a microdialysis study of 223 patients; Brain 2011 Feb;134(Pt 2):484–94.

69. Verweij BH, Muizelaar JP, Vinas FC, Peterson PL, Xiong Y, Lee CP. Impaired cerebral mitochondrial function after traumatic brain injury in humans. J Neurosurg 2000;93:815–20.

70. Vespa P, Bergsneider M, Hattori N, Wu HM, Huang SC, Martin NA, et al. Metabolic crisis without brain ischemia is common after traumatic brain injury: a combined microdialysis and positron emission tomography study. J Cereb Blood Flow Metab 2005;25:763–74.

71. Vespa PM, O'Phelan K, McArthur D, Miller C, Eliseo M, Hirt D, et al. Pericontusional brain tissue exhibits persistent elevation of lactate/pyruvate ratio independent of cerebral perfusion pressure. Crit Care Med 2007;35:1153–60.

72. Vespa PM, McArthur D, O'Phelan K, Glenn T, Etchepare M, Kelly D, et al.Persistently low extracellular glucose correlates with poor outcome 6 months after human traumatic brain injury despite a lack of increased lactate: a microdialysis study. J Cereb Blood Flow Metab 2003;23:865–77.

73. Tokutomi T, Morimoto K, Miyagi T, Yamaguchi S, Ishikawa K, Shigemori M. Optimal temperature for the management of severe traumatic brain injury: effect of hypothermia on intracranial pressure, systemic and intracranial hemodynamics, and metabolism. Neurosurgery. 2007 Jul;61(1 Suppl):256–65; discussion 265–6.

74. Tokutomi T, Morimoto K, Miyagi T, Yamaguchi S, Ishikawa K, Shigemori M. Optimal temperature for the management of severe traumatic brain injury: effect of hypothermia on intracranial pressure, systemic and intracranial hemodynamics, and metabolism. Neurosurgery. 2003 Jan;52(1):102–11; discussion 111–2.

75. Huschak G, Hoell T, Hohaus C, Kern C, Minkus Y, Meisel HJ. Clinical evaluation of a new multiparameter neuromonitoring device: measurement of brain tissue oxygen, brain temperature, and intracranial pressure. J Neurosurg Anesthesiol. 2009 Apr;21(2):155–60. doi: 10.1097/ANA.0b013e31818f2eac.

76. Chunyan Li, Pei-Ming Wu, WooSeok Jung, Chong H. Ahn, Lori A. Shutter and Raj K. Narayan A novel lab-on-a-tube for multimodality neuromonitoring of patients with traumatic brain injury (TBI), Lab Chip 2009,1988;9.

77. Raabe A, Grolms C, Keller M, Dohnert J, Sorge O, Seifert V. Correlation of computed tomography findings and serum brain damage markers following severe head injury. Acta Neurochir. (Wien) 1998;140:787–91.

78. Romner B, Ingebrigtsen T, Kongstad P, Borgesen SE. Traumatic brain damage, serum S-100 protein measurements related to neuroradiological findings. J. Neurotrauma. 2000;17:641–7.

79. Woertgen C, Rothoerl RD, Metz C, Brawanski A. Comparison of clinical, radiologic, and serum marker as prognostic factors after severe head injury. J. Trauma 1999;47:1126–30.

80. Raabe A, Grolms C, Sorge O, Zimmermann M, Seifert V. Serum S-100B protein in severe head injury. Neurosurgery 1999;45:477–83.

81. Rothoerl RD, Woertgen C, Holzschuh M, Metz C, Brawanski A. S-100 serum levels after minor and major head injury. J. Trauma 1998;45:765–7.

82. Herrmann M, Curio N, Jost S, Wunderlich MT, Synowitz H, Wallesch CW. Protein S-100β and neuron specific enolase as early neurobiochemical markers of the severity of traumatic brain injury. Restor. Neurol. Neurosci 1999;14:109–14.

83. McKeating EG, Andrews PJ, Mascia L. Relationship of neuron specific enolase and protein S-100 concentrations in systemic and

jugular venous serum to injury severity and outcome after traumatic brain injury. Acta Neurochir. Suppl 1998;71:117–9.

84. Pelinka LE, Kroepfl A, Leixnering M, Buchinger W, Raabe A, Redl H. GFAP versus S-100β in serum after traumatic brain injury, relationship to brain damage and outcome. J. Neurotrauma 2004;21:1553–61.

85. Woertgen C, Rothoerl RD, Holzschuh M, Metz C, Brawanski A. Comparison of serial S-100 and NSE serum measurements after severe head injury. Acta Neurochir. (Wien) 1997;139:1161–64.

86. Rothoerl RD, Woertgen C. High serum S100β levels for trauma patients without head injuries. Neurosurgery 2001;49:1490–1.

87. Anderson RE, Hansson LO, Nilsson O, Dijlai-Merzoug R, Settergren G. High serum S100β levels for trauma patients without head injuries. Neurosurgery 2001;48:1255–8.

88. Romner B, Ingebrigtsen T. High serum S-100β levels for trauma patients without head injuries. Neurosurgery 2001;49:1490–3.

89. Jonsson H, Johnsson P, Backstrom M, Alling C, Dautovic-Bergh C, Blomquist S. Controversial significance of early S100B levels after cardiac surgery. BMC Neurol 2004;4:24.

90. Woertgen C, Rothoerl RD, Metz C, Brawanski A. Comparison of clinical, radiologic, and serum marker as prognostic factors after severe head injury. J. Trauma 1999;47:1126–30.

91. Raabe A, Grolms C, Sorge O, Zimmermann M, Seifert V. Serum S-100β protein in severe head injury. Neurosurgery 1999;45:477–483.

92. Rothoerl RD, Woertgen C, Holzschuh M, Metz C, Brawanski A. S-100 serum levels after minor and major head injury. J. Trauma 1998;45:765–7.

93. Berger RP, Dulani T, Adelson PD, Leventhal JM, Richichi R, Kochanek PM. Identification of inflicted traumatic brain injury in well-appearing infants using serum and cerebro-spinal markers, a possible screening tool. Pediatrics 2006;117:325–32.

94. Piazza O, Storti MP, Cotena S, et al. S100B is not a reliable prognostic index in pediatric TBI. Pediatr. Neurosurg 2007;43:258–64.

95. Kövesdi E, Lückl J, Bukovics P, Farkas O, Pál J, Czeiter E, Szellár D, Dóczi T, Komoly S, Büki A. Update on protein biomarkers in traumatic brain injury with emphasis on clinical use in adults and pediatrics. Acta Neurochir (Wien) 2010 Jan;152(1):1–17.

96. Marangos PJ, Schmechel DE. Neuron specific enolase, a clinically useful marker for neurons and neuroendocrine cells. Annu. Rev. Neurosci 1987;10:269–95.

97. Vos PE, Lamers KJ, Hendriks JC, et al. Glial and neuronal proteins in serum predict outcome after severe traumatic brain injury. Neurology 2004;62:1303–10.

98. Pelinka LE, Hertz H, Mauritz W, et al. Nonspecific increase of systemic neuron-specific enolase after trauma, clinical and experimental findings. Shock 2005;24:119–23.

99. Eng LF, Vanderheghen JJ, Bignami A, Gerstl B. An acidic protein isolated from fibrous astrocytes.Brain Res 1971;28:351–4.

100. Eng LF. Proteins of the Nervous System. Raven Press; NY, USA 2010; pp. 85–117.

101. Eng LF, Ghirnikar RS, Lee YL. Glial fibrillary acidic protein: GFAP-thirty-one years (1969–2000) Neurochem. Res 2000;25:1439–51.

102. Missler U, Wiesmann M, Wittmann G, Magerkurth O, Hagenstrom H. Measurement of glial fibrillary acidic protein in human blood: analytical method and preliminary clinical results. Clin. Chem 1999;45:138–41.

103. Pelinka LE, Kroepfl A, Schmidhammer R, et al. Glial fibrillary acidic protein in serum after traumatic brain injury and multiple trauma. J. Trauma 2004;57:1006–12.

104. van Geel WJ, De Reus HP, Nijzing H, Verbeek MM, Vos PE, Lamers KJ. Measurement of glial fibrillary acidic protein in blood, an analytical method. Clin. Chim. Acta 2002;326:151–4.

105. C-tau biomarker of neuronal damage in severe brain injured patients: association with elevated intracranial pressure and clinical outcome. Zemlan FP, Jauch EC, Mulchahey JJ, Gabbita SP, Rosenberg WS, Speciale SG, Zuccarello M.Brain Res 2002 Aug 23; 947(1):131–9.

106. Magnoni S, Esparza TJ, Conte V, Carbonara M, Carrabba G, Holtzman DM, Zipfel GJ, Stocchetti N, Brody DL (November 2011). "Tau elevations in the brain extracellular space correlate with reduced amyloid-β levels and predict adverse clinical outcomes after severe traumatic brain injury". Brain 2012 April;135:1268–80.

107. Pike BR, Flint J, Dave JR, et al. Accumulation of calpain and caspase-3 proteolytic fragments of brain-derived áII-spectrin in cerebral spinal fluid after middle cerebral artery occlusion in rats. J. Cereb. Blood Flow Metab 2004;24:98–106.

108. Riederer BM, Zagon IS, Goodman SR. Brain spectrin (240/235) and brain spectrin (240/

235E): two distinct spectrin subtypes with different locations within mammalian neural cells. J. Cell Biol 1986;102:2088–97.

109. Wang KK, Posmantur R, Nath R, et al. Simultaneous degradation of αII- and βII-spectrin by caspase-3 (CPP32) in apoptotic cells. J. Biol. Chem 1998;273:22490–7.

110. Ringger NC, O'Steen BE, Brabham JG, et al. A novel marker for traumatic brain injury, CSF αII-spectrin breakdown product levels. J. Neurotrauma 2004;21:1443–56.

111. Pineda JA, Lewis SB, Valadka AB, et al. Clinical significance of αII-spectrin breakdown products in cerebrospinal fluid after severe traumatic brain injury. J. Neurotrauma 2007;24:354–66.

112. Mondello S, Robicsek SA, Gabrielli A, Brophy GM, Papa L, Tepas J, Robertson C, Buki A, Scharf D, Jixiang M, Akinyi L, Muller U, Wang KK, Hayes RL. αII-spectrin breakdown products (SBDPs): diagnosis and outcome in severe traumatic brain injury patients. J Neurotrauma 2010 Jul; 27:1203–13.

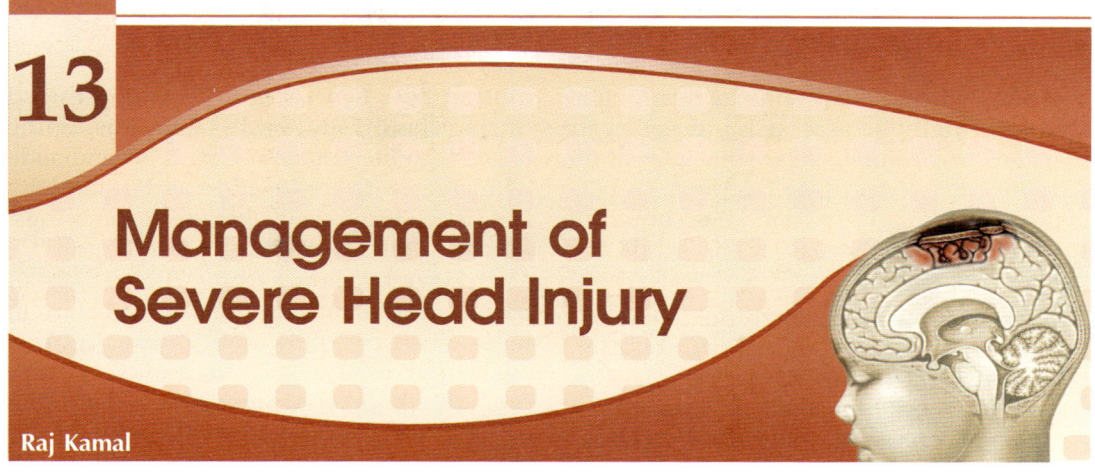

13

Management of Severe Head Injury

Raj Kamal

INTRODUCTION

Severe traumatic brain injury remains a major health care problem worldwide. Although major progress has been made in understanding of the pathophysiology of this injury, this has not yet led to substantial improvements in outcome. Patients with severe head injury should be transported directly to a facility that is better equipped to manage any patient with multiple injuries. The definitive management of major trauma is best possible at centers where all major specialities are present, including neurosurgery.

Patients with moderate to severe injuries are likely to receive treatment in an intensive care unit. In the acute stage the primary aim of the medical personnel is to stabilize the patient and focus on preventing secondary injury because little can be done to reverse the initial damage caused by trauma. Resuscitation should begin while shifting the patient to neurosurgical center. Quick neurological assessment and urgent CT scan of head should be top priority. Certainly following a standardized protocol with emphasis on early diagnosis and evacuation of intracranial mass lesions by craniotomy, artificial ventilation, control of increased intracranial pressure, and aggressive medical therapy improves outcome in severe head injury. These protocols, by preventing or reversing secondary cerebral insults, enables some patients who would have died to make a good recovery without increasing the proportion of severely disabled patients.

INITIAL MANAGEMENT OF ACUTE CLOSED HEAD INJURY AT THE ACCIDENT SITE AND DURING TRANSIT

Life saving measures should be started at the site of the accident. Usually, these prehospital care is managed by trained paramedics. The aims of this emergency service are:

1. Resuscitation
2. Prevention of second accident
3. Preparation of the injured for transport
4. Maintenance of optimum condition possible during transport until the patient is taken care of in the hospital.

The "ABC" system, where A = Airway, B = Breathing, and C = Circulation, is aimed at rapidly assessing and initiating the life supports urgently needed, followed by more detailed diagnostic examination and adjustment of treatment. Usually the head injured patients come quickly under the care of police and sometime under the ambulance services. Until the patient arrives at hospital care must be taken to see that the airway is clear. It is reported that approximate 50% severe head injury patients are hypoxic at the site of injury, which is associated with an increased mortality.[1,2] A control study had suggested prehospital intubation was associated with significant reduction of mortality.[3]

Adults who have sustained a head injury should initially be assessed and their care managed according to clear principles of the Advanced Trauma Life Support (ATLS) course.[4] Ambulance paramedics should be fully trained in the use of the adult and pediatric versions of the GCS.

Early hypotension or hypoxia greatly increase morbidity and mortality from severe head injury.[3, 5] At present, defining level of hypotension and hypoxia is unclear in these patients. However, ample class II evidence exists regarding hypotension (*refer* to page 180) defined as a single observation of a systolic blood pressure of < 90/mm Hg, or hypoxia, defined as apnea/cyanosis in the field or a PaO_2 < 60 mm Hg by arterial blood gas analysis, to warrant the formation of guidelines stating that these values must be avoided, if possible, or rapidly corrected in severe head injury patients.[5] A significant proportion of adult and pediatric TBI patients are discovered to be hypoxemic or hypotensive in the pre-hospital setting. Patients with severe head injury that are intubated in the pre-hospital setting appear to have better outcomes. Strong class II evidence suggests that raising the blood pressure in hypotensive, severe head injury patients improves outcome in proportion to the efficacy of the resuscitation.

Patients who have sustained a head injury and having impaired consciousness should be assumed to have spinal injury until proved otherwise. In conscious patients having neck pain possibility of spinal injury is high. Accordingly a rigid cervical collar and spinal board should be attached to all patients with suspected spinal injury.

While shifting the patient **"log rolling"** technique, keeping the position of head constant in relation to the trunk while turning, should be used. Cervical spine immobilization should be maintained until full risk assessment including clinical assessment (and imaging if deemed necessary) indicates it is safe to remove the immobilization device. However,

motion between C5 and C6 was reduced during the lift-and-slide technique. Spine boards can be removed using a lift-and-slide maneuver with less motion and potentially less risk to the patient's long-term neurologic function than expected using the log roll.[6,7]

Primary transport from accident site to trauma center should be done immediately, in most cases by road ambulance. Injuries sustained in remote areas may require properly equipped air ambulances (Helicopter or fixed wing aircraft). Air transfer should consider a few important effects of altitude on transport. The partial pressure of oxygen reduce with increasing altitude. Also gases expand in cavities at higher altitude. Hence an undrained pneumothorax and pneumo-cephalous (intracranial air) will expand at higher altitude.

INITIAL MANAGEMENT OF AIRWAY

Initial management of airway involves clearing the upper airway of vomitus, blood, secretions, and foreign bodies such as false or loose teeth. If possible an airway should be placed and oxygen should be given by mask. Initial attempts to establish an airway include chin-lift and jaw-thrust maneuver. If there is any doubt about the airway, intubate, especially if the patient is unconscious or has facial injuries. Special attention should be given to the possibility of a fracture of the cervical spine. Where multiple injuries are suspected and particularly in the case of fractures of the spine, the pelvis, a femur or a tibia, transport by stretcher is advised. Some authors have advised pulse oxymetry during transport of patient.[8,9]

It is reported that approximately 50% severe head injury patients are hypoxic at the site of injury, which is associated with an increased mortality.[1,2]

Management in the Casualty Room

In emergency room, the patient should be examined carefully and quickly. The airway patency and blood pressure should be checked again. Associated injuries should be identified and recorded. Reassessment of the patient is done by trauma team. The trauma team normally comprises general surgeon, orthopedician, neurosurgeon, and intensive care specialist.

If a patient airway cannot be obtained with simple oral or nasopharyngeal tubing, the patient should be intubated. Breath sounds should be evaluated, and, if the patient is intubated, the position of the endotracheal tube should be assessed to insure that it has not become dislodged during transport. In patients suspected to have cervical injury, intubation should be performed cautiously. Intubation should be done preferably by an anesthetist or by a qualified doctor to do so. If due to any reason intubation is not possible or delayed, an immediate tracheostomy should be done in patient who are having respiratory obstruction. The intensive care unit (ICU) management of patients with traumatic injuries presents a variety of challenges.

Patients with severe head injury may frequently have other traumatic injuries to internal organs, lungs, limbs, or the spinal cord. Thus, the management of the patient with severe head injury is often complex and requires a multidisciplinary approach.

Patients usually have been evaluated by an emergency physician and/or a general or trauma surgeon prior to transfer to the ICU. However, patients remain at risk for deterioration due to unrecognized injuries, iatrogenic complications of initial diagnostic studies and therapy, and general complications of critical care.

Early recognition and management of complications along with aggressive treatment of underlying medical conditions are necessary to minimize morbidity and mortality in this patient population. The management of traumatically injured patients will be reviewed here.

The trauma patient transferred to the ICU from the emergency department or operating room warrants full reassessment by the receiving medical personnel in accordance with advanced trauma life support (ATLS) guidelines.[4] Immediate attention should be given to the airway, breathing, and circulation.

The first hour or 'golden hour' following severe trauma will largely determine the patient's eventual outcome. Rapid resuscitation is essential. In the presence of significant hypovolemia, blood is redirected to the so-called vital organs—the brain, heart and kidneys. The so-called non-vital organs suffer relative ischemia. This has important implications for the splanchnic circulation. Hypoperfusion of the gastrointestinal tract predisposes to bacterial translocation and endotoxin absorption across a compromised mucosal barrier. This is compounded by ischemia of the reticuloendothelial system, particularly the liver, which otherwise would filter bacteria and toxins from the portal circulation. It has been proposed that bacterial translocation predisposes to the multiorgan failure (MOF) frequently seen after multi-trauma. It is crucial, therefore, to rapidly restore the circulation. This means not only maintaining a normal blood pressure (BP) but also guaranteeing perfusion to the non-vital organs, particularly the GIT.[10,34]

The neurological evaluation includes neurological evaluation of the level of consciousness as determined by the GSC (Table 13.1),[11,12] pupillary examination for size and reactivity, to assess potential or impending herniation. External evaluation of the head may reveal signs of basal skull fracture, mastoid ecchymosis (Battle's sign), periorbital ecchymosis (racoon eyes), and CSF otorrhea or rhinorrhea. Head injury can be classified as mild, moderate and severe according to Glasgow Coma Scale (GCS).

Mild head injury—GCS score 13 to 15
Moderate head injury—GCS score 9 to 12
Severe head injury — GCS score < 8

A CT scan is indicated immediately in all patients with moderate and severe head injury to rule out any intracranial mass lesion

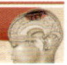

Table 13.1: Glasgow Coma Scale	
A. Eye opening	
Spontaneous	4
To speech	3
To pain	2
No eye opening	1
B. Best motor response	
Obeys command	6
Localizes to pain	5
Withdraws from stimulation (Flexion)	4
Abnormal flexion	3
Extension	2
No motor response	1
C. Best verbal response	
Oriented	5
Confused	4
In appropriate words	3
In comprehensible sounds	2
No verbal response	1

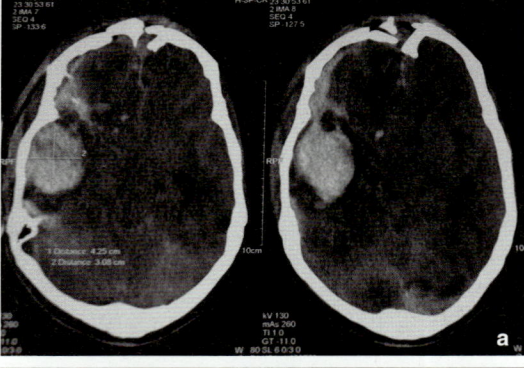

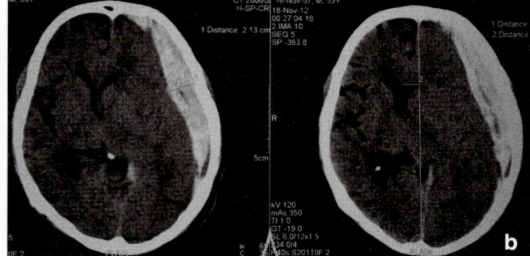

Fig. 13.1: CT scan showing intracranial hematoma with mass effect (a) large contusion hematoma, (b) acute subdural hematoma

(Fig. 13.1). CT scan of the brain is the cornerstone test in the evaluation of traumatic brain injury The primary approach to a large extradural hematoma or subdural hematoma with significant midline shift is surgical removal. In contrast, for patients with diffuse head injury and compressed cisterns should be treated in an ICU with a systematic protocol that includes intracranial pressure (ICP) monitoring and control, management of respiratory and cardiovascular parameters and cerebral metabolic control. Furthermore, an abnormal CT scan increases the risk of subsequent intracranial hypertension; 60% of patients with a closed head injury who have an abnormal CT scan developed increased ICP compared with only 13% of those with similar injuries but a normal presenting CT scan.[13] The literature generally supports the use of CT scanning for all cases of mild traumatic brain injury (MTBI) in which at least one of the following is present: loss of consciousness; post-traumatic amnesia (PTA); confusion or impaired alertness.[14,15] Stein and Ross[15] retrospectively studied patients admitted with GCS of 13 to 15 and loss of consciousness or

amnesia and showed that a significant percentage of these patients had abnormalities on CT scan. Studies of patients who may be categorized as "talk and deteriorate" also support the practice of scanning all mild traumatic brain injury patients.[16–21] In this manner, finding significant lesions on CT may allow earlier treatment prior to deterioration or allow close observation of patients who may otherwise have been discharged home. Although delayed neurological deterioration is more likely with a lower initial GCS, cases of fatal deterioration from GCS of 15 have been reported.[22,23] For those patients with a GCS of 15, no neurologic or cognitive abnormalities, and a normal brain CT, including absence of skull fracture, it is reasonable to discharge them home with a reliable adult.

As stated earlier systematic arterial blood pressure should be monitored and kept in normal range to maintain cerebral perfusion pressure (CPP). Crystalloid solution should be

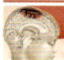

infused through a good intravenous line. Hypotonic solutions should not be used as they can produce or aggravate brain edema by lowering serum osmolality. Any patient presenting with hypotension, the source of internal bleeding must be sought. In unconscious patients with hypotension, hemopneumothorax, abdominal trauma, pelvic fracture should be carefully ruled out. Abdominal paracentesis is useful for diagnosing hemoperitoneum, but a negative tap does not exclude the diagnosis. Diagnostic peritoneal lavage may be done for diagnosing hemoperitoneum.

Subsequently, CT scan of abdomen should be planned in doubtful abdominal injury. X-ray films of the chest, pelvis may determine pneumohemothorax and fractured pelvis respectively. Cervical injury may also lead to hypotension. A failure to detect these injuries in an unconscious patient can result in drastic consequences.

Miller et al[9, 29] found additional systemic injuries in 49 percent cases of severe head injuries, the most common being limb fracture (30 percent). Chest injury occurred in 29 percent, abdominal injuries in 17 percent and spinal injuries in 6 percent of cases.[24]

The practical essential steps to be taken when a patient of severe head injury arrives in casualty.[25]

1. Maintenance of airway
   - Nasopharyngeal tube
   - Intubation
   - Tracheostomy.
2. Breathing (ventilation)
3. Circulation
   - Maintenance of systematic BP
   - Good intravenous line
   - CVP line
   - Crystalloid infusion
   - Blood transfusion, if required
4. Foley's catheterization and nasogastric intubation
5. Neurological assessment
   - GCS score

   - Pupillary size reaction
   - External injuries
6. Investigation
   - X-ray skull AP/Lat.
   - X-ray chest
   - X-ray cervical spine AP/Lat.
   - CT scan head.

If required, X-ray pelvis, X-ray abdomen, or CT abdomen arterial blood gases (ABG).

Intensive Care Unit Management

The intensive care unit (ICU) management of patients with traumatic injuries presents a variety of challenges. Patients usually have been evaluated by an emergency physician and/or a general or trauma surgeon prior to transfer to the ICU. However, patients remain at risk for deterioration due to unrecognized injuries, iatrogenic complications of initial diagnostic studies and therapy, and general complications of critical care. Intensive care unit management of both surgically treated and non-surgical patients is similar. Management of severe head injury is targeted at optimizing cerebral perfusion, oxygenation and avoiding secondary insults to brain (Table 13.2). for the management of CPP/ICP, Addenbrook's neurocritical care unit (NCCU) protocol[56] can be followed as given in Fig 13.4. Potentially treatable factors such as **hypoxia, hypotension, hyperthermia** and intracranial hypertension should be identified and treated accordingly. The outcome from severe head injury to a large extent depends on recognition and early treatment of the preventable secondary damage.

In the ICU following parameters can be monitored simultaneously systemic physio-

Table 13.2: Principles in management of head injury
The management of head injury are basically based on following principles
1. Measures to prevent secondary damage to brain; maintaining optimum CPP and by decreasing ICP
2. Increase oxygen delivery and reduce oxygen consumption of brain
3. Controlling volume of brain, blood and CSF

logic monitoring—**blood pressure and oxygenation,** neurological assessment, intracranial pressure (ICP) and cerebral perfusion pressure (CPP).

These parameters will guide in proper medical and surgical management.

1. *Neurological monitoring:* Periodic good neurological assessment will help in detecting early deterioration, improvement or static nature during therapy. No investigation can substitute for good neurological assessment.

2. Intracranial pressure (ICP) and cerebral perfusion pressure (CPP).

Normally, resting ICP is 5 to 15 mm. Transient elevations of ICP occurs normally with straining, coughing or the trendelenburg position. A sustained ICP greater than 20 mm Hg is clearly abnormal. An ICP between 20 and 40 mm Hg is considered moderate intracranial hypertension. An ICP greater than 40 mm Hg represents severe, usually life threatening intracranial hypertension.[27] About 50% of the patients with severe head injury will develop increased intracranial pressure. Increased ICP occurs in 50–70% of patients even after evacuation of intracranial hematoma.

The cranium and the vertebral canal, along with the relatively inelastic dura, form a rigid container, such that the increase in any of its contents; brain, blood, or CSF, will tend to increase the ICP. In addition, any increase in one of the components must be at the expense of the other two; this relationship is known as the Monro-Kellie doctrine. Rigid bony skull offers excellent protection to brain but allows little tolerance for additional volume. The intracranial contents include brain 1400 gm of which 80% is water, 75 ml of CSF mostly in ventricles, 75 ml of blood mostly in post capillary venous circulation.

Brain parenchyma account for most of the intracranial content. A 4-yr-old boy is least able to accommodate mass lesion than an elderly man. Apart from removing brain tissue or shrinking it with diuretics, the cell mass cannot be decreased.

Small increases in brain volume do not lead to immediate increase in ICP because of the ability of the CSF to be displaced into the spinal canal, as well as the slight ability to stretch the falx cerebri between the hemispheres and the tentorium between the hemispheres and the cerebellum. As the intracranial volume increases, compensation takes place and the ICP remains stable up to a point at which decompensation begins to occur, and then the ICP rises dramatically (Fig. 13.2). On that part of the intracranial compliance curve where the pressure suddenly increases, a small rise in volume will cause a dramatic increase in the ICP and will further reduce cerebral perfusion. Similarly, meticulous care of a patient who is functioning on this part of the curve can be rewarding. Any small decrease in intracranial volume that can be achieved, e.g. by sitting the patient up, keeping the head straight, using adequate sedation) can have a dramatic effect in bringing the ICP down. **Meticulous nursing care is crucial to outcomes for patients with increased ICP.**

The cerebral perfusion pressure (CPP) is equivalent to the mean arterial pressure (MAP) minus the ICP.

$$CPP = MAP - ICP$$

Cerebral ischemia is the single most important secondary factor that influences the

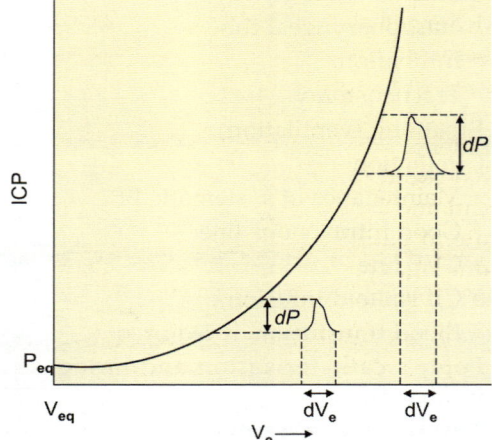

Fig. 13.2: Volume–pressure relationship

outcome after the TBI.[52] The outcome after severe head injury improved if the CPP was maintained above 70 mm Hg.[53] The compliance (C) describes the volume-dependent increase of the pressure in the craniospinal space and can be used for the assessment of the cerebrospinal space reserves. The inversion is termed elastance (E).

Marmarou, et al.[28] demonstrated that the non-linear craniospinal volume–pressure relationship could be described as a straight line segment relating the logarithm of pressure to volume, which implies a monoexponential relationship between volume and pressure. Marmarou termed the pressure–volume index (PVI) which is the imaginary volume required to raise ICP tenfold. PVI is calculated from pressure changes by injecting or withdrawing CSF. Higher values of PVI indicates higher brain compliance. Practically this means that withdrawing 10–15 ml of CSF through ventriculostomy could reduce ICP significantly.

For example, an increase in lesion volume (e.g. epidural hematoma) will be compensated by the downward displacement of CSF and venous blood. These compensatory mechanisms are able to maintain a normal ICP for any change in volume less than approximately 100–120 ml.

The association between the severity of intracranial hypertension and a poor outcome after severe head injury is well recognised. Miller, et al.[9] reported that mortality rate increased from 18 to 92% and the frequency of good outcomes decreased from 74 to 3% in patients with normal ICP compared with patients who had intracranial hypertension that could not be reduced below 20 mm Hg. Saul and Ducker[30] reported a 69% mortality rate in patients with an ICP greater than 25 mm Hg, compared with a mortality rate of 15% if ICP remained less than 25 mm Hg.[30]

Indications for ICP Monitoring in Head Injury Patients

Brain Trauma Foundation (BTF) guidelines[31, 41] (Table 13.3) suggest that ICP monitoring is primarily used when there is difficulty in clinical assessment of the patient or if there is a high risk of increased ICP. ICP monitoring is not necessary in the awake patient, in whom clinical assessment of neurological status is possible, and is contraindicated in the patient with a bleeding diathesis. In the latter case, all effort should be made to correct this if ICP monitoring is required. Patients with head injury not requiring ICP monitoring: Patients less than 40 years without evidence of abnormal motor activity, with normal pupillary examinations, with no significant history of secondary brain insults, and with CT scans showing no pathology and open basilar cisterns. These patients may be managed without ICP monitoring if they can undergo continuous neurological observation in the intensive care unit.[9] Furthermore, an abnormal CT scan increases the risk of subsequent intracranial hypertension; 60% of patients with a closed head injury who have an abnormal CT scan developed increased ICP compared with only 13% of those with similar injuries but a normal presenting CT scan.[13]

Brain Trauma Foundation[31] Recommends ICP Monitoring (Table 13.3)

1. All patients with severe TBI (GCS between 3–8 after resuscitation) and an abnormal CT scan that reveals hematomas, contusions, swelling, herniation or compressed cisterns (level II recommendation) (Table 13.4).
2. Patients with severe TBI with normal CT Scan if two or more features are noted at admission: age over 40 years, unilateral or bilateral motor posturing, or systolic BP < 90 mm of Hg (level III recommendation).

Methods

Two types of ICP monitoring devices are available (Table 13.4)

1. Fluid coupled
2. Non-fluid coupled

The fluid coupled devices are placed in ventricles, subarachnoid space or the subdural spaces and are connected to a

Table 13.3: Recommendations by brain trauma foundation[31] in the management of severe head injury

Level II recommendations

- Blood pressure should be monitored and hypotension (systolic blood pressure 90 mm Hg) avoided.
- Mannitol is effective for control of raised intracranial pressure (ICP) at doses of 0.25 g/kg to 1 g/kg body weight. Arterial hypotension (systolic blood pressure 90 mm Hg) should be avoided
- Periprocedural antibiotics for intubation should be administered to reduce the incidence of pneumonia. However, it does not change length of stay or mortality. Early tracheostomy should be performed to reduce mechanical ventilation days. However, it does not alter mortality or the rate of nosocomial pneumonia.
- Intracranial pressure (ICP) should be monitored in all salvageable patients with a severe traumatic brain injury (TBI; Glasgow Coma Scale [GCS] score of 3 to 8 after resuscitation) and an abnormal computed tomography (CT) scan. An abnormal CT scan of the head is one that reveals hematomas, contusions, swelling, herniation, or compressed basal cisterns
- Treatment should be initiated with intracranial pressure (ICP) thresholds above 20 mm Hg
- Aggressive attempts to maintain cerebral perfusion pressure (CPP) above 70 mm Hg with fluids and pressures should be avoided because of the risk of adult respiratory distress syndrome (ARDS)
- Prophylactic administration of barbiturates to induce burst suppression EEG is not recommended. Patients should be fed to attain full caloric replacement by day 7 post-injury
- Prophylactic hyperventilation ($PaCO_2$ of 25 mm Hg or less) is not recommended

Level III recommendations

- Oxygenation should be monitored and hypoxia (PaO_2 60 mm Hg or O_2 saturation 90%) avoided
- Restrict mannitol use prior to ICP monitoring to patients with signs of transtentorial herniation or progressive neurological deterioration not attributable to extracranial causes
- Pooled data indicate that prophylactic hypothermia is not significantly associated with decreased mortality when compared with normothermic controls. However, preliminary findings suggest that a greater decrease in mortality risk is observed when target temperatures are maintained for more than 48 h. Prophylactic hypothermia is associated with significantly higher Glasgow Outcome Scale (GOS) scores when compared to scores for normothermic controls
- Routine ventricular catheter exchange or prophylactic antibiotic use for ventricular catheter placement is not recommended to reduce infection. Early extubation in qualified patients can be done without increased risk of pneumonia
- Graduated compression stockings or intermittent pneumatic compression (IPC) stockings are recommended, unless lower extremity injuries prevent their use. Use should be continued until patients are ambulatory. Low molecular weight heparin (LMWH) or low dose unfractionated heparin should be used in combination with mechanical prophylaxis. However, there is an increased risk for expansion of intracranial hemorrhage
- ICP monitoring is indicated in patients with severe TBI with a normal CT scan if two or more of the following features are noted at admission: age over 40 years, unilateral or bilateral motor posturing, or systolic blood pressure (BP) 90 mm Hg
- A combination of ICP values, and clinical and brain CT findings, should be used to determine the need for treatment. CPP of < 50 mm Hg should be avoided
- Jugular venous saturation (50%) or brain tissue oxygen tension (15 mm Hg) are treatment thresholds. Jugular venous saturation or brain tissue oxygen monitoring measure cerebral oxygenation.
- High-dose barbiturate administration is recommended to control elevated ICP refractory to maximum standard medical and surgical treatment. Hemodynamic stability is essential before and during barbiturate therapy.
- Propofol is recommended for the control of ICP, but not for improvement in mortality or 6 month outcome. High-dose propofol can produce significant morbidity.
- Prophylactic use of phenytoin or valproate is not recommended for preventing late post-traumatic seizures (PTS)

Contd.

Table 13.3: Recommendations by brain trauma foundation[31] in the management of severe head injury (*Contd.*)

- Anticonvulsants are indicated to decrease the incidence of early PTS (within 7 days of injury). However, early PTS is not associated with worse outcomes
- Hyperventilation is recommended as a temporizing measure for the reduction of elevated intracranial pressure (ICP)
- Hyperventilation should be avoided during the first 24 hours after injury when cerebral blood flow (CBF) is oftencritically reduced
- If hyperventilation is used, jugular venous oxygen saturation (SjO_2) or brain tissue oxygen tension ($PbrO_2$) measurements are recommended to monitor oxygen delivery

Level I recommendations

The use of steroids is not recommended for improving outcome or reducing intracranial pressure (ICP). In patients with moderate or severe traumatic brain injury (TBI), high-dose methylprednisolone is associated with increased mortality and is contraindicated

Table 13.4 Intracranial pressure monitoring catheters[33]		
Method	*Advantages*	*Disadvantages*
Intraventricular	• Gold standard • Measures global values • Allows drainage of CSF • *In vivo* calibration	• Insertion may be difficult • Most invasive method • Risk of hematoma
Microtransducer system	• Intraparenchymal/subdural placement • Low complication risk • Low infection risk	• Small zero drift over time • No *in vivo* calibration • Measures local pressure
Epidural catheter	• Easy to insert • No penetration of dura • Rarely used	• Limited accuracy

CSF: Cerebrospinal fluid

pressure transducer through a fluid filled line. The ventriculostomy catheter remains the standard against which all of the newer monitors are compared. Ventricular catheter also allows cerebrospinal fluid drainage for therapeutic purposes. It can be placed easily and quickly in most patients with head trauma, even those with mass effect. Disadvantages of ventricular catheter include infection rate of 8 to 10% and 1 to 2% risk of intracranial hemorrhage.[41] **Subdural bolt (Richmond Screws)** which is placed in subdural space is less invasive. Subdural and epidural devices are comparatively less reliable and higher rate of blockage.

A ventricular catheter connected to an external strain gauge is the most accurate and low cost method for ICP monitoring. It also allows periodic re-zeroing. Presently, most common method of ICP monitoring is probably intraparenchymal catheters. Contemporary intraparenchymal transducers may be classified as solid state, based on silicon chips with pressure sensitive resistores forming Wheatstone bridge, or of fiberoptic design. Both systems are accurate but they have been reported to zero-drift over 4–5 days. Most neurosurgeons use ICP only for short time, hence these shortcomings may become irrelevant. The Codman ICP express monitoring system is one such system readily available and gives real time accurate ICP readings, so one can make timely decisions on surgical or medical aspects, contributing to good outcome.[32,66]

Non-fluid coupled system such as the Camino intraparenchymal monitor is placed within the parenchyma, and therefore, is not subjected to the discontinuities of pressure transmission afforded by the subarachnoid or dural layers and it is not prone to clogging. This system is expensive and the risks involved are similar to the fluid compiled systems.

Management of Raised ICP

Higher mortality and morbidity rates were observed in those patients whose ICP was persistently > 20 mm Hg.[34,36] Several studies done in past have shown the poorer outcomes associated with the failure to control ICP beyond certain ICP threshold.[35–39] It has been suggested that early initiation of treatment, before the ICP reaches 20 mm Hg, results in better ICP control. The duration of intracranial hypertension also contributes to outcome.[40] The tolerated threshold may also be related to the nature of the injury, with the results of an early study suggesting that those patients with mass lesions may tolerate higher ICP increases (< 40 mm Hg) and still obtain good outcomes, whereas those patients with diffuse brain injury may have poor outcomes with smaller increases in ICP (< 10 mm Hg).[5] Nevertheless, most centers initiate treatment when the ICP is more than 20 to 25 mm Hg, and the BTF guidelines support the initiation of treatment when ICP is ≥ 20 mm Hg.[31,38]

SURGICAL OPTIONS

An **intracranial hematoma** which is causing significant mass effect should be removed as soon as possible. Intracranial mass requiring expedient surgical removal is given in Table 13.4.

Decompressive craniectomy has been found to be useful if done early. Brain trauma foundation guidelines recommended timely evacuation of mass lesions (Table 13.5), however decompressive craniectomy is cautiously recommended as a possible option in selected patients (Fig. 13.5). Cooper et al[39,43] for the decompressive craniectomy trial concluded that, in patients with severe diffuse traumatic brain injury and increased intracranial pressure that was refractory to first-tier therapies, the use of craniectomy, as compared with standard care, decreased the mean intracranial pressure and the duration of both ventilatory support and the ICU stay but was associated with a significantly worse outcome at 6 months, as measured by the score on the extended Glasgow Outcome Scale. Timofeev et at[40] supported the theory that decompressive craniectomy leads to sustained reduction in ICP and improved cerebral pressure–volume compensation. He concluded that following decompressive craniectomy, adequate CPP levels can be achieved at lower MAP levels. This may reduce the load on the cardiovascular system and the risks associated with aggressive CPP

Table 13.5: Mass lesions requiring expedient surgical removal[44]

- *Acute extradural hematoma:* Volume > 30 cm^3 as measured on CT scan
- *Acute subdural hematoma:* Thickness > 10 mm *or* midline shift > 5 mm as measured on CT scan
- *Acute subdural hematoma:* Thickness < 10 mm or midline shift < 5 mm *but* GCS score < 9, which decreased by ≥ 2 points between injury and admission *and/or* presenting with fixed dilated pupils *and/or* ICP > 20 mmHg
- *Intraparenchymal lesion:* CT evidence of mass effect *or* increased ICP refractory to medical treatment *or* progressive neurological deterioration referable to lesion
- *Frontal/temporal contusion:* Volume > 50 cm^3 as measured on CT scan *or* GCS score 6–8 and volume > 20 cm^3 and midline shift > 5 mm/compression of cisterns
- *Posterior fossa lesion:* Mass effect on CT *or* neurological deterioration *or* deterioration referable to lesion
- Lesions not fulfilling these criteria may be conservatively managed along with serial imaging and close monitoring

CT: computed tomography; GCS: Glasgow Coma Scale; ICP: intracranial pressure

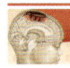

augmentation. Nevertheless, concurrent derangement in cerebrovascular pressure reactivity also occurred in most patients.

There are at present two prospective randomized controlled trials aimed at providing class I evidence on the role of DC in the treatment of intracranial hypertension following severe TBI. The decompressive craniectomy (DECRA) trial is a multicenter prospective randomized trial designed to evaluate the effect of early DC on neurological function in patients with severe TBI. It was based on the theory that early DC can improve long-term neurological outcome in patients with severe TBI and intracranial hypertension which is refractory to conventional management. DECRA stduy fail show a clinica benefit with the use of early decompressive craniectomy (details in chapter 18).[39, 43] Randomized evaluation of surgery with craniectomy for uncontrollable elevation (RESCUE) of ICP (RESCUEicp) is another prospective, randomized international multicentre trial aimed at providing class I evidence as to whether DC is effective for the management of patients with refractory intracranial hypertension following TBI as compared with medical management alone.[42]

Ventricular CSF drainage significantly reduces ICP. Its principal is based on the non-linear craniospinal volume–pressure relationship which Marmarou[28] termed the pressure–volume index (PVI) which is the imaginary volume required to raise ICP tenfold. Generally, a few milliliters of fluid are drained from the ventricle at a time resulting in an immediate decrease in ICP. However, ventricular space is often compressed due to associated brain swelling, which limits the potential for drainage as a stand alone therapy for ICP control[44] (James et al, 1976). The potential risk of ventricular drainage is ventricular catheter infection.

Standard practice has been to avoid lumbar drainage for fear of transtentorial or tonsillar herniation, however, technological improvements have renewed interest in its potential

for reducing ICP in patients refractory to other treatments (Tuettenberg et al, 2009).[45]

Hence, therapeutically, reducing cerebral blood volume (head-up positioning, hyperventilation and barbiturates); reducing CSF volume (CSF drainage) and reducing brain tissue volume (osmotic diuretics and glucocorticoids). Other conventional treatments, such as neuromuscular blockage, sedation and analgesia exert less specific effects.

MEDICAL MANAGEMENT (Figs 13.3 and 13.4)

Position of the patient's head: Ventilated head injured patients should be nursed with 15 to 30° from horizontal and the head should be maintained in neutral position.[31] This enhances cerebral venous drainage. This is an effective method of decreasing ICP and also may decrease the likelihood of subsequent ICP spikes. Care should be taken to note the level of the external auditory meatus, which is the zero reference point for the calibration of ICP monitors.

Hyperventilation: Hyperventilation to produce an arterial PCO_2 of 25 to 30 mm Hg will reduce ICP by promoting cerebral vasoconstriction and subsequent reduction of cerebral blood flow (CBF). $PaCO_2$ is a major determinant of cerebral vessel diameter, with its reduction causing cerebral vasoconstriction, and therefore, a reduction in cerebral blood volume and ICP. The onset of action is within 30 seconds and peaks within 8 minutes after PCO_2 drops to desired range.[46–50] In most patients hyperventilation lowers the ICP significantly; if the patient does not rapidly respond, the prognosis for survival is generally poor. Prolonged hyperventilation probably loses its effectiveness, and therefore, is of limited value beyond acute phase.[49,50] The partial pressure of carbon dioxide should not fall below 25 mm Hg because this may cause profound vasoconstriction and ischemia in normal and injured areas of brain. It can worsen regional ischemia, particularly in the first 24 h after TBI.[31,33,65] The routine application of hyperventilation is discouraged and a

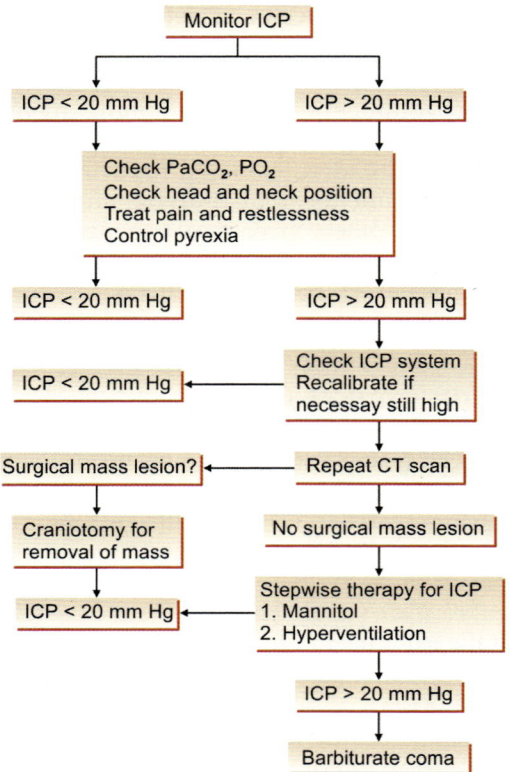

Fig. 13.3: Algorithm for management of raised intracranial pressure

$PaCO_2$ target of 30–35 mm Hg should be used in the first instance. The major difficulty with managing hyperventilation is the difficulty in assessing its effect on CBF metabolism matching. Hyperventilation to lower levels should always be carried out in association with cerebral oxygenation monitoring to avoid cerebral ischemia. One useful approach to this problem is the use of jugular venous saturation monitoring.[33] If hyperventilation is used, jugular venous oxygen saturation (SjO_2) or brain tissue oxygen tension ($PbrO_2$) measurements are recommended to monitor oxygen delivery and it should be avoided during the first 24 hours after injury when cerebral blood flow (CBF) is often critically reduced (level III recommendation, Table 13.3).[31]

Gopinath et al[51] found that hypocapnia (< 30 mm Hg) increased the incidence of cerebral desaturation [decreased jugular bulb oxygen saturation ($SjvO_2$) J. Current data supports the concept of optimized hyperventilation ($PaCO_2$ 30–35 mm Hg). $PaCO_2$ is a major determinant of cerebral vessel diameter, with its reduction causing cerebral vasoconstriction, and therefore, a reduction in cerebral blood volume and ICP.

Sedation

Sedation is often indicated in agitated or uncontrollable patient movement resulting from pain related to trauma, diagnostic or therapeutic maneuvers resulting in increased ICP. Sedation and analgesia are two important variables in the management of head injury. They reduce agitation and also reduce cerebral metabolic rate. A variety of different sedating agents have been used to facilitate ventilation, e.g. diazepam, midazolam, opiates and propofol. Propofol is a widely used sedative agent because it reduces ICP, has profound cerebral metabolic suppressive effects, allows easy control of sedation levels and ICP, and permits rapid wake-up.[54,50]

OSMOTIC AGENTS; MANNITOL AND HYPERTONIC SALINE

Mannitol is commonly used to control raised ICP following head injury. The osmotic effects of mannitol occur within minutes of its administration and peak at about 60 minutes after the bolus has been administered. The ICP-lowering effects of a single bolus may last for 6 to 8 hours. Mannitol (0.25 to 1.0 g/kg) can effectively reduce cerebral oedema by producing an osmotic gradient that draws tissue water into the vascular space.[55–58]

Hyperosmolar solutions (mannitol and hypertonic saline) are effective in reducing elevated intracranial pressure through 2 distinct mechanisms firstly, by plasma expansion with a resultant decrease in blood hematocrit, reduced blood viscosity, and decreased cerebral blood volume. Mannitol improves CBF by reducing blood viscosity and

Addenbrooke's NCCU: ICP/CPP management algorithm

All patients with or at risk of intracranial hypertension must have invasive arterial monitoring, CVP line, ICP monitor, and Rt SvO_2 catheter at admission to NCCU.

this algorithm should be used in conjunction with the full protocols for patient management.
Aim to establish multimodality monitoring within the first 6 h of NCCU stay
Interventions in stage III to be targeted to clinical picture and multimodality monitoring.
CPP 70 mm Hg set as initial target, but CPP >> 60 mm Hg is acceptable in most patients.
If brain chemistry monitored, $PtO_2 > 1$ kPa and LPR < 25 are 2° targets (*see* full protocol)

Evacuate significant SOLs and drain CSF before escalating medical Rx.
Rx in italics and grades IV and V only after approved by NCCU consultant.

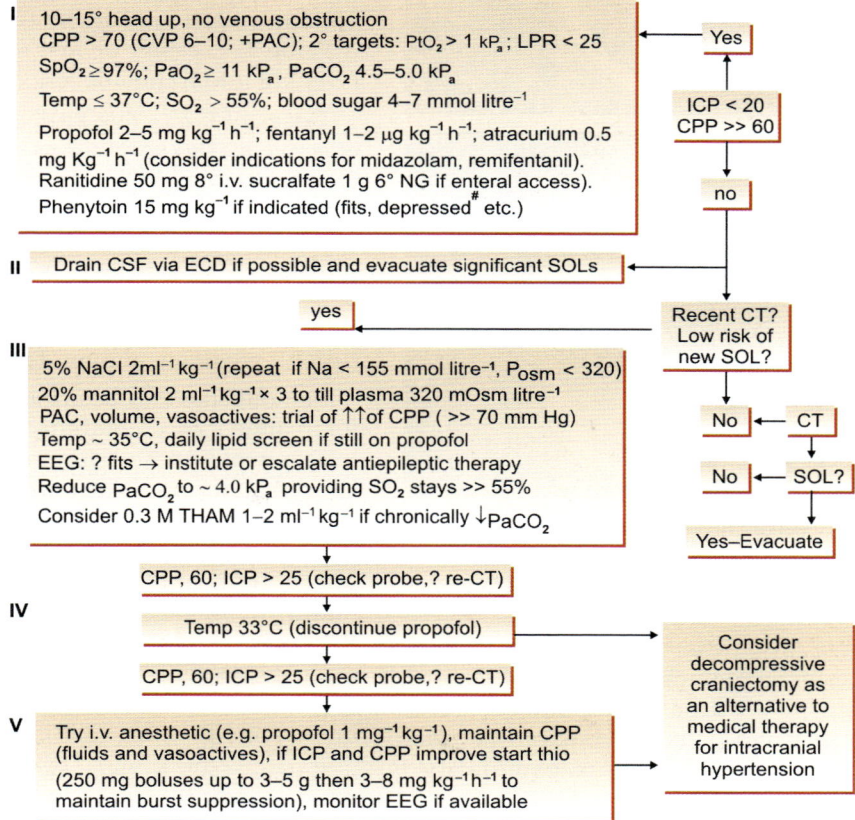

I 10–15° head up, no venous obstruction
CPP > 70 (CVP 6–10; +PAC); 2° targets: $PtO_2 > 1$ kPa; LPR < 25
$SpO_2 \geq 97\%$; $PaO_2 \geq 11$ kPa, $PaCO_2$ 4.5–5.0 kPa
Temp ≤ 37°C; $SO_2 > 55\%$; blood sugar 4–7 mmol litre^{-1}
Propofol 2–5 mg kg^{-1} h^{-1}; fentanyl 1–2 µg kg^{-1} h^{-1}; atracurium 0.5 mg Kg^{-1} h^{-1} (consider indications for midazolam, remifentanil).
Ranitidine 50 mg 8° i.v. sucralfate 1 g 6° NG if enteral access).
Phenytoin 15 mg kg^{-1} if indicated (fits, depressed# etc.)

II Drain CSF via ECD if possible and evacuate significant SOLs

III 5% NaCl 2ml^{-1} kg^{-1} (repeat if Na < 155 mmol litre^{-1}, $P_{osm} < 320$)
20% mannitol 2 ml^{-1} kg^{-1} × 3 to till plasma 320 mOsm litre^{-1}
PAC, volume, vasoactives: trial of ↑↑of CPP (>> 70 mm Hg)
Temp ~ 35°C, daily lipid screen if still on propofol
EEG: ? fits → institute or escalate antiepileptic therapy
Reduce $PaCO_2$ to ~ 4.0 kPa providing SO_2 stays >> 55%
Consider 0.3 M THAM 1–2 ml^{-1} kg^{-1} if chronically ↓$PaCO_2$

IV CPP, 60; ICP > 25 (check probe,? re-CT)
Temp 33°C (discontinue propofol)
CPP, 60; ICP > 25 (check probe,? re-CT)

V Try i.v. anesthetic (e.g. propofol 1 mg^{-1}kg^{-1}), maintain CPP (fluids and vasoactives), if ICP and CPP improve start thio (250 mg boluses up to 3–5 g then 3–8 mg kg^{-1}h^{-1} to maintain burst suppression), monitor EEG if available

Yes

ICP < 20
CPP >> 60

no

Recent CT?
Low risk of
new SOL?

No ← CT
No ← SOL?
Yes–Evacuate

Consider decompressive craniectomy as an alternative to medical therapy for intracranial hypertension

#Mean fracture

Fig. 13.4: The intracranial pressure (ICP)/cerebral perfusion pressure (CPP) management algorithm for the neuro critical care center in Addenbrooke's Hospital, 56 Cambridge, UK. CT: computed tomography; CVP: central venous pressure; MAP: mean arterial pressure; NCCU, neurological intensive care unit; OGT: oral gastric tube; PAV, pulmonary artery catheter; (Rt) SvO_2: (right) jugular bulb oxygen saturation; TCD: transcranial Doppler; SpO_2: oxygen saturation as measure by pulse oximetry

microcirculatory resistance. It reduces RBC deformity, and therefore, improves oxygen delivery. These effects may explain why mannitol reduces ICP within a few minutes of its administration, and why its effect on ICP is most marked in patients with low CPP (< 70 mm Hg).[59–62]

Secondly, the creation of an osmotic gradient that draws cerebral edema fluid from brain tissue into the circulation. In effect, this

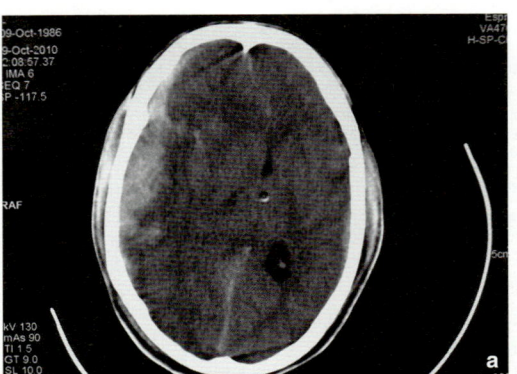

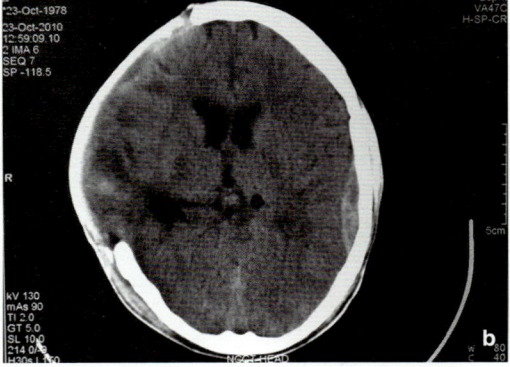

Fig. 13.5: Preoperative (a) and postoperative (b) CT scan following decompressive craniectomy. Midline shift is better and ventricles and sulci have opened up

reduces brain volume. The effect of mannitol depends on the dose, rate of infusion, serum osmolality and patient's state of hydration. The upper limit of serum osmolality is 320 mOsm/L.

Mannitol has neuroprotective properties. It is an effective free radical scavenger, reducing the concentration of oxygen free radicals that may promote cell membrane lipid peroxidation. Mannitol also promotes CBF by reducing blood viscosity and microcirculatory resistance. It reduces RBC deformity, and therefore, improves oxygen carrying capacity.

Mannitol can induce hypovolemic hypotension. Repeated doses of mannitol increases serum osmolality. This reduces the effectiveness of mannitol, may cause dilutional

hyponatremia, and may precipitate acute renal failure. Also repeated episodes of diuresis may wash out the renal medullary concentration gradient and thereby interfere with the ability of the kidneys to concentrate the urine. As mannitol enters areas of damaged blood–brain barrier (BBB), mannitol may concentrate within brain tissue, producing reverse osmotic effect.[57] By reducing brain volume, tamponade of extra-axial hematoma may be decreased or lost, allowing more bleeding into traumatic lesion.

Doses of 0.25 g/kg appear to be equally effective as 1 g/kg in terms of effect on ICP. Serum osmolality should not be allowed to increase beyond 320 mOsm/L). Mannitol is effective for control of raised intracranial pressure (ICP) at doses of 0.25 g/kg to 1 g/kg body weight. Arterial hypotension (systolic blood pressure 90 mm Hg) should be avoided (level II recommendation, Table 13.3).

Mannitol has long been the "gold standard" for treatment of cerebral edema and refractory intracranial hypertension in traumatic brain injury, subarachnoid hemorrhage, and stroke. Studies performed in animals have shown that hypertonic saline (HS), in doses ranging from 3% to 10%, may be more effective than mannitol in treating these populations. Recently, randomized clinical trials have evaluated the efficacy and safety of HS versus mannitol in the treatment of elevated intracranial pressure (ICP).[59]

Kamel et al[61] in their meta-analysis found that hypertonic saline is more effective than mannitol for the treatment of elevated intracranial pressure. Their meta-analysis comprised of five trials comprising 112 patients with 184 episodes of elevated intracranial pressure . In random-effects models, the relative risk of intracranial pressure control was 1.16 (95% confidence interval, 1.00–1.33), and the difference in mean intracranial pressure reduction was 2.0 mm Hg (95% confidence interval, 1.6 to 5.7), with both favoring hypertonic saline over mannitol. A mild degree of heterogeneity was present

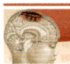

among the included trials. There were no significant adverse events reported. Theses findings suggested that hypertonic saline may be superior to the current standard of care and argue for a large, multicenter, randomized trial to definitively establish the first-line medical therapy for intracranial hypertension. Proposed beneficial effects of HTS in TBI may arise from several mechanisms. The permeability of the BBB to sodium is low.[63,64] HTS administration produces an osmotic gradient between the intravascular and intracellular/ interstitial compartments, leading to shrinkage of brain tissue (where BBB is intact), and therefore, a reduction in ICP. The reflection coefficient (selectivity of the BBB to a particular substance) of NaCl is more than that of mannitol, making it potentially a more effective osmotic drug.[62,64] HTS augments volume resuscitation and increases circulating blood volume, mean arterial blood pressure (MAP), and CPP.[65] Other beneficial effects include restoration of the neuronal membrane potential, maintenance of the BBB integrity, and modulation of the inflammatory response by reducing adhesion of leukocytes to endothelium.[66–68]

Furosemide is a loop diuretic often used in patients with head injury. It also can lead to significant dehydration and hypokalemia. Evidence exists that furosemide works synergistically with mannitol in lowering ICP.[69]

Barbiturates

Barbiturates are effective in lowering ICP. Second tier therapy with barbiturates is required in select group of patients with refractory intracranial hypertension.[52,70]

Barbiturates have a potent depressant effect on cerebral electrical activity and metabolism, with the degree of depression being related to the anesthetic depth.[71] Because barbiturates decrease cerebral metabolism and thus the need for oxygen delivery. They are vasoconstrictors thereby decreasing cerebral blood flow (CBF) and ICP. In patients with intracranial hypertension, barbiturates caused the greatest reduction in ICP in those patients whose initial ICP was abnormally high. This decrease in ICP is often associated with an increase in cerebral perfusion pressure (CPP). Barbiturates lower ICP by many mechanisms and, although there is no good evidence that they improve outcome after TBI,[72] there has been a resurgence of interest in the use of high-dose barbiturate therapy for the treatment of refractory intracranial pressure.[53] Hypotension is a frequent complication of treatment, and drug accumulation leads to delayed recovery and difficulties in rapid clinical assessment when the drug is discontinued. Continuous EEG monitoring can be used to titrate barbiturate infusion and minimize side effects. Prophylactic administration of barbiturates to induce burst suppression EEG is not recommended (level II recommendation, Table 13.3).

Beneficial effects
- Decreases $CMRO_2$ and CBF
- Vasoconstriction
- Inhibits free radicals

Side effects
- Hypotension
- Myocardial depression

Thiopental, a short acting barbiturate, is most commonly used to control intracranial hypertension.

Thiopental should be given only in patients admitted to an intensive care unit capable of intensive neurosurgical care. Barbiturate therapy should be accomplished with a loading dose of 10 mg/kg of **thiopental** given during 30 minutes. This dose should be followed by an infusion of 5 mg/kg/hr during the next 3 hours. The maintenance dose should be started on a 1 mg/kg/hr. During administration of loading dose, if the patient's blood pressure decreases, the intravascular volume should be increased and pressures such as **dopamine** should be started.

Propofol

Propofol is a relatively new sedative-hypnotic with a very rapid onset and short duration of action. The intravenous anesthetic agent propofol has many advantages as an agent for treating raised ICP. It reduces $CMRO_2$ and CBF. It also reduces systemic BP usually results in net decrease in cerebral perfusion pressure (CPP). This decrease is usually not significant. At least two studies have shown a beneficial effect on ICP in head injury patients treated with this agent[73–75] infusion. Propofol is recommended for the control of ICP, but not for improvement in mortality or 6 month outcome. High-dose propofol can produce significant morbidity. (level II recommendation, Table 13.3). Other drugs which reduce ICP (action similar to **propofol) are: Etomidate and Lidocaine.**

Hypothermia: Hypothermia reduces cerebral metabolism and hence prevents hypoxic and ischemic damage. Hypothermia induced very early after traumatic brain injury (TBI) does not, in general, lead to improved outcomes compared with normothermia, but might be beneficial in a subgroup of patients who undergo surgery to treat large traumatic hematomas.[76] Moderate hypothermia (33–35°C) has efficient neuroprotective effects in animal studies but human trials have been disappointing, mainly because of infection. We must control this morbidity, which is not that simple, before using it again in humans. In addition, high temperatures are associated with worse outcomes after TBI and are the most important cause of secondary brain injury. Core temperature and cerebral temperature should be continuously monitored and pyrexia must be prevented and aggressively treated.

SEIZURE PROPHYLAXIS

Up to 9% of all patients who sustain blunt head trauma suffer from **early post-traumatic seizures.**[76,77] The incidence of early post-traumatic seizure approaches 42% in patients who have sustained penetrating head trauma.[21] Although the occurrence of seizures in the immediate post-trauma period has no predictive value for future epilepsy, early seizures can cause **hypoxia, hypercarbia, release of excitatory neurotransmitters** and increased ICP, which can worsen secondary brain injury. Therefore, all paralyzed head injured patients should have prophylactic anticonvulsant therapy in the acute phase. If the patient is actively seizing, **benzodiazepines** are effective rapidly acting **anticonvulsants.**

Diazepam: 0.1 mg/kg, up to 5 mg IV, every 5 minutes up to a total of 20 mg.

For a long-term anticonvulsant activity, phenytoin is given:

Loading dose: 15 mg/kg IV is given slowly at 50 mg/minute
Maintenance dose: 5 mg/kg.

Corticosteroids and control of ICP: Steroids are highly effective in controlling brain edema when it is tumor associated, but there is no convincing evidence of their efficacy in head injury, intracerebral hematoma or stroke.[79–81]

There is level I evidence that the use of steroids is not recommended for improving outcome or reducing intracranial pressure (ICP). In patients with moderate or severe traumatic brain injury (TBI), high-dose methylprednisolone is associated with increased mortality and is contraindicated.

CEREBRAL PERFUSION PRESSURE (CPP) MONITORING

When ICP monitoring is used as a guide to the therapy of acutely brain injured patients, its main value is in preserving cerebral perfusion pressure (CPP).

CPP represents the pressure gradient across the intracranial compartment and is defined as the mean arterial pressure (MAP) minus the ICP. The major role of ICP monitoring lies in determination of CPP.

$$CPP = MAP - ICP$$

Measures to Maintain MAP

1. Administration of crystalloid, colloids and blood products to maintain euvolemia.

2. Administration of inotropes; dopamine, dobutamine, norepinephrine and epinephrine, phenylephrine HCl.

Recent work suggested that CPP should be kept above 60 mm Hg. If CPP is sustained above 60 mm Hg then long-term outcome improves significantly[53,82] while attempting to reduce ICP. Hence, mean arterial pressure (MAP) should be maintained. Rosner et al in 1995,[53] had laid down the protocol for CPP management and reported good outcome when CPP was more than 70 mm of Hg. However, CPP management can be possible following proper guidelines.[83] It consisted of vascular expansion, systemic vasopressors, cerebrospinal fluid (CSF) drainage through ventriculostomy, and mannitol to maintain a CPP of at least 70 mm Hg. All patients had an ICP monitor. An oxygen saturation greater than 90% and a $PaCO_2$ of 35 mm Hg was maintained in all patients. Hyperventilation was used only when ICP was raised. Fluid management was aimed at maintaining euvolemia or moderate hypervolemia. Albumin infusions were used to mobilize the extracellular water into intravascular compartment in patients who were well- or over-hydrated. Packed red cells were transfused with hemoglobin and hematocrit values as targets. Serum sodium and potassium levels were maintained within normal limits.

A CPP of 70 mm Hg was targeted initially, by draining CSF until the ICP decreased to 15 mm Hg. In addition, CSF was continuously drained whenever CPP dropped to below 70 mm Hg. If still the CPP did not increase to 70 mm Hg, vasopressors are added. Phenylephrine or norepinephrine with or without dopamine were used to achieve the required MAP. Mannitol in a dose of 0.5–1.0 g/kg was used whenever CPP decreased to below 70 mm Hg due to ICP elevation. Following the initial studies that showed better outcomes than other contemporary series, a number of studies tried to define the critical CPP in TBI. The threshold values suggested by these studies varied widely between 50 mm Hg and higher than 70 mm Hg.

Side effects of CPP therapy; ARDS and increase in ICP are main problems faced when CPP is increased. Robertson et al[84] compared a CBF-targeted protocol (CPP higher than 70 mm Hg and normocapnic ventilation) with an ICP management protocol (with a target ICP of less than 20 mm Hg and a CPP greater than 50 mm Hg). Hyperventilation was permitted to treat elevated ICP in the latter group. There was a substantial reduction in ischemic episodes in the CBF-targeted group. This was, however, associated with a fivefold increase in the incidence of acute respiratory distress syndrome (ARDS). Further analysis of the same data[85] revealed that the use of epinephrine and high dose dopamine to maintain CPP greater than 70 mm Hg was the main risk factor for the development of ARDS.

Hypertensive therapy can be expected to increase ICP and cause poor outcome.[85,86] The effect of artificial blood pressure elevation on ICP and CBF has been studied by Bouma and Muizelaar.[87] In 35 patients with TBI, they found that elevation of the mean arterial blood pressure from 92 ±10 to 123 ± 8 mm Hg led to only an insignificant increase in ICP in those patients with intact autoregulation.[87] In the group with defective autoregulation, there was actually a decrease in mean ICP. Bruce et al found that artificially increasing the systolic blood pressure by 30 mm Hg caused an average increase in ICP of only 4 mm Hg, and in 3 cases the ICP actually decreased.[88]

Nutritional Support to Severely Head-Injured Patients

Severe head injury results in a hypercatabolic state. Starting early enteral nutrition helps in establishing integrity of gastric mucosa, which has a beneficial effect on immunocompetence and helps in metabolic response to stress[89–91] Patients should be fed to attain full caloric replacement by day 7 post-injury [level II recommendation, Table 13.3). Some meta analysis have shown the comparison of initiation of enteral nutrition within 36 hours

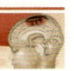

and beyond. Early enteral nutrition showed 55% reduction in risk of infection. Parenteral nutrition must be avoided, as it is associated with profound metaboli immunologic and GI changed and increases the mortality. There is increased gastric emptying time in head injured patients.[91] Immune enhancing nutrition formula through nasogastric tube 20–30 ml per hour is started to achieve the nutritional goal.[89,91] Well planned and balanced nutritional replacement reduces the mortality by reducing risk of infection.

CONCLUSIONS

The management of severe head injury should aim toward prevention of secondary brain damage and maintenance of an optimum cerebral perfusion pressure and low ICP for adequate neuronal recovery. Prevention of secondary brain damage can help to reduce mortality and morbidity. Recommendations of BTF should be kept in mind while treating severe patients. Factors which ultimately play a role in outcome are hypoxia, hypotension, intracranial hematoma, diffuse injury, ICP > 20 mm Hg, level of cerebral perfusion pressure and associated medical problems. Any effort to maintain the above factors within normal limits will prevent secondary damage, hence outcome.

REFERENCES

1. Stocchetti N, Furlan A, Volta F. Hypoxemia and arterial hypotension at the accident scenie in head injury. J. Trauma 1996;40:764–7.

2. Witchall RJ, Hoyt DB. Endotracheal intubation in the field improves survival in patients with severe head injury. Arch Sury 1977;132:592–7.

3. White RJ. Programmed management of severe head injuries revisited. J Trauma 1975;15:779–84.

4. Kortbeek JB, Al Turki SA, Ali J, Antoine JA, Bouillon B, Brasel K, Brenneman F, Brink PR, Brohi K, Burris D, Burton RA, Chapleau W, Cioffi W, Collet e Silva Fde S, Cooper A, Cortes JA, Eskesen V, Fildes J, Gautam S, Gruen RL, Gross R, Hansen KS, Henny W, Hollands MJ, Hunt RC, Jover Navalon JM, Kaufmann CR, Knudson P, Koestner A, Kosir R, Larsen CF, Livaudais W, Luchette F, Mao P, McVicker JH,
Meredith JW, Mock C, Mori ND, Morrow C, Parks SN, Pereira PM, Pogetti RS, Ravn J, Rhee P, Salomone JP, Schipper IB, Schoettker P, Schreiber MA, Smith RS, Svendsen LB, Taha W, van Wijngaarden-Stephens M, Varga E, Voiglio EJ, Williams D, Winchell RJ, Winter R. J Trauma. Advanced trauma life support, 8th edition, the evidence for change 2008;64:1638–50.

5. The Brain Trauma Foundation. The American Association of Neurological Surgeons. The Joint Section on Neurotrauma and Critical Care. Resuscitation of blood pressure and oxygenation. J Neurotrauma 2000;17:471–8.

6. Conrad BP, Horodyski M, Wright J, Ruetz P, Rechtine GR 2nd. Log-rolling technique producing unacceptable motion during body position changes in patients with traumatic spinal cord injury. J Neurosurg Spine 2007;6: 540–3.

7. Horodyski M, Conrad BP, Del Rossi G, DiPaola CP, Rechtine GR 2nd. Removing a patient from the spine board: is the lift and slide safer than the log roll? J Trauma 2011;70:1282–5.

8. Silverston P. Pulse oxymetry at the road side a study of pulse oxymetry in immediate care. BMJ 1989;298:711–3.

9. Miller JD, Butlerworth JF, Gudeman SK. et al. Further experience in the management of severe head injury. J Neurosurg 1981;54:289–99.

10. Ken Hillman and Gillian Bishop. Trauma. In Clinical Intensive Care and Acute Medicine Second Edition. Cambridge university press 2004;224–63.

11. Teasdale, G. and B. Jennett. "Assessment of coma and impaired consciousness. A practical scale." Lancet 1974;2(7872):81–84.

12. Teasdale, G. and B. Jennett. "Assessment and prognosis of coma after head injury." Acta Neurochir (Wien) 1976;34:45–55.

13. Narayan RK, Kishore PRS, Becker DP, Ward JD, Enas GG, Greenberg RP, Domingues Da Silva A, Lipper MH, Choi SC, Mayhall CG, Lutz HA III., Young HF. Intracranial pressure: to monitor or not to monitor? J Neurosurg 1982;56:650–9.

14. Shackford SR, Wald SL, Ross SE, et al. The clinical utility of computed tomographic scanning and neurologic examination in the management of patients with minor head injuries. J Trauma 1992;33:385–94.

15. Stein SC, Ross SE. Mild head injury: A plea for routine early CT scanning. J Trauma 1992;33:11–13.

16. Livingston DH, Loder PA, Koziol J, Hunt CD. The use of CT scanning to triage patients

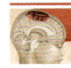
requiring admission following minimal head injury. J Trauma 1991;31:483–9.

17. Stein SC, Ross SE. The value of computed tomographic scans in patients with low-risk head injuries. Neurosurgery 1990;26:638–40.

18. Dacey RG Jr, Alves WM, Rimel RW, Winn HR, Jane JA. Neurosurgical complications after apparently minor head injury. Assessment of risk in a series of 610 patients. J Neurosurg 1986;65:203–10.

19. Reilly PL, Graham DI, Adams JH, Jennett B. Patients with head injury who talk and die. Lancet 1975;2:375–7.

20. Rockswold GL, Pheley PJ. Patients who talk and deteriorate. Ann Emerg Med 1993;22:1004–1007.

21. Rockswold GL, Leonard PR, Nagib MG. Analysis of management in thirty-three closed head injury patients who "talked and deteriorated". Neurosurgery 1987;21:51–55.

22. Gomez PA, Lobato RD, Ortega JM, De La Cruz J. Mild head injury: Differences in prognosis among patients with a Glasgow Coma Scale score of 13 to 15 and analysis of factors associated with abnormal CT findings. Br J Neurosurg 1996;10:453–60.

23. Riesgo P, Piquer J, Botella C, Orozco M, Navarro J, Cabanes J. Delayed extradural hematoma after mild head injury: Report of three cases. Surg Neurol 1997;48:226–31.

24. Michael DB, Guyot DR, Darmody WR Coincidence of head and cervical spine injury. J Neurotrauma 1989;6:177–89.

25. Initial assessment and management Advanced trauma life support for doctors: Students course manual Chicago II American college of surgeon 1997;21–46.

26. Zaloga CP, Marik P. Promotility agents in the intensive care unit. Crit Care Med 2000;28:265–9.

27. Lundberg N, Troupp H, et al. Continuous recording of the ventricular fluid pressure in patients with severe acute traumatic brain damage. J Neurosurg 1965;22:581–90.

28. Marmarou A, Maset AL, Ward JD, et al. Contribution of CSF and vascular factors to elevation of ICP in severely head-injured patients. Journal of Neurosurgery 1987;66:883–90.

29. Miller JD, Becker DP, et al. Significance of intracranial hypertension in severe head injury. J Neurosurg 1977;47:501–16.

30. Saul TG, Ducker TB; Effect of intracranial pressure monitoring and aggressive treatment on mortality in severe head injury. J Neurosurg 1982;56:498–503.

31. Brain Trauma Foundation; American Association of Neurological Surgeons; Congress of Neurological Surgeons; Joint Section on Neurotrauma and Critical Care, AANS/CNS, Bratton SL, Chestnut RM, Ghajar J, McConnell Hammond FF, Harris OA, Hartl R, Manley GT, Nemecek A, Newell DW, Rosenthal G, Schouten J, Shutter L, Timmons SD, Ullman JS, Videtta W, Wilberger JE, Wright DW . Guidelines for the management of severe traumatic brain injury. VIII. Intracranial pressure thresholds. J Neurotrauma 2008;24: S55–8.

32. Gupta DK, Mahapatra AK, Kumar H. Monitoring in Patients with Traumatic Brain Injury: an Experience of 98 cases. Indian Journal of Neurotrauma 2006;3:31–36.

33. Flavio M.B. Maciel, Central Nervous System Monitoring, In Antonino Gullo, José Besso, Philip D. Lumb, Ged F. Williams (Eds.) Intensive and Critical Care Medicine WFSICCM World Federation of Societies of Intensive and Critical Care Medicine 2009;135–43.

34. Juul N, Morris GF, Marshall SB, Marshall LF. Intracranial hypertension and cerebral perfusion pressure: influence on neurological deterioration and outcome in severe head injury. J Neurosurg 2000;92:1–6.

35. STICH (Trauma) Trial. Balestreri M, Czosnyka M, Hutchinson P, Steiner LA, Hiler M, Smielewski P, Pickard JD. Impact of intracranial pressure and cerebral perfusion pressure on severe disability and mortality after head injury. Neurocrit Care 2006;4:8–13.

36. Miller JD, Butterworth JF, Gudeman SK, Faulkner JE, Choi SC, Selhorst JB, Harbison JW, Lutz HA, Young HF, Becker DP ;Further experience in the management of severe head injury. J Neurosurg 1981;54:289–99.

37. Marshall LF, Smith RW, Shapiro HM. The outcome with aggressive treatment in severe head injuries. Part I: The significance of intracranial pressure monitoring. J Neurosurg 1979;50:20–5.

38. Treggiari MM, Schutz N, Yanez ND, Romand JA. Role of intracranial pressure values and patterns in predicting outcome in traumatic brain injury: a systematic review. Neurocrit Care 2007;6:104–12.

39. Cooper DJ., Rosenfeld JV, Murray L, Arabi YM, MD, Davies AR, D'Urso P, Kossmann T, Ponsford J, Seppelt I, Reilly P and Wolfe R, for the DECRA Trial Investigators and the Australian and New Zealand Intensive Care Society Clinical Trials Group, Decompressive

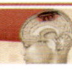

Craniectomy in Diffuse Traumatic Brain Injury. N Engl J Med 2011; 364:1493–1502.

40. Timofeev I, Czosnyka M, Nortje J, Smielewski P, Kirkpatrick P, Arun Gupta A, and Hutchinson P, Effect of decompressive craniectomy on intracranial pressure and cerebrospinal compensation following traumatic brain injury J Neurosurg 2008;108:66–73.

41. Luerssen T, Chestnut R, et al. Post traumatic cerebrospinal fluid infections in the Traumatic Coma Data Bank : The influence of type ad management of ICP monitors. In: Avezaat C, Van Eyndhoven J, Mass A, et al., eds. Intracranial pressure VIII. Berlin : Springer-Verlag 1993;157–63.

42. Hutchinson PJ, Corteen E, Czosnyka M, Mendelow AD, Menon DK, Mitchell P, Murray G, Pickard JD, Rickels E, Sahuquillo J, Servadei F, Teasdale GM, Timofeev I, Unterberg A, Kirkpatrick PJ. Decompressive craniectomy in traumatic brain injury: the randomized multicenter RESCUEicp study (www. RESCUEicp.com). Acta Neurochir Suppl 2006;96:17–20.

43. Cooper DJ, Rosenfeld JV, Murray L, Wolfe R, Ponsford J, Davies A, D'Urso P, Pellegrino V, Malham G, Kossmann T. Early decompressive craniectomy for patients with severe traumatic brain injury and refractory intracranial hypertension: a pilot randomized trial. J Crit Care 2008;23:387–93.

44. James HE, Langfitt TW, & Kumar VS. Analysis of the response to therapeutic measures to reduce intracranial pressure in head injured patients. J.Trauma 1976;16:437–41.

45. Tuettenberg J, Czabanka M, Horn P, Woitzik J, Barth M, Thome C, et al. Clinical evaluation of the safety and efficacy of lumbar cerebrospinal fluid drainage for the treatment of refractory increased intracranial pressure. J Neurosurg 2009;110:1200–8.

46. Marshall LF, Smith RW, Shapiro HM: The outcome with aggressive treatment in severe head injury. The significance of intracranial pressure monitoring, J Neurosurg, 1979;50:20–25.

47. Mendelow AD, Teasdale G, Jennett B, et al. Risks of intracranial haematoma in head injured adults, Br Med J 1983;287:1173–6.

48. Greenberg MS. Head trauma. In Handbook of Neurosurgery. Fla, Greenberg Graphics, 1994.

49. Muizelaar JP, Marmaror A, Ward JD, et al. Adverse effects of prolonged hyperventilation : A randomized clinical trial. J Neurosurg 1991;75:731.

50. Michelle H Biros. Head Trauma. In Rosen P, Barkin R (eds) : Emergency Medicine, Concepts and Clinical Practice 4th Ed., Mosby, 1998.

51. Gopinath SP, Robertson CS, et al. Jugular venous desaturation and outcome after head injury. J Neurol Neurosurg Psychiatry 1994;57:717–23.

52. Marshall LF. Treatment of brain swelling and brain edema in man Adv Neurol, 1980;28:459–69.

53. Rosner MJ, Rosner SD, John Son AH. Cerebral perfusion pressure. Management protocol and clinical results. J Neurosurg 1995;83:949–62.

54. Citerlo G, Cormio M. Sedation in neurointensive care: Advances in understanding and practice. Curr Opin Crit Care 2003;9:120–6.

55. Berger S, Schurer L, Hartl R, et al. Reduction of post-traumatic intracranial hypertension by hypertonic/hyperoncotic saline/dextran and hypertonic mannitol. Neurosurgery 1995; 37:98–107. Ovid Full Text ExternalResolverBasic Bibliographic Links [Context Link].

56. Helmy A, Vizcaychipi M, Gupta AK (2007) Traumatic brain injury: Intensive care management. Br J Anaesth 99:32–4.

57. Kaufmann AM, Cardoso ER. Aggravation of vasogenic edema by multiple-dose mannitol. J Neurosurg 1992;77:584–9.

58. Bullock R. Mannitol and other diuretics in severe neurotrauma. New Horizons, Crit Care Med 1995;3:448–52.

59. Knapp JM. Hyperosmolar therapy in the treatment of severe head injury in children: mannitol and hypertonic saline. AACN Clin Issues 2005;16:199–211.

60. Brain Trauma Foundation; American Association of Neurological Surgeons; Congress of Neurological Surgeons; Joint Section on Neurotrauma and Critical Care, AANS/CNS, Bratton SL,Chestnut RM, Ghajar J, McConnell Hammond FF, Harris OA, Hartl R, Manley GT, Nemecek A, Newell DW, Rosenthal G, Schouten J, Shutter L, Timmons SD, Ullman JS, Videtta W, WilbergerJE, Wright DW . Guidelines for the management of severe traumatic brain injury. VIII. Hyperosmolar therapy J Neurotrauma 2007;24 Suppl 1:S14–20.

61. Kamel, Hooman MD; Navi, Babak B. MD; Nakagawa, Kazuma MD; Hemphill, J. Claude III MD, MAS; Ko, Nerissa U. MD; Hypertonic saline versus mannitol for the treatment of elevated intracranial pressure: A meta-analysis of randomized clinical trials. Critical Care Medicine 2011;39:554–9.

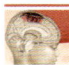

62. Fenstermacher JD, Johnson JA. Filtration and reflection coefficients of the rabbit blood–brain barrier. Am J Physiol 1966;211:341–6.

63. Betz AL. Sodium transport in capillaries isolated from rat brain. J Neurochem 1983;41:1150–7.

64. Zornow MH. Hypertonic saline as a safe and efficacious treatment of intracranial hypertension. J Neurosurg Anesthesiol 1996;8: 175–7.

65. Schmoker JD, Shackford SR, Wald SL, Pietropaoli JA. An analysis of the relationship between fluid and sodium administration and intracranial pressure after head injury. J Trauma 1992;33:476–81.

66. Cross JS, Gruber DP, Gann S, et al. Hypertonic saline attenuates the hormonal response to injury. Ann Surg 1989;209:684–91; discussions 91–2.

67. Hartl R, Medary MB, Ruge M, et al. Hypertonic/hyperoncotic saline attenuates microcirculatory disturbances after traumatic brain injury. J Trauma 1997;42:S41–7.

68. Hartl R, Schurer L, Schmid-Schonbein GW, del Zoppo GJ. Experimental antileukocyte interventions in cerebral ischemia. J Cereb Blood Flow Metab 1996;16:1108–19.

69. White PF, Schlobohm RM, et al. A randomized study of drugs for preventing increases in intracranial pressure during endotracheal suctioning. Anesthsiology 1982;57:242–4.

70. Rea G, Rockswold G. Barbiturate therapy in uncontrolled intracranial hypertension. Neurosurgery 1983;12:401–04.

71. Michen felder JD. The interdependency of cerebral functional and metabolic effects following massive doses of thiopental in the dog. Anesthesiology 1974;41:231.

72. Roberts I. Barbiturates for acute traumatic brain injury. Cochrane Database Syst Rev, 2000.

73. Farling PA, Johnston JR, et al. Propofol infusion for sedation of patients with head injury in intensive care: a preliminary report. Anesthesia 1989;44:222–6.

74. Hartung HJ. Intracranial pressure after propofol and thiopental administration in patients with severe head trauma. Anaesthetist 1987;36:285–7.

75. Moss E, Powell D, Gibson RM. Effect of etomidate on intracranial pressure and cerebral perfusion pressure. Br J Anaesth 1979;51:347–51.

76. Kennedy CR, Freeman JM. Post-traumatic seizures and post-trauma tic epilepsy in children, J Head Trauma Rehab 1986;1:66.

77. Heather Wood Traumatic brain injury: Is hypothermia beneficial in TBI? Nature Reviews Neurology March 2011;7:127.

78. Temkin NR, Dikmen SS, Winn HR. Post-traumatic seizures, Neurosurg Clin North Am, 1991;2:425.

79. Todd NV, Teasdale GM. Steroids in human head injury. In : Capildeo R, ed. steroids in Diseases of the Central Nervous system. John Wiley, 1989;151–9.

80. Knietowicz Z. Trial of steroids for treating head injury begins BMJ 1999;318:1441.

81. Bullock MR, Chestnut RM, Clifton GL, et al. Role of steroids. J. Neurotrauma 2000;17:531–5.

82. Chan KH, Miller JD, et al. The effects of changes in cerebral perfusion pressure upon middle cerebral artery blood flow velocity and jugular bulb venous oxygen saturation after severe brain injury. J Neurosurg 1992;77:55–61.

83. Guidelines for cerebral perfusion pressure J. Neurotrauma 2000;17:507–11.

84. Robertson CS, Valadka AB, Hannay HJ, Contant CF, Gopinath SP, Cormio M. Prevention of secondary ischemic insults after severe head injury. Crit Care Med 1999;27:2086–95.

85. Contant CF, Valadka AB, Gopinath SP, Hannay HJ, Robertson CS. Adult respiratory distress syndrome: a complication of induced hypertension after severe head injury. J Neurosurg 2001;95:560–8.

86. Marshall WJS, Jackson JLF, Langfitt TW: Brain swelling caused by trauma and arterial hypertension. Arch Neurol 1969;21:545–53.

87. Bouma GJ, Muizelaar JP: Relationship between cardiac output and cerebral blood flow in patients with intact and with impaired autoregulation. J Neurosurg 1990;73:368–74.

88. Bruce DA, Langfitt TW, Miller JD, Schultz H, Vapalhti MP, Stanek A, et al: Regional cerebral blood flow, intracranial pressure, and brain metabolism in comatose patients. J Neurosurg 1973;38:131–44.

89. K lodell CT, Carroll M, Carrillot, et al. Routine intragastric feeding following traumatic brain injury is safe and well tolerated. Am J. Surg 2000;179:168–71.

90. Marik PE, Zaloga GP. Early enteral nutrition in acutely ill patients: a systemic review. Crit Care Med 2001;29:2264–70.

91. Kao CH. Changlai SP, Chieng PU, et al. Gastric emptying in head-injured patients. Aue J. Gastroenterol 1998;93:1108–12.

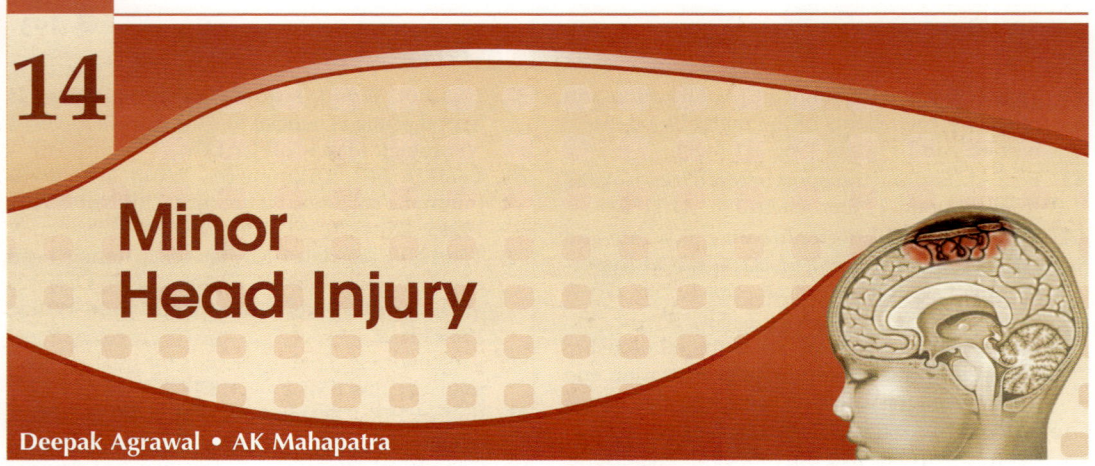

14

Minor Head Injury

Deepak Agrawal • AK Mahapatra

INTRODUCTION

'Minor head injury', also known as 'Mild traumatic brain injury' or 'concussion' has been the subject of intense investigation in recent years as it is being increasing realized that in spite of an apparently normal CT head (Fig. 14.1), there might be subtle organic brain damage, which may be associated with distressing neuropsychological sequelae in these patients.[1]

Epidemiology

Head injuries are amongst the most common types of trauma seen in developing as well as developed countries. Minor head injuries in turn, form the bulk of these head injuries ranging from 80 to 90%. A typical review of head injured patients admitted to a neuro-surgical service found that 5% were 'severe' (GCS score < 8), 11% were 'moderate' (GCS score 8 to 12) and 84% were 'minor' (GCS score 13 to 15).[2]

Clinical Features

The most widely used definition of minor head injury is a set of criteria published by the members of the Mild Traumatic Brain Injury Interdisciplinary Special Interest Group (BISIG) of the American Congress of Rehabilitation Medicine (Handbook 16)[3] which states that:

1. Loss of consciousness should not exceed 30 minutes.

2. After 30 minutes the initial GCS score should be between 13 and 15.

3. Post-traumatic amnesia does not exceed 24 hours.

Following minor head injury, a syndrome called **'postconcussion syndrome'** has been reported to occur in up to 80% of the patients.[4] This syndrome includes symptoms such as headache, irritability, poor concentration, memory disturbances, dizziness, anxiety and depression. Persistent postconcussion syndrome, defined as persistence of symptoms of postconcussion syndrome beyond three months, is seen in more than 30% of the patients, and up to 15% may have persistent, disabling symptoms beyond six months.[5] To assist with the diagnosis of postconcussion syndrome, the International Statistical Classi-fication of Diseases and related Health Problems, 10th edition (ICD-10),[6] published a set of guidelines based on epidemiological studies in several countries and regions. Here postconcussion syndrome was defined as history of head trauma with loss of conscious-ness that precedes symptom onset by a maximum of four weeks with three or more symptoms of the following:

- Headache, dizziness, malaise, fatigue, noise intolerance.

- Irritability, depression, anxiety, emotional liability.

- Subjective concentration, memory or intellectual difficulties without neuropsychological evidence of marked impairment.
- Insomnia.
- Reduced alcohol tolerance.
- Preoccupation with above symptoms and fear of brain damage without hypochondriacal concern and adoption of sick role.

Pathophysiology

The clue to suspected structural damage in minor head injuries might be found in experimental studies, in which pathological evidence of damage to the medial temporal lobes after mild or moderate head injury has been documented. Smith et al[7] found that bilateral dentate hilar neuron loss was a consistent finding two weeks after minor head injury and was uniformly associated with memory dysfunction. In a related study, Kotapka et al[8] delivered mild acceleration type experimental head injuries to nonhuman primates and found hippocampal lesions in virtually all animals injured in the lateral plane. The hippocampus, a key structure in the medial temporal lobe, is located within the hippocampal formation, a collection of cytoarchituraly distinct subdivisions that also includes the dentate gyrus, subicular complex, and entorhinal cortex.[9] The hippocampus is especially vulnerable to mechanically induced head injury and to other types of insults such as ischemia, hypoxia, and seizures,[10] and the extent of hippocampal damage may be correlated with severity of memory impairment.[11]

Even more revolutionary is the study by Nakatomi et al[12] which provides the first evidence of functional neurogenesis. Using a rat model of transient forebrain ischemia, the authors evaluated whether they could manipulate and enhance ischemic injury induced endogenous neurogenesis. They administered fibroblast growth factor-2 (FGF-2) and epidermal growth factor (EGF) intraventricularly and found that it resulted in an increased repopulation of CA1 hippocampal neurons lost following ischemic insult. More importantly, growth factor treated rats demonstrated improved functional outcome as compared to control ischemic rats. It is tempting to speculate that humans may similarly be affected with neuronal loss in hippocampus after minor head injury, which in future may be reversible. However, as practical considerations preclude histopathological analysis in this group of patients, newer investigative modalities such as SPECT and PET due to their high sensitivity appears as an attractive proposition for studying structural damage in such patients. At a study conducted at AIIMS using SPECT in children with persistent postconcussion syndrome and abnormal SPECT brain (unpublished data), all children showed medial temporal (86%) or frontal (13%) hypoperfusion, and no patient showed hyperperfusion (Figs 14.2 and 14.3). This finding of areas of hypoperfusion in minor head injury has been described previously[17–19] and may result from vasospasm, direct vascular injury and perfusion changes due to alterations in remote neuronal activity (diaschisis).[13] There is evidence to show that brain is more vulnerable to ischemic injury after minor head injury[14] and it has been hypothesized that SPECT findings representing hypoperfusion may in fact lead to secondary ischemic injury.[13] TCD study also shows defect in blood flow velocity.

Investigations

In the recent years, with its widespread availability, the use of CT for minor head injury has become increasingly common (Fig. 14.1). However, there is considerable disagreement in the literature as to the indications for CT in the large number of head trauma cases classified as 'minor.[15] Some studies have tried to derive algorithms to identify a subset of patients in whom CT may be avoided.[15,16] These studies fail to address the basic issue of CT having a abysmally low sensitivity of less than 10% in the so-called 'minor head injuries'.[17,18] Because of this, various modalities ranging from neuropsychological testing, evoked potential and P_{300} testing, to newer

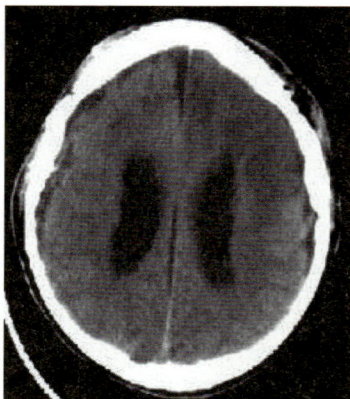

Fig. 14.1: CT scan of a minor head injury

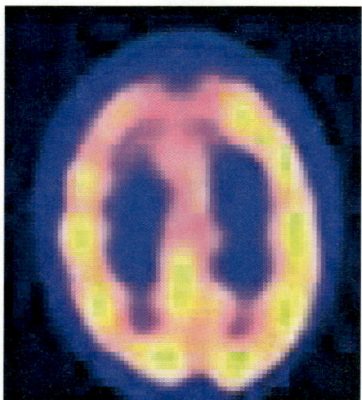

Fig. 14.2: SPECT of the same patient as in CT scan Fig. 14.1

radiological techniques such as PET, SPECT and MRI have been investigated as tools to correlate cerebral dysfunction with symptoms in cases of minor head injuries.[19,20] Umile et al[21] tried to correlate dynamic imaging (PET and SPECT) findings with static imaging (CT and MRI) as well as with neuropsychological testing in 19 patients with minor head injury and postconcussion syndrome and found that 90% had abnormal findings on PET or SPECT imaging. Though PET is slightly superior to SPECT in terms of spatial resolution however, SPECT is much more affordable and widely available making it attractive as a costeffective investigative and diagnostic tool in postconcussion syndrome. In our study SPECT has shown a sensitivity of 80% which is excellent when compared to abysmally poor sensitivities of 9% for CT and 46% for MRI scan recorded by others.[17,18] As our own studies show, perfusion abnormalities seen on SPECT do not correct spontaneously over a long time in a significant number of patients, and changes in cerebral perfusion have been found to persist for as long as one year following mild traumatic brain injury.[18, 22]

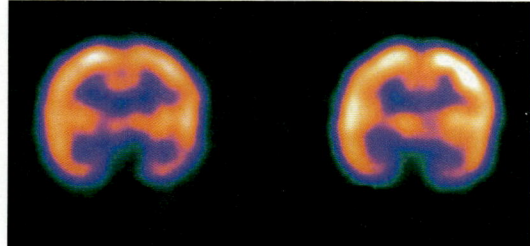

Fig. 14.3: SPECT coronal section showing medial temporal hypoperfusion

Management

Management of minor head injury revolves around two broad issues: Firstly, the use of investigative procedures such as SPECT, PET and neuropsychological testing as a means of prognostication and secondly, treatment strategies for postconcussion syndrome.

Investigative tools such as SPECT, PET and neuropsychological assessment help in prognostication, especially in preschool children (less than five years of age) as there is good evidence that even minor head injury, if occurring at an age that is critical for the development of a certain skill, may cause persisting deficits.[21] Wrightson et al[23] prospectively studied the effect of minor head injury on preschool children using neuropsychological tests and found that injury in the preschool years seemed to affect the process of learning to read. The authors stressed that if early identification and diagnosis of these children could be made, teachers could be made aware of this and remedial teaching could be made available to them.

Despite new insights gained in the pathophysiology of mild traumatic brain injury and the realization that there may be profound brain perfusion abnormalities existing behind a seemingly normal CT head of such 'minor' head injury patients with postconcussion syndrome, most neurosurgeons can do little except giving reassurance and prescribing analgesics and anti-vertigo medication. Recently, a neurotropic agent, piracetam has been tried in such patients. Piracetam has a unique mode of action that though not entirely clear, may be explained by its neuroprotective properties, mediated through effects on the cell membrane.[24] Piracetam improves membrane bound cell functions including ATP production[25,26] and secondary messenger activity.[25] It also has been shown that piracetam has beneficial effects on the cerebral blood flow, by decreasing the adhesivity, aggregation, and deformability of erythrocytes along with flow thrust tension of the blood.[27] We conducted a randomized controlled trial with found that low dose of piracetam successfully reversed cerebral perfusion deficits and resulted in accelerated symptomatic improvement in patients with postconcussion syndrome (Figs 14.1a and b). However, as the study number was small, before recommending piracetam for clinical use in postconcussion syndrome, placebo-controlled trials using larger number of patients are required.

REFERENCES

1. Watson MR, Fenton GW, McClelland RJ, Lumsden, Headley M, Rutherford WH. The postconcussion state: Neurophysiological aspects. Br J Psychiatry 1995;167:514–21.

2. Miller JD. Minor, moderate and severe head injury. Neurosurg Rev 1986;9:135–9.

3. Mild Head Injury Interdisciplinary Special Interest Group of the American Congress of Rehabilitation Medicine. Definition of mild traumatic brain injury. J Head Trauma Rehabil 1993;8:86–88.

4. Hugenholtz H, Stuss DT, Stethem BA, Richard MT. How long does it take to recover from a mild concussion? Neurosurgery 1998;22:853–8.

5. Alexander MP. Mild traumaic brain injury: Pathophysiology, natural history, and clinical management. Neurology 1995;45:1253–60.

6. World Health Organization: International Statistical Classification of Diseases and related Health Problems, 10th edn. Geneva, Switzerland, World Health Organization, 1992.

7. Smith DH, Lowensteifi DH, Gennarelli DI, McIntosh TK. Persistent memory dysfunction is associated with bilateral hippocampal damage following experimental brain injury. Neurosci Lett 1994;168:151–4.

8. Kotapka MJ, Gennareli TA, Graham DI, et al. Selective vulnerability of hippocampal neurons in acceleration-induced experimental head injury. J Neurotrauma 1991;8:247–58.

9. Zola-Morgan S. Squire LR, Amaral DG. Human amnesia and the medial temporal region: Enduring memory impairment following a bilateral lesion limited to field CAT of the hippocampus. J Neurosci 1986;6:2950–67.

10. Hicks RR, Smith DH, Lowenstein DH, Saint Marie R, McIntosh TK. Mild experimental brain injury in the rat induces cognitive deficits associated with regional neuron loss in the hippocampus. J Neurotrauma 1998;10:405–15.

11. Rempel-Clower NL, Zola SM, Squire LR, Amaral DG. Three cases of enduring memory impairment after bilateral damage limited to the hippocampal formation. J Neurosci 1996; 16:5233–55.

12. Nakatomi H, Kuriu T, Okabe S, et al. Regeneration of hippocampal pyramidal neurons after ischemic brain injury by recruitment of endogenous neural progenitors. Cell 2002:110: 429–41.

13. Hofman PAM, Stapert SZ, van Kroonenburgh MJPG, Jolles J, de Kruijk Jelle, Welmink JT. MR imaging, Single-photon emission CT, and neurocognitive performance after mild traumatic brain injury. AJNR 2001;22:441–9.

14. Jenkins LW, Lu Y, Johnston WE, Lyeth BG, Prough DS. Combined therapy affects outcomes differentially after mild traumatic brain injury and secondary forebrain ischemia in rats. Brain Res 1999;817:132–44.

15. Steill IG, Lesiuk H, Wells GA, et al. The Canadian CT head rule study for patients with minor head injury: rationale, objectives and methodology for phase I (derivation). Ann Emerg Med 2001;38: 160–9.

16. Haydel MJ, Preston CA, Mills T}, et al. Indications for computed tomography in patients with minor head injury. N eng J Med 2000;343:100–5.

17. Kant R, Smith-Seemiller L, Isaac G, Duffy J. Tc-HMPAO SPECT in persistent postconcussion syndrome after mild head injury: comparison with MRI/CT. Brain Inj 1997;11:115.

18. Jacobs A, Put E, Ingels M, Bossuyt A. One-year follow up of technitium-99m-HMPAO SPECT in mild head injury. J Nucl Med 1996;37:1605–09.

19. Jain KC, Mahapatra AK, Walia. BS. Objective assessment of post minor head injury Syndrome. A P_{300} and blood flow velocity study. Clinical Neurology and Neurosurg 1997;99:574 (abstract).

20. Jain KC, Mahapatra AK. Central blood flow velocity P_{300} studies in patients with minor head injury: A preliminary study. In : Brain protection and Neural Trauma. VK Khosla, VK Kal and BS Sharma (eds). Narosa publishers, New Delhi, 2000;298–305.

21. Umile EM, Sandel E, Alavi A, Terry CM, Plotkin RC. Dynamic imaging in mild traumatic brain injury: support for the theory of medial temporal vulnerability. Arch Phys Med rehabil 2002;83: 1506–13.

22. Agrawal D, Naveen K, Bal CS, Mahapatra AK. Postconcussion vertigo: Is the cause central?

Correlation with single photon emission computed tomography. Neurosciences Today 2003;7:33–36.

23. Wrightson P, McGinn V, Gronwall D. Mild head injury in preschool children: evidence that it can be associated with persisting cognitive defect. J Neurol Neurosurg Psychiatry 1995;59:375–80.

24. Peuvot J, Schanck A, Deleers M, et al. Piracetam-induced changes to membrane physical properties: a combined approach by 31P nuclear magnetic resonance and conformational analysis. Biochem Pharmacol 1995;50:1129–34.

25. Nickolson VJ, Wolthuis OI. Effect of acquisition-enhancing drug Piracetam on rat cerebral energy metabolism: comparison with naftidofuryl and metamphetamine. Biochem Pharmacol 1975;25: 2241–4.

26. Benzi G, Pastoris O, Villa RF, et al. Influence of aging and exogenous substances on cerebral energy metabolism in post hypoglycemic recovery. Biochem Pharmacol 1985;34:1477–83.

27. Vernon E. Piracetam a nootropil analogue. In: Gouliaev AH, Seening A (eds). :Piracetam and other structurally related neurotropic. Brain research reviews 1991;19:180.

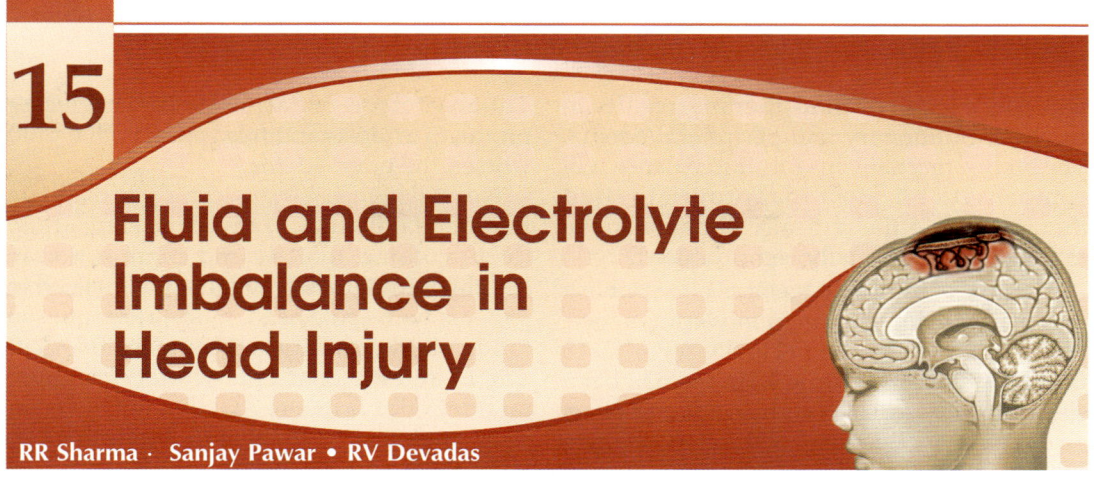

15

Fluid and Electrolyte Imbalance in Head Injury

RR Sharma · Sanjay Pawar • RV Devadas

INTRODUCTION

The past few years have witnessed important advances in our understanding of the aetiology and pathogenesis of acute head injury as well as development and use of new novel treatment strategies to improve overall outcome in such cases. The Advanced Trauma Life Support (ATLS) protocol has come a long way since its inception nearly 4 decades ago. The goals of this historical perspective are to revisit its orgin, review what changes have lead to the changes of the ATLS system, and determine its affect on today's global health care environment in the trauma setting, particularly the development of scoring systems and their applicability in triaging and predicting outcomes.[1,2] Of particular note amongst these advances are active resuscitative measures as used in primary survey of ATLS, the introduction of GCS for initial and subsequent clinical evaluations, controlled ventilation, use of computerized tomography (CT scan) to study intracranial status on periodic basis, emergency neurosurgical interventions, NICU (neurointensive care unit) care and ICP (intracranial pressure) and CPP (cerebral perfusion pressure) monitoring for physiologic management. However, arterial blood gases, coagulation profile, fluid and electrolyte balances are also of paramount importance in the day-to-day management of these patients. Controversy regarding crystalloids or colloids for resuscitation has existed for over five decades, and large numbers of clinical trials have failed to resolve the controversy. The saline versus albumin fluid evaluation (SAFE) study compared the effect of fluid resuscitation with albumin or saline on mortality in a heterogeneous population of patients in intensive care units (ICUs).[2,3,6] Overall, the study showed no significant difference in the risk of death among patients who received albumin as compared to those who received saline. There was evidence of heterogeneity of treatment effects among patients who did and those who did not have a diagnosis of trauma; this evidence resulted from an increased number of deaths among patients with traumatic brain injury who received albumin.[2,3]

The field of acute head injury research is moving rapidly. In order to keep abreast of new discoveries and current thinking, we review our experiences in the area of fluid and electrolyte imbalance in head injury patients including therapeutic options.

GENERAL CONSIDERATIONS

In severe head injury patients, maintenance of precise fluid balance is of paramount importance in preventing hypovolaemia, electrolyte imbalance and intravascular coagulation. Inadequate fluid therapy results in hypotension and underperfusion of the vital organs, whereas excessive fluid therapy results in cerebral, pulmonary and peripheral edema. The body's mechanisms for fluid balance will compensate for most inappropriate fluid therapy, but in the critically ill patients, the mechanisms are usually compromised.

The goal of fluid management is to establish and maintain euvolemia to moderate hypervolemia (CVP = 8–10 mm Hg; PCWP = 12–15 mm Hg)[4] Negative fluid balance has been shown to be associated with an adverse effect on outcome, independent of its relationship to ICP, MAP, or CPP.[5] Isotonic crystalloids should be used for fluid management, and normal saline (NS) is the recommended solution. Aggressive fluid resuscitation with NS may result in hyperchloremic metabolic acidosis, a predictable and important consequence of large-volume, saline-based intravenous fluid administration, with different clinical implications. Hypotonic solutions, such as 1/2 NS, ¼ NS, Dextrose 5% in water (D5%W), D5% 1/2 NS, or D5% ¼ NS should be avoided. Ringer's lactate solution is slightly hypotonic and is not preferred for fluid resuscitation in severe TBI patients, particularly for large volume resuscitation, as it may decrease serum osmolarity.[4] Glucose containing solutions, as above or D10%W should be avoided in the first 24 to 48 hours, unless the patient develops hypoglycemia in the absence of nutritional support. In addition to the detrimental effects of hyperglycemia in TBI, anaerobic cerebral metabolism of glucose produces acidosis and free water; both would worsen the brain edema.[4]

Normal homeostatic mechanisms maintain intracellular fluid (ICF) and extracellular fluid (ECF) volume, tonicity and composition in healthy individuals (Table 15.1). However, in patients with acute head injury, alterations in fluid volume, tonicity and composition occur due to an emergent neuroendocrine surge (antidiuretic hormone, ADH) to retain water, renin-angiotensinogen II-aldosterone to retain sodium, and catecholamines to support vascular system which is mainly aimed at maintaining an effective intravascular volume for adequate cerebral blood flow at the expense of ICF and ECF fluid tonicity and composition (Na^+, K^+, HCO_3^- and H^+).[6–9]

Disturbances of ICF/ECF fluid tonicity and composition are often associated with a worsening neurological status. Excessive capillary leakage in the brain is well recognized for acute cerebral swelling and its association with high mortality and morbidity. Inappropriate fluid therapy is therefore potentially harmful in such patients with acute cerebral trauma. The maintenance of a stable ionic concentration in the body fluids is necessary for normal cellular metabolism.[10,11] Many of these potentially serious complications due to improper fluid therapy are largely preventable and therefore should be recognized early and treated in time.

Sr. No.		Ions	ECF (plasma)	ECF (ISS)	ICF
Cations	1.	Na^+	135–145	135–140	5–10
	2.	K^+	4.5–5.5	4.5–5.5	156–160
	3.	Others	2–3	2–3	14
Anions	1.	Cl^-	101–105	115–120	3–4
	2.	HCO_3^-	26–28	26–28	10
	3.	PO_4 and others (non-diffusible)	1	1	106
	4.	Protein (non-diffusible)	15–17	0	64–66
		Total	292	302	368

Table 15.1: Composition of intracellular space (ICF) and extracellular space (ECF) (mmol/L)

Serum electrolyte imbalances in patients with severe head injury more often present with diagnostic dilemma and therefore a list of diagnosis is resolved by investigations. A 70 kg person has 42 litres of body water; 28 litres (66%) in intracellular space (ICF) and 14 litres in extracellular space (ECF). 10.5 litres in interstitial space and 3.5 litres in plasma. Water is obtained from the diet (1.5 to 2.1 L/day) and oxidative metabolism (400 mL/day) and is lost (2–2.5 L/day) through the kidneys (sensible loss of 1.5 L/day), lungs, gut and skin (sum total insensible loss of 1 L/day). Its distribution in ICF and ECF is determined by the osmolalities of these compartments. Normally, ICF and ECF are isotonic. Any change in osmolarity of a compartment results in the net to and fro movement of water between the ECF and ICF to restore isotonicity. The minimum volume of urine necessary for normal excretion of metabolic waste products is about 500 ml/day {20 ml/hr} and minimum daily dietary water intake is about 1100 ml.

Majority of exchangeable sodium is extracellular: The normal ECF sodium concentration is 135–145 mmol/L, while that of the ICF is only 4–10 mmol/L. Most cell membranes are permeable to sodium and the gradient is maintained by active pumping of sodium from ICF to ECF by Na^+-K^+ ATPase pump. The normal daily intake of sodium is about 100–200 mmol/day. But daily obligatory loss is less than 10 mmol/day. Sodium balance is maintained by regulations of its renal excretions, 70% of glomerular filtrate is absorbed in the proximal convoluted tubule, 25% in the loop of Henle and 5% in the distal convoluted tubules and collecting ducts (renin-angiotensin II-aldosterone mechanism).[1–5]

Na^+ requirement is usually calculated by the following equation:

0.6 × body wt × serum Na^+ deficit = mmol of sodium × 0.05 = gm of salt required.

1 gm of NaCl gives 44 mmol of Na^+.

Na^+ deficit in mmol × 2 = ml of 3% saline. One ml of 3% saline provides 0.5 mmol of Na^+.

The osmolarities of the ECF is normally maintained in the range 280–295 mmol/kg of water. Increase in ECF osmolality in comparison to ICF osmolality causes three main effects:[8–12]

1. Stimulation of hypothalamic thirst center promoting dietary water intake.
2. Movement of water from ICF to ECF in order to maintain isotonicity.
3. Stimulation of hypothalamic osmoreceptors causing the release of ADH for effective renal water reabsorption and minimizing urinary water output and therefore resulting in a concentrated (low water and high solute) urine.

Osmoreceptors are highly sensitive to increased ECF osmolality even by 1% more than the ICF osmolarity resulting in release of ADH in the circulation.[9–14] They are located outside the blood–brain barrier in the anteroventral region of the third ventricle in the hypothalamus. If the ECF osmolality falls, there is no sensation of thirst; ADH secretion is inhibited (and a dilute urine is produced) allowing renal water loss to restore ECF osmolality (by raising it) to a normal level. If an increase in ECF osmolality occurs as a result of a solute such as urea, which readily diffuses across cell membranes, the ICF osmolality is also increased. In such cases, the ECF and ICF remain isotonic and therefore osmoreceptors are not stimulated.

A significant hypovolemia (10%), is a powerful stimulus (via angiotensinogen, arterial and venous baroreceptors and volume receptors) to ADH release to restore effective ECF volume even though there is a decrease in osmolality.[2–4,7–10] Maintenance of volume takes precedence over the maintenance of serum osmolarity. ADH is synthesized in the supraoptic nuclei of the hypothalamus and pass down the nerve axons into the posterior pituitary from where it is released into the circulation.[7–10]

ADH is essential for life as it maintains serum osmolarity by enhancing renal water reabsorption as it increases the permeability of the renal collecting tubules to water in response to increase in ECF osmolarity (above 285 mmol/kg), however, if ECF osmolarity is below 285 mmol/kg, ADH secretion is strongly inhibited.[8–10,16–18]

Mechanism of action of ADH on renal tubules is interesting.[16,19] ADH attaches to a specific vasopressin receptor on the contra-luminal side of the renal medullary tubular cell. This attachment activates renal (medul-lary tubular) cellular adenyl cyclase. The latter stimulates production of cyclic AMP. Abundant cellular cyclic AMP then activates a protein kinase on the luminal side of the cell causing phosphorylation of membrane protein leading to an increased permeability of the tubular cell to water, facilitating its transport into the renal medullary circulation and then back into the general circulation. Steroid replacement therapy lowers plasma ADH to normal and inhibits the secretary activity of the supraoptic neurons, and therefore has some role in SIADH (syndrome of inappropriate ADH secretion).

ADH plays a vital role in the control of the tonicity of the ECF[8,14] and hence indirectly of the ICF and therefore overall of water balance. Excessive secretion results in dilutional hyponatraemia (SIADH) with a risk of water intoxication while decreased secretion results in excessive renal water loss (diabetes insipidus-DI) causing hypernatremia with a risk of severe dehydration (Table 15.2).

In head injury, SIADH occurs when there is no direct damage to the pituitary gland, whereas DI is commonly due to hypothalamo-pituitary axis disturbance/damage.[7–12,20,21] Damage to the posterior pituitary may also cause temporary failure of ADH secretion.

In head injury patients, ADH is released in response to the clinical status (raised ECF osmolarity, raised ICP, hypovolemia, noci-ceptive stimuli, emotional stress), drug therapy (barbiturates, morphine, carbamaze-pine, chlorpropamide, angiotensin, thyroxin, glucocorticoids, cholinergic and beta adre-nergic stimulation) and mechanical ventilation (positive airway pressure); whereas ADH is suppressed by phenytoin, ethanol, anti-cholinergics, atropine alpha adrenergic stimulation, reserpine, chlorpromazine besides increased plasma volume (hypervolaemia) and reduced plasma osmolarity.[8–10,13–16,18–20] Steroid replacement therapy lowers plasma ADH to normal and permits the normal diuretic response to hydration by inhibiting

Sr. No.	Organic systems/clinical state	Hyponatremia	Hypernatremia
1.	Neurological	Cerebral edema, disorientation, lethargy, apathy, impairment of consciousness, seizures, coma, Chyne-Stokes respiration, hypothermia	Cerebral dehydration, restlessness, irritability, disorientation, ataxia, seizures, coma, hemorrhage, intracranial
2.	Muscular	Cramps, hypotonic weakness, depressed reflexes, rhabdomyolysis	Increased muscle tone, hyperreflexia
3.	Renal	Oliguria, concentrated urine or hypertonic urine	Polyuria, diluted urine or hypotonic urine
4.	Gastrointestinal	Loss of appetite, nausea, vomiting	Thirst

Table 15.2: Clinical manifestations of Na+ imbalance

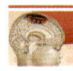

the secretory activity of the supraoptic neurons (a weak response).[3–5] Antinatriuretics catecholamines, renin angiotensin-II-aldosterone, cortisol attempts at volume restitution or expansion following trauma.

Atrial natriuretic peptide (ANP) and brain natriuretic peptide (BNP) (largely of cardiac ventricular origin) have similar biological effects on the control of blood volume, blood pressure and electrolyte composition. ANP/BNP induces natriuresis through direct tubular effects or by inhibition of the renin-angiotensin-aldosterone mechanism.[21–23]

Hypervolemia is also kept under check as there is no appreciable ADH secretion in such circumstances and the excess of water is therefore lost from the kidneys. It is routinely measured by central venous pressure monitoring. Moreover, natriuretic peptide hormone (ANP, a 28-amino acid peptide) is produced by the cardiac atria when hypervolemia exerts excessive stretch on the sensitive atrial stretch receptors. It antagonizes renin-angiotensin II-aldosterone mechanism and causes natriuresis and hypovolemia.[23–25]

In clinical practice the serum osmolarity is routinely measured using following equation:

$$\text{Osmolarity} = 2 \times [\text{Na}^+] + [\text{Urea}] + \text{glucose} \quad [\text{all in mmol/L}]$$

Osmolality is a measure of solute concentrate per kilogram of solvent; whereas osmolarity is a measure of solute concentrate per litre of solution.[9] In clinical practice, the difference between osmolality and osmolarity is negligible (Table 15.3).

In head injury patients abnormalities of serum sodium (<125 or >150 mEq/L) and serum osmolality (<260 or >320 mOsm/L) should be avoided. Overhydration *per se* will not cause brain edema if the serum sodium value is normal (135–145 mEq/L); however, it can cause brain edema at brain injury sites only when it is combined with hyponatremia (<130 mEq/L) because ECF water shifts to ICF compartment in an attempt to maintain ECF/ICF isotonicity.

The loss of fluid and electrolytes without protein loss will cause rise in the hematocrit and plasma protein concentration.[5–11,14–17]

Sr. No.	Name	Concentration	Na⁺	Cl⁻	K⁺	HCO₃	Ca²⁺	Calculated mmol /L
			Na^+	Cl^-	K^+	HCO_3	Ca^{2+}	
1.	Normal saline	NaCl 0.9 %	154	154	—	—	—	300
2.	Hartman's solution (Ringer lactate)	Saline + K⁺ + HCO₃–	131	111	4	2.0	—	280
3.	5% Glucose	5% dextrose	—	—	—	—	—	280
4.	Dextrose saline	4% glucose, 0.18% saline	30	30	—	—	—	286
5.	Half normal saline	NaCl 0.45%	75	75	—	—	—	150
6.	Human plasma protein fraction	HPPF mol. wt. 69000	150	150	5	—	2	314 or more
7.	Hemaccel polygeline	Degraded gelatin mol. wt. 24500	145	145	5.1	—	6.25	310 or more
8.	Succinylated gelatin	Gelofusine (4%) molecular wt 22600	154	154	0.4	—	0.4	310
9.	Hetastarch	Hydroxyethyl starch 6% in saline mol. wt. 70000	154	154	—	—	—	310 or more
10.	Blood	Whole blood constituents	140	102	4	26	2.4	285

Table 15.3: Characteristics of parenteral fluid therapy

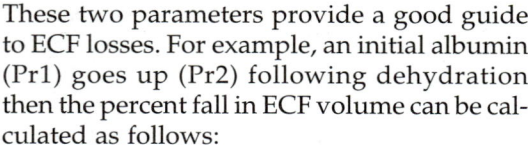

These two parameters provide a good guide to ECF losses. For example, an initial albumin (Pr1) goes up (Pr2) following dehydration then the percent fall in ECF volume can be calculated as follows:

% fall in ECF volume = (1 – Pr1/Pr2) × 100.

A fall in plasma volume can be more precisely calculated with the initial (Hct 1) and subsequent (Hct 2) hematocrit readings:

% fall in plasma volume:

$$100 \left[1 - \left(\frac{Hct\ 1}{100 - Hct\ 1} \times \frac{100 - Hct\ 2}{Hct\ 2} \right) \right]$$

where Hct, in initial hematocrit, Hct 2 is after plasma loss.

Hematocrit and plasma albumin are therefore more useful in the assessment of plasma and ECF losses than the Na^+ (measurements) which although being lost does not change in its serum concentration (CSWS) 7–11.[19,25]

By invasive hemodynamic monitoring, a low pulmonary capillary wedge (PCWP) pressure (< mm Hg) or low CVP < 6 mm Hg) implies volume depletion. Clinical evidence of dehydration, weight loss, orthostatic hypotension, CVP < 6 mm Hg and negative water balance are noted in CSWS. Moreover, elevation of hematocrit, the serum creatinine and serum protein concentration point to dehydration in CSWS. Increased natriuresis and elevated serum K^+ also suggest CSWS.[20, 23,26]

Using isotope dilution techniques, a decreased plasma volume (< 35 ml/kg) and a decreased total blood volume (< 60 ml/kg) are central features of CSWS.[22]

In water loading test, an increased free water reabsorption suggests increased ADH secre tion.[19,22,27] Appropriate or inappropriate ADH secretion can be differentiated from one another by examining the urine volume, creatinine clearance, osmotic clearance and fractional water excretion.[22] If overall results suggest dehydration, then the increased free water reabsorption points to an appropriate ADH secretion. On the other hand, the increased free water reabsorption in the absence of dehydration suggests an inappropriate ADH secretion in SIADH. Normal or reduced free water reabsorption, with dehydration (reduced creatinine clearance, polyuria, high fractional or osmotic diuresis) and inappropriate natriuresis (sodium excretion of > 0.001 mmol hour which is inappropriate in the presence of severe hyponatremia) are central features of CSWS. Disproportionate fractional water clearance relative to the free water clearance suggests an osmotic diuresis. In DI there is a disproportionate free water clearance.[17–20,22,26–29]

It is essential that appropriate fluid and electrolyte studies be done early in the course of management of the head injured patient. Therapy is directed primarily towards the underlying cause of the fluid and electrolyte abnormality. In the potentially salvagable patient optimal correction may occur spontaneously or may require cautious use of medical therapy to achieve a good outcome (Table 15.4).

MAINTENANCE OF VOLUME IN HYPONATREMIC STATES

Hyponatremia (a low serum sodium concentration) is a common finding in NICU as a secondary phenomenon reflecting the presence of dysregulation of hypothalamo hypophyseal axis, metabolic response to trauma or a sick cell syndrome requiring principally the management of underlying cause.[5–11,18–21,28–31,32] It is commonly due to water excess than to sodium loss. Significant hyponatremia is relatively common after the head injury occurring in about 8 to 15% of patients with moderate and severe head injuries.In a recent prospective study by Schirmer-Mikalsen, et al.[33] the incidence of hyponatremia was 34.6%.[33] Hyponatremia is detrimental and major secondary systemic brain insult in patients with severe TBI, as it leads to exacerbation of brain edema and an increase in ICP. It is usually secondary to cerebral salt wasting syndrome,[4] or to the syndrome of inappropriate anti-diuretic

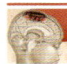

Table 15.4: Clinical characteristics of common causes of Na⁺ imbalance in head injuries

S.r. No.	Clinical features	Hyponatremia SIADH	Hypernatremia CSWS	Hypernatremia Solute diuresis	Hypernatremia DI
1.	Intravascular volume	Hypervolemia	Hypovolemia	Hypervolemia	Hypovolemia
2.	Dehydration features	Absent	Present	Absent	Present
3.	Body weight	Increased	Decreased	Increased	Decreased
4.	CVP	Increased	Decreased	Increased	Decreased
5.	Hematology:		Increased or		
	(i) PCWP	Decreased	Normal	Variable	Increased
	(ii) Hematocrit	Decreased	Increased	Decreased	Increased
6.	Biochemical parametres:				
	(i) S. osmolarity	Decreased	Incr/normal	Increased	Increased
	(ii) S. protein	Decr/normal	Increased	Variable	Increased
	(iii) BUN/creatinine	Decreased	Incr/normal	Variable	Incr/normal
	(iv) S. uric acid	Decreased	Normal	Decr/normal	Normal
	(v) S. Na⁺	Decreased	Decreased	Increased	Increased
	(vi) Urine Na⁺	Incr/normal	Increased	Increased	Decreased
	(vii) Urine osmolarity	Increased	Increased	Increased	Decreased
7.	Management	Fluid restriction, salt replacement, loop diuretics, phenytoin, demeclocycline, lithium, fludrocortisone, diuretics, hemodialysis	Fluid replacement with isotonic fluid therapy, blood transfusions fludrocortisone	Fluid replacement with hypotonic fluid, treatment of cause	Fluid replacement with hypotonic fluids, vasopressin, chlorpropamide clofibrate, thiazide carbamazepine, steroids, Hemofiltration

Incr: increased, Decr: decreased, CSWS: cerebral salt wasting syndrome, SIADH: syndrome of inappropriate ADH secretion, DI: diabetes insipidus, PCWP: pulmonary capillary wedge pressure

hormone secretion (SIADH).[34,35] Hyponatremia is divided into three categories: mild ($Na^+ <$ 135 to 125 mEq/L); moderate (Na^+ 120–124 mEq/L) and severe ($Na^+ >$120 mEq/L).

Aetiopathogenesis: The risk of developing hyponatremia increases in the presence of severe head injuries, fracture of skull base and subdural haematoma.[18,27,29,31]

Following acute injury, the body retains water and sodium as a consequence of an acute neuroendocrine surge in an attempt to maintain an effective extracellular volume and thereby intravascular volume. As the water content of ECF increases as compared to its solute concentration, a dilutional hyponatremia results.

Hyponatremia lowers the seizure threshold, exacerbates cerebral oedema and causes impairment of the level of consciousness.[4,13,27] However, the degree of brain dysfunction depends upon the rapidity of the development of hyponatraemia; the serum sodium level of 115 mmol/L may be asymptomatic if developing slowly over a period whereas rapidly developing serum sodium level of 120–130 mmol/L may have severe neurological disturbance. In the setting of hypervolemia with hyponatremia, initially the brain cells (glia and neurons) swell due to an increase in cell volume due to movement of ECF water to ICF compartment because of the fall in ECF osmolality as compared to ICF osmolarity.

Later, a gradual adaptive down regulatory volume reduction is achieved by loss of intracellular ions such as K^+, Cl^-, taurine, phosphocreatine and amino acids including excitatory neurotransmitters (glutamine, glutamate); with consequent neurologic impairment.[1–6] Hyponatremia ultimately lead to cerebral edema and raised ICP with their deleterious consequences.

Wu et al[36] found that BNP (basic natriuretic peptide also known as B-type natriuretic peptide) plasma concentrations increase rapidly after severe TBI. Atrial natriuretic peptide (ANP), is a hormone secreted from atria which regulates the homeostatic balance of body fluid and BP. ANP like immuno-reacting is also present in the brain known as BNP (basic natriuretic peptide) patients but not in mild and moderate TBI. The peak of BNP level was measured at 703.9 pg/ml ± 179.1 pg/ml on day 3 after injury, which was correlated to the severity of TBI. Among patients with severe TBI, plasma NT-proBNP concentrations in patients with hyponatremia were statistically higher than those without hyponatremia ($p < 0.05$). In addition, we found plasma NT-proBNP concentrations in patients with ICP > 15 mm Hg were significantly higher than those in patients with ICP 15 mm Hg ($p < 0.01$).

Water retention (not the natriuresis) is a marked feature of ADH excess whereas natriuresis (not the water retention) is a prominent feature of ANP (atrial natriuretic peptide) excess therefore the volume expansion is a prominent feature of SIADH, and the concomitant volume depletion with natriuresis is a marked feature of CSWS (cerebral salt wasting syndrome). ANP can suppress ADH secretion while ADH may itself stimulate ANP secretion.

In SIADH water retention (hyponatremic hypervolemia) inhibits aldosterone secretion and therefore relative natriuresis continues. In SIADH and CSWS, there is an increase in ADH secretion. In SIADH, water retention occurs due to high ADH. Whereas CSWS have high natriuresis due to high ANP/BNP and a low aldosterone activity.[18,19,21–23,26–31]

In a study, Bettinelli et al[37] found hypotonic hyponatremia, a serious and recognized complication of an intracranial disorder, results from extracellular fluid volume depletion, inappropriate antidiuresis or renal salt-wasting. The putative mechanisms by which intracranial disorders might lead to renal salt-wasting are either a disrupted neural input to the kidney or the elaboration of a circulating natriuretic factor. The key to diagnosis of renal salt-wasting lies in the assessment of extracellular volume status: the central venous pressure is currently con-sidered the yardstick for measuring fluid volume status in subjects with intracranial disorders and hyponatremia. Approximately 110 cases have been reported so far in subjects ≤ 18 years of age (male: 63%; female: 37%): intracranial surgery, meningoencephalitis (most frequently tuberculous) or head injury were the most common underlying disorders. Volume and sodium repletion are the goals of treatment, and this can be performed using some combination of isotonic saline, hyper-tonic saline, and mineralocorticoids (fludro-cortisone).[37]

Differential diagnosis: Various hypona-tremic syndromes in head injured patients may be differentiated primarily on the clinical grounds.[5–12, 17–20,30,31,38–41]

In low dietary intake, depletion of both ICF and ECF solute can lead to hyponatremia. In true sodium depletion due to nutritional neglect, hyponatremia is accompanied by an evidence of a contracted blood volume (low blood pressure, decreased skin turgor and elevated hematocrit). In dilutional hypo-natremia due to excessive hypotonic fluid infusion, peripheral edema is a prominent feature and in addition, there may be an evidence of cerebral oedema, congestive heart failure or hepatic disease. Urinary sodium concentration is less than 10 mmol/L in both aforementioned conditions: Chronic dietary salt depletion and dilutional hyponatremia due to hypotonic fluid therapy.

Pseudohyponatremia may result due to a decreased fractional water content of plasma in cases of hyperproteinemia (two times the normal values) and hyperlipidemia. An increase in positively charged paraproteins or a decrease in negatively charged albumin concentrations in plasma can displaces Na^+ from the plasma to the ICF compartment causing hyponatremia. Factitious hyponatremia therefore requires no special treatment.

Hyperosmolar hyponatremia: Hyperglycemia may also result in hyponatremia. When plasma solute concentrations (glucose) are increased, a shift of water from the ICF to the ECF causes dilutional hyponatremia. In addition, an increased serum osmolarity causes direct stimulation of osmoreceptors and ADH release leading to renal water retention that further worsens the hyponatremia. Moreover, such increase in ECF volume inhibits volume receptors controlling aldosterone secretion leading to renal loss of sodium (natriuresis). Following mannitol infusion (osmotic diuretic increases ECF volume and reduces ICF volume to treat cerebral edema), hyponatremia occurs due to the sum total effects of the aforementioned mechanisms.

The persistence of dilutional hyponatremia implies either SIADH or renal impairment (acute tubular necrosis). Dilutional hyponatremia (low serum proteins and low serum urea) indicates SIADH. In normal subjects, osmolarity of the maximally dilute urine is about 50 mmol/kg. In SIADH, osmolarity of urine is more than 50 mmol/kg, and peripheral edema is not a prominent feature whereas dilutional hyponatremia with a dilute urine with peripheral edema indicates renal impairment. Sodium depletion is seldom due to inadequate input (nutritional restriction) but more often due to excessive renal loss of sodium (CSWS or due to high ANP levels or urinary sodium loss in diuretic therapy). The clinical features of sodium depletion are primarily as a result of decrease in ECF

volume. The plasma sodium will be normal if fluid is lost isotonically (bleeding) and increased if it is lost hypotonically (excessive sweating in hyperpyrexia, mechanical ventilation, or gastrointestinal hyperkinesia). Thus the plasma sodium concentration in sodium depletion may be variable (low, normal or high). Sodium loss never occurs alone but is always accompanied by some water loss. The fluid lost may be isotonic or hypotonic with respect to the plasma.

Hyponatremia is common after infusion of hypotonic fluids (5% dextrose or dextrose saline), when ability of the body to excrete water is depressed.

THE COMMON HYPONATREMIC STATES IN HEAD INJURY PATIENTS: CSWS AND SIADH

Initially, cerebral salt wasting syndrome (CSWS) was recognized in the early 1950s and later the syndrome of inappropriate (excess) antidiuretic harmone (SIADH) in 1957 by Schwartz.[10,42–44] Majority of head injury patients with hyponatremia present with CSWS or SIADH. In a few cases, both conditions may coexist. CSWS and SIADH, both are characterized by hyponatremia, hyperosmolar urine and hypernatriuresis in patients with normal renal, suprarenal and thyroid functions. The major distinction among these conditions is the volume status of the patient. In CSWS, the ECF volume is contracted and the patient appears dehydrated; whereas in SIADH the ECF volume is expanded and a clinical picture of fluid overload is often seen. Patients with CSWS respond to fluid and sodium administration while those with SIADH respond to fluid restriction. In neurosurgical patients, CSWS is common than SIADH.

A. Syndrome of Inappropriate ADH Secretion (SIADH)[5,7–17,18–20,27,44]

It usually begins in first or second week after head injury and with appropriate therapy, lasts no more than one to two weeks. In SIADH, there is a continuous secretion of

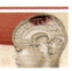

ADH despite hyponatremia, hypo-osmolar serum and hypervolemia.

It is defined by the hyponatremia and hypo-osmolality resulting from inappropriate continued secretion of ADH despite normal or increased plasma volume.

The typical clinical features of SIADH are hyponatremia, with concomitant hyper-volemic hypo-osmolar ECF, relative hyper-natriuresis with hyperosmolar urine and absence of clinical evidence of volume depletion (normal skin turgor, blood pressure). The clinical symptoms include anorexia, nausea, vomiting, irritability, personality changes and neurological signs (bulbar or pseudobulbar palsy, stupor, muscular weakness, loss of reflexes, positive Babinski sign and convulsions.

B. Cerebral Salt Wasting Syndrome (CSWS)[5,7–10,21–24, 41–43]

This syndrome is due to an unregulated release of atrial natriuretic peptide. It presents with hyponatremia, with concomitant hypo-volemic hyposmolar ECF, hypernatriuresis with hyperosmolar urine and presence of clinical evidence of volume depletion. Persistence of high salt loss in the urine despite fluid restriction differentiates this condition from SIADH where salt loss depends on a liberal fluid intake. The estimation of intravascular volume (by CVP) and urinary sodium usually differentiates salt retaining states (SIADH) from salt losing states (CSWS). Peters et al[41] and Cort[40] described CSWS as a condition with hyponatremia with natriuresis and believed that the CNS normally influences the ability of the kidneys to reabsorb sodium in the proximal tubule and that a defect in this regulatory function can lead to natriuresis. Many workers have reported a reduction in the red cell mass in patients with CSWS. Vingerhoets and de Tribolet[34] distinguished between two clinical syndromes of hypo-natremia and natriuresis, which differed in the interval between the neurological insult and the emergence of hyponatremia: The acute syndrome (< 3 days) and the delayed syndrome

(> 1 week). They found elevated serum ADH levels in patients with acute syndrome and depressed or normal in chronic syndrome. SIADH is commonly seen in acute and CSWS in chronic syndrome.

The main diagnostic criteria of SIADH and CSWS are outlined in Table 15.4.

Management

Hyponatremia is basically treated according to the underlying disease process, serum osmolality and clinical estimate of total body sodium. The cornerstone of therapy in SIADH is fluid restriction whereas in CSWS the volume replacement and correction of the hematocrit.[5–19,22,45–48].

SIADH:[5–11,14–19,21–23,45–48] The patients with SIADH are basically treated with fluid restriction usually below 1 L/day until serum Na+ returns to normal levels with some salt supplement or replacements. The free water restriction should be sufficient to decrease total body water by 0.5 to 1.0 L/day. The resultant reduction in glomerular filtration rate enhances proximal tubular reabsorption of salt and water and stimulates aldosterone secretion.

Mild cases (Na+ > 125 mEq/L), are best treated with fluid restriction whereas moderate cases (Na+ < 125 mEq/L to 120 mEq/L) with water restriction 600 to 800 ml 5% dextrose in 0.45% saline per 24 hrs, with or without normal saline; diuresis usually occurs in 36 to 48 hours. Patients with severe hyponatremia (Na+ < 120 mEq/L) or in coma or with seizures may require hypertonic saline, with furosemide 20 to 40 mg.[24] The diuretic therapy is used with utmost caution and monitoring to promote water loss. When hypertonic saline therapy is considered then it should be given only to restore Na+ concentration to levels that no longer represent a hazardous state. The end point of hypertonic saline therapy is generally a serum Na+ of 120 mEq/L or absence of overt symptoms. Initially plasma Na+ may be increased by 1 to 2 mEq/L/hr. Care should be

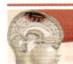

taken to avoid hypematrnemia by cautious correction so that the plasma Na$^+$ should not be increased more than 12 mEq/L in 24 hours or 25 mEq/L in 48 hours, or to a concentration greater than 130 mEq/L.[4,17,39] Demeclocycline (anti-ADH synthetic hormone) antagonizes the action of ADH on the renal collecting ducts and therefore may be used (600 to 1200 mg/day) to induce nephrogenic resistance to ADH.[8,11,22,47] Phenytoin is used as an anti-epileptic drug with an added benefit as an anti-ADH agent.[46] Fludrocortisone (0.3 to 3 mg daily) to inhibit action of ADH on aldosterone mechanism and helps in raising serum Na$^+$ levels.[51]

CSWS[5–11,19–25,41–44,52] The principles of the management of hyponatremia associated with CSWS consists of the treatment of an underlying cause, restriction of intravascular volume, isotonic fluid (normal saline, plasma, blood) infusion and fludrocortisone in CSWS.[18–22,51–54] These measures are effective without jeopardizing ICP control in most cases.

The patients with CSWS are best managed with salt containing fluid orally, enterally or intravenously to maintain CVP around 10–12 mm of Hg. Patient's hemoglobin and hematocrit levels are measured daily and if needed packed cell with isotonic fluid or whole blood is given as per requirement.

Rapid correction of chronic hyponatremia[13,18,19,50,53] has been associated with fatal central pontine and extrapontine myelinolysis; on the other hand, severe acute hyponatremia can cause fatal cerebral edema (tentorial herniation) and status epilepticus. Despite such concerns, the management of hyponatremia with diuretic therapy (furosemide) and saline (isotonic/hypertonic) is safe.

MAINTENANCE OF VOLUME IN HYPERNATREMIC STATES

Hypenatremia (a high serum sodium concentration) is much less frequent in head injured patients than hyponatremia and is much more frequent of clinical significance. It is caused by either (1) water loss or (2) sodium excess.

Etiopathogenesis:[2–12,19–22,30,31] In hypernatremic head injury patients, water depletion occurs due to increased water loss as in diabetes insipidus (lack of ADH), renal-diabetes insipidus (ADH insensitivity), mannitol (osmotic diuresis), glycosuria (osmotic diuresis), prolonged hyperpyrexia (increased sweating); hyperventilation (increased insensible loss), antibiotics related diarrhea and due to decreased dietary water intake. The neurological causes include cerebral trauma, cerebral tumors (craniopharyngioma, secondary deposits, pituitary tumors), vascular disorders (Sheehan's syndrome, SAH or cerebral aneurysm), meningoencephalitis, surgery and idiopathic. Despite the frequent pathological demonstration of pituitary and hypothalamic damage in head injury, the incidence of DI is relatively less. However, DI is a mortel sign in patients with massive brain injuries, uncontrollable intracranial hypertension.

In clinical practice, excessive water loss without much sodium loss is unusual except in diabetes insipidus. Pure water loss is borne by the total body water and not just the ECF, and therefore signs of a reduced ECF volume are not usually present. Severe water depletion causes cerebral dehydration that stimulates intracellular mechanisms for brain cells to synthesize osmotically active compounds and acute cerebral edema may then follow rapid fluid replacement with deleterious consequences. Severe water depletion is therefore corrected in cautious manner by 5% dextrose or hypotonic saline (2/3 deficits in the first 24 hours and 1/3 in next 24 hour).

Differential diagnosis:[1,2,6–13,17–26,40] The differential diagnosis of serum hyperosmolarity and polyuria following trauma in the region of hypothalamopituitary axis may be different due to the presence of variety of overlapping causes.

Polydipsia (thirst leading to increased intake) and polyuria are hallmark of DI. The differential diagnosis includes other conditions causing polyuria and polydipsia, i.e. renal diabetes insipidus, diabetes mellitus, chronic renal failure, hypercalcemia, hypokalemia and psychogenic polydipsia. Simple biochemical tests will easily eliminate many of these possibilities. Solute diuresis in hyperglycemia, uremia, osmotic or loop diuretics and aldosterone deficiency presents with a normal or slightly decreased serum sodium with only an occasional change in thirst mechanism. The urine specific gravity remains between 1.009 and 1.035 mOsm/kg and urine osmolarity between 250 and 320 mOsm/kg whereas water diuresis (diabetes insipidus) presents with a normal or increased serum sodium levels and intense thirst and polyuria. The urine remains between 50 and 150 mmol/kg. Whereas a normal (water deprived) individual will concentrate his urine with urine output of 0.5 ml/min and urine osmolarity of greater than 750 mOsm/kg. In diabetes insipidus decreased ADH secretion results in uncontrolled renal water loss (a dilute urine) with a dehydrational hypernatremia. Renal diabetes insipidus is due to renal insensitivity to ADH despite increased ADH levels in serum and urine, and psychogenic polydipsia-polyuria is due to a compulsive desire to drink. These conditions are differentiated with the help of either water deprivation tests or serum and urine ADH assays. Diabetes mellitus (hyperglycemia), hypercalcemia, chronic renal failure and hypokalemia may also cause polyuria and polydipsia but are easily differentiated from central diabetes insipidus by routine biochemical tests. If it is due to demeclocycline (anti-ADH agent) this should be discontinued. If a random urine osmolality is greater than 750 mmol/kg, diabetes insipidus is basically excluded.

Diabetes insipidus:[1–8,13,15,16,18,21,29,44,45] Diabetes insipidus is a common phenomenon after craniofacial injury and basilar skull fractures, and can be permanent or transient disappearing in a few days or weeks. Trauma, hypoxia, hemorrhagic shock, surgery, fat embolism, drug overdose, etc. may cause diabetes insipidus. Hypothalamo hypophyseal injury poses a particular risk of developing transient or permanent diabetes insipidus. It is transient in majority of patients lasting for 3–5 days, however, in one-fourth to one-third of cases, it may be permanent.

Some patients show a triphasic response manifested by early diabetes insipidus, followed by return of normal urinary functions for 1–3 weeks and then relapse leading to permanent diabetes insipidus.

CLINICAL MANIFESTATIONS OF DIABETES INSIPIDUS[3–5,8,29,44,45]

Polyuria, (>2–3 L/day), polydipsia, hypernatremia with hypovolemia, high serum osmolality (320–330 mOsm/kg), low urine osmolarity and a dilute urine (specific gravity less than 1005) and a urine to serum osmolarity ratio of less than one, implying a negative water balance are characteristic features of DI.

Diagnostic tests:[1–4,13,44,45] Serum and urine ADH assays and/or a water deprivation test are performed. A normal person on water deprivation for 8 hours will have urine output 0.5 ml/min and will concentrate urine to preserve water. Urine osmolarity will rise and become greater than 500 mOsm/kg. Patients with diabetes insipidus fail to concentrate their urine and the water loss continues as a dilute urine.

During the water deprivation testing, in diabetes insipidus, the urine does not become concentrated and the serum osmolarity rises during the eight hour test period, whereas a normal person will maintain serum osmolarity below 295 mmol/kg during this period. Serum osmolarity above 285 mmol/kg is a strong stimulus for ADH release to maintain serum osmolarity in normal range by retaining more water. On administration of desmopressin in patients suspected of DI, if the urine becomes concentrated and the serum osmolarity falls then the diagnosis of DI will be confirmed.

Measurement of ADH levels in urine and serum in relation to plasma osmolality is far more desirable than the water deprivation test

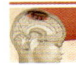
in acute head injury patients as the latter may be highly inappropriate in many of these patients. If the ADH essays are not available then a therapeutic trial with desmopressin is highly indicated to resolve the diagnostic dilemma.

Management[1-8,13-16,18-21,29,44,45]

Daily measurements of body weight, fluid intake/output, hemoglobin, hematocrit, renal function tests (serum creatinine, BUN, sugar, electrolytes), serum osmolarity, urine specific gravity and urine osmolarity are performed. Treatment of hypernatremia by water loss basically consists of water replacement as well as repletion of associated deficits of sodium and other electrolytes. Hypernatremia is corrected slowly because of the risk of neurologic sequelae such as seizures and cerebral edema. The water deficit is corrected over 24–48 hours and plasma Na^+ is gradually reduced by 1–2 mEq/L/hr.

The aim of the fluid therapy is to replace hourly urine output with the usual estimate for the insensible loss with hypotonic fluids. The volume depletion leads to reduction in the mean systemic arterial pressure and subsequently a reduction in the cerebral perfusion pressure and therefore needs cautious correction.

Regardless of its cause, hypernatremia should initially be treated by administration of hypotonic fluids such as water (orally) or 5% dextrose (parenterally). The antidiuresis is enhanced by low sodium intake and diminished by high sodium. Urine output in DI may exceed 10 L/day although less than this is more usual. Adequate fluid replacement, desmopressin [Desmopressin (1-desamino-D-arginine-vasopressin) is a synthetic analogue of ADH] for severe cases and chlorpropamide (oral hypoglycemic agent) 50 to 200 mg/day or carbamazepine (antiepileptic agent 600 mg/day) for mild cases of DI may be used. Desmopressin is indicated if urine output exceeds 6 to 7 L/day, or urinary output remains more than 250 ml/hr for two to four consecutive hours or the patient is unable to maintain fluid balance and the normal intravascular volume. Treatment with vasopressin should not be withheld in verified cases of DI. There are many preparations of vasopressin which are highly effective:

a. Aqueous vasopressin (5–10 IU IM/IV, 4 to 6 hourly)

b. Vasopressin Tannate-in-oil (5 IU IM/ daily as initial therapy once in 2–3 days).

c. Lysine vasopressin nasal spray (21 IU/ spray, 6–8 hourly).

d. DDAVP (l-deamino-8-D-arginine vasopressin)-10–20 mg intranasally on OD or BD basis.

Care must be exercised during the active treatment of DI/hypernatremia to prevent water intoxication (lethargy, confusion, seizures and coma) due to excessive desmopressin administration, hypoglycemia due to chlorpropamide therapy, and significant hypovolemia following diuretics therapy (by further contracting ECF volume). While controlling post-traumatic seizures, Carbamazepine stimulates ADH release in patients with diabetes insipidus. In patients with dangerously high serum sodium, the peritoneal dialysis/hemodialysis/hemofiltration to remove excess serum sodium may have to be considered. In terminal hypernatremia, the patient does not respond to any treatment and has the worst prognosis. Hemofiltration employs a filter containing a membrane with characteristics similar to those of capillary endothelial endothelial cells, in that water and smaller molecules (with a molecular weight ≤ 20,000) can pass freely across it. The filter is connected to arterial and venous lines and the ECF across the cell membrane. Hemofiltration in NICU has advantages over the conventional hemodialysis in fine control of fluid and electrolyte balance and removal of water soluble waste products and drugs.

CONCLUSIONS

Significant head injury results in marked hypermetabolism and hypercatobolism.

Patients with injury to central neuraxis including the brainstem and hypothalamo-hypophyseal system causes the greatest response. Majority of the patients with head injury show no appreciable fluid and electrolyte abnormalities; however, a subset of significant head injury patients suffer from fluid and electrolyte disturbances. Neurological recovery in such patients occur rapidly if they are treated in time with adequate fluid and electrolyte therapy. To institute an appropriate therapy, a proper understanding of the aetiopathological mechanisms their diagnostic parameters and treatment protocols is necessary. Failure to execute such responsibility may lead to increased morbidity and mortality which may be avoidable in many of these critically ill head injury patients.

REFERENCES

1. Evolution and Development of the Advanced Trauma Life Support (ATLS) Protocol: A Historical Perspective. David S. Radvinsky, MD; Richard S. Yoon, MD; Paul J. Schmitt, MD; Charles J. Prestigiacomo, MD; Kenneth G. Swan, MD; Frank A. Liporace, Orthopedics 2012;35:305–11.

2. American College of Surgeons. *Advanced trauma life support for doctors ATLS: manuals for coordinators and faculty*. 8th ed. Chicago, IL: American College of Surgeons; 2008.

3. The SAFE Study Investigators. A comparison of albumin and saline for fluid resuscitation in the intensive care unit. N Engl J Med 2004;350:2247–56.

4. Haddad SH, Arabi YM. Critical care management of severe traumatic brain injury in adults; Scandinavian Journal of Trauma, Resuscitation and Emergency Medicine 2012:3;20:12.

5. Cerdà-Estevea M, Cuadrado-Godiab E, Chillarona JJ, Pont-Sunyerb C, Cucurellab G, Fernándeza M, Godaya A, Cano-Péreza JF, Rodríguez-Campellob A, Roquerb J, Cerebral salt wasting syndrome: Review European Journal of Internal Medicine, 2008;19(4): 249–54.

6. Saline or Albumin for Fluid Resuscitation in Patients with Traumatic Brain Injury, The SAFE Study Investigators, N Engl J Med 2007;357:874–84.

7. Gill GV, Flear CTG. Hyponatraemia. Recent advances in clinical biochemistry 1985;3:149–59.

8. Marshall WJ. Water and sodium. In 'Clinical Chemistry. WJ Marshall (ed) IInd edition, Mosby Yeaf Book, Europe Limited 1993;10–28.

9. Morgan DB (ed). Electrolyte disorders. Clinics in Endocriology and Metabolism 1984;13:231–434.

10. Welt LG, Seldin DW, Nelson WP. Role of the central nervous system in metabolism of electrolytes water. Am J Med 1952;90:355–78.

11. Young B, Ott L, Twyman D, et al. The effect of nutritional support outcomes from severe head inju J Neurosurg 1987;67:668–76.

12. Bacic A, Gluncic I, Gluncic V. Disturbances in plasma sodium in patients with war head injuries. Med 1999;164:214–7.

13. Darby JM, Nelson PB. Fluid electrolyte and acid base balance. In: Neurosurgical Intensive Ca, Andrews BT (ed). McGraw-Hill Inc. Baltimore 1993;133–43.

14. Guggiari M, Georgrschu H. The injured brain. Basis for hydroelectrolyte and hemodynami resuscitation. Ann Fr Anesth Reanim 1994;13:98–104.

15. Maclaurin RL, King LR. Recognition and treatment of metabolic disorders after head injuries. Clinical Neurosurg 1972;19:281–95.

16. Orlof F J, Handler JS. Cellular mode of action of antidiuretic hormone. Am J Med 1964;36:686–97.

17. Bakay RAE, Ward AA. Enzymatic changes in serum and cerebrospinal fluid in neurological injury. J Neurosurg 1983;58:27–37.

18. Lolin K, Jackowski A. Hyponatraemia in neurosurgical patients: Diagnosis using derived parameter of sodium and water homeostasis. Brit J Neurosurg 1992;6:457–66.

19. Crompton MR. Hypothalamic lesions following closed head injury. Brain 1971;94:165–69.

20. Griffin JM, Hartley JH, Crow RW, et al. Diabetes insipidus caused by craniofacial trauma. J Trauma 1976;16:979–984.

21. Amer M, Hasse J, Holmegaard SN, Djurberg H. Cerebral salt wasting syndrome and syndrome of inappropriate antidiuretic hormone secretion in subarachnoid haemorrhage caused by ruptured berry aneurysms. Pan Arab Journal of Neurosurgery 2000;4:25–31.

22. Weinand ME, Boynick PL, Goetz KL. A study of serum antidiuretic hormone and atrial natriuretic peptide levels in a series of patients with intracranial disease and hyponatremia. Neurosurg 1990;25:751–85.

23. Decauy G, Waaterlot Y, Genette F, et al. Treatment of the syndrome of inappropriate secretion

of antidiuretic hormone with furosemide. N Eng J Med 1981;304:329–30.

24. Ibarra-de-la-Rosa I, Perez Navero JL, Palocios Cordoba A, Montero Schiemann C, Montilla Lopez P, Ramanos Lezcano A. Inadequate secretion of atrial natriuretic peptide in children with acute brain injury. An EspPediatr 1999;51: 27–32.

25. Brigham WF. The limits of cerebral dehydration in the treatment of head injury. Surg Neurol 1986;25:340–4.

26. Sivakumar V, Rajshekhar V, Chandy MJ. Management of Neurosurgical patients with hyponatraemia and natriuresis. Neurosurgery 1994;34:269–74.

27. Padilla G, Leake JA, Castro R, et al. Vasopressin levels and pediatric head trauma. Pediatrics 1989;97:62.

28. Steinbok P, Thompson GB. Metabolic disturbances after head injury. Abnormalities of sodium and water balance with special reference to the effects of alcohol intoxication. Neurosurgery 1978;3:9–16.

29. Becker RM, Daniel RK. Increased antidiuretic hormone production after trauma to the craniofacial complex. J Trauma 1973;13:112–115.

30. Simma B, Burger R, Falk M, Sacher P, Fanconi S. A prospective, randomized and controlled study of fluid management in children with severe head injury: Lactated Ringer's solution versus hypertonic saline. Crit Care Med 1998;26:1265–70.

31. Diringer M, Ladenson PW, Stern BJ, Schleimer J, Hanley DF. Plasma atrial natriuretic factor and subarachnoid haemorrhage. Stroke 1988;19: 1119–24.

32. Wright WL. Sodium and fluid management in acute brain injury. Curr Neurol Neurosci Rep 2012;12:466–73.

33. Schirmer-Mikalsen K, Moen KG, Skandsen T, Vik A, Klepstad P. Intensive care and traumatic brain injury after the introduction of a treatment protocol: a prospective study. Acta Anaesthesiol Scand 2013;57:46–55.

34. Helms O, Freys G, Pottecher T. Severe hypophosphatemia and grave head injury. Ann Fr Anesth Reanim 2002;21:525–9.

35. Polderman KH, Bloemers FW, Peerdeman SM, et al. Hypomagnesemia and hypophosphatemia at admission in patients with severe head injury. Crit Care Med 2000, 28:2022–25.

36. Wu X, Sha H, Sun Y, Gao L, Liu H, Yuan Q, Zhang T, Zhu J, Zhou L, Hu J N-terminal pro-B-type natriuretic peptide in patients with isolated traumatic brain injury: a prospective cohort study. J Trauma 2011;71:820–5.

37. Bettinelli A, Longoni L, Tammaro F, Faré PB, Garzoni L, Bianchetti MG. Pediatr Nephrol. Renal salt-wasting syndrome in children with intracranial disorders 2012;27:733–9.

38. De Foer F, Mahler C, Dua G, et al. Post-traumatic diabetes insipidus. Acta Anesthesiol Belg 1987;38:297–302.

39. Ganong CA, Kappy MS. Cerebral salt wasting in children. The need for recognition and treatment Am J Dis Child 1993;147:167–9.

40. Cort JH. Cerebral salt wasting. Lancet 1954;1: 752–4.

41. Peters JP, Welt LG, Sims EAH. A salt wasting syndrome associated with cerebral disease. Trans Assoc Am Physicians 1950;63:57–64.

42. Schwartz WB, Bennett W, Curelop S. A syndrome of renal sodium loss and hyponatraemia probably resulting from inappropriate secretion of antidiuretic hormone. Am J Med 1957;23:529–42.

43. Vingerhoets F, de Tribolet N. Hyponatraemia hypo-osmolarity in neurosurgical patients. Appropriate secretion of ADH and cerebral salt wasting syndrome. Acta Neurochir (Wien) 1988;91:50–54.

44. Fichman MP, Kleeman CR, Bethume JE. Inhibition of antidiuretic hormone secretion by diphenyl hydantoin. Arch Neurol 1970;22:45–53.

45. Forrest JN, Cox M, Hong C, et al. Superiority of demeclocycline over lithium in the treatment of chronic syndrome of inappropriate secretion of antidiuretic hormone. N Eng J Med 1978;298: 173–7.

46. Fox JL, Falik JL, Shahoub RJ. Neurological hyponatraemia: The role of inappropriate anti-diuresis. J. Neurosurg 1971;34:506–14.

47. Robertson CS, Narayan RK, Gokaslan ZL, et al. Cerebral arteriovenous oxygen difference as an estimate of cerebral blood flow in comatose patients. J Neurosurg 1989;70:222–30.

48. Cluitmans FAM, Meinders AE. Management of severe hyponatraemia: Rapid or slow correction? Am J Med 1990;88:161–66.

49. Ishikawa S, Saito T, Kaneko K, Okada K, Kuzuya T. Hyponatraemia response to fludrocortisone acetate in elderly patients after head injury. Am Intern Med 1987;16:707–11.

50. Aviram A, Pfau A Czaczkes JW, et al. Hyperosmolality with hyponatremia caused by inappropriate administration of mannitol. Am J Med 1967;42:648–50.

51. Swales JD. Dangers in treating hyponatraemia. BMJ 1987;294:261–2.

52. Yamakki T, Tano-oka A, Takahashi A, Imaizumi T, Suetake K, Hashi K. Cerebral salt wasting syndrome distinct from the syndrome of inappropriate secretion of anti-diuretic hormone (SIADH). Acta Neurochir (Wien) 1992;115:156–62.

53. Norman DD, Mortek MA, Moses AM. Permanent diabetes insipidus following head trauma: Observation on ten patients and an approach to diagnosis. J Trauma 1980;20:599–602.

54. Sucart W A, Jackson I. Management of diabetes insipidus in neurosurgical patients. J Neurosurg 1976;44:65–71.

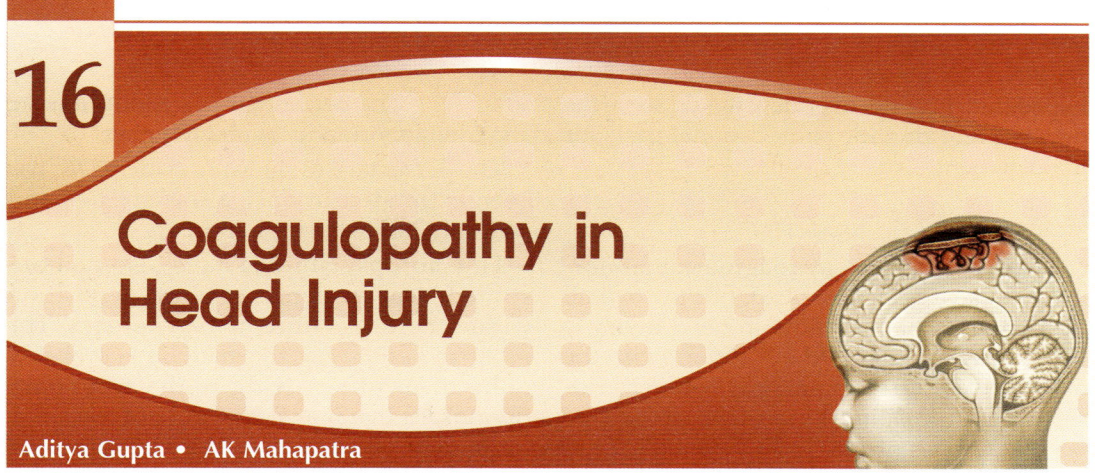

16

Coagulopathy in Head Injury

Aditya Gupta • AK Mahapatra

INTRODUCTION

Several reports have described coagulation abnormalities in patients with head trauma.[1-8] Starting with preliminary reports in the 60s,[9-11] many reports have attempted to define the precise disturbances in the coagulation system. Similar reports have highlighted dysfunction of various coagulation components in other situations of brain injury as well as other neurological disorders.[1-9] Abnormalities consistent with a state of disseminated intravascular coagulation (DIC) have been shown to occur after acute head injury. The other abnormalities noted include alterations in platelet numbers and function.[12] Additionally, "defibrination" has been reported in numerous reports and mainly refers to the consumption coagulopathy that follows severe DIC.

It has been frequently suggested that the primary reason for development of DIC in head-injured patients is the release of brain thromboplastin. Additional factors as well as the evolving secondary events in these critically ill patients are certainly of much relevance in the development of fresh abnormalities and worsening of pre-existing ones. A good proportion of these patients require brain surgery mainly for decompressive purposes, especially when a lesion responsible for raised intracranial pressure (ICP) is evident. This adds the further confounding factor of general anesthesia and operative trauma and stress, all of which may very likely play a role. It is also recognized that coagulopathy can lead to delayed and progressive hematomas in patients with brain injury. After surgery, these patients may develop recurrent haematomas that are extremely difficult to treat and carry a high morbidity and mortality.[13-15]

The mechanisms responsible for the spectrum of coagulation abnormalities following head trauma are varied and some continue to be controversial. There is similarly no consensus on the exact evaluation protocol for the detection of coagulation abnormalities in head-injured patients. There is also no agreement as to whether any prophylaxis for the impending coagulopathy is of any benefit to these patients. With the increasing trend of high velocity and missile injuries, it is possible that the neurosurgeon may encounter this kind of coagulopathy more frequently. Even otherwise, we feel that this kind of coagulation abnormality needs to be better recognized. We feel that this complication of head injury has been erroneously labelled as "rare" by numerous authors, without much more than anecdotal data. It is, therefore, of relevance to be aware of the various coagulation abnormalities, the mechanisms and the therapy in a neurosurgical setting. This review aims at discussing the above mentioned aspects with regard to the current state of knowledge. It is

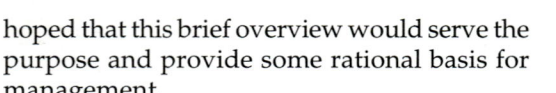

hoped that this brief overview would serve the purpose and provide some rational basis for management.

Incidence of Coagulopathy

An entire spectrum of coagulation abnormalities have been described, but the overall incidence of coagulopathy in head injury is difficult to estimate. Many reports cite the incidence as "rare" in passing, and very few reports exist detailing the incidence from large neurotrauma centres.

In the late 1960s, single case reports described this complication. From that time, many other reports are available. None of these systematically try to estimate the true magnitude of the problem.

There are two major approaches to address this issue: incidence based on laboratory test abnormalities, and based on autopsy studies. Laboratory test abnormalities (later detailed) are a common feature in trauma patients.[13] These frequently are not associated with any clinical evidence of overt or occult bleeding. It should be realized that whereas normal values for these laboratory parameters are known, the exact cutoff values for the definition of DIG are still not well defined.[13] Further limitations include an inhomogeneous battery of various tests by various authors, in order to justify a diagnosis of DIC. It is also clear that only gross alterations (decline 20–30% of normal) in coagulation factor levels lead to abnormal test results.[14,15] With these limitations in mind we can now place the available data in the correct perspective. It has been said that abnormal coagulation parameters are "common" in head-injured patients.[13–16] Several other reports cite the occurrence of abnormal coagulation parameters (suggestive of DIC) anywhere between 17 and 76%.[3–5,7,8,15,17,18] The most obvious reason for this vast range is primarily the varying criteria used for the diagnosis of DIC. Review of the larger series with some homogeneity as to the criteria for the diagnosis of DIC reveal that the actual range may lie somewhere between 20 and 50%.[5–7,15,17] The percentage of patients having a milder abnormality is much higher.

The percentage of clinically evident DIC has been estimated in only a few studies and probably lies between 1 and 24%.[3–15, 17]

Few autopsy studies have also demonstrated clear evidence of fibrin deposition within the vasculature in many organs. The problem here is that this method is probably quite insensitive owing to the secondary fibrinolysis that may occur and not leave any fibrin deposits in tissues. It is also clear that routine autopsy surveys would markedly under report the microthrombi and special stains are required for this purpose. However, few available autopsy reports do give a clear indication of the existence of this syndrome, but are far too anecdotal to convey any idea about incidence of this complication.[1,19]

Pathogenesis

It is an often quoted fact that brain tissue has been frequently used as a rich source of tissue thromboplastin in performing the prothrombin time (PT) examination. Human brain tissue extract was used in the one stage method standardized by quick as early as 1935. This leads us to probably the most important link in the pathogenesis of coagulopathy following head injury. It is now generally agreed that the most important factor leading to coagulopathy following head injury is the release of tissue thromboplastin from the brain tissue into the circulation, which then activates the coagulation cascade mainly through the extrinsic system.

The role of tissue thromboplastin was supported by the experiment of Cooper et al[20] who produced DIG in dogs after infusing canine brain thromboplastin. This was implicated also in solitary case reports in 1970s[1–7] and later has been confirmed in several large studies.[3,6,8,17–19] In a report by Clark et al, the case reported developed florid DIC following head injury. The patient succumbed to the injuries, and autopsy revealed traumatized brain tissue within

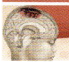

lacerated dural sinus. The authors implicated that thromboplastin may have reached the systemic circulation by this route. In another interesting study,[22] patient with a ventriculo-atrial shunt sustained head injury and later developed DIC. The patient had traumatic intraventricular hemorrhage, and the authors postulate that the ventriculoatrial shunt may have drained the tissue thromboplastins into the general circulation. While we agree that the head injury and DIC in the above two cases were causally linked, we feel that the postulated route of entry of thromboplastins into the general circulation in both the above cases are over simplifications. It is clear that trauma leads to widespread blood–brain barrier alterations and these are then sufficient to allow leakage of tissue thromboplastin into the circulation. Other indications as to the truth of above statements come from various other clinical studies. It is worthwhile to highlight an important study by Goodnight et al.[3] They studied 13 patients each of head injury with and without obvious brain tissue destruction. The authors found highly significant differences between coagulation parameters in both the groups, with 9 of 13 patients with obvious brain tissue destruction having "defibrination". Other studies have also correlated the severity of the coagulo-pathy with the severity of head injury.[7,8,15,17,19] On the other hand, review of a report by Simmons and co-workers[23] reveals that among 240 combat casualties with extensive wounds but without head injuries, there were minor abnormalities of coagulation in a few cases.

While the role of tissue thromboplastin is important, the possible mechanisms of patho-genesis of DIC are mainly three:

- *Endothelial cell injury:* Leading to activation of the Hageman factor and then the intrinsic system.
- *Tissue injury:* Leading to thromboplastin release and activation of the extrinsic system.
- Red cell or platelet injury with release of procoagulant phospholipids.

The second pathway would seem to be the most important in our setting. So far, there is a general agreement as to the pathogenesis. There is controversy as to the exact triggering mechanism and few reports even deny the existence of coagulopathy following head injury. In two such reports, the first one[24] concluded that the authors could not identify any instance of DIC in 34 patients with moderate and severe head injury. These authors were able to identify a mild activation of the coagulation system. In the second report[25, 40] trauma patients were studied, of which 15 had DIC. The authors stated that from their data, head injury did not significantly affect post-trauma coagulation or fibrinolysis. These authors feel that in general blood coagulation activity is enhanced and fibrinolytic activity is promoted on the day of trauma, but inhibited thereafter. This has found general acceptance, and most now believe that head injury initially induces a hypercoagulable state, which is then followed by fibrinolysis. A particular study demons-trated that the extent of fibrinolytic activity measured as early as 1 hour after injury correlates well with the extent of brain damage.[26] Another recent study has attempted to address some of these controversies.[6] The authors studied 20 patients having isolated severe head injury with 4 patients having isolated bone fracture (control group). They performed sampling of both the central venous as well as jugular bulb blood samples. As in other reports, there was a significant difference in fibrinogen levels and platelet counts compared to the control group. Similarly, thrombin-antithrombin complex, prothrombin fragment and soluble fibrin concentrations were all higher in the head injury group. An important finding was that all but the latter concentrations were signi-ficantly higher in the cerebrovenous blood, thus indicating the source. On the other hand, as there was no difference in D-dimer and soluble fibrin levels between cerebral and central venous blood, it indicates the likely systemic source of these two coagulation factors. The authors therefore, state that there seems to be a marked activation of the systemic coagulation system following head injury, as a result of procoagulant influences from the brain tissue. This may "spark" DIC in some such head injury patients.

Apart from DIC, other coagulation abnormalities do exist. Platelet counts have been shown to be less in head trauma patients in numerous reports.[3,5–8,14,15,17,19] The exact mechanism is not clear, but this finding may be also of equal importance from therapeutic aspect. Disturbances of platelet function have been reported in head injury patients.[12] In the study, authors studied ADP-induced platelet aggregation for 6 weeks in 34 head-injured patients. In all 8 patients dying within 24 hours of injury, the platelet aggregation was markedly reduced. In 17 patients that remained unconscious for 4 or more days, the platelet function was decreased and remained so for 9 days. Even the remaining 9 patients with mild decline in consciousness demons-trated subnormal function, which returned to normal by fourth day. This has important implications, as it implies the existence of neurohumoral factors that can directly influence platelet function. The authors postulate that serotonin or other catecholamine levels that rise after head injury may exert some influences on platelet functions through platelet p receptors. A recent study has attempted to define the differences between patients having symptomatic versus asymptomatic DIC after head injury.[27] The authors found that neutrophil elastase was significantly higher in the symptomatic DIC group. Neutrophil elastase is well known to mediate DIC after sepsis and causes tissue destruction and multi-organ failure. The authors suggest that monitoring neutrophil elastase early after head injury may help in identifying patients at risk for developing symptomatic DIC. Another valuable suggestion is that although laboratory parameters may reveal a DIC-like picture, the disorder may not truly be DIC as overall only very few patients become symptomatic, and neutrophil elastase elevation is present in only these patients.

Laboratory Evaluation

Reliable laboratory evaluation of coagulopathy is the cornerstone of diagnosing it, as it is the only available tool for identifying clinically silent abnormalities. However, the laboratory assessment has many limitations, which need to be understood. Firstly, the routine evaluation tests are quite insensitive to even substantial declines in coagulation factor levels. These become abnormal only when the levels decline 20–30% of normal. This also means that abnormal parameters cannot be completely disregarded, even though the patient may not be symptomatic. The other problem is that head injury being a dynamic pathological state, one-time assessments may frequently be fallacious. The previous section has already told us the hypercoagulable state that exists in head-injured patients, with frequently coexistent fibrinolysis.

Prior to laboratory assessment, the following considerations merit attention:

- *Clinical status of the patient:* Time of injury; degree of blood loss and any replacement prior to sample collection; prior coagulation abnormality or history suggestive of it; intake of anti-inflammatory drugs or anticoagulants; existence of liver disease.
- *Careful collection of specimens:* Wrong dilutions or non-optimal amount of reagent in collection tubes may all affect test results.
- Timely delivery of specimens to the laboratory.
- Assessment of test results by an experienced hematologist.

Six basic tests of coagulation function assessment are routinely recommended for any health care organization:

- Prothrombin time (PT)
- Activated partial thromboplastin time (APTT)
- Thrombin clotting time (TT)

- Platelet count
- Fibrinogen essay
- Fibrin degradation product essay (FDP)

In cases where hemodilution is suspected, concomitant performance of hematocrit should be done. This may be of importance in polytrauma patients, with significant blood loss. Taking into conjunction all these evaluations, different centres have devised their own grading systems for the diagnosis of DIG. There is yet no final consensus. In the absence of any underlying disease that could alter hemostasis, any abnormal result implies some coagulopathy. Abnormal PT mainly implies a derangement of the extrinsic system, and abnormal APTT implies a dysfunction of the intrinsic system. DIG usually causes prolongation of PT, APTT and TT accompanied by a low platelet count and elevation of FDP levels. The exact cut-off values are still controversial. For more details, a few grading scales are referred to.[28,29]

Certain specialized tests can be under some circumstances to better define the exact underlying mechanism[6,12,13,19,25-29] and may provide some input of therapeutic significance:

- Fibrinopeptide A and B
- D-dimer
- Thrombin-antithrombin complex
- Protamine sulphate test
- Prothrombin fragment assay
- Platelet function tests

Therapeutic Considerations

The therapy should be primarily based on clinical grounds and needs, and should not necessarily rely only on the biochemical evidence of a coagulopathy. The various parameters to be taken into consideration are:

- Active bleeding from skin, mucosae and other puncture sites.
- Clinical and neurological state of the patient.
- Severity of the intracranial injury and intracranial pressure.
- Need for urgent operative decompression or repair.

- Any underlying disease or drug intake predisposing to coagulopathy.

It is clear that patients having active bleed need urgent correction of the underlying coagulation abnormality. Any patient with clinically or biochemically evident coagulopathy needing urgent decompression should similarly undergo replacement of clotting factors prior to surgical intervention. This is of importance as operative stres, operative trauma including that to the brain tissue may further aggrabate the existing coagulopathy. It has been clearly documented that these head-injured patients with coagulopathy are at risk for developing delayed and recurrent postoperative hematomas.[13,16,30-33] At the same time, it would be imprudent to make a patient with a large hematoma (especially an epidural hematoma) wait for decompression after obtaining a full report and correcting the abnormality as these patients can deteriorate rather rapidly. This can only be decided as per the merits of a particular case, however, in these patients we do perform simple bedside tests such as evaluations of bleeding and clotting times and start therapy as required by the urgency of the clinical situation. In such case, occasionally the replacement therapy and surgery may have to be done simultaneously. Surgically, in such a patient one should take care to minimize the time taken and further blood loss. The least extensive procedure should be planned in these patients. Adequate replacements of clotting factors should be available and transfusion of these should be continued throughout the procedure. In case of any doubt about adequacy of hemostasis, a drain should readily be left. Similarly, the same tube could be used to monitor the intracranial pressure after surgery. Postoperatively, check of the coagulation status should be carried out and replacement done to maintain adequate levels of coagulation function.

The line of therapy for the actively bleeding patient and for the one requiring surgery is quite clear. Controversy exists regarding the optimal management of patients that are

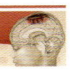

asymptomatic and do not require surgery. It has been previously stated that the biochemical coagulopathy only mimics DIC and is usually self-limiting. In this context, if only a minority of these patients is to develop full-blown DIC, it may not be cost-effective to treat all such patients with precious coagulation factors. It is also not clear whether in these patients therapy will be rewarded with improved outcome. It is possible that the DIC may only reflect the severity of the injury and thus appear to be associated with poor outcome without any benefit even if it is reversed. With all this in mind because DIC parallels outcome and it seems prudent to prevent further hemorrhagic complications in these critically ill patients we follow an aggressive approach. Some do not even agree to treat all abnormal coagulation parameteres,[34] but this remains a matter of debate. On the other hand, some recommend that the replacement therapy should be started on clinical grounds even before coagulation results are available.[3,13, 35] May et al, in their patients have a greater mortality and hospital stay. Of their patients, 81% of those with GCS of or below 6 were coagulopathies, compared to none with GCS above that. In such patients, the neurosurgical intervention was also delayed, which even included the placement of an ICP monitor. They recommend that empiric replacement therapy should be considered in patients with GCS of or below 6, as waiting for a full coagulation profile involves a delay of at least 1 to 1.5 hours. Our recommendations are to treat all abnormal coagulation tests and these abnormalities have also been shown to occur in patients with mild injuries and to affect outcomes even in these patients. We do not routinely infuse coagulation factors prior to obtain at least simple bedside estimates of hemostasis such as bleeding time and clotting time. If these indicate obvious abnormality and there is enough clinical evidence for coagulopathy or need for urgent correction, we do go ahead and replace clotting factors prior to obtain a full evaluation. We feel that these clotting factors are too valuable a

resource to be wasted to patients who do not need them urgently and without firm justi- fication.

The mainstay of the therapy is to replace the depleted coagulation factors, in adequate doses. Fresh frozen plasma (FFP) and platelet concentrates are the preparations of choice. If fresh frozen plasma is not available or fibrino- gen level is extremely low, cryoprecipitate should be infused. It should be noted that fresh frozen plasma is a rich source of Factor V and cryoprecipitate of fibrinogen and Factor VIII. In their study, Goodnight et al replaced 12 bags of cryoprecipitate and 2–4 units of fresh frozen plasma while waiting for results of coagulation tests. The authors opinion was that the replacement was of benefit in the survival of at least two patients. Advice should certainly be sought from an experi- enced hematologist as to the replacement of these blood factors and should be titrated depending on the existing levels of these factors, with performance of repeat estima- tions. Platelets may not be required unless the count is below 75,000 per cubic mm. If the patient requires neurosurgical operation, the count should be kept at 100,000. As a general rule, the aim should be to administer the following doses:

- *Platelets:* 1 concentrate pack per 10 kg weight
- *Fibrinogen:* 50 mg/kg

Most authors do not advise the administra- tion of either procoagulant medications such as epsilon aminocaproic acid (EACA) as it may cause unchecked thrombosis to occur, given the overall coagulation activation following head injury. Moreover, it may precipitate renal failure by preventing lysis of fibrin in glomerular capillaries.[36] The use of heparin is also to be avoided. In other situations, heparin is routinely used in the management of DIG. In case of active bleed and in any patient with head injury heparin should probably not be used except as a last resort. No controlled studies are available in this regard. It is generally agreed that in head-injured patients some degree of disruption of the vascular tree can be assumed, and further intracranial hemorrhage has to be avoided.

Prognostic and Outcome Considerations

It has been shown in many studies that the presence of coagulopathy in head-injured patients is of definite prognostic value; coagulopathy has been shown to be linked to the extent of brain injury as well as the consciousness status of these adult and pediatric patients.[3,5,7,8,11,14,15,17,26,27,37,38] The problem therefore, is whether the presence of a coagulopathy is an independent prognostic factor or not. If not, then it may just appear to associate with prognosis and outcome as it is closely related to the severity of the injury. To address this issue, a few studies have used the statistical tool of multivariate analysis. In one such study,[37] the authors concluded that even a single abnormality in the FT or APTT within the first day of admission was significantly related to the mortality. Mortality was 80% in patients with coagulopathy and 7.4% in those without. The corresponding p value was less than 0.001 and odds ratio was 50. In the other study,[15] DIG was seen in 24% of patients overall and the highest incidence was in the acute subdural hematoma group. The mortality rate for patients with DIG was 58%. This study reveals two additional important points. Firstly, APTT value was the single most important predictor of survival in their study, even more than the GCS. This highlights the prognostic significance of DIG, if it is present in a head-injured patient. Other studies report that presence of coagulopathy was the second important predictive factor of survival, after GCS.[38,39] Secondly, in the patients in the DIG group, the fibrinogen level was the most important predictive factor for their survival. Another study has utilized logistic regression analysis to prove the independent predictive value of coagulopathy in survival of head-injured patients.[17] The authors noted that 38% of their patients had coagulation derangements, and for any particular value of GCS, the APTT, FDP and DIG scores had

independent predictive value. In patients with GCS,[13–15] the FDP scores were significant predictors. In the GCS,[6-12] subgroup, APTT and DIG scores were important predictors. Similarly, van der Sande and co-workers[7] reported on 150 patients with head injury among whom 60 had deranged coagulation. They felt that FDP levels correlated most accurately with the extent of brain damage and outcome. In some cases, the FDP levels were better indicators of prognosis than the GCS. They cite example of two cases that were initially conscious but later deteriorated; both had deranged coagulation parameters. This finding bears striking similarity to that in the report quoted prior[4] to this[17] and to the report by Olson et al.[29] The adverse prognostic impact of coagulopathy has also been studied in pediatric head injury,[38,40,41] pediatric abusive head trauma[42] and as a predictor of fetal mortality in trauma to pregnant patients.[43]

From the above discussion, it is clear that coagulopathy is an independent predictor of poor outcome in head injury patients. The mortality, morbidity, hospital stay and poor outcome as assessed by the GOS are all much more in head-injured patients with coagulopathy. Another point to stress is the validity of this prognostic indicator even in alert and seemingly well patients. The mortality rate of patients once DIG is present is remarkably high, as mentioned and lies in the range of 40–60%.

CONCLUSIONS

From the preceding review, it appears that coagulopathy after head injury is a common phenomenon than is routinely recognized. The mechanisms may vary, but the abundance of tissue thromboplastin in the brain is certainly of importance. This triggers the coagulation cascade and later fibrinolysis ensues. The coagulopathy itself is usually self-limiting and only a few patients are symptomatic for this. Despite this, reliable evaluation of basic coagulation parameters should be performed as early as possible. The therapy should be urgently initiated and further decisions taken considering the presence of active bleeding or the need for a neurosurgical procedure. Even otherwise, any abnormal coagulation parameter should be treated, but there does not seem to be any clear role at present for prophylactic administration of clotting factors prior to establishing coagulopathy. There does not seem to be any indication for administration of other procoagulant or anticoagulant agents at present, such as EACA or heparin. Evaluation and therapy should be urgent because the presence of coagulopathy appears to have significant independent predictive value for the prognosis and survival of such patients and correcting it may have a beneficial effect on survival. The latter is more an expression of hope rather than a proven fact, and it is hoped that future studies would give us firmer indications and guidelines for management. At present, the mortality of DIG associated with head injury remains alarmingly high.

REFERENCES

1. Preston FE, Malia RG, Sworn MJ, Timperley WR, Blackburn EK. Disseminated intravascular coagulation as a consequence of cerebral damage. J Neurol Neurosurg Psychiatry 1974;37:241–8.

2. Vardi Y, Streifler M, Schujman E, Lowenthal M. Diffuse intravascular clotting associated with a primary brain tumor. J Neurol Neurosurg Psychiatry 1974;37:987–90.

3. Goodnight SH, Kenoyer G, Rapaport SI, Patch MJ, Lee JA, Kurze T. Defibrination after brain-tissue destruction: A serious complication of head injury. N Engl J Med 1974:1043–7.

4. Pondaag W. Disseminated intravascular coagulation related to outcome in head injury. Acta Neurochir Suppl (Wien) 1979;28:98–102.

5. Miner ME, Kaufman HH, Graham SH, Haar FH, Gildenberg PL. Disseminated intravascular coagulation fibrinolytic syndrome following head injury in children: frequency and prognostic implications. J Pediatr 1982;100:687–91.

6. Scherer RU, Spangenberg P. Procoagulant activity in patients with isolated severe head trauma. Crit Care Med 1998;26:149–56.

7. Van der Sande JJ, Veltkamp JJ, Boekhout Mussert RJ, Bouwhuis-Hoogerwerf ML. Head injury and coagulation disorders. J. Neurosurg 1978; 49:357–65.

8. Auer L. Disturbances of the coagulatory system in patients with severe cerebral trauma. I. Acta Neurochir (Wien) 1978,43:51–9.

9. Bang NU, McDowell F. Cerebral infarction and blood clotting. Trans Am Neurol Assoc 1966;91:84–6.

10. Innes D, Sevitt S. Coagulation and fibrinolysis in injured patients. J Clin Path 1964;17:1–13.

11. Obrzut A, Jarzyna A, Skrzydiewski S. Thromboelastographical evaluation of the coagulative system of blood and fibrinolysis in craniocerebral injuries. Minerva Neurochir 1967; 11:42–6.

12. Vecht CJ, Minderhoud JM, Sibinga CT. Piatelet aggregability in relation to impaired consciousness after head injury. J Clin Pathol Oct 1975; 28:814–20.

13. Kaufman HH, Timberlake G, Voelker J, Pait TG. Medical complications of head injury. Med Clin North Am 1993;77:43–60.

14. Kaufman HH, Moake JL, Olson JD, Miner ME, duCret RP, Pruessner JL, Gildenberg PL. Delayed and recurrent intracranial hematomas related to disseminated intravascular clotting and fibrinolysis in head injury. Neurosurgery 1980;7:445–9.

15. Kumura E, Sato M, Fukuda A, Takemoto Y, Tanaka S, Kohama A. Coagulation disorders following acute head injury. Acta Neurochir (Wien) 1987;85:23–8.

16. Mattson J, Hoots K, Contant C, et al. Influence of coagulopathy on prognosis in head injured patients: A study of 2032 consecutive cases (abstract). Blood 1983; 62(suppl):276a.

17. Selladurai BM, Vickneswaran M, Duraisamy S, Atan M.Coagulopathy in acute head injury - a study of its role as a prognostic indicator. Br J Neurosurg 1997;11:398–404.

18. Anzil AP. Letter: Defibrination after head trauma.N Engl J Med 1974;291:632–3.

19. Kaufman HH, Hui KS, Mattson JC, Borit A, Childs TL, Hoots WK, Bernstein DP, Makela ME, Wagner KA, Kahan BD, et al. Clinicopathological correlations of disseminated intravascular coagulation in patients with head injury. Neurosurgery 1984; 15:34–42.

20. Cooper HA, Bowie EJW, Owen CA. Chronic induced intravascular coagulation in dogs. Am J Physiol 1973; 225:1355–58.

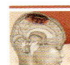

21. Clark JA, Finelli RE, Netsky MG. Disseminated intravascular coagulation following cranial trauma. Case report. J Neurosurg 1980;52:266–9.

22. Tinnemans JG, Gerritsen SM. A fibrinogenemia and blunt head injury. Intensive Care Med. 1980;6:211–3.

23. Simmons RL, Collins JA, Heistercamp CA III, et al. Coagulation disorders in combat casualties. I. Acute changes after wounding. II. Effects of massive transfusion. III. Post-resuscitative changes. Ann Surg 1969;169:455–482.

24. Vecht CJ, Sibinga CT, Minderhoud JM. Disseminated intravascular coagulation and head injury. J Neurol Neurosurg Psychiatry 1975;38:567–71.

25. Gando S, Tedo I, Kubota M. Post-trauma coagulation and fibrinolysis. Crit Care Med 1992;20:594–600.

26. Takahashi H, Urano T, Takada Y, Nagai N, Takada A. Fibrinolytic parameters as an admission prognostic marker of head injury in patients who talk and deteriorate. Neurosurgery 1997;86:768–72.

27. Takahashi H, Urano T, Nagai N, Takada Y, Takada A. Neutrophil elastase may play a key role in developing symptomatic disseminated intravascular coagulation and multiple organ failure in patients with head injury. J Trauma 2000;49:86–91.

28. Kaufman HH, Mattson JC. Coagulopathy in head injury. In Becker DP, Povlishock JT (eds): Central Nervous System Trauma Status Report. Richmond, William Byrd Press 1985;187–206.

29. Olson JD, Kaufman HH, Moake J, O'Gorman TW, Hoots K, Wagner K, Brown CK, Gildenberg PL. The incidence and significance of hemostatic abnormalities in patients with head injuries. Neurosurgery 1989;24:825–32.

30. Kaufman HH. Delayed post-traumatic intracerebral hematoma. In Kaufman HH (ed): Intracerebral hematomas. Etiology, Pathophysiology, Clinical presentation and Treatment. New York, Raven Press, 1992,173–80.

31. Mellion BT, Narayan RK. Delayed traumatic intracerebral hematomas and coagulopathies. In Barrow DL (ed): Complications and sequelae of head injury. Park Ridge, IL, American Association of Neurological Surgeons Publications Committee 1992; 51–9.

32. Stein SC, Young GS, Talucci RC, Greenbaum BH, Ross SE. Delayed brain injury after head trauma: significance of coagulopathy. Neurosurgery 1992;30:160–5.

33. Touho H, Hirakawa K, Hino A, Karasawa J, Ohno Y. Relationship between abnormalities of coagulation and fibrinolysis and postoperative intracranial hemorrhage in head injury. Neurosurgery 1986;19:523–31.

34. Winter JP, Plummer D, Bottini A, Rockswold GR, Ray D. Early fresh frozen plasma prophylaxis of abnormal coagulation parameters in the severely head-injured patient is not effective. Ann Emerg Med 1989;18:553–5.

35. May AK, Young JS, Butler K, Bassam D, Brady W. Coagulopathy in severe closed head injury: is empiric therapy warranted? Am Surg 1997; 63:233–6; discussion 236–7.

36. McKay DG, Muller-Berghaus G. Therapeutic implications of disseminated intravascular coagulation. Am J Cardiol 1967;20:392–410.

37. Shaffrey ME, Polin RS, Phillips CD, et al. Classification of craniocerebral gunshot wounds: A multivariate analysis predictive of mortality. J Neurotrauma 1992; 9 (suppl 1): S279–85.

38. Vavilala MS, Dunbar PJ, Rivara FP, Lam AM. Coagulopathy predicts poor outcome following head injury in children less than 16 years of age. J Neurosurg Anaesthesiol 2001;13:13–8.

39. Polin RS, Shaffrey ME, Phillips CD, Germanson T, Jane JA. Multivariate analysis and prediction of outcome following penetrating head injury. Neurosurg Clin N Am 1995;6:689–99.

40. Keller MS, Fendya DG, Weber TR. Glasgow Coma Scale predicts coagulopathy in pediatric trauma patients. Semin Pediatr Surg 2001; 10:12–6.

41. Chiaretti A, Pezzotti P, Mestrovic J, Piastra M, Polidori G, Storti S, Velardi F, Di Rocco C. The influence of hemocoagulative disorders on the outcome of children with head injury. Pediatr Neurosurg 2001;34:131–7.

42. Hymel KP, Abshire TC, Luckey DW, Jenny C. Coagulopathy in pediatric abusive head trauma. Pediatrics 1997;99:371–5.

43. Ali J, Yeo A, Gana TJ, McLellan BA. Predictors of fetal mortality in pregnant trauma patients. J Trauma 1997; 42:782–5.

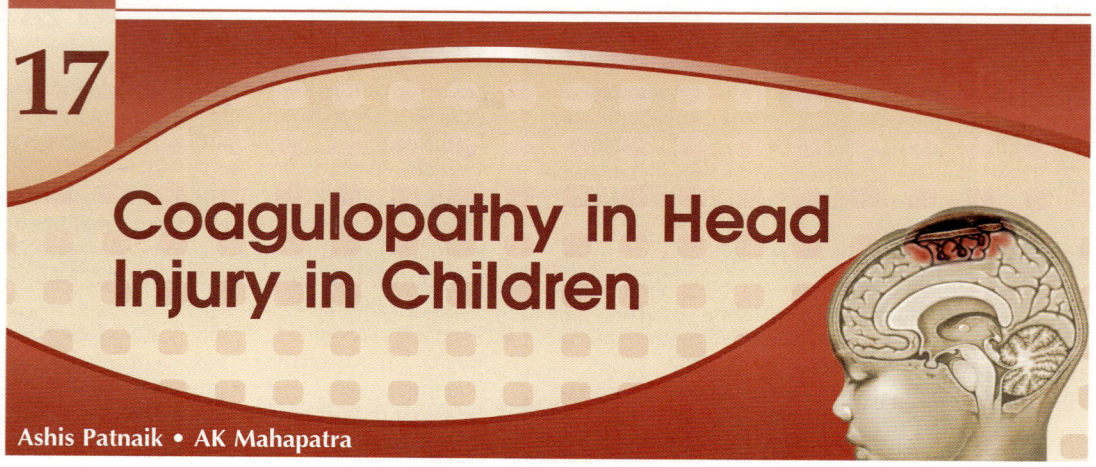

17

Coagulopathy in Head Injury in Children

Ashis Patnaik • AK Mahapatra

INTRODUCTION

Coagulopathy is an underreported problem following head injury. In the recent years, it is being diagnosed more frequently, with easy and wide availability of coagulation tests. Brain injury results in release of brain tissue thromboplastins, which stimulates the coagulation cascade. This is followed by a brief period of fibrinolysis and the overall process leads to a full-fledged syndrome of disseminated intravascular coagulation (DIC). Many of these head injury patients require urgent neurosurgical interventions mainly for decompressive purposes, when a lesion causing significant raised intracranial pressure is present. Effect of general anesthesia, operative trauma and stress further destabilise the already compromised coagulation system, thus exposing the patient to life-threatening bleeding. In addition to DIC, alteration in platelet function and numbers also add to the coagulation problems in head injury. This coagulopathy can also lead to delayed, progressive and recurrent hematomas in patients who have undergone cranial surgery which are extremely difficult to treat and carry high morbidity and mortality. Overall, the presence of coagulopathy is an independent predictor of high morbidity and mortality after head injury.[1–7] This association between abnormalities in coagulation system and poor outcome of patients with head injury was first reported by Pondaag.[8] But the exact mechanisms of coagulation abnormality after head injury are not known. Similarly, there is no consensus regarding the evaluation protocol for detecting coagulation abnormalities and prophylaxis for preventing such catastrophes. Treatment for such problem is also controversial with no single treatment protocol being ideal. However, early recognition of coagulopathy is of value in predicting the occurrence of delayed brain injury and may contribute to prevention of bleeding disorders.[1] This chapter aims at reviewing various aspects of coagulopathy in head injury and tries to give the current state of knowledge.

Incidence of Coagulopathy in Head Injury

Abnormal blood coagulation following brain injury was first reported by Penick and McLendon in a newborn during delivery.[9] Now it is known that abnormalities in coagulation system are very common in head injury as coagulation tests are routinely being used.[10–13]

Overall incidence of coagulopathy is difficult to estimate. Many reports cite the incidence as "rare" whereas very few reports exist detailing the incidence from large neurotrauma centres. Although laboratory test abnormalities are quite common feature in head injury patients, these are not associated with any clinical evidence of overt

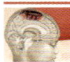

or occult bleeding. Exact cut off values of for defining DIC has not been established clearly. Again various authors and series have utilised inhomogeneous battery of coagulation tests which adds to difficulty in comparing the test results. Only gross alterations in coagulation factors (decline up to 20–30% of normal) lead to abnormal test results. All these limitations make the exact calculation of incidence of coagulopathy in head injury difficult. Several reports cite the occurrence of abnormal coagulation parameters in form of DIC anywhere between 15 and 100% depending upon the severity of trauma.[1-4,14–19] This wide range is caused by varying criteria to diagnose DIC. The number of patients showing milder abnormality will be quite high. The percentage of clinically evident DIC has been estimated to lie between 1 and 24%.[20–23]

Pathogenesis

Coagulopathy after traumatic brain injury includes hypercoagulable and hypocoagulable states that can lead to secondary injury by either the induction of microthrombosis or the progression of hemorrhagic brain lesions. Multiple hypotheses have been proposedto explain this phenomenon, including the release of tissue factor,[20,24–31] disseminated intravascular coagulation,[11,23,32–36] hyperfibrinolysis, hypoperfusion with protein C

activation,[37,38] and platelet dysfunction.[4,39–41] Current evidence suggests that it is a dynamic process involving a state of hypercoagulability followed by a bleeding diathesis.[11,17,24,32,33] The loss of equilibrium among the tightly regulated coagulation factors can lead either to hypercoagulable states with microthrombosis and ischemia or to hypocoagulable states with possible progression of hemorrhagic lesions (Fig. 17.1).

Overall, the possible mechanisms of pathogenesis of coagulopathy after head injury are mainly three:

1. *Tissue injury:* Leading to thromboplastin release and activation of extrinsic system of coagulation.

2. *Endothelial injury:* Leading to activation of Hageman factor and then the intrinsic system.

3. *Red cell or platelet injury:* Results in release of procoagulant phospholipids.

Release of brain tissue thromboplastins into the circulation and activation of coagulation process is the most acceptable mechanism for post head injury coagulopathy. Trauma to the brain leads to widespread breakdown of blood–brain barrier (BBB) and leakage of tissue thromboplastins into the circulation. It leads to a hypercoagulable state, which is then followed by fibrinolysis. Takahashi et al[42]

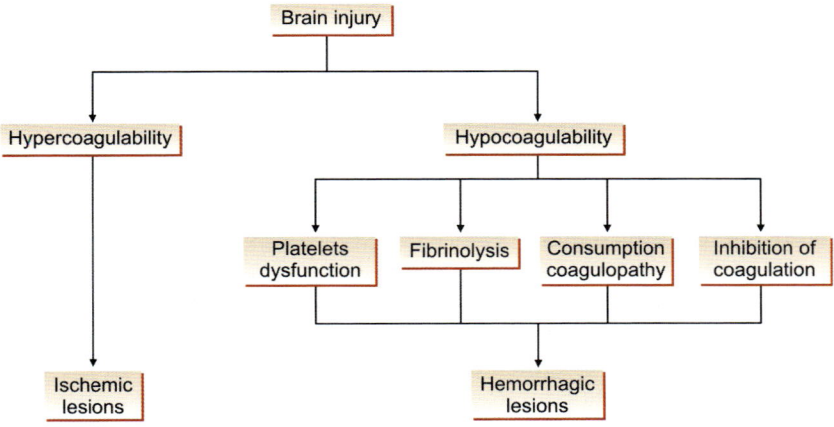

Fig. 17.1: Development of coagulopathy after traumatic brain injury

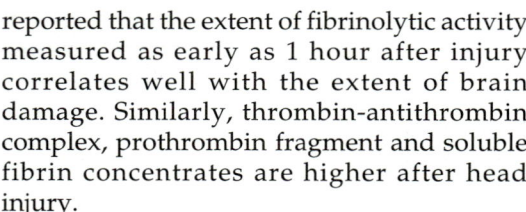

reported that the extent of fibrinolytic activity measured as early as 1 hour after injury correlates well with the extent of brain damage. Similarly, thrombin-antithrombin complex, prothrombin fragment and soluble fibrin concentrates are higher after head injury.

In addition to DIC, other coagulation abnormalities do exist in head injury. Platelet counts have been shown to be less in head injury patients.[20,43,44] Disturbances in platelet function have been reported in head injury patients.[21] After head injury, levels of serotonin or other catecholamines rise which may play a role in disturbance of platelet function through their effect on platelet? receptors. Neutrophil elastase, which is a well-known factor mediating DIC after sepsis and causes tissue damage and multiorgan failure, also increases significantly after head injury and may be a potential cause for DIC in head injury.

Laboratory Evaluation

Reliable laboratory evaluation of coagulopathy is important in head injury as it is the only available means to diagnose clinically silent abnormalities. However, this evaluation has many limitations such as:

1. Routine coagulation tests are insensitive to mild to substantial decline in coagulation factor levels and they become abnormal only when the levels decline to 20–30% of normal.

2. As head injury is a dynamic pathological state, one time laboratory evaluation has little value in management of DIC after head injury. Hypercoagulable state frequently co-exists or is followed by fibrinolysis in DIC after head injury. Hence single assessment often gives fallacious reports.

Routine tests of bloodcoagulation are able to identify the earliest signs of coagulopathy, assess its severity, monitor its course, and predict the short-term and long-term outcome in patients with severe head trauma.[45,46]

Routine determination of the coagulation status, should be performed in all patients with traumatic brain injury.[3]

Basic coagulation tests which should be done in head injury scenario are:
1. Prothrombin time (PT)
2. Activated partial thrmboplastin time (APTT)
3. Thrombin clotting time (TT)
4. Platelet count
5. Fibrinogen assay
6. Fibrin degradation product assay (FDP)
7. International normalised ratio (INR)

DIC usually causes prolongation of PT, APTT and TT with low platelet count and elevated FDP levels. Exact cut-off values to diagnose DIC in head injury is controversial. Apart from the basic coagulation parameters, some of the other specialised tests can be done under some circumstances to better define the exact underlying mechanism:
1. Fibrinopeptide A & B.
2. D-dimer.
3. Thrombin-antithrombin complex.
4. Protamine sulphate test.
5. Prothrombin fragment assay.
6. Platelet function tests.

Overall, the laboratory evaluation of coagulopathy in head injury can be divided into 3 categories to detect any hypercoagulable or hypocoagulable states (Table 17.1):
1. Tests measuring enzymatic coagulation.
2. Tests measuring platelet function.
3. Tests measuring fibrinolysis system.

THROMBOELASTOGRAPHY

It is a recently introduced coagulation test which measures the overall viscoelastic properties of blood and allows realtime assessment of both hypocoagulable and hypercoagulable states in a single test. It provides information on the kinetics of clot formation and its stability by assessing viscoelastic properties of blood during dynamic blood clot formation. It also provides

Table 17.1: Laboratory tests to assess coagulopathy		
Enzymatic coagulation	*Fibrinolysis*	*Platelets*
INR/PT	D-Dimer	Platelet count
PTT	Fibrinogen degradation product	Bleeding time
Fibrinogen	Plasminogen activator inhibitor-1	Platelet function analyser
Thrombin time	Thromboelastography	Rapid platelet function assay
Thrombin-antithrombin III complex		Whole-blood impedence aggregometry
Prothrombin cleavage fragments		Thromboelastography
Thromboelastography		

information on the effect of transfusion on coagulation system and has been used in neurosurgical operation theatres.[47,48] It has been reported that the proper use of this test can lower down the morbidity and mortality associated with blood transfusions in trauma patients.[49–52] The most advantage part of thromboelastography in coagulopathy patients is that it assesses the hypercoagulable state, which is difficult to do with other tests.

Therapeutic Considerations

Treatment of coagulopathy after head injury should be based on clinical features and needs rather than only on the biochemical evidence of coagulopathy. The following factors should be taken into consideration during planning of therapy for coagulopathy:

- Active bleeding from skin, mucosae, wounds or other puncture sites.
- Clinical and neurological state of the patient.
- Severity of intracranial injury, status of intracranial pressure and need for any urgent operative procedure.
- Any underlying disease or drug intake predisposing to coagulopathy.

The line of therapy for patients having active bleeding or requiring urgent neurosurgical intervention is rather quite clear. In patients having active bleeding, coagulation factor transfusion should be given as soon as possible to raise their level to normal. Patients requiring surgical procedures cannot wait for long periods so that their coagulation parameters become normal by transfusion. In these patients, coagulation factor level should be raised to a minimum level so that operative procedure can safely be carried out. Only simple bed side coagulation tests can be done and therapy started depending upon the urgency of the situation. Replacement of coagulation factors, blood and surgery can be carried out simultaneously. Surgically, least extensive procedure should be planned and in case of doubt regarding haemostasis, a drain should be left. Postoperatively coagulation profile should be regularly checked and any deficit should be replaced to maintain adequate levels of coagulation function.

Management of patients those are asymptomatic and do not require surgery is debatable. As only a minority of patients who show biochemical abnormality develop DIC, hence correcting their abnormality through transfusion of coagulation factors will not be cost effective. Again it is not clear whether prophylactic transfusion will improve their overall outcome. Once DIC develops in head injury, the overall prognosis becomes poor. Hence in critically ill patients such as those with low GCS, aggressive approach should be adopted in correcting the abnormal coagulation parameters.

Role of fresh frozen plasma (FFP): It is the preparation of choice to replace the depleted coagulation factors. But its prophylactic administration in head injury patients has not been proven tobe beneficial in correcting the coagulopathy or improving the overall outcome.[53] Etemadrezaie et al[54] reported increasein mortality of severe head injury patients those have received early empirical infusion of FFP. It should be administrated only when there is evidence of coagulation abnormalities.

In case of non-availability of FFP or fibrinogen level is extremely low, cryoprecipitate should be infused. FFP is a good source of factor V and cryoprecipitate of fibrinogen and factor VIII. Platelet concentrates may not be required unless the count is below 75000 per cubic mm. If the patient requires neurosurgical operation, the count should be kept at 100,000 per cubic mm. As a general rule, the aim should be to administer the following doses:

- *Platelets:* 1 concentrate pack per 10 kg weight
- *Fibrinogen:* 50 mg/kg

Antifibrinolytic medications: Clinical randomisation of an antifibrinolytic in significant hemorrhage (CRASH-2) study showed the usefulness of tranexamic acid after general trauma, but it had no benefits in terms of reduced mortality in head injury patients.[55] Similarly the beneficial effect of aprotinin, an antifibrinolytic agent is questionable.[56]

Recombinant factor VIIa: It initiates thrombus formation by binding to exposed tissue factor. It has beneficial effect in arresting life-threatening hemorrhage caused by severe coagulopathy in trauma patients. It rapidly corrects abnormal INR in comparison to FFP. It also restricts the progression of hemorrhagic lesions in high-risk patients and allows quicker neurosurgical intervention.[57–62]

Procoagulant medications such as epsilon aminocaproic acid (EACA) are not advisable as they can cause unchecked thrombosis and renal failure. Heparin should also be avoided in coagulopathy in head injury unless as a last resort.

Treatment for hypercoagulation stage: Unlike the hypocoagulable stage, hypercoagulable conditions do not have satisfactory treatment protocols. Treatment with antithrombin concentrate, a procoagulant blocker,[63] heparin, antiplatelet therapy are not beneficial.

Outcome

It has been reported by many studies that the coagulopathy in head injury is associated with poor outcome in terms of mortality, morbidity, hospital stay, GOS score.[4–6,45] Although coagulopathy has been associated with more severe head injury and less initial GCS score, multivariate analysis studies have shown that the coagulopathy itself is an independent prognostic factor for the overall poor outcome of head injury patients.[3,22,64–66] The mortality rate of patients once DIC is present is very high, and lies in the range of 40–60%. Engström et al[67] reported a significant fall in platelet counts after severe head trauma was related to prolonged mechanical ventilation. The platelet count of $229 \times 10^3/\mu l$ or less (sensitivity, 78.8%; specificity, 78.9%), PT of 13.8 seconds or more (sensitivity, 57.9%; specificity, 63.3%), PTT of 33.5 seconds or more (sensitivity, 63.2%; specificity, 81.8%), and INR of 1 or greater (sensitivity, 73.7%; specificity, 72.7%) were the best cutoff points in prediction of mortality in the series of patients reported by Salehpour et al.[45] Values above this in initial 3 hours period were associated with increased mortality rates.

CONCLUSIONS

Coagulopathy after head injury is a common phenomenon than is routinely recognised. Various mechanisms may play in triggering the abnormal coagulation process but release of tissue thromboplastins from injured brain tissue is certainly the main mechanism. Coagulopathy starts with the hypercoagulable state and then fibrinolysis, consumption coagulopathy in form of frank DIC follows. Mild forms of coagulopathy are self-limiting and a few patients become symptomatic. However, evaluation of basic coagulation parameters should be performed in each head injury patients to rule out any abnormality. In presence of biochemically proven coagulopathy, with active bleeding or need for a urgent neurosurgical procedure, therapy should be urgently started. Even otherwise,

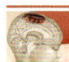

any abnormal coagulation parameter should be treated, but at present there is no clear cut consensus regarding prophylactic administration of clotting factors prior to establishing coagulopathy. Fresh frozen plasma, cryoprecipitates for diminished coagulation factors and platelet concentrates for low platelet count are reasonable therapy. In gross DIC, fibrinogen administration is advisable. There is no need for administration of procoagulant or anticoagulant such as EACA or heparin at present. Evaluation and therapy should be done promptly, as presence of coagulopathy is a significant independent negative prognostic factor for prognosis of head injury patients and once the DIC develops, mortality grossly increases.

REFERENCES

1. Stein SC, Young GS, Talucci RC, Greenbaum BH, Ross SE. Delayed brain injury after head trauma: significance of coagulopathy. Neurosurgery 1992;30:160–5.

2. Piek J, Chesnut RM, Marshall LF, van Berkum-Clark M, Klauber MR, Blunt BA, et al. Extracranial complications of severe head injury. J Neurosurg 1992;77:901–7.

3. Harhangi BS, Kompanje EJ, Leebeek FW, Maas AI. Coagulation disorders after traumatic brain injury. ActaNeurochir (Wien) 2008;150:165–75.

4. Laroche M, Kutcher ME, Huang MC, Cohen MJ, Manley GT. Coagulopathy after traumatic brain injury. Neurosurgery 2012;70:1334–45.

5. Talving P, Benfield R, Hadjizacharia P, Inaba K, Chan LS, Demetriades D. Coagulopathy in severe traumatic brain injury: a prospective study. J Trauma 2009;66:55–61; discussion 61–2.

6. Wafaisade A, Lefering R, Tjardes T, et al. Acute coagulopathy in isolated blunt traumatic brain injury. Neurocrit Care 2010;12:211–9.

7. Stein SC, Spettell C, Young G, Ross SE. Delayed and progressive brain injury in closed-head trauma: radiological demonstration. Neurosurgery 1993;32:25–30; discussion 30–1.

8. Pondaag W. Disseminated intravascular coagulation related to outcome in head injury. Acta Neurochir Suppl (Wien) 1979;28:98–102.

9. Penick GD, McLendon WW. Disorders of the hemostatic mechanism. Int Rec Med 1960;173:491–6.

10. Goodnight Jr SH. Defibrination following head injury. Compr Ther 1977;3:25–8.

11. van der Sande JJ, Veltkamp JJ, Boekhout-Mussert RJ, Bouwhuis-Hoogerwerf ML. Head injury and coagulation disorders. J Neurosurg 1978;49:357–65.

12. Auer L. Disturbances of the coagulatory system in patients with severe cerebral trauma. Acta Neurochir (Wien) 1978;43(1–2):51–9.

13. Auer LM, Ott E. Disturbances of the coagulatory system in patients with severe cerebral trauma II. Platelet function. Acta Neurochir (Wien) 1979;49:219–26.

14. Sawada Y, Sadamitsu D, Sakamoto T, Ikemura K, Yoshioka T, Sugimoto T. Lack of correlation between delayed traumatic intracerebral haematoma and disseminated intravascular coagulation. J Neurol Neurosurg Psychiatry 1984;47:1125–7.

15. Sorensen JV, Jensen HP, Rahr HB, Borris LC, Lassen MR, Fedders O, et al. Haemostatic activation in patients with head injury with and without simultaneous multiple trauma. Scand J Clin Lab Invest 1993;53:659–65.

16. May AK, Young JS, Butler K, Bassam D, Brady W. Coagulopathy in severe closed head injury: is empiric therapy warranted? Am Surg 1997;63:233–6.

17. Scherer RU, Spangenberg P. Procoagulant activity in patients with isolated severe head trauma. Crit Care Med 1998;26:149–56.

18. Jacoby RC, Owings JT, Holmes J, Battistella FD, Gosselin RC, Paglieroni TG. Platelet activation and function after trauma. J Trauma 2001;51:639–47.

19. Murshid WR, Gader AG. The coagulopathy in acute head injury: comparison of cerebral versus peripheral measurements of haemostatic activation markers. Br J Neurosurg 2002;16:362–9.

20. Goodnight SH, Kenoyer G, Rapaport SI, Patch MJ, Lee JA, Kurze T. Defibrination after brain-tissue destruction: A serious complication of head injury. N Engl J Med 1974;290:1043–7.

21. Vecht CJ, Minderhoud JM, Sibinga CT. Platelet aggregability in relation to impaired consciousness after head injury. J Clin Pathol 1975;28:814–20.

22. Vavilala MS, Dunbar PJ, Rivara FP, Lam AM. Coagulopathy predicts poor outcome following head injury in children less than 16 years of age. J Neurosurg Anesthesiol 2001;13:13–8.

23. Kaufman HH, Moake JL, Olson JD, Miner ME, duCret RP, Pruessner JL, Gildenberg PL.

Delayed and recurrent intracranial hematomas related to disseminated intravascular clotting and fibrinolysis in head injury. Neurosurgery 1980;7:445–9.

24. Stein SC, Smith DH. Coagulopathy in traumatic brain injury. Neurocrit Care 2004;1:479–88.

25. Astrup T. Assay and content of tissue thromboplastin in different organs. Thromb Diath Haemorrh 1965;14:401–16.

26. Keimowitz RM, Annis BL. Disseminated intravascular coagulation associated with massive brain injury. J Neurosurg 1973;39:178–80.

27. Fleck RA, Rao LV, Rapaport SI, Varki N. Localization of human tissue factor antigen by immunostaining with monospecific, polyclonal anti-human tissue factor antibody. Thromb Res 1990;59:421–37.

28. Gando S, Nanzaki S, Kemmotsu O. Coagulofibrinolytic changes after isolated head injury are not different from those in trauma patients without head injury. J Trauma 1999;46:1070–6; discussion 1076–7.

29. Pathak A, Dutta S, Marwaha N, Singh D, Varma N, Mathuriya SN. Change in tissue thromboplastin content of brain following trauma. Neurol India 2005;53:178–82.

30. Halpern CH, Reilly PM, Turtz AR, Stein SC. Traumatic coagulopathy: the effect of brain injury. J Neurotrauma 2008;25:997–1001.

31. Nemerson Y, Giesen PL. Some thoughts about localization and expression of tissue factor. Blood Coagul Fibrinolysis 1998;9(suppl 1):S45–47.

32. Dietrich WD, Alonso O, Busto R, et al. Widespread hemodynamic depression and focal platelet accumulation after fluid percussion brain injury: a double label autoradiographic study in rats. J Cereb Blood Flow Metab 1996;16:481–89.

33. Maeda T, Katayama Y, Kawamata T, Aoyama N, Mori T. Hemodynamic depression and microthrombosis in the peripheral areas of cortical contusion in the rat: role of platelet activating factor. Acta Neurochir (Suppl) 1997;70:102–5.

34. Kaufman HH, Hui KS, Mattson JC, et al. Clinicopathological correlations of disseminated intravascular coagulation in patients with head injury. Neurosurgery 1984;15:34–42.

35. Cortez SC, McIntosh TK, Noble LJ. Experimental fluid percussion brain injury: vascular disruption and neuronal and glial alterations. Brain Res 1989;482:271–82.

36. Dietrich WD, Alonso O, Halley M. Early microvascular and neuronal consequences of traumatic brain injury: a light and electron microscopic study in rats. J Neurotrauma 1994;11289–301.

37. Brohi K, Cohen MJ, Davenport RA. Acute coagulopathy of trauma: mechanism, identification and effect. Curr Opin Crit Care. 2007;13:680–85.

38. Cohen MJ, Brohi K, Ganter MT, Manley GT, Mackersie RC, Pittet JF. Early coagulopathy after traumatic brain injury: the role of hypoperfusion and the protein C pathway. J Trauma 2007;63:1254–61; discussion 1261–2.

39. Carrick MM, Tyroch AH, Youens CA, Handley T. Subsequent development of thrombocytopenia and coagulopathy in moderate and severe head injury: support for serial laboratory examination. J Trauma 2005;58:725–9; discussion 729–30.

40. Nekludov M, Bellander BM, Blomback M, Wallen HN. Platelet dysfunction in patients with severe traumatic brain injury. J Neurotrauma 2007;24:1699–706.

41. Schnuriger B, Inaba K, Abdelsayed GA, et al. The impact of platelets on the progression of traumatic intracranial hemorrhage. J Trauma 2010;68:881–5.

42. Takahashi H, Urano T, Takada Y, Nagai N, Takada A. Fibrinolytic parameters as an admission prognostic marker of head injury in patients who talk and deteriorate. J Neurosurg 1997;86:768–72.

43. Miner ME, Kaufman HH, Graham SH, Haar FH, Gildenberg PL. Disseminated intravascular coagulation fibrinolytic syndrome following head injury in children: frequency and prognostic implications. J Pediatr 1982;100:687–91.

44. Selladurai BM, Vickneswaran M, Duraisamy S, Atan M. Coagulopathy in acute head injury–a study of its role as a prognostic indicator. Br J Neurosurg 1997;11:398–404.

45. Salehpour F, BazzaziAM, Porhomayon J, Nader ND. Correlation between coagulopathy and outcome in severe head trauma in neurointensive care and trauma units. J Crit Care 2011;26:352–6.

46. Lustenberger T, Talving P, Kobayashi L, Inaba K, Lam L, Plurad D, Demetriades D. Time course of coagulopathy in isolated severe traumatic brain injury. Injury 2010;41:924–8.

47. Abrahams JM, Torchia MB, McGarvey M, Putt M, Baranov D, Sinson GP. Perioperative

assessment of coagulability in neurosurgical patients using thromboelastography. Surg Neurol 2002;58:5-11; discussion 11–2.

48. El Kady N, Khedr H, Yosry M, El Mekawi S. Perioperative assessment of coagulation in paediatric neurosurgical patients using thromboelastography. Eur J Anaesthesiol 2009;26:293–7.

49. Gonzalez E, Pieracci FM, Moore EE, Kashuk JL. Coagulation abnormalities in the trauma patient: the role of point-of-care thromboelastography. Semin Thromb Hemost 2010;36:723–37.

50. Park MS, Martini WZ, Dubick MA, et al. Thromboelastography as a better indicator of hypercoagulable state after injury than prothrombin time or activated partial thromboplastin time. J Trauma 2009;67:266–75; discussion 275–6.

51. Kashuk JL, Moore EE, Sabel A, et al. Rapid thrombelastography (r-TEG) identifies hyper-coagulability and predicts thromboembolic events in surgical patients. Surgery 2009;146: 764–72; discussion 772–4.

52. Plotkin AJ, Wade CE, Jenkins DH, et al. A reduction in clot formation rate and strength assessed by thromboelastography is indicative of transfusion requirements in patients with penetrating injuries. J Trauma 2008;64:S64–S68.

53. Winter JP, Plummer D, Bottini A, Rockswold GR, Ray D. Early fresh frozen plasma prophylaxis of abnormal coagulation parameters in the severely head injured patient is not effective. Ann Emerg Med 1989;18:553–5.

54. Etemadrezaie H, Baharvahdat H, Shariati Z, Lari SM, Shakeri MT, Ganjeifar B. The effect of fresh frozen plasma in severe closed head injury. ClinNeurolNeurosurg 2007;109:166–71.

55. Shakur H, Roberts R, Bautista R, et al. Effects of tranexamic acid on death, vascular occlusive events, and blood transfusion in trauma patients with significant haemorrhage (CRASH-2): a randomised, placebo-controlled trial. Lancet. 2010;376:23–32.

56. Mangano DT, Rieves RD, Weiss KD. Judging the safety of aprotinin. N Engl J Med 2006;355:2261–2.

57. Roitberg B, Emechebe-Kennedy O, Amin-Hanjani S, Mucksavage J, Tesoro E. Human recombinant factor VII for emergency reversal of coagulopathy in neurosurgical patients: a retrospective comparative study. Neurosurgery 2005;57:832-6; discussion 832–6.

58. Bartal C, Freedman J, Bowman K, Cusimano M. Coagulopathic patients with traumatic intra-cranial bleeding: defining the role of recombinant factor VIIa. J Trauma 2007;63:725–2.

59. Brown CV, Foulkrod KH, Lopez D, et al. Recombinant factor VIIa for the correction of coagulopathy before emergent craniotomy in blunt trauma patients. J Trauma 2010;68:348–52.

60. McQuay N Jr, Cipolla J, Franges EZ, Thompson GE. The use of recombinant activated factor VIIa in coagulopathic traumatic brain injuries requiring emergent craniotomy: is it beneficial? J Neurosurg 2009;111:666–71.

61. Stein DM, Dutton RP, Kramer ME, Handley C, Scalea TM. Recombinant factor VIIa: decreasing time to intervention in coagulopathic patients with severe traumatic brain injury. J Trauma 2008;64:620–7; discussion 627–8.

62. Stein DM, Dutton RP, Kramer ME, Scalea TM. Reversal of coagulopathy in critically ill patients with traumatic brain injury: recombinant factor VIIa is more cost-effective than plasma. J Trauma 2009;66:63–72; discussion 73–5.

63. Grenander A, Bredbacka S, Rydvall A, et al. Antithrombin treatment in patients with traumatic brain injury: a pilot study. J Neurosurg Anesthesiol 2001;13:49–56.

64. Shaffrey ME, Polin RS, Phillips CD, Germanson T, Shaffrey CI, Jane JA. Classification of civilian craniocerebral gunshot wounds: a multivariate analysis predictive of mortality. J Neurotrauma 1992;9:S279–85.

65. Kumura E, Sato M, Fukuda A, Takemoto Y, Tanaka S, Kohama A. Coagulation disorders following acute head injury. Acta Neurochir (Wien) 1987;85:23–8.

66. Polin RS, Shaffrey ME, Phillips CD, Germanson T, Jane JA. Multivariate analysis and prediction of outcome following penetrating head injury. Neurosurg Clin N Am 1995;6:689–99.

67. Engström M, Romner B, Schalén W, Reinstrup P. Thrombocytopenia predicts progressive hemorrhage after head trauma. J Neurotrauma 2005;22:291–6.

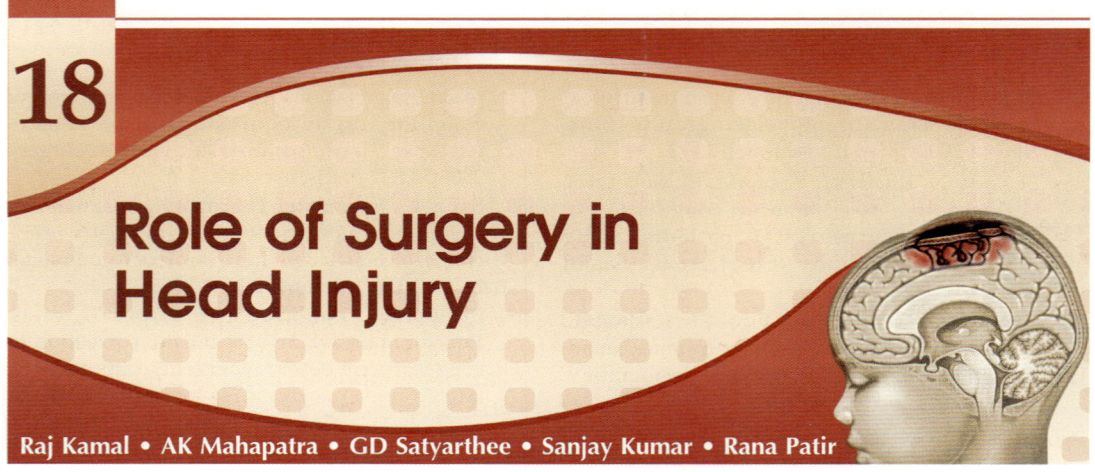

18

Role of Surgery in Head Injury

Raj Kamal • AK Mahapatra • GD Satyarthee • Sanjay Kumar • Rana Patir

INTRODUCTION

Mortality and morbidity due to head injury is high even with present neuro ICU care and monitoring. It is also correct that the majority deaths are due to intracranial hematoma, leading to intracranial hypertension, hypoperfusion and ischemia. However, in significant number of cases, death is preventable[1-6] if the diagnosis is made early and surgery is carried out timely. It is also right at this time to re-emphasize that head injury does not necessarily mean hematoma nor intracranial haematoma means surgery and more importantly, surgery does not mean cure. All these terminologies are not synonymous. Hence, there is a need for clear understanding, what is an intracranial hematoma? What are the indications for surgery? Having removed a hematoma, what is the expected outcome? Decisions regarding removal of hematomas, particularly contusions and intracerebral hematomas, may be difficult, especially so when surgery is prophylactic and intended to prevent deterioration. An uncontrolled increase in intracranial pressure (ICP) is a poor prognostic factor in closed head injuries. Studies have consistently reported a decrease in both survival and proportion of good outcomes in those patients whose increase in ICP could not be managed.[7-11] A poor prognosis is especially associated with an increase in ICP within the first 24 hours after injury[3] and secondary (3–10 days post-trauma) increases in ICP.[12,13] The causes of such ICP increases are numerous and not solely associated with the nature of the original injury (Table 18.1).[14, 15] To assess the use, benefits, and complications of decompressive craniectomy (DC) on ICP control and long-term outcome has been conducted. The RESCUEicp[16] and DECRA[17,18] trials are 2 multicenter investigations into the use of DC as a second-tier therapy for control of ICP following head injury. The DECRA study failed to show a clinical benefit with the use of early/neuroprotective decompressive

Table 18.1: Raised ICP following head injury and causes[14,15]

- Cerebral edema
- Hyperemia
- Mass lesion: epidural hematoma; subdural hematoma; hemorrhagic contusions; depressed skull fracture; foreign body
- Cerebral vasodilation
- Systemic hypertension
- Hydrocephalus
- Venous sinus thrombosis or any other obstruction
- Post-traumatic seizure activity (status epilepticus, subclinical seizures)
- Increased intrathoracic or intra-abdominal pressure, caused by mechanical ventilation, agitation, or abnormal motor posturing
- Hyperthermia or febrile states
- Lightening from coma with inadequate sedation

craniectomy following diffuse TBI, whereas trial of RESCUEicp is still going on.

Another trial, surgical trial in traumatic intra-cerebral hemorrhage [STITCH (Trauma)][19,20] is going on to determine whether a policy of early surgery in patients with TICH [traumatic intracerebral hemorrhage] improves outcome compared to a policy of initial conservative treatment. The details of these studies will be discussed in this chapter.

INDICATIONS FOR SURGERY IN HEAD INJURY (Table 18.2)

Basically, aims of the surgery in acute head injury are probably two:

a. First one is to remove a sizable intracranial hematoma producing mass effect, raised pressure and removal of hematoma is to

reduce the intracranial pressure[21,22] (Figs 18.1a and b, 18.2a and 18.3a).

b. The second aim is to operated open compound head injury to prevent CSF leak and meningitis[6,23] (Figs 18.4a and b). Thus the indications for definite surgery in acute head injuries are given in Tables 18.2 and 18.3. Surgery is also required for placing external ventricular drain/intraparenchymal catheter/subdural bolt for the purpose of ICP monitoring or CSF drainage.[24]

Brain trauma foundation[25] recommends ICP monitoring in

1. All patients with severe TBI (GCS between 3–8 after resuscitation) and an abnormal CT scan that reveals hematomas, contusions, swelling, herniation or compressed cisterns. (Level II recommendation). (Table 13.5 from Chapter 13).

2. Patients with severe TBI with normal CT scan if two or more features are noted at

Table 18.2: Indications for surgery in head injury

A. In acute head injury
  1. Large intracranial hematoma producing mass effect and raised ICP (Figs 18.1a and b, 18.2a, 18.3a)
     - Patient is not improving
     - Patient is deteriorating
     - Patient having shown improvement then deteriorating
  2. Compound head injury (Fig. 18.4)
     - Scalp laceration with compound communated fracture with CSF leak or CSF leak and oozing of brain tissue
     - Surgery for foreign body; bullet, splinters, knife, spear or sword, penetrating woodpiece, broken pencil or pen
     - Profuse CSF rhinorrhea or otorrhea not controlled on conservative management in 2–3 weeks time
  3. Surgery for ICP monitoring
     For ICP monitoring indications are given above
B. Surgery in chronic head injury
  Chronic SDH
  Subdural effusion
  Post-traumatic hydrocephalus
  CSF fistulae
  Cranial defect or growing skull fracture
  Hydrocephalus
  Osteomyelitis, brain abscess

Table 18.3: Mass lesions requiring expedient surgical removal[26]

- *Acute extradural hematoma:* Volume > 30 cm³ as measured on CT scan
- *Acute subdural hematoma:* thickness > 10 mm or midline shift > 5 mm as measured on CT scan
- *Acute subdural hematoma:* Thickness < 10 mm or midline shift < 5 mm but GCS score < 9, which decreased by ≥ 2 points between injury and admission and/or presenting with fixed dilated pupils and/or ICP > 20 mm Hg
- *Intraparenchymal lesion:* CT evidence of mass effect or increased ICP refractory to medical treatment or progressive neurological deterioration referable to lesion
- *Frontal/temporal contusion:* Volume > 50 cm³ as measured on CT scan or GCS score 6–8 and volume > 20 cm³ and midline shift > 5 mm/compression of cisterns
- *Posterior fossa lesion:* Mass effect on CT or neurological deterioration or deterioration referable to lesion
- Lesions not fulfilling these criteria may be conservatively managed along with serial imaging and close monitoring

CT: computed tomography; GCS: Glasgow Coma Scale; ICP: intracranial pressure

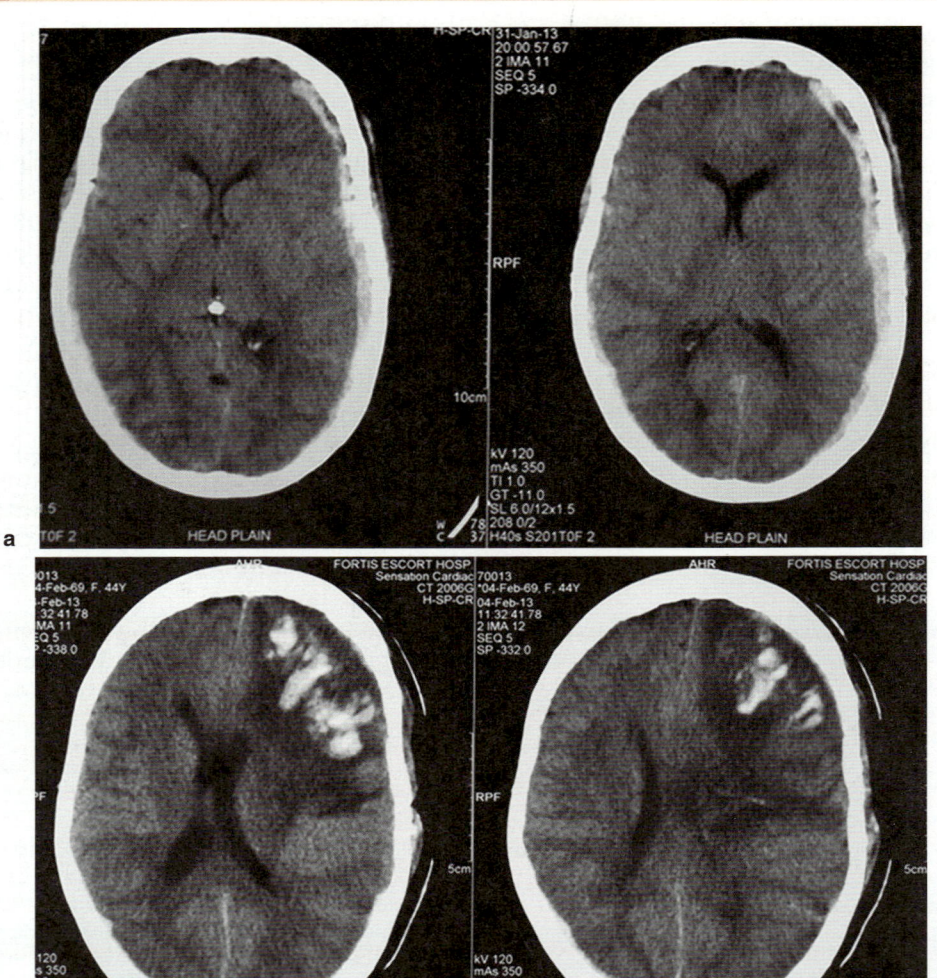

Figs 18.1a and b: CT head showing thin acute SDH (a) later on developed left frontal contusion requiring surgery (b)

admission: Age over 40 years, unilateral or bilateral motor posturing or systolic BP < 90 mm of Hg (Level III recommendation).

Surgery for Intracranial Hematomas

Large intracranial hematomas produce significant mass effect and raised ICP. The patients with severe intracranial hypertension are mostly comatose and do not show signs of clinical improvement.[23,26–29] Not infrequently, patients following initial coma improved and have a varying period of lucid interval.[3,30] During this period patients fully or partially improve in their conscious state and give a false impression that they are normal. These patients subsequently deteriorate in neuro- logical status and may die if the hematoma is not evacuated timely and adequately. Thus, there are several situations:

a. Patients of head injury in coma from the time of injury and not showing signs of improvement.

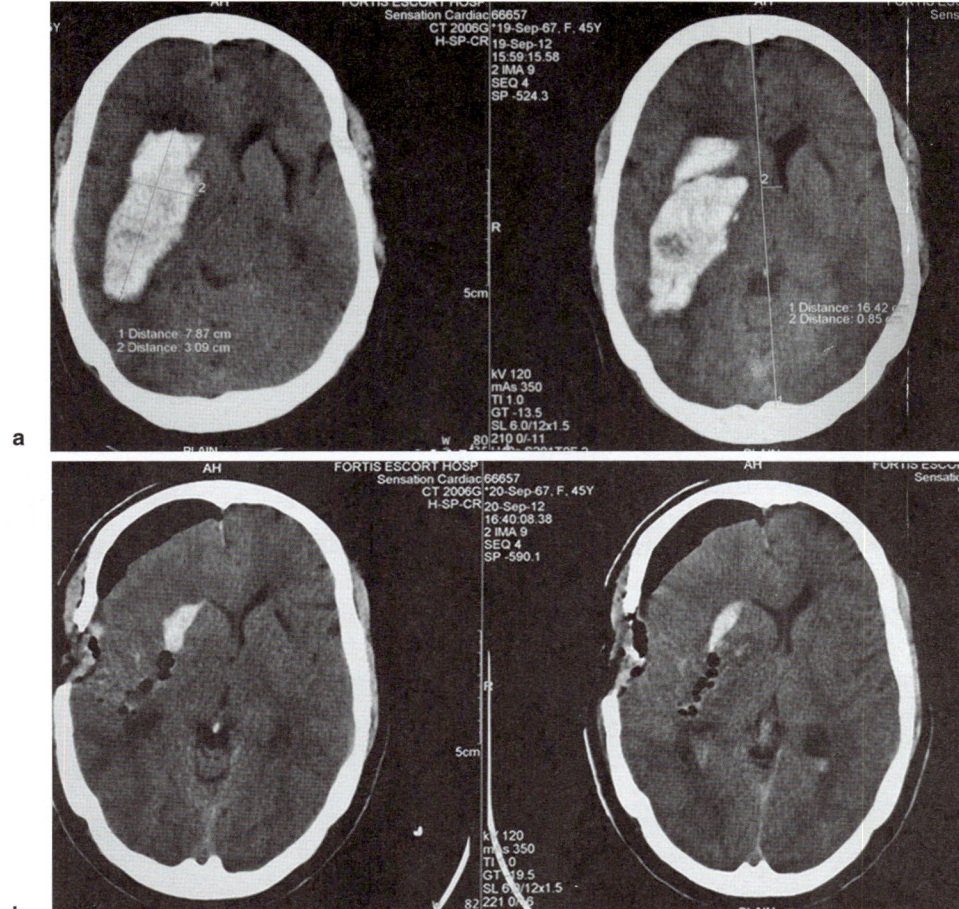

Figs 18.2a and b: Pre- and postoperative CT scan showing good evacuation. Patients survived with good outcome score

b. Patients of head injury in coma from the time of injury but the level of coma is deteriorating, for example, motor scale 5 deteriorated to 3 or 4 (GCS from 6 or 7 deteriorated to scale 5, 4 or 3)

c. Patients with classical lucid interval, during which they are completely or partially lucid.[3,29,30] This means, patients following initial coma improved in conscious state, subsequently deteriorated again.

As an intracranial hematoma keeps on increasing in size, the conscious state goes on deteriorating (Figs 18.1a and b). The deterioration is unpredictable, can be slow or rapid.

These types of patients are the maximum priority group for surgery. Because, quick evacuation of hematoma is likely to result in good outcome. **One must also remember that the surgery becomes futile if the evacuation of hematoma is significantly delayed**[30,31] **during which patients may deteriorate to either GCS 3 or brain death. It indirectly means severe deterioration might have resulted in irreversible brain damage.**

On the other hand, some percentage of patients with intracranial hematomas are well, may be even conscious and oriented. This, happens more frequently in young children

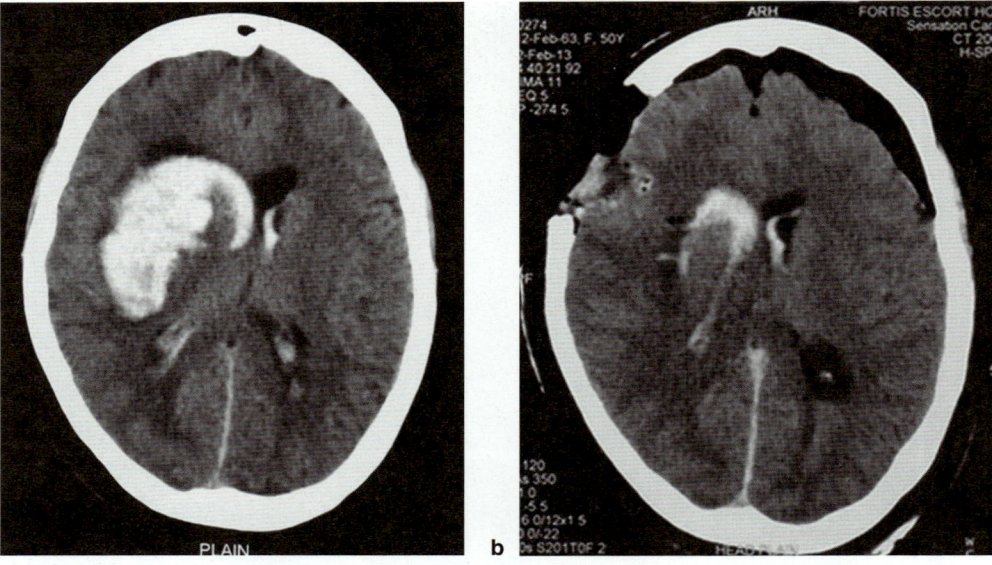

Figs 18.3a and b: Role of good surgical evacuation; pre- and postoperative CT scan showing good evacuation of traumatic basal ganglia hemorrhage

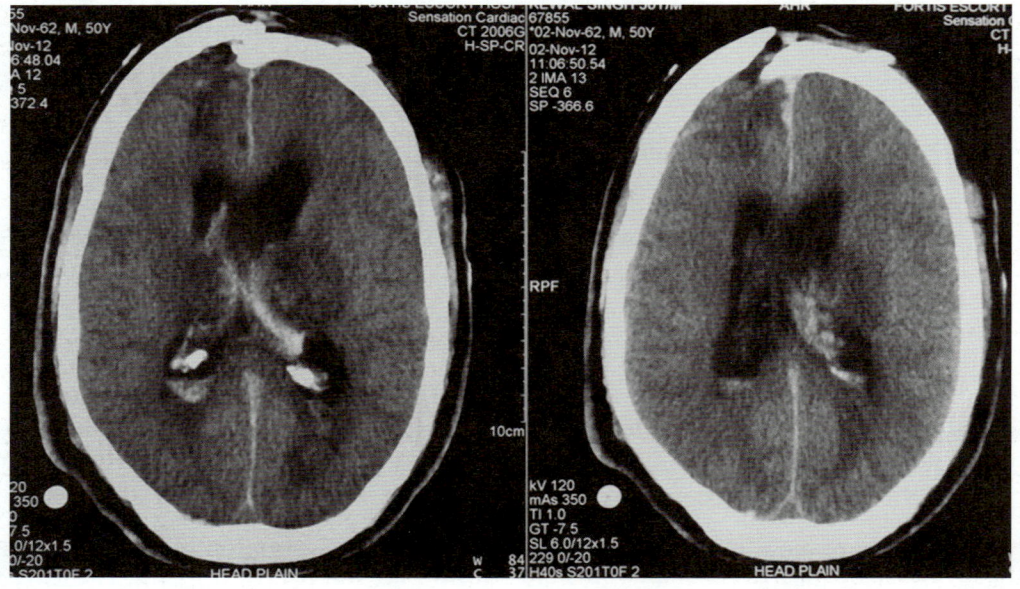

Figs 18.4a and b: Compound head injury requiring surgery

and elderly, in whom a large hematoma in brain can be accommodated without manifesting signs of raised ICP.[32,33] No doubt, these patients need close observation and may require ICP monitoring depending on the case. Close watch, repeat CT and clinical monitoring can avoid unnecessary surgery (Table 18.4). Recently, large number of papers

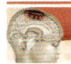

have been published, reporting conservative treatment of intracranial hematomas.[34–36]

Surgery in intracranial hematoma is aimed to reduce raised ICP. While it is possible to totally remove an extradural hematoma and acute subdural hematoma, it may not be always possible to remove entire contusion or large intracerebral hematoma. Hence, the aim of surgery is to remove as much as possible, to achieve a significant lowering of ICP. At operation, one can adjudge adequate removal by a lax and pulsating brain. After the evacuation of hematoma in temporal lobe, one must incise the tentorial edge to relieve the transtentorial herniation.

INDICATIONS FOR REOPERATION OR SECOND SURGERY

Indications for reoperation are many (Table 18.5). Firstly, while removing contusion or intracerebral hematoma at the first operation, it is difficult to be sure about the amount of contusion/hematoma left. Surgeon stops when he feels adequate amount of pathological lesion is removed to provide significant reduction in raised ICP. However, it is not unusual to see in repeat CT, the residual haematoma increased in size and producing significant mass effect. In such a situation if the ICP is high or patient not showing satisfactory improvement, a reoperation must be undertaken to remove the residual pathology to reduce raised ICP.

Secondly, reaccumulation of hematoma may be possible, which does not allow the patient to improve or ICP to normalise. There are two reasons for reaccumulation of hematoma.

a. Inadequate or improper hemostasis during 1st surgery,

b. Bleeding abnormality resulting from severe head injury or due to excessive blood loss during first surgery. Hence, in such a situation, before 2nd surgery, careful hematological evaluation is necessary, and if warranted fresh blood, platelet or fresh frozen plasma should be infused prior to second surgery and during surgery.

Also, it is well known and repeatedly reported that a small hematoma elsewhere in the brain, may increase in size after removal of a large hematoma (Figs 18.1a to c). It is also possible to have a fresh hematoma at a distant site to the first operation (Figs 18.2a and b). The chance is more if the first operation is performed within 6 hours of injury, and CT scan is performed even earlier, when second hematoma was not formed.[37,38]

Surgery for Compound Head Injury

There are various types of compound head injuries.

1. *Open compound head injury:* It may be due to blunt injury or penetrating injury like bullet, splinter injury[39,40] or injury due to sharp weapons. The aim of surgery in such

Table 18.4: Conservative management of intracranial hematoma
A. Patients with good GCS (mostly small children or elderly)   Showing progressive   Improvement   Static with normal coma score
B. Patients with hematoma with poor GCS   ICP shows normal pressure
C. Multiple small contusion or hematoma   None of them individually producing mass effect
D. Patients with hematoma in brain death impending brain death

Table 18.5: Indications for reoperation
A. Operation for same hematoma   • Recollection of hematoma   • Inadequate evacuation and patient not showing improvement, CT showing significant clot   • ICP remaining high postoperative
B. Following removal of one hematoma   • Patient may develop a new hematoma which is large   • Smaller hematoma increased in size following evacuation of larger one   • Infected wound or bone flap
Postoperative abscess.

situations, is to convert an open injury to a close system by debriding the scalp, removing the bone fragments and damaged brain.[41] Sometimes, bone pieces are embedded in the damage brain tissue, which should also be removed. In bullet or splinter injury, the metallic foreign bodies should be removed. Adequate debridement and dura closure can prevent CSF leak and meningitis, to a great extent.[41] However, controversies exist when patients with compound injury come after 24 hours. Generally it is believed that a wound is infected after 24 hours. When a patient comes after 24 hours he might already have wound infection or meningitis. Hence, antibiotics in antimeningitic dosage must be administered intravenously and observed.

2. *Closed compound injury:* These are the patients in whom there is no scalp laceration nor oozing brain tissue or CSF leak. The compound injury is because of CSF leak though paranasal sinuses or mastoid. The fracture of skull base also allow air entering into the cranial cavity, thus make it a closed compound head injury. When there is continuous CSF leak, there is chance of meningitis.[41] Frequently, CSF rhinorrhea or otorrhea stops in few days time, following injury. However, in small number of cases CSF leak may continue even after 2 weeks of conservative treatment. When CSF rhinorrhea or otorrhea persists, there is need for an operation to repair the dural defect in anterior cranial fossa floor, which is most frequent site for post-traumatic CSF rhinorrhea. In 90–95% cases CSF leak stops following surgery.

Role of Evacuation of Hematoma/ Decompressive Craniectomy

An intracranial hematoma which is causing significant mass effect should be removed as soon as possible. Intracranial mass requiring expedient surgical removal is given in Table 18.3.

Surgical trial in traumatic intracerebral hemorrhage [STITCH (Trauma)][19,20] is going on to determine whether a policy of early surgery in patients with TICH (traumatic intracerebral hemorrhage) improves outcome compared to a policy of initial conservative treatment. Intracranial hemorrhage occurs in over 60% of severe head injuries in one of three types: extradural (EDH); subdural (SDH); and intraparenchymal (TICH). Prompt surgical removal of significant SDH and EDH is established and widely accepted. However, TICH is more common and is found in more than 40% of severe head injuries. It is associated with a worse outcome but the role for surgical removal remains undefined. Surgical practice in the treatment of TICHs differs widely around the world. The aim of early surgery in TICH removal is to prevent secondary brain injury. Trial will include a health economics component and carry out a subgroup analysis of patients undergoing invasive monitoring. There have been trials of surgery for spontaneous ICH (including the STITCH II trial[20, 43, 44]), but none so far of surgery for TICH.

This is an international multicenter pragmatic randomized controlled trial. Patients are eligible if: they are within 48 h of injury; they have evidence of TICH on CT scan with a confluent volume of attenuation significantly raised above that of the background white and grey matter that has a total volume > 10 ml; and their treating neurosurgeon is in equipoise.

Patients will be ineligible if they have: a significant surface hematoma (EDH or SDH) requiring surgery; a hemorrhage/contusion located in the cerebellum; three or more separate hematomas fulfilling inclusion criteria; or severe pre-existing physical or mental disability or severe co-morbidity which would lead to poor outcome even if the patient made a full recovery from the head injury.

Decompressive craniectomy has been found to be useful, if done early (Figs 18.5a to d).

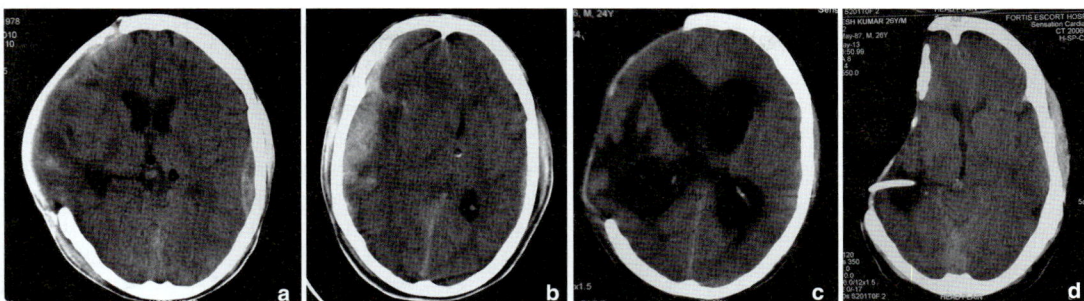

Figs 18.5a to d: Role of surgery: (a) Preoperative; (b) postoperative CT scan following decompressive craniectomy. Midline shift is better and ventricles and sulci have opened up; (c) CT showing development of severe ventriculomegaly; (d) CT following VP shunt

Severe refractory intracranial hypertension in absence of focal intracranial pathology still remains a challenging situation. Craniectomy conducted in the past for severe brain swelling was proven to be useless.

Brain trauma foundation guidelines[25] recommended timely evacuation of mass lesions (Table 18.2), however, decompressive craniectomy is cautiously recommended as a possible option in selected patients.

Timofeev et al supported the theory that decompressive craniectomy leads to sustained reduction in ICP and improved cerebral pressure-volume compensation. He concluded that following decompressive craniectomy, adequate CPP levels can be achieved at lower MAP levels. This may reduce the load on the cardiovascular system and the risks associated with aggressive CPP augmentation. Nevertheless, concurrent derangement in cerebrovascular pressure reactivity also occurred in most patients. There are at present two prospective randomised controlled trials aimed at providing Class I evidence on the role of DC in the treatment of intracranial hypertension following severe TBI.

From 2002 to 2004, two multicentre randomized trials (Table 18.6) started to assess decompressive craniectomy (DC) following TBI,: the DECRA trial and the RESCUEicp trial. The decompressive craniectomy (DECRA) trial was a multicentre prospective randomised trial designed to evaluate the effect of early DC on neurological function in patients with severe TBI. It is based on the theory that early DC can improve long-term neurological outcome in patients with severe TBI and intracranial hypertension which is refractory to conventional management.[17] Randomised evaluation of surgery with craniectomy for uncontrollable elevation of ICP (RESCUEicp)[16,44] is another prospective, randomised international multicentre trial aimed at providing Class I evidence as to whether DC is effective

Table 18.6: The hypotheses and result of two trials	
DECRA Cooper et al[17]	RESCUEicp[16,53]
Early/neuroprotective bifrontal DC can improve outcomes following diffuse TBI	Decompressive craniectomy can improve outcomes as a last-tier therapy for refractory post-traumatic intracranial hypertension
Result: The DECRA study failed to show a clinical benefit with the use of early/neuroprotective decompressive craniectomy following diffuse TBI	Result still awaited The study is ongoing and has now recruited more than 85% of the required sample size. The required sample size is 400 patients have been recruited from more than 40 units in 17 different countries

for the management of patients with refractory intracranial hypertension following TBI as compared with medical management alone.

Cooper et al,[17] for the DECRA trial concluded that, in patients with severe diffuse traumatic brain injury and increased intracranial pressure that was refractory to first-tier therapies, the use of craniectomy, as compared with standard care, decreased the mean intracranial pressure and the duration of both ventilatory support and the ICU stay but was associated with a significantly worse outcome at 6 months, as measured by the score on the extended Glasgow Outcome Scale.

Among adults with severe diffuse traumatic brain injury and refractory intracranial hypertension in the ICU, Cooper et al found that decompressive craniectomy decreased intracranial pressure, the duration of mechanical ventilation, and the time in the ICU, as compared with standard care. In the craniectomy group, the duration of the hospital stay was unchanged, and the rate of surgical complications was low. However, patients in the craniectomy group had a lower median score on the extended Glasgow Outcome Scale and a higher risk of an unfavorable outcome (as assessed on that scale) than patients receiving standard care.

Their findings were contrary to the initial hypothesis that in patients with severe traumatic brain injury, decompressive craniectomy would decrease intracranial pressure, improve functional outcomes, and decrease the proportion of survivors with severe disability. Despite the positive clinical signs in the ICU, decompressive craniectomy instead increased the likelihood of a poor outcome. They concluded that it is unlikely that findings were due to an increased rate of survival of severely injured patients in a vegetative state (grade 2 on the extended Glasgow Outcome Scale), because even though the number of such patients increased after craniectomy, the rates of death were similar in the two study groups. Decom-

pressive craniectomy instead shifted survivors from a favorable outcome to an unfavorable outcome (i.e. dependence on assistance to complete activities of daily living). One possible explanation is that craniectomy allowed expansion of the swollen brain outside the skull and caused axonal stretch[18,45] which *in vitro* causes neural injury.[46–48] Alterations in cerebral blood flow and metabolism may also be relevant.[42]

Another possible explanation for the inferior outcomes with craniectomy concerns the characteristics of the surgical procedure. Some surgeons prefer a unilateral procedure, with studies (in retrospective, nonrandomized series with mixed causes of brain injury) suggesting that the bilateral approach may have more complications.[10,49,50] Some surgeons divide the sagittal sinus and falx cerebri, which is a component of the original Polin procedure,[49] but others do not. Complications are possible with both alternatives (Fig. 18.5c). Craniectomy or cranioplasty may also have had other harmful complications, including hydrocephalus (Table 18.7).[50–52]

In conclusion, in patients with severe diffuse traumatic brain injury and increased intracranial pressure that was refractory to first-tier therapies, the use of craniectomy, as compared with standard care, decreased the mean intracranial pressure and the duration of both ventilatory support and the ICU stay but was associated with a significantly worse outcome at 6 months, as measured by the score on the extended Glasgow Outcome Scale.

In general, with better understanding of CPP and availability of very good imaging facilities there is insurgence of interest in decompressive craniotomy.[17,51] It is generally believed that such type of surgery may save life but increase the number of vegetative or severely disable.

RESCUEicp trial[16,53] (randomised evaluation of surgery with craniectomy for uncontrollable elevation of ICP) is an international multicentre randomised trial comparing decompressive

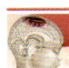

craniectomy with optimal medical management (including barbiturate therapy). Inclusion criteria are: TBI, age 10 to 65, ICP (> 25 mm Hg for 1 to 12 hours, refractory to first-line treatment). Exclusion criteria are: treatment with barbiturates prerandomisation, primary decompression (during evacuation of mass lesion), bilateral fixed and dilated pupils, bleeding diathesis, devastating injury unlikely to survive > 24 hours. In this study, patients are managed on ICUs using a standard protocol. The major objective of this protocol is to maintain ICP < 25 mm Hg by applying treatment measures in a number of stages. The total number of patients will be 400 (200 in each arm of the study) for a 15% difference in outcome (power = 80%, P = 0.05). The primary outcome measure was extended Glasgow Outcome Score at 6 months. Over 280 patients have been recruited to date from more than 40 centres in 17 countries. The follow-up rate at 6 months is 96%. To date, evaluation of the first 182 patients shows equal distribution of characteristics between the two arms, i.e. DC and medical management.

CONCLUSIONS

Prompt and adequate evacuation of haematoma are key points in surgery and overall outcome.

Uncontrolled ICP is associated with higher mortality, morbidity, and worse long-term outcomes after TBI. The importance of CPP as a treatment target should not be neglected in treatment. Two surgical interventions, in addition to primary evacuation of mass lesions, are principally used: ventricular catheterization and DC. The debates about the efficacy of DC is going on. The DECRA study failed to show a clinical benefit in this aspect. It is hoped that the findings of the RESCUEicp trial will clarify the role of this operation in patients with TBI.

Surgery in head injury is required in small percentage of patients. The aim of the surgery is to remove intracranial haematoma to reduce raised ICP or to operate open compound injury to prevent CSF leak and meningitis. Rarely, reoperation is also indicated if the residual hematoma is significant or a sizeable hematoma is encountered elsewhere.

Table 18.7: Complications following decompressive craniectomy[50–52]

Subdural hygroma (16–50%)

Progression of hemorrhage/contusion (5–58%)

Intracranial infection (2–6%)

Contralateral SDH/EDH (6–28%)

Hydrocephalus (2–29%)

Herniation through skull defect (26% in 1 case study defining herniation as brain tissue in the center of the defect 1.5 cm above plane of normal outer table of skull[83])

Syndrome of the trephined: a late complication consisting of headaches, confusion, dizziness, memory difficulties, mood disturbances, and sometimes motor disturbances, consisting of progressive contralateral upper limb weakness not previously affected by injury (10 of 38 patients in 1 case series[84]). In many cases, this syndrome can be reversed by cranioplasty; all patients developing motor symptoms in the case series experienced full and rapid motor recovery within days of their cranioplasty

Paradoxical herniation has been reported as occurring as a result of lumbar puncture after large decompressive craniectomy[85,86]

Complications of subsequent cranioplasty

Bone flap resorption/sinking after cranioplasty (1.6–12%)

Infection (11.3%)

Status epilepticus (1.6%): Note that seizures after neurosurgical procedures are a well-recognized occurrence

REFERENCES

1. Rose J, Valtonen S, Jennett B. Avoidable factors contributing to death after head injury. Br Med J 1977;2:615–18.
2. Kohi YM, Mendelow AD, Teasdale GM, et al. Extracranial insults and outcome in patients with acute head injury-relationship to GCS. Injury, 1984;16:25–6.
3. Mahapatra AK. Lucid interval in fatal head injury. Ind J Surg, 1991.
4. Campbell S, Watkin G, Kreis D. Preventable death in a self-designated trauma system. Am Surg 1989;55:478–80.

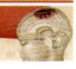

5. Wilson D, MC Elligott Fielding L. Identification of preventable trauma death. Confounded inquiries? J Trauma 1992;32:45–51.

6. Mahapatra AK. Management of Head injury. Neurosciences Today 1997;1:197–204.

7. Miller JD, Butterworth JF, Gudeman SK, Faulkner JE, Choi SC, Selhorst JB, Harbison JW, Lutz HA, Young HF, Becker DP. Further experience in the management of severe head injury. J Neurosurg 1981;54:289–99.

8. Marshall LF, Smith RW, Shapiro HM. The outcome with aggressive treatment in severe head injuries. Part I: The significance of intracranial pressure monitoring. J Neurosurg 1979;50:20–5.

9. Juul N, Morris GF, Marshall SB, Marshall LF. Intracranial hypertension and cerebral perfusion pressure: influence on neurological deterioration and outcome in severe head injury. J Neurosurg 2000;92:1–6.

10. Jiang JY, Gao GY, Li WP, Yu MK, Zhu C. Early indicators of prognosis in 846 cases of severe traumatic brain injury. J Neurotrauma 2002;19:869–74.

11. Treggiari MM, Schutz N, Yanez ND, Romand JA. Role of intracranial pressure values and patterns in predicting outcome in traumatic brain injury: a systematic review. Neurocrit Care 2007;6:104–12.

12. Unterberg A, Kiening K, Schmiedek P, Lanksch W. Long-term observations of intracranial pressure after severe head injury. The phenomenon of secondary rise of intracranial pressure. Neurosurgery 1993;32:17–24.

13. Stocchetti N, Colombo A, Ortolano F, Videtta W, Marchesi R, Longhi L, Zanier ER. Time course of intracranial hypertension after traumatic brain injury. J Neurotrauma 2007,24(8):1339–46.

14. Rangel-Castillo L, Gopinath S, Robertson CS. Management of intracranial hypertension. Neurol Clin 2008;26:521–41.

15. Badri S, Chen J, Barber J, Temkin NR, Dikmen SS, Chestnut RM, et al. Mortality and long term functional outcome associated with ICP after TBI, Intensive Care Med 2012; 38(11):1800–9.

16. PJ, Kolias AG, Timofeev I, E Corteen E, Czosnyka M, DK Menon DK, Pickard JD, and Kirkpatrick PJ; Update on the RESCUEicp decompressive craniectomy trial; Crit Care 2011; 15(Suppl 1): 312.

17. Cooper DJ, Rosenfeld JV, Murray L, Arabi YM, Davies AR, D'Urso, Kossmann T, Ponsford J, Seppelt I, Reilly P, Wolfe R, for the DECRA Trial Investigators and the Australian and New Zealand Intensive Care Society Clinical Trials Group; N Engl J Med 2011;364:1493–502.

18. Cooper PR, Hagler H, Clark WK, Barnett P. Enhancement of experimental cerebral edema after decompressive craniectomy: implications for the management of severe head injuries. Neurosurgery 1979;4:296–300.

19. Gregson BA, Rowan EN, Patrick M Mitchell, Unterberg A, McColl EM, Iain R Chambers, Paul McNamee, Mendelow AD. Surgical trial in traumatic intracerebral hemorrhage [STITCH (Trauma)]: study protocol for a randomized controlled trial. Trials 2012;13:193. Published online 2012.

20. Mendelow AD, Gregson BA, Mitchell PM, Murray GD, Rowan EN, Gholkar AR, STICH II Investigators. Trials. 2011. Surgical trial in lobar intracerebral haemorrhage (STICH II) protocol.

21. Miller JD, Becker DP, Ward JD, et al. Significance of intracranial hypertension in severe head injury. J Neurosurg 1977;47:503–76.

22. Marshall LF, Gautille T, Klauber MR, et al. Outcome of severe closed head injury. J Neurosurg 1991;75:528–36.

23. Mahapatra AK. Current management of head injury. Asian Arch Anae Rescu 1996;25:1–10.

24. Ghajar JB, Hariri RJ, Patterson RH. Improved outcome from traumatic coma using only venticular CSF drainage for ICP control (Class III) Adv Neurosurg 1993;21:173–7.

25. Brain Trauma Foundation; American Association of Neurological Surgeons; Congress of Neurological Surgeons; Joint Section on Neurotrauma and Critical Care, AANS/CNS, Bratton SL, Chestnut RM, Ghajar J, McConnell Hammond FF, Harris OA, Hartl R, Manley GT, Nemecek A, Newell DW, Rosenthal G, Schouten J, Shutter L, Timmons SD, Ullman JS, Videtta W, WilbergerJE, Wright DW. Guidelines for the management of severe traumatic brain injury. VIII. Intracranial pressure thresholds. J Neurotrauma 2008;24:S55–8.

26. Bullock MR, Chesnut R, Ghajar J, Gordon D, Hartl R, Newell DW, Servadei F, Walters BC, Wilberger JE. Guideline for the surgical management of traumatic brain injury. Neurosurgery 2006;58 (suppl 3).

27. Mahapatra AK, Tandon PN, Bhatia R, Banerji AK. Bilateral decerebration in head injury. Surg Neurol 1985;23:436–9.

28. Gentleman D, Nath F, MaCpherson P. Diagnosis and management of delayed traumatic intracerebral haematoma. Brit J Neurosurg 1989;3:367–72.

29. Jennett B, Teasdale G, Galbraith S, et al. Severe head injury in three countries. J Neurol Neurosurg Psychiat 1977;40:291–95.

30. Marshall LF, Toole B, Bower S. The National Traumatic coma Data Bank. Part II. Patient who talk and deteriorate. Implication for treatment. J Neurosurg 1983;59:285.

31. Reilly PL, Adams JH, Graham DI, Jennett B. Patients with head injury who talk and die. Lancet 1975;2:375–77.

32. Choux M, Grisoli F, Peragut JC. Extradural haematomas in children. Child's Brain, 1975; 1:337.

33. Choux M, Lena G, Geniton L. Intracranial haematoma. In Raimondi AJ (ed): Head injury in Newborn and Infants. Springer-Verlag, New York 1986:203.

34. Bullock R, Smith RM, van Dellen JR. Non-operative management of extradural haematoma. Neurosurgery 1985;16:602–6.

35. Pozzati E, Togmetti F. Spontaneous healing of acute extradural haematomas: A study of twenty-two cases. Neurosurgery, 1986;18:696–700.

36. Knuckey NW, Gelbard S, Epstein MH. The management of "asymptomatic epidural haematomas". A prospective study. J Neurosurg, 1989;70:392–96.

37. Werner A. Diagnostic technique. In: NIMS. Basic and Clinical Approaches—Head injury Clinical Management and Research. E Frost (ed) AIREN, Geneva, Switzerland 1990; 2:151–9.

38. Yague LG, et al. Contralateral extradural haematoma following craniotomy for traumatic intracranial lesion. Case report. J Neurosurg Sci 1991;35:107–9.

39. Carey ME, Young HF, Mathis JD. The neuro-surgical treatment of craniocerebral missile wound in Vietnam. Surg Gynaecol Obstet 1972;13:386.

40. Carey ME, Sarna GG, Farrell JB, et al. Experimental missile wound to brain. J Neurosurg 1989;71:754.

41. Carey ME. Therapeutic Management. In: NINS Head injury Clinical Management and Research. E Forst (ed) AIREN, Geneva, Switzerland, 1990;2:171–6.

42. Timofeev I, Czosnyka M, Nortje J, et al. Effect of decompressive craniectomy on intracranial pressure and cerebrospinal compensation following traumatic brain injury. J Neurosurg 2008;108:66–73.

43. Mendelow AD, Gregson BA, Fernandes HM, Murray GD, Teasdale GM, Hope DT, Karimi A, Shaw MD, Barer DH. STICH investigators. Early surgery versus initial conservative treatment in patients with spontaneous supratentorial intracerebral haematomas in the International Surgical Trial in Intracerebral Haemorrhage (STICH): a randomised trial. Lancet 2005 Jan 29 to Feb 4; 365(9457):387–97.

44. Gregson BA, Murray GD, Mitchell PM, Rowan EN, Gholkar AR, Mendelow AD. Trials. Update on the Surgical Trial in Lobar Intracerebral Haemorrhage (STICH II): statistical analysis plan 2012 Nov 21; 13:222. Epub 2012 Nov 21.

45. Stiver SI. Complications of decompressive craniectomy for traumatic brain injury. Neurosurg Focus 2009;26:E7-E7.

46. Chung RS, Staal JA, McCormack GH, et al. Mild axonal stretch injury in vitro induces a progressive series of neurofilament alterations ultimately leading to delayed axotomy. J Neurotrauma 2005;22:1081–91.

47. Staal JA, Dickson TC, Gasperini R, Liu Y, Foa L, Vickers JC. Initial calcium release from intracellular stores followed by calcium dysregulation is linked to secondary axotomy following transient axonal stretch injury. J Neurochem 2010;112:1147–55.

48. Tang-Schomer MD, Patel AR, Baas PW, Smith DH. Mechanical breaking of microtubules in axons during dynamic stretch injury underlies delayed elasticity, microtubule disassembly, and axon degeneration. FASEB J 2010;24:1401–10.

49. Polin RS, Shaffrey ME, Bogaev CA, et al. Decompressive bifrontal craniectomy in the treatment of severe refractory posttraumatic cerebral edema. Neurosurgery 1997;41:84–92.

50. Gooch MR, Gin GE, Kenning TJ, German JW. Complications of cranioplasty following decompressive craniectomy: analysis of 62 cases. Neurosurg Focus 2009;26:E9-E9.

51. Aarabi B, Hesdorffer DC, Ahn ES, Aresco C, Scalea TM, Eisenberg HM. Outcome following decompressive craniectomy for malignant swelling due to head injury. J Neurosurg 2006; 104:469–79.

52. Yang XF, Wen L, Shen F, Li G, Lou R, Liu WG, Zhan RY. Surgical complications secondary to decompressive craniectomy in patients with a head injury: a series of 108 consecutive cases. Acta Neurochir (Wien) 2008;150:1241–8.

53. RESCUEicp Study. http://www.rescueicp.com.

19

The Role of Stereotactic Surgery in Head Injury

RR Sharma • SJ Pawar • RV Devadas • SD Lal

INTRODUCTION

Even in the current era of minimally invasive neurosurgery, majority of post-traumatic intracranial lesions are routinely managed with conventional neurosurgical procedures. Despite many limitations in conventional neurosurgical approaches, they remain preferred methods of managing acute post-traumatic intracranial mass lesions in many neurosurgical institutions around the globe.

Their familiarity and immediate availability overshadow their limitations. During such undertakings neurosurgeons are not infrequently faced with the task of attempting to reconstruct sequential two dimensional CT or MR images into a three dimensional 'mental image' of intracranial surgical targets. Not so in large post-traumatic lesions in the superficial intracranial sites; but determining the exact cranial site of entry, and cerebral trajectory to reach the deeper subcortical or basal ganglionic or brain stem lesions may be frustrating. In such situations, the neurosurgeons consider exploration when planning osteoplastic craniotomy flaps and can find themselves searching for the post-traumatic lesion during the brainsurgery. More brain destruction/manipulation, though preventable by stereotactic neurosurgical procedures is largely inevitable in such circumstances. It is therefore increasingly realized that the intraparenchymal cerebral manipulations be minimized and be guided.[1,2]

GENERAL CONSIDERATIONS

In this modern era of microstereotactic neurosurgery, the precision of stereotactic localization removes the uncertainty commonly associated with conventional neurosurgical approaches in selected cases of acute and chronic post-traumatic intracranial lesions.[1–4]

Such **stereotactic procedures provide an elegant solution by marking the chosen trajectory from the scalp to the desired intracranial target such as deep basal ganglionic hematoma.** Therefore, the neuroimaging directed stereotactic neurosurgery is currently being increasingly employed in a selected subset of, post-traumatic intracranial lesions.[4,5]

Among neurosurgical centres, those who can obviously afford image guided stereotactic (frame-based or frame-less) neurosurgery, the management of a selected subset of post-traumatic intracranial lesions should preferably be done with the aid of stereotaxy.[5–8] Free hand approaches and exploratory craniotomies are highly undesirable in the modern era of stereotactic precision.[1] *Stereotactic burr hole procedures* offer a safe, rapid, easily reproducible accurate craniocortical entry, transit and targeting whether it is a deep-seated hematoma or a pinched cerebral ventricle. Whereas image guided precise *stereotactic minicraniotomy* is appropriate for conditions such as deep basal ganglionic hematoma and minimizes operative craniocerebral entry and transit[7] trauma in an already traumatized brain parenchyma. Those patients whose advanced age, associated medical illnesses or severe neurological disability pose unacceptable risks of conventional neurosurgical interventions under general anesthesia, will certainly be benefited with a minimal interference by using image guided stereotactic burr hole procedures under local anaesthesia. If a craniotomy is required than the *image guided stereotactic trephine craniotomy procedures* permit a small scalp incision, precise placement of a small bone flap, minimal dural opening and a controlled cerebral trauma. The neurosurgeon will have advantage of choosing the cranial site of entry, the operating cerebral trajectory and knowing the surgical target. In order to preserve functions, minimal surgical manipulations may then be performed using microsurgical techniques. Image guided stereotactic procedures achieve low morbidity and mortality, rapid convalescence and a short hospital stay when compared with the conventional neurosurgical procedures.[1,8] There are many stereotactic devices, all of which provide precise localization. The one used by an individual neurosurgeon is largely a matter of his training and experience.

The Spectrum of Post-traumatic Lesions: Conventional Neurosurgery vs Stereotaxy

Neurosurgical aspects in the management of significant head injury consist of dealing with a wide spectrum of injuries of the scalp, skull and intracranial contents. According to the current practice, image guided stereotactic neurosurgery is superflush in the former two (scalp and skull) and useful in some subsets of the last group (intracranial contents).

A general outline of the current neurosurgical practice in a variety of post-traumatic intracranial lesions is as follows:

Acute Post-traumatic Intracranial Injuries

These are subdivided into two major groups: focal injuries and diffuse injuries.

1. Focal Injuries

a. Intracranial hemorrhage with and without significant cerebral contusion includes:

  i. *Meningeal hemorrhage (EDH/SDH, SAH):* EDH/SDH are best treated by the emergency conventional neurosurgical approaches and SAH by conservative surgical and medical therapy.

  ii. *Cerebral hemorrhage [ICH/IVH]:*
  - Superficial cortical and subcortical lesions are managed with emergency conventional neurosurgical techniques.
  - Deep subcortical, basal ganglionic, thalamic and brainstem hematomas are best approached by stereotactic procedures.
  - IVH is best treated with external ventricular drainage.

b. Cerebral contusions/lacerations are best managed by conventional neurosurgical approaches.

c. Impairment injuries are best treated by conventional neurosurgical approaches and only a select subset may need stereotactic surgery.

d. Bullet injuries are best treated by conventional neurosurgical approaches and only a select subset will need stereotactic surgery.

2. Diffuse Injuries

Concussion: Intensive neurosurgical observation (masterly inactivity and cat like observations).

Diffuse axonal injury: Intensive neurosurgical observations and neurointensive care.

Diffuse hypoxic encephalopathy: Intensive neurosurgical observations and neurointensive care.

Diffuse brain swelling: NICU care-stereotactic placement of intraventricular catheter

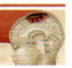

for ICP monitoring and CSF diversion/drainage, care to protect brain.

Subacute and Chronic Post-traumatic Intracranial Injuries

Septate subdural hematoma: Conventional neurosurgery vs stereotactic surgery.

Intracerebral hematoma: Stereotactic burr hole aspiration.

Sino-dural fistula with CSF leak: Stereotaxy guided endoscopic packing.

Sequelae of Head Injury

Post-traumatic movement disorders: Stereotactic thalamic/subthalamic lesions or stimulations.

Post-traumatic cerebellar syndrome: Stereotactic lesion/stimulations.

Post-traumatic intracerebral abscess: Stereotactic burr hole/minitrephine aspiration or removal of an abscess.

Post-traumatic spasticity: Antispasmodic drug therapy (dantrolene, baclofen, clonazepam, diazepam), Botox injection, intraspinal baclofen pump and spinal cord stimulation.

Definitive Indications of Stereotactic Neurosurgical Procedures in Significant Post-traumatic Intracranial Lesions/Disorders

Remarkable achievements have occurred in modern image guided Stereotaxy during the past decade. Most importantly, the scientific concepts of this common modality are assimilated across the neurosurgical disciplines. The new facts and ideas developed in this arena of neurosurgery are having great impact on the concepts, important to other neurosurgical fields. The area of head injury also remained no exception to this important technique.

Currently, the image guided stereotactic procedures are indicated in the following post-traumatic intracranial lesions:

1. Stereotactic removal/aspiration of intracranial hematomas:
   a. Acute post-traumatic space occupying intracerebral contusion hematomas, basal ganglionic hematomas thalamic hematomas and brainstem hematoma.
   b. Chronic septate subdural hematomas or chronic intracerebral hematoma.
2. Stereotactic ventriculostomy in severe generalized brain oedema with small cerebral ventricle for ICP monitoring and CSF diversion/drainage.
3. Stereotactic removal of intracranial foreign body.
4. Stereotactic guided deep brain stimulation (DBS) or lesions for post-traumatic involuntary movements:
   a. Stereotactic thalamic lesions for post-traumatic resting tremors/Parkinson's syndrome.
   b. Stereotactic thalamic lesions for post-traumatic acute myoclonic syndrome.
   c. Stereotactic thalamotomy for hemidystonia due to focal post-traumatic basal ganglionic lesion.
   d. Stereotactic ventral intermediate thalamotomy for post-traumatic hemiballismus.
   e. Stereotaxic lesions for post-traumatic cerebellar syndrome.
5. Stereotactic guided surgical closure of post-traumatic cranio-sinus fistula in the sella turcica.
6. Stereotactic neurosurgery in post-traumatic intracerebral hematomas.

Traumatic intracerebral hemorrhage is a common neurosurgical emergency and an important cause of disability and death in head injured patient.[9–11] It may begin as a primary event at the time of impact but its effects manifest later on and therefore it is usually considered as a secondary complication of head injury. Hematomas manifesting in 24 hours following head injury are considered delayed. Traumatic bleeding may occur singly or in combination with cerebral contusion, laceration and hemorrhage in other areas (EDH/SDH/SAH/IVH).

Traumatic primary ICHs in their pure forms occur within the brain parenchyma and are not in contact with the surface of the brain. They occur in about 25% of severe head injury patients and are frequently multiple (20%). In

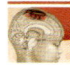

about one-third to two-thirds of cases they are associated with EDH and in one-third to one-fourth of patients with SDH. They make up at least 30–40% of all intracranial hematomas being more common (80%) in the frontal and temporal regions and in the deep cerebral/locations. Small deep ICHs (usually less than 1 cm) are associated with diffuse axonal injuries. These can secondarily progress to large hematomas. Similarly secondary intracranial haematomas may result from damage to cerebral cortical vessels in the focus of cerebral contusions or lacerations in about 25–50% of cases. Multiple contusion hematomas occur in one-third of such patients and solitary ones in two-thirds. In the burst cerebral lobe (frontal and temporal polar regions) there is a coexisting cerebral contusion-laceration, intracerebral hematoma and subdural hematoma.

Deep ICHs arise due to rupture of intrinsic vessels deep in the brain at the time of injury and often penetrate ventricular system.[5] Post-traumatic basal ganglionic hematomas, thalamic hematomas and brainstem hematomas in head injury were thought to be uncommon entities in the past and their mechanisms have not been revealed clearly.

Traumatic deep basal ganglionic ICHs are probably secondary to the rupture of lenticulostriate or anterior choroidal branches. Thalamic hematomas due to posterior choroidal vessels and brainstem hematomas due to posterior perforating vessel, which are damaged by shearing forces in high velocity acceleration/deceleration injuries. The anterior and posterior perforating arteries are end arteries. Especially, the intermediate and lateral lenticulostriate arteries pursue an S-shaped course from their origin in the middle cerebral artery and enter the anterior perforated substance at an acute angle. The vessels are susceptible to damage where there is a transition from a fixed to a mobile segment; the perforators being more susceptible because of their redundant/S-shaped course and entry into the anterior perforated

substance at an acute angle, during the *acceleration-deceleration* movements.[11]

Traumatic basal ganglia hematomas commonly occur as a part of the spectrum of lesions that may be seen in diffuse axonal injury (DAI) which is almost always related to the mechanisms of injury in which the rotational acceleration produces shear and tensile strains of high magnitude.[4,5] Most studies indicate that traumatic basal ganglia hematoma is a primary event and its identification in an early CT scan of the head suggests that the patient has sustained a severe diffuse brain damage at the time of impact. It would appear that the acceleration-deceleration forces are such that both the axons and the blood vessels in the brain are damaged simultaneously at the time of injury. Basal ganglia hematomas occurring in isolation are rare and occur especially in impacts along the long axis of the skull producing shear injury between the perforating vessels and the basal ganglias.

The prognosis differs markedly between the two entities.[12] Whereas the traumatic basal ganglia hematomas associated with DAI carries a very poor prognosis with mortality reaching 40–50%, the isolated hematomas in the basal ganglia usually carries a good prognosis, suggesting that the mortality is associated with the injuries produced in other parts of the brain.[12,13]

The CT scan is the method of choice to diagnose various characteristics of an acute ICH. It differentiates ICH from cerebral contusions, cerebral edema, cerebral infarction and diffuse axonal injuries.

The management of ICH depends on the clinical characteristics.[4,5,12,15]

- The patients with isolated ICH even though large but not causing raised ICP, brain shift, unconsciousness or progressive focal neurological deficits are managed on the expectant conservative lines with a close ICU monitoring and periodic CT brain scans. Multiple small ICHs involving hypothalamopituitaty axis, basifrontal

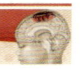

lobes and basal ganglia irrespective of the level of consciousness are best treated expectantly in majority of the cases.

- Patients with GCS of 10/15 and above, ICH of less than 4 cm and the absence of clinical as well as computed tomographic signs of brainstem compression are managed with non-operative treatment.
- The lobar haematomas greater than 5 cm in diameter should be removed surgically if they are responsible for altered consciousness, focal neurological deficits and a shift of the midline structures.
- If removal of ICH is expected to make a significant reduction in the intractable raised ICP then it should be removed.
- *Various operative procedures are commonly used:*[13–17]

Osteoplastic trephination and encephalotomy' is the principle surgical method. Burr hole and needle aspiration may be resorted to if more than three-fourths of the volume of the hematoma can be aspirated. The stereotactic method is recommended for the removal of traumatic ICH situated in the region of basal ganglia, thalamus or brainstem with minimum risk and high accuracy. The potential usefulness of this surgery is positively suggested in the management of deep cerebral hematomas. Patients may show dramatic recovery with remarkable improvement in neurological deficits. Even in patients with disturbed level of consciousness in the absence of focal neurological deficits, the large basal ganglia hematomas are treated rewardingly by CT guided stereotactic aspiration. Stereotactic removal of ICH is particularly useful in hematomas affecting several cerebral/lobes simultaneously or in case of symmetrical hematomas.[14]

The stereotactically aimed treatment of ICH is an advance for the patient's benefit. The evacuation cannula is safely inserted to its target from a transcutaneous drill hole of the skull and thus the patient is spared the surgical trauma associated with a large craniotomy and further brain damage. If necessary, the focus of hemorrhage can be reached again by puncture *via* the channel in the bone, which navigates the cannula. The surgery under local anesthesia is rapid and the results are promising.[13] In a series of 37 traumatic ICH evacuated by a simplified stereotactic surgical procedure, the mortality was 80% in patients with Glasgow Coma Scale (GCS) scores of 3–5 and 25% in patients with scores of 6–7. There were no deaths in patients with GCS of 8 or more. The results were better than those achieved by wide craniotomy. The importance of reduced operative trauma in patients with ICHs which are often associated with multifocal or diffuse brain injuries[16] cannot be overemphasized. However, the stereo tactic procedures are still rarely used. In Schneider et al series of 318 patients with severe head injury, 161 patients had cerebral contusion, and in about 90% of cases it was co-existing with other lesions (EDH 24 cases, SDH 29 cases, depressed skull fractures in 6 and traumatic SAH in 37 cases).[12] In their series, 10 patients underwent operative removal of their contusions-hematomas by trephination and only 2 others by stereotactic burr hole puncture aspiration.[12]

Chronic Septated SDH/ICH[18–20]

Chronic SDH are well delineated collections of fluid (blood) between duramater and the arachnoid membrane. Two forms of encapsulated chronic SDH can be distinguished: the non-septated and the septated form. The non-septated form can be treated easily using the burr hole-drainage method, whereas treatment of septated chronic subdural hematoma remains a therapeutic problem. The main concern is about the division of the hematoma by neomembranes into compartments, which hinder the efflux of the hematoma fluid through one or two burr holes. In such situation a relatively large loculi can be well localized using the stereotaxy and then operated on using flexible stereable endoscopes through a burr hole approach. The flexible endoscopes may be fixed and guided as needed. For resection of neomembranes

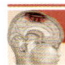
small microscissors or micro forceps may be used. This technique avoids blunt rupture of the membranes, which may cause bleeding. A closed drainage system is applied temporarily to guarantee the efflux of the remaining hematoma. Majorities of such patients have satisfactory evacuation of septated SDH.[19]

Stereotactic Ventriculostomy

In patients with severe head injury, the severe generalized brain swelling or edema and small cerebral ventricles are frequent CT findings. The raised intracranial pressure in these patients is invariably present. Therefore ICP monitoring as well as CSF drainage form the diagnostic and therapeutic measures to treat these cases. In such pinched/small ventricles, stereotaxy is unquestionably beneficial to place the ventricular catheter in the lateral ventricles for ICP monitoring and CSF drainage.[1,2]

Stereotactic Removal of Foreign Body

Removal of a foreign body lodged in the deep brain tissue may need stereotactic approach without causing a significant brain injury. Using a stereotactic system any point in the intracranial compartment[21–27] and around the craniofacial skeleton[23–31] can be reached exactly with pre-calculated precision. Thus a foreign body can be exposed and subsequently removed by a surgical approach that gives minimal discomfort and carries low risk. The target probe serves the surgeon as a guide bar whilst the tissue is dissected.[29] Kojima et al[23] reported an interesting case of a patient with air-gun bullets in the third ventricle associated with delayed ventricular hemorrhage. Through an anterior transcallosal approach they successfully removed the bullets without causing any significant permanent sequelae although they had to undertake a major craniotomy procedure. Hitchcock and Cowie reported the removal of air-gun pellet in the temporal lobe with the help of stereotaxy.[22]

Retained ventricular catheters are usually well tolerated but when infection is present then their removal becomes imperative because such catheters serve as a nidus for persistent infection. Minimally invasive methods for their removal are desirable. The removal of such catheters using stereotactic guided endoscopic surgery is a well proven minimally invasive technique.[21]

Stereotactic techniques certainly allow safe removal of a foreign body from a deep cerebral location with minimal traumal to the brain.[25]

STEREOTACTIC NEUROSURGERY IN POST-TRAUMATIC MOVEMENT DISORDERS

The sphere of stereotactic neurosurgery covers various post-traumatic intractable movement disorders, which are not controlled with maximal medicinal efforts.[32–34] The diagnosis is much more straightforward in these cases as compared to their idiopathic counterparts. The history of on-set of movement disorder following head injury, progression during the convalescence period and the characteristics of the clinical features of the particular type of involuntary movement, provide reasonable clue for an accurate diagnosis of a specific post-traumatic movement disorder. Movement disorders commonly occur due to the injury to the extrapyramidal system, therefore the neurosurgical interventions are mainly directed at various portions of the extra-pyramidal system.[32–35] However, indications of the stereotactic procedures with their implications (benefits, limitations and risks) must be carefully evaluated, expressed and discussed before these undertakings.

As widely recognized, extrapyramidal pathways concerning movement disorders are mainly two interlocking neuronal pathways involving the basal ganglia.[32–37] In the first pathway, the neurons of the corpus striatum (caudate and putamen) project to the globus pallidus, which gives two fibre bundles to the anterior nucleus of the thalamus. One fibre bundle (fasciculus) runs above the subthalamic nucleus of Luiz and other (ansa lenticularis) below the subthalamic nucleus of Luiz. Both bundles join above the subthalamic nucleus to form pallidothalamic bundle (thalamic fasciculus HI) in the Forel's field-H to reach to the ventral anterior thalamic nucleus. From here, the thalamic projections go to the supplementary motor cortex (which lies just anterior to the motor cortex) which in turn projects to the caudate nucleus to complete the pathways (caudate-putamen-globus pallidus-ventral anterior thalamus-supplementary motor cortex caudate). In the second pathway, the dentate nucleus of the cerebellum projects to the red nucleus then to ventrolateral thalamus from where the fibre projection goes to primary and secondary motor cortex. From these cortical areas corticopontine projection goes to pontine nuclei and then to cerebellar cortex which in turn projects to the dentate nuclei (dentato-rubro-thalamo-cortico-pontine-cerebellar-dentate pathways).

Currently, in intractable movement disorders, stereotactic neurosurgical procedures are utilized to interrup neuronal pathways in the Forel's field (compotomy campus foreli),[35–37] ventrolateral nucleus of thalamus (thalamotomy)[35–37] or in the dentate nucleus for cerebellar syndrome (dentatotomy).[38]

Following intractable disabling post-traumatic movement disorders are treated with stereotactic procedures:

Hemiballism[36–37]

In an awake patient, constant irregular, hurling, frequently violent exhaustive *movements of the shoulder and proximal arm occur. Hemiballism is due to a partial lesion in the subthalamic nucleus* with a tendency to resolve spontaneously (1 to 3 months) in some patients. It may be effectively controlled with stereotactic surgery in up to two-thirds of cases *by making a lesion in the ventrolateral thalamic* nucleus thalamotomy or in the Forel's field (campotomy).

Myoclonus[39]

It is characterised by *sudden unpredictable synchronous* severely disabling contractions of *the functionally synergestic muscles*. It causes a sudden jerk of a segment of the limb, head or part of the trunk. The movements involve mainly the proximal muscles and are usually bilateral and may be precipitated by any form of external stimuli but generally disappear during the sleep. Most of the time, *the dentate or olivary nuclei show abnormality*. Serotoninergic system may be involved. The stereotactic target is the *ventrolateral nucleus of the thalamus (thalamotomy)* or *Forel's field (campotomy) contralateral to the more severe movement disorder* with reasonably good results in majority of the cases.

Post-traumatic Resting Tremors[32–37]

Resting tremors are commonly presented in Parkinson's syndrome. Parkinson's syndrome is well known since 1817 and is characterized by tremor, rigidity, bradykinesia and disturbances of postural adjustment: pill-rolling tremor of the hand present at rest and usually stop at intention. Simultaneous contraction of the opposing muscles without hyper-reflexia causes rigidity. However, bradykinesia is the most disabling and contributes to the characteristic gait. The characteristic posture is due to the changes in the postural reflexes. Mask like face with loss of autonomic facial statement occurs.

Parkinson's disease is usually an idiopathic disorder but Parkinson's syndrome may occur due to ischemic cerebral atherosclerotic disorder, post-encephalitic syndrome or as a post-traumatic sequelae. At autopsy, commonly there is a loss of pigmented cells in the zona compacta of the substantia nigra and of the locus ceruleus. There is a deficiency of dopamine inbasal ganglia, particularly in the substantia nigra. L-dopa (the precursor of dopamine) is administered orally which after absorption in the circulation crosses the blood–brain barrier to enter the brain where it is converted into dopamine to-correct the deficiency. Carbidopa is given to avoid systemic and gastrointestinal side effects of the L-dopa. The disadvantages of the long-term medical treatment are well known, but many patients respond best to the medical therapy. However, for intractable cases, stereotactic surgery has been employed with some success. It relieves the tremor at best (after stereotactic campotomy or thalamotomy), rigidity next and bradykinesia least.

A combination of medical and surgical therapy maybe optimal in many patients. Stereotactic pallidotomy is considered for severe bradykinesia.

Stereotactic surgery basically involves interruption of the extrapyramidal pathways in Forel's field (campotomy), in the ventrolateral or ventrointermediate nucleus of the thalamus (thalamotomy for tremors) or in the globus pallidus (pallidotomy for rigidity and bradykinesia). About 80–90% of the patients report relief in their tremors and 50–60% in rigidity and some in bradykinesia. Morbidity occurs in about 5% cases (changes in mentation, speech and equilibrium) and mortality in less than 1% cases.

Post-traumatic Intention Tremors[40–43]

Among the variety of post-traumatic movement disorders especially following severe head injury, a moderate to severe intention tremor is often the major source of disability for the patients.[42]

Intention tremors occur in the distal part of the extremity as it approaches its target or when it performs fine distal movements. It is frequently due to cerebellar lesion. In Parkinson's syndrome, tremors occur at rest and are suppressed by action, whereas action/postural tremors is an exaggeration of the physiological tremors (benign essential tremors) and occur when the muscles of a limb are contracted as and when the arms are outstretched (exaggerated by anxiety, thyrotoxicosis, alcohol withdrawal).

Intention tremors usually occur in Wilson's disease, multiple sclerosis, ischemic atherosclerotic cerebrovascular disorder, encephalitis or trauma. Beta-adrenergic receptors may be involved. Propanolol (if not con-

traindicated for the patient) helps. Stereotactic thalamotomy (ventrolateral nucleus or ventrointermediate nucleus) or campotomy usually result in relief in about 80% cases in non-progressive disorders.

Tremors following cerebellar trauma or stroke respond very well. However, the tremors should be severe enough to cause disability and show no response to medication.

The target for cerebellar tremor/essential tremor is same as for the Parkinson's tremor. Best results are obtained with a lesion in the ventrointermediate nucleus of the thalamus just in front of the sensory area for the hand as identified by intraoperative stimulation. Marks[42] reported the results of stereotactic ablation of the ventralis intermedius thalamic nucleus in seven patients with post-traumatic cerebellar syndrome, and found a good relief of their tremor in six patients and no appropriate benefit in one. For post-traumatic cerebellar syndrome, the conservative treatment is usually ineffective but in appropriately selected cases, Stereotactic thalamotomy has a high degree of clinical success.

Thalamic targets in the treatment of involuntary movements usually include the lateral and the intermediate ventral nuclei. Destruction of their afferents in Forel's fields (campotomy) provides the same therapeutic results but the size of the lesion must then be very small due to the proximity of essential structures particularly corpus luysi. Efficacy of treatment depends partly on the etiology of the involuntary movement; however, tremors of all types are usually improved or suppressed.

The CT stereotactic dentatotomy is well described by Weigel and Mundinger.[38] According to these authors, with modern CT imaging, ventriculography or pneumonencephalography is no longer needed to determine the target point.

In addition due to the direct representation of the anatomic structures in the CT, abnormal positions of the dentate nucleus may be taken into consideration in the determination of the target point and approach for the coagulation probe with reasonable good results.

Chorea[32-37]

Choreiform movement of an extremity progressively involves the other limbs. Despite medication if chorea is disabling, then Stereotactic thalamotomy may offer some relief.

Dystonia[44-46]

In dystonia there is a sustained increase in the muscle tone without hyper-reflexia. There is a limitation of voluntary activity. Asymmetrically increased tone in the opposing muscles gives a distorted posture. In dystonia musculorum deformans it involves mainly the trunk and extremities, whereas spasmodic torticollis involves the neck muscles, and in tardive dystonia only extremities are involved. In most dystonias, the aetiology remains unknown and it is rarely due to trauma. Dystonia musculorum deformans and tardive dystonia, however, respond to the stereotactic thalamotomy whereas spasmodic torticollis to the spinal cord stimulation. If there is a poor response to spinal cord stimulation then anterior rhizotomy or selective neurectomy may be tried. Stereotactic guided surgical closure of post-traumatic craniosinus CSF fistula in the sella turcica.[47-50]

CSF leak may arise as a complication of trauma, transsphenoidal surgery, endoscopic sinus surgery or hydrocephalus, or may occur spontaneously without any identifiable cause. CSF leakage following head injury is a significant complication with a risk of meningitis and pneumocephalus especially in patients with fractures of the sella turcica or ethmoid bone. CT stereotaxy guided intrasphenoidal/ethmoidal packing or injection of fibrin sealant through a 12 gauge needle or fibroendoscopic packing is a simple alternative to the conventional neurosurgical management of CSF fistula. This procedure avoids a large

bifrontal craniotomy, preserves olfaction and avoids the risk of frontal lobe damage. Location and size of the leak, cause, technique and choice of the packing material used for the repair do not significantly affect the surgical outcome. However, the presence of hydrocephalus influences the outcome utmost. Many patients with increased intraventricular pressure required a ventricular shunt in addition to a second endoscopic repair. Certainly the endoscopic repair of CSF rhinorrhea is a promising alternative to conventional surgical repair techniques. Since sphenoid/ethmoid sinuses have multiple septa and therefore may behave like a maze. Stereotaxy may be used to localize precisely and identify a particular sinus compartment if needed. The endoscopic repair of CSF rhinorrhoea is a safe and effective approach that can be improved with stereotactic localization techniques. Proper graft placement is critical and lumbar drainage is an important adjunct in some cases. Following proper localization of the leak, repair is safely performed in most of the cases by endonasal route with the help of free mucoperiosteal flaps taken from the inferior or middle turbinates. CSF leakage bears high risk of meningeal or intracranial infection and therefore should be repaired as soon as it is recognized that the conservative treatment has failed. The sphenoid sinus CSF fistula may be closed successfully using fascia, muscle and gelfoam or fibrin glue and gelfoam.

Where the skull base defect is accessible to the stereotactic-assisted endoscopic surgery, it should be considered as the preferred method. Its high success rate, low rate of morbidity and good long-term results recommend endonasal duroplasty as a primary treatment modality for frontobasal dural lesions. For extended traumatic frontobasal dural lesions, the conventional intracranial dural repair is preferred, however, the endonasal approach should then be reserved for the closure of the additional sphenoid sinus leaks in such cases. The excellent visualization and a traumatic surgical techniques of endoscopic sinus surgery combined with stereotactic localization results in successful outcome in majority of these complicated cases.

IMPLICATIONS OF STEREOTACTIC SURGERY

The benefits of stereotactic surgery are enormous and the risk of morbidity and mortality is certainly low as compared to the conventional neurosurgical procedures ranging between 1 and 5%. However, post-operative hemorrhage, infection and neuronal damage may still occur.[1,2,51–53]

The postoperative artifacts should also be well recognized following stereotactic surgery if confusion is to be avoided.[54] The extent of resection bed usually does not change during the first week after operation and reduction of the size of artifact then began and continued up to 3–6 months. Mass effect and edema show no change during the first 4 days; then they regress gradually. Pneumocephalus is found in about half of the cases.

In the first three weeks. Benign surgically induced cerebral enhancement usually appears at the margins of the encephalotomy (and on the surface of the brain at the retractor site if used) at the end of the first postoperative week. It becomes more prominent during the following weeks and lasts up to 3–5 months. In many cases, such cerebral enhancement may prevent recognition of a residual lesion. Dural enhancement at the site of surgery is also noted in early postoperative period and may last for up to one year period.

CONCLUSIONS

The value of image guided stereotactic systems is directly dependant on the ease and speed of their use. In the past, most stereo-tactic techniques were complicated and time consuming to set up. They were exclusively used either for biopsing neoplasms[55–58] or for functional neuro-surgery.[31–37] However, current systems equipped with advanced registration techniques are much simpler and faster to employ and indications for their use are rapidly increasing and certainly embrace head injury.[4,5,12–16,31,47–49]

REFERENCES

1. Sharma RR, Da vis CHG, Lynch PG, Keogh AJ. Minimally invasive neurosurgery using CRW-3 Stereotaxy. Ann Saudi Med 1994;14:507–10.

2. Sharma RR, Lad SD, Pawar SJ, Sousa J, Mishra GP, Netalkar AS, Athale SD. The scope of image guided Leksell Stereotactic neurosurgery in Oman. Oman Medical Journal 1999;15:14–26.

3. Pawar SJ, Lad SD, Sharma RR, et al. CT guided Stereotactic neurosurgery experience in Oman (Abstract). Pan Arab J Neurosurg 1999;3:73–4.

4. Delmendo A. Stereotaxy in head injuries and strokes in Oman. In Sharma RR, Pawar SJ, Mishra GP (eds).Illustrated Synopsis: Helical CT guided microstereotactic neurosurgery in Oman. National Printers, Muscat, Oman June 1999;28.

5. Devadas RV, Mahapatra AK, Sharma RR, Lad SD. Traumatic primary Basal Ganglia Haematomas. In Sharma RR, Pawar SJ, Lad SD (eds) Illustrated Synopsis: Management of Head Injury in Oman. AL Zahra Printers, Muscat, Oman April 2000;97–8.

6. Brown AP, Dacey RG. New management techniques in neurosurgery. Curr Opin Neurol Neurosurgery 1992;5:799–807.

7. Bucholz RD, Greco D. Image guided surgical Techniques for infections and trauma of the central nervous system Neurosurg Clin N Am 1996;7:187–200.

8. Ko K, Ghajar J, Hariri RJ. A method for monitoring intracranial temperature via tunneled ventricular catheter: technical note. Neurosurgery 1994;34:927–30.

9. Broseta J, Gonzalez-Darder J, Barcia-Saloria JL. Stereotactic evacuation of intracerebral hematomas. Appl Neurophysiol 1982;45:443–8.

10. Hondo H, Matsumoto K. CT guided stereotactic evacuation of hypertensive and traumatic intracerebral haematomas experiences with 35 cases. No Shinkei Geka (Jap) 1983;1:35–48.

11. Jaykumar PN, Kolluri VR, Basavakumar DG, Arya BY, Das BS. Prognosis in traumatic basal ganglia haematoma. Acta Neurochir (Wien) 1989;3–4:114–6.

12. Schneider R, Mauer UM, Waldbaur H, Oldenkott P. Surgical indications in space occupying contusion haemorrhage. Unfallchirurg (German) 1993;96:191–200.

13. Fadrus P, Maca K, Smrcka V, Nadvornic P. Minimally invasive treatment of traumatic cerebral haematoma. Further experience with Stereotactic evacuation. Rozhl Chir (Czech) 1998; 77:441–4.

14. Chrastina J, Smrcka V, Nadvornik P, Zborilova E. Stereotactic therapy of post-traumatic cerebral haemorrhage. Rozhl Chir (Czech) 1996;75:330–3.

15. Yamamoto F, Eguchi G, Yoshimura K, Shigemori M, Kuramoto S. Massive traumatic haematoma localized in the basal ganglia: Treatment by CT - guided Stereotactic aspiration surgery. No Shinkei Geka (Japanese) 1990;18:563–5.

16. Coraddu M, Floris F, Nurchi G, Meleddu V, Lobina G, Marcucci M. Evacuation of traumatic intracerebral haematomas using a simplified stereotactic procedure. Acta Neurochir (Wien) 1994;129:6–10.

17. Potapov AA, Lantukh AV, Likhterman LB, Loshakov VA, Kravchuk AD, Melikian VG. The differentiated treatment of traumatic intracranial hematomas. Zh Vopr Neirokhir Im NN Burdenko (Russian) 1992;1:5–10.

18. Helling D, Kuhn TJ, Bauer BL, List-Hellwig E. Endoscopic treatment of septated chronic subdural haematoma. Surg Neurol 1996; 45:272–7.

19. Hellwig D, Bauer BL. Minimally invasive neurosurgery by means of ultra thin endoscopes. Acta Neurochir Suppi (Wien) 1992:54:63–68.

20. Karakhan VB. End of ibroscopic intracranial stereotopography and end of iberscopic neurosurgery. Acta Neurochir Suppi (Wien) 1992:54:11–25.

21. Blacklock JB, Maxwell RE. Stereotactic removal of a migrating ventricular catheter. Neurosurgery 1985;16:230–1.

22. Hitchcock E, Cowie R. Stereotactic removal of intracranial foreign bodies: Review and case report. Injury 1983;14:471–5.

23. Kojima T, Waga S, Kubo Y, Sbimazu T. Successful removal of air gun bullets from the third ventricle. Neurosurgery 1987;20:322–5.

24. Kosary IZ, Shacked Y, Ouaknine G. Removal of intracerebral foreign bodies with the aid of a stereotoxic procedure. Harefuah (Hebrew) 1971,80:243–4.

25. Muhammad AK, Maruno M, Maeda N, Kato A, Yoshimine T. Syringe needle located deep in the brain: Image guided removal. Surg Neurol 2000; 54:458–63.

26. Schorf F. Stereotactic removal of foreign bodies form the visceral cranium. Fotschr Kiefer Gesichtschir (German) 1976:21:280–1.

27. Yoshijima S, Murayama Y, Matsumoto K. A case of successful removal of a deep-seated bullet in the brain by stereotactic approach. No Shinkei Geka (Jap) 1979:7:989–94.

28. Eschler J, Scharf F, Rucker. A Localization and planned removal of foreign bodies in the maxillo-facial region by means of a new stereotactic device. Disch Zahn Mund Kieferheilkd Zentralbl Gesamte (German) 1966;46:425–34.

29. Hailing F, Merten HA, Dieckmann G, Luhr HG. Stereotactic removal of foreign bodies in the maxillofacial area. Dentomaxillofac Radiol 1991;20:100–4.

30. Horton CE, McFadden JT. Stereotactic localization of a facial foreign body. Case report. Plast Reconstr Surg 1971;47:598–9.

31. McFadden JT, Horton CE. Stereotaxic localization of extracranial foreign bodies in the head. Am Surg 1971;37:353–6.

32. Bullard DE, Nashold BS. Stereotaxic thalamotomy for treatment of post-traumatic movement disorders. J Neurosurg 1984;61:316–21.

33. Derome PJ, Jedynak CP, Visot A, Delalande 0. Treatment of abnormal movements by thalamic lesions. Rev Neurol (Paris) 1986;142(4):391–7.

34. Nizuma H, Kwak R, Ohyama H, Ikeda S, Ohtsuki T, Suzuki J, Sago S. Stereotactic thalamotomy for postapoleptic and post-traumatic involuntary movements. Appi Neurophysiol 1982;45:295–8.

35. Tasker RR, Dostrovsky JO, Dolan EJ. Computerized Tomography (CT) is just as accurate as ventriculography for functional stereotactic thalamotomy. Stereotact Funct Neurosurg 1991;57:157–66.

36. Levesque MF, Markham CH. Ventral intermediate thalamotomy for post-traumatic hemiballismus. Stereotact Funct Neurosurg 1992; 58:26–9.

37. Levesque MF, Markham CH, Makasato N. MR-guided ventral intermediate thalamotomy for post-traumatic hemiballismus. Stereotact Funct Neurosurg 1992;58:88–9.

38. Weigel K, Mundinger F. Computerized tomography-guided stereotactic dentatotomy. Appl Neurophysiol 1986;49:301–6.

39. Eiras J, Garcia Cosamalon J. Post-traumatic myoclonic syndrome. Effectiveness of the thalamic lesions on the action of myoclonus. Arch Neurobiol (Madr) 1980;43:17–28.

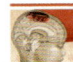
40. Andrew J, Fowler CJ, Harrison MJ. Tremor after head injury and its treatment by stereotactic surgery. J Neurol Neurosurg Psychiatry 1982; 45:815–9.

41. Fox JL, Kurtzke JF. Trauma Induced intention tremor relieved by stereotactic thalamotomy. Arch Neurol 1966;15:247–51.

42. Marks PV. Stereotactic surgery for posttraumatic cerebellar syndrome: An analysis of seven cases. Stereotact Funct Neurosurg 1993; 60(4):157–67.

43. Van Manen J. Stereotaxic operations in cases of hereditary and intention tremor. Acta Neurochir (Wien) 1974; Suppl 21:49–55.

44. Andrew J, Fowler C, Harrison MJ. Hemidystonia due to focal basal ganglia lesion after head injury and improved by stereotactic thalamotomy. J Neurol Neurosurg Psychiatry 1982;45:276.

45. Andrew J, Fowler CJ, Harrison MJ. Stereotactic thalamotomy in 55 cases of dystonia. Brain 1983; 106 (pt 4):

46. Krauss JK Mohadjer M, Braus DF, Wakhloo AK, Nobbe F, Mundinger F. Dystonia following head trauma: A report of nine patients and review of the literature. Mov Disord 1992;7:263–72.

47. Fraioli B, Pastore FS, Floris R, Vagnozzi R, Simonetti G, Liccardo G, Giuffre R. Computed tomography-guided trans-sphenoidal closure of post-surgical cerebrospinal fluid fistula: A transmucosal needle technique. Surg Neurol 1997;48(4):409–13.

48. Petr R. Surgical closure of a cranisinus fistula of iatrogenic origin in the area of the sella turcica. Rozhl Chir (Czech) 1966;45(11):731–4.

49. Zervas NT. Stereotaxic thermal pituitary ablation. Acta Neurochir (Wien) 1974; Suppl 21: 165–8.

50. Kurzeja A, Wenzel M, Korves B, Mosges R. Decompression of the optic nerve after fractures of the rhinobasal skull with computer assisted surgery. Laryngorhinology (German) 1994; 73:274–6.

51. Lafia DJ. Acute subdural haematoma as a complication of Stereotaxic thalamotomy. Cofin Neurol 1965;26:441–4.

52. Nashold BS. Operative complications due to stereotactic surgery. Confin Neurol 1968;30: 325–36.

53. Zarsi S, Sierpinski S, Mempel E, Pilipowska T. Intracranial haemorrhage as complications of stereotactic operations. Neurol Neurochir Pol 1971;5:29–35.

54. Herman M, Pozzi-Mucelli RS, Skrap M. CT and MR1 findings after stereotactic resection of brain lesions. Eur J Radiol (Czech) 1996;75:330–3.

55. Pa war SJ, Lad SD, Sharma RR, et al. CT guided stereotactic neurosurgery experience in Oman (Abstract). Annual Meeting of the Egyptian Society of Neurological Surgeons, Cairo, Egypt 8–12th March 1999.

56. Sharma RR, Davis CHG. The impact of CT Stereotaxy on tumour surgery for the 90s. Paper presented at the 12th Annual Meeting of the British Neuro-Oncology Group, 25–26 Juen 1992,Bristol, UK (Abstract) p-8.

57. Sharma RR, Davis CHG, Lynch PG. Management of intrathird ventricular craniopharyngioma using Cosman-Roberts-Wells (CRW-III) Stereotaxy. Surgical Neurology 1994;42:551–2.

58. Sharma RR, Parekh HC, Davis CHG. The impact of CT Stereotaxy on tumour surgery for the 1990s. Abstract of the 12th Annual Meeting of the British Neuro-Oncology Group. Br J Neurosurg 1993;7:105–6.

20

Endocrinal Abnormalities Following Head Injury

AK Mahapatra • Raj Kamal • N Barua

INTRODUCTION

Despite of numerous case reports of patients with post-traumatic endocrinal distur-bances,[1–5] prospective studies or even large retrospective studies are not available, dealing with trauma induced pituitary dysfunction. Moreover, pituitary function studies are infrequently considered in acute stage or even in long-term management of patients with traumatic brain injury, even though it is almost a well known fact that severe head injury offers considerable risk to pituitary function. Earlier autopsy studies had demon-strated anterior pituitary necrosis in as high as one-third fatal head-injured patients.[6–8] However, inspite of development of neuro-imaging and well established laboratory for neuroendocrinal assessment, the incidence, clinical significance and degree of risk due to endocrinal deficits, in head-injured patients are not well known.

Hypopituitarism is not an uncommon complication of head trauma, with a pre-valence of at least 25% among patients who were studied months or years following injury. This remarkably high frequency has changed the traditional concept of hypo-pituitarism being a rare complication of TBI, and suggests that most cases of post-traumatic hypopituitarism remain undiagnosed and untreated in clinical practice.[9]

The prevalence of hypopituitarism in children with traumatic brain injury is unknown. Most cases of post-traumatic hypopituitarism remain undiagnosed and untreated in the clinical practice, and it may contribute to the severe morbidity seen in patients with traumatic brain injury. In the acute phase of brain injury, the diagnosis of adrenal insufficiency should not be missed.[10] Determination of morning serum cortisol concentration is mandatory, because adrenal insufficiency can be life-threatening. Morning low serum cortisol (normal range from 8 AM to 12 Noon is 138–690 nmol/L) strongly suggests adrenal insufficiency. A complete hormonal investigation should be performed after one year of the trauma. Isolated growth hormone deficiency is the most common deficiency after traumatic brain injury. Sports-related chronic repetitive head trauma (because of boxing, kickboxing, football and ice hockey) may also result in hypopituitarism.

PATHOGENESIS OF ENDOCRINAL ABNORMALITIES

The exact incidence of pituitary dysfunction following head injury is not known. **Partial or complete pituitary dysfunction affects 33–50% of all traumatic brain injury (TBI) survivors and is a significant contributor to the overall disability burden.**[11] The hypo-physeal vessels are anatomically vulnerable to

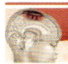

shearing injuries, raised intracranial pressure and anterior base of skull fractures, and pituitary ischemia or hemorrhage is a common finding at autopsy. Post-traumatic hypopituitarism (PTHP) can affect all grades of severity of injury and is often difficult to diagnose, as its features largely overlap with common post-concussive symptoms. **In a review article the pooled prevalences of hypopituitarism in the chronic phase after traumatic brain injury was 27.5%** (95% confidence interval [CI], 22.8–28.9%).[12]

Schneider et al[13] studied the prevalence of hypopituitarism in a total of 1242 patients based on different definitions of laboratory values and stimulation tests. The prevalence of hypopituitarism in the chronic phase (at least 5 months after the event) by laboratory values, physician diagnoses, and stimulation tests, was 35%, 36%, and 70%, respectively. Hypopituitarism was less common in the acute phase. According to the frequency of endocrine dysfunction, pituitary hormone secretion was impaired in the following sequence: **ACTH, LH/FSH, GH, and TSH.** TBI patients with abnormal stimulation tests had suffered from more severe TBI than patients with normal stimulation tests.

The endocrinal problem could result either due to pituitary or from hypothalamic damage following the head injury. No doubt, pituitary is highly vulnerable due to its location in sella turcica, and delicate infundibular hypothalamic structures. Autopsy studies in sixties had shown pituitary gland necrosis in one-third of fatal head injuries. Cohan et al[18] showed that **acute adrenal insufficiency occurs in 50% of moderate and severe TBI victims, and is associated with lower blood pressure and higher vasopressor requirements.** Acute thyroid dysfunction has also been demonstrated in TBI victims and in other critically ill patients in intensive care units[14] (Fig. 20.1).

It is generally believed that the **pituitary dysfunction** following head injury is by and large due to diffuse swelling, hypotension or hypoxic insult.[16] However, primary pituitary

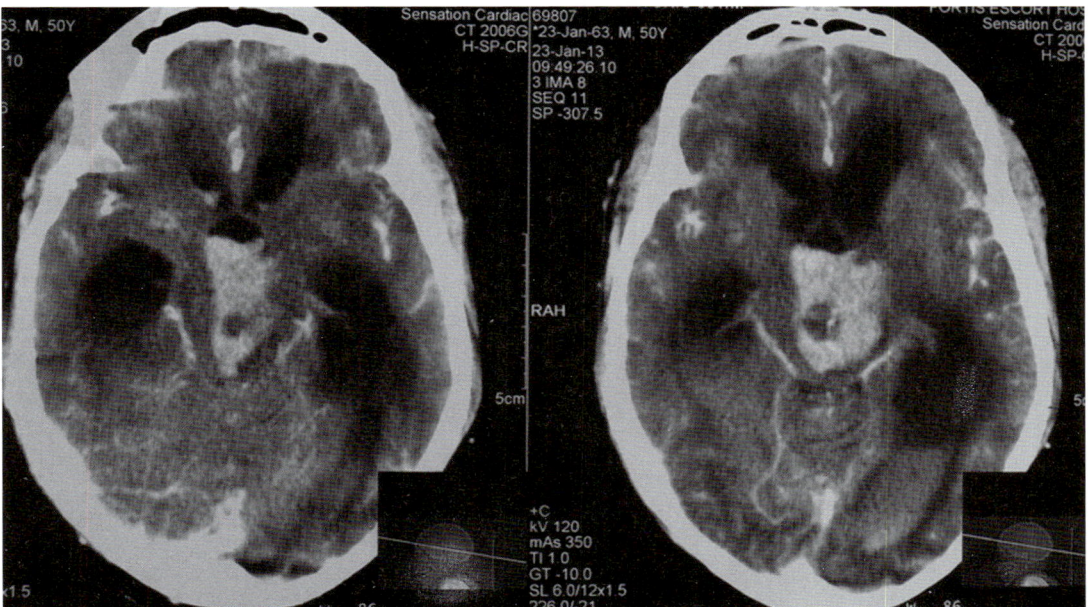

Fig. 20.1: CT scan head of a patient of post-traumatic intraventricular bleed with hydrocephalus. Contrast given to rule out any other cause of bleed

damage is well described.[6,8] Prior to CT scans most of the evidences were autopsy based. In autopsy studies, pituitary abnormality is recorded in almost 75%.[8] **The significant primary abnormalities include capsular hemorrhage in over 50%, followed by posterior lobe and stalk hemorrhage in 30% and 20% cases approximately.** Next to the hemorrhages, **necrosis** is another important finding. The common site of necrosis is anterior lobe followed by pituitary stalk (Table 20.1). In an autopsy study, Kornblum and Fisher in 1969,[8] had reported anterior pituitary necrosis in 35% patients of fatal head injuries those who had survived longer than 12 hours. Necrosis patterns always corresponds to the blood supply of the long **hypophyseal portal veins.** Long portal veins pass through diaphragma sella, where they are vulnerable to mechanical compression from swollen brain and swollen pituitary gland.[2,6–8,15,16] Long hypophyseal portal veins supply 70% blood to anterior pituitary. The somatotrophs and gonadotrophs are laterally placed, hence more frequently involved.[3] This anatomical arrangements very well explains the long-term hormonal insufficiency.

Direct stalk injury in form of stalk transection and stalk hemorrhage (Fig. 20.2) also lead to immediate and long-term hypopituitarism.[1,17–19] This can result due to fracture of the sella turcica.[1] With the advent of CT and MRI it is possible to demonstrate rupture of the pituitary stalk.[18,19]

Hypothalamic injury also can lead to hypopituitarism following severe head injury. By and large these patients do not survive to have long-term hypothalamic problems. Crompton in 1971[20] had described hypothalamic lesions in closed head injury. Recently, with improved imaging such lesions are more frequently diagnosed radiologically.[15,16,18] Traumatic SAH with or without vasospasm also contribute to hypothalamic and pituitary dysfunction (Fig. 20.3).

CLINICAL PROBLEM

Clinical problem in head injury varies from acute stage to chronic problems. In acute stage there is likely have cortisol and ADH deficiency which can manifest persistent hypotension in absence of any obvious cause, as patients cannot withstand stress in presence of acute pituitary failure. **Diabetes insipidus (DI)** is not uncommon in severe head injury. Failure of posterior pituitary lead to fall of plasma ADH resulting in DI and easily diagnosed as patients pass large volume of urine which is of low specific gravity, serum osmolality is high and urinary osmolality is low.[19,20] **Syndrome of inappropriate ADH (SIADH)** secretion in severe head injury is not rare and can be diagnosed on the biochemical parameters of serum and urine.

Pituitary dysfunctions are also reported in minor or moderate head injury. Ziaber et al[21] reported plasma cortisol and beta endorphin abnormality in minor head injury.

Table 20.1: Pathology in pituitary gland follow head injury			
	Type of pathology	*Site*	*%*
Primary	Hemorrhage	• Capsular	50–55%
		• Posteriorl lobe	30%
		• Stalk	15
	Necrosis	• Anterior pituitary	20%
		• Stalk	3%
Secondary	Hypoxia		—
	Edema		—
Direct stalk injury	Rupture of stalk		—
	Transection of stalk		—
	Stalk hemorrhage		—

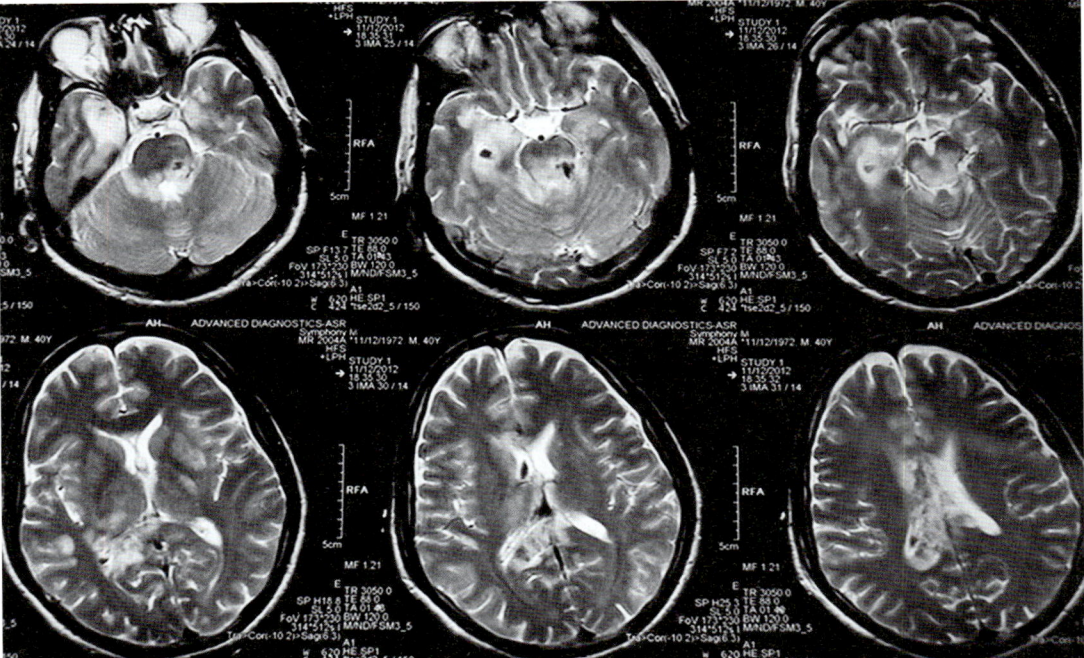

Fig. 20.2: MRI brain of a patient (who developed severe SIADH on fourth day) showing the presence of multifocal areas of abnormal signal (bright on T_2-weighted images) at the white matter in the temporal or parietal corticomedullary junction, in the splenium of the corpus callosum and the dorsolateral rostral midbrain and the corona radiata. There is suspected injury to pituitary stalk

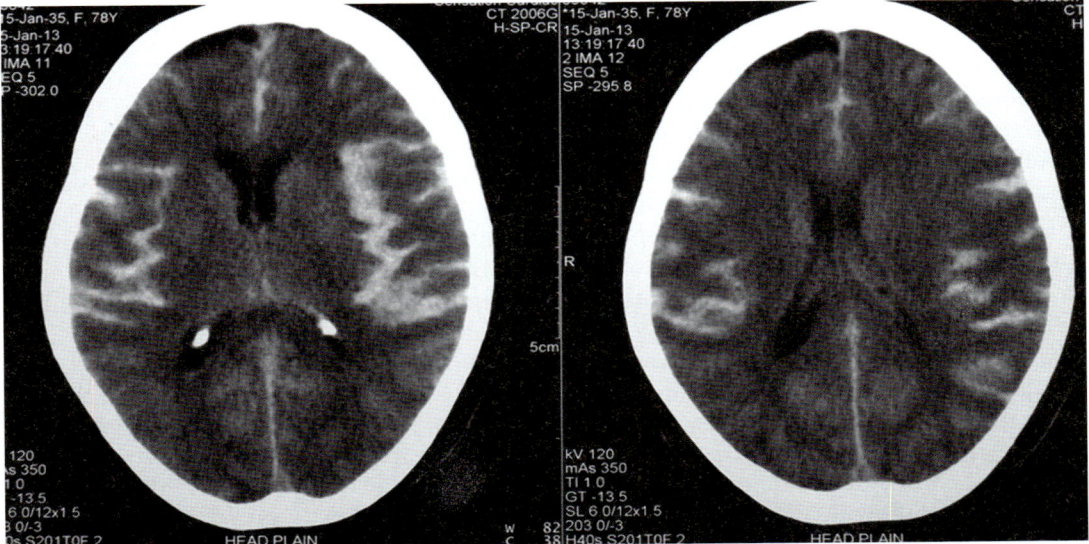

Fig. 20.3: CT scan showing post-traumatic SAH. This patient had pituitary hypofunction

Diabetes insipidus is an important clinical problem in severe head injury.[19,20,22] In addition to DI, SIADH is not uncommon.[23] These clinical problems are also to be differentiated from patients with **cerebral salt wasting** (CSW). In these patients, serum sodium is low and 24 hours urinary sodium secretion is very high. For above reasons, only, a careful electrolyte balance should be monitored in severe head injury patients up to two weeks.[23] Electrolyte and plasma osmolality abnormalities are more frequent in patients with diabetes mellitus and chronic alcoholism.

Clinically, significant **hypogonadism** is not uncommon in major head injury.[24–26] The hypogonadism could be transient[25] or long-term. Clark et al[24] in 1988 reported 33 male patients with major head injury in whom total free testosterone was significantly lower on third day. However, persistent hypogonadism was only reported in five of these 21 patients in whom the test were performed between 3 and 6 months after injury. They suggested repeated endocrinal assessment in patients with severe head injury. Woolf et al in 1986[25] reported transient hypogonadism following head injury. They included both severe and moderate head injury patients. They studied 31 male patients in whom testosterone and other hormonal assessments were performed shortly after injury and on the fourth day. They observed good correlation between severity of head injury and sex hormone abnormalities.

Precocious puberty is another rare problem following severe head injury.[3,37] The precise mechanism is not still clear. Some authors have hypothesized extrahypothalamic involvement.

Neurobehavioral impact of hypopituitarism is significant. Chronic behavioral problems are recorded in significant number of patients with brain injury.[28–31] Both behavioral and cognitive defects are noticed even one year following injury.[4–30] Saatmari et al[31] in 1997 demonstrated cognitive abnormality in experimental brain injury. It is generally believed that the deficiency of growth hormone or insulin-like growth factor[1] deficiency results in neurobehavioral and **cognitive** deficit.[31,32] Saatman et al[31] reported improvement in incognitive function by supplementing insulin-like growth factor. Loss of memory, higher anxiety level, impaired motor skill and lower quality of life is also attributed to growth hormone deficiency.[33,34] Sex hormone deficiency also lead to mood disturbances and behavioral problems.

Investigations

Both anterior and posterior pituitary functions are tested (Table 20.2), when there is high degree suspicion of hypopituitarism:[36] (a) insulin tolerance test is a simple test to find out corticotroph and somatotroph secretion by measuring GH and cortisol level, (b) A TRH stimulation test is important to assess the level of TSH and prolactin, (c) GnRH stimulation test is necessary to assess gonadotroph function. Blood is tested 30 minutes prior to record the baseline hormone level followed by stimulation. Blood samples are collected every 30 minutes for the next two hours. For assessment of pituitary reserve combined anterior pituitary test (CAP)[35] is done by injecting: GHRH: 1.5 µg/kg; GnRH: 2.5 µg/kg (up to 100 µg maximum); TRH: 7 µg/kg (500 µgm maximum), CRH: 1.5 µg/kg IV sequentially over 30 seconds using separate syringes. Blood samples of ACTH, GH, LH, FSH, TSH and prolactin at baseline were measured at 15, 30, 60, 90 and 120 minutes. Failure to respond to stimulation test indicates pituitary hypofunction.

Stimulation tests for the corticotropic and somatotropic axes were performed in 26% and 22% of the patients, respectivly.[13] The prevalence of hypopituitarism in the chronic phase (at least 5 months after the event) by laboratory values, physician diagnoses, and stimulation tests, was 35%, 36%, and 70%, respectively. Hypopituitarism was less common in the acute phase. According to the frequency of endocrine dysfunction, pituitary

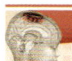

	Test	Method	Normal adult level
Table 20.2: Hormonal assessment			
GH	Insulin tolerance test (ITT)	RIA	0.5–17.0 ng/ml
ACTH	Insulin tolerance	RIA	6–76 pg/ml
TSH	TRH stimulation	Immunochemo-luminescences assay	0.3–4.25 mIU/L
Free thyroxin		RIA	10.3–21.9 pmol/L
FSH (H)	GnRH stimulation test	Fluroimmunometric assay	Female Follicular: 3.0–20.0 mIU/ml Ovulatory: 9.0–26.0 mIU/ml Luteal: 1.0–12.0 mIU/ml Postmenopausal: 18–153.0 mIU/ml Male: 1.0–12.0 mIU/ml
Serum Testosterone	GnRH stimulation test	RIA	270–1070 ng/dl (male) 6–86 ng/dl (female)

hormone secretion was impaired in the following sequence: ACTH, LH/FSH, GH, and TSH. TBI patients with abnormal stimulation tests had suffered from more severe TBI than patients with normal stimulation tests.[13]

Posterior pituitary function is not of less importance, realizing the problem of fluid electrolyte imbalance, problems of DI and SIADHs. Hence, measurement of serum sodium, blood urea, nitrogen, creatinine and osmolality of plasma and urine are important (Table 20.3). In addition, a regular check in urinary specific gravity and 24 hours urinary sodium excretion is also carried out to differentiate one from the other. Assessment of serum ADH level is also important.[15]

Overall growth hormone insufficiency is reported in 85% and **gonadotrophin** in 95%. Approximately 30% patients developed DI during their illness. Isolated or combined somatotroph and gonadotroph dysfunction is most common as compared to corticotroph, thyrotroph and posterior pituitary dysfunctions.

Treatment of Hypopituitarism

No doubt endocrinal abnormality, be it in acute phase of head injury or chronic state require careful evaluation and replacement therapy. In acute stage patients with DI, or SIADH or cerebral salt wasting need treatment to correct the deficiency. The treatment may be long-term or short-term depending on the need, in an individual patient. DDA-VP nasal spray, arginine vasopressin and pitressin injections are widely used.[15,19,20]

Desmopressin acetate injection 4 mcg/ml is available as a clear colorless sterile solution as 4 mcg/ml. The usual dosage range in adults is 0.5 ml (2 mcg) to 1 ml (4 mcg) daily, administered intravenously or subcutaneously, usually in two divided doses. The dosage for intranasal spray is 5 to 40 mcg spray twice a day The morning and evening doses should be separately adjusted for an adequate diurnal rhythm of water turnover. Several studies

Table 20.3 : Biochemical test	
Serum	Na+, creatinine
	Blood urea nitrogen
	Osmolality
Urine	Osmolality
	Specific gravity
	24 hours Na excretion

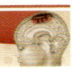

dealing with GH deficient patients showed beneficial role of GH replacement, which include improved memory, attention, comprehension and vocabulary. Improvement also included general well-being of mood and reduction in depression and anxiety state.[32–35] GH also helps in increasing muscle mass. Some authors have used insulin like growth factor I and shown improvement in various cognitive functions.[31,32]

Other important replacement therapy include the deficiency of testosterone. Testosterone replacement in men helps in normalization of libido and sexual function, helps in bone formation and increases the muscle mass.[38,39] Overall, sex hormone replacement be it testosterone or estrogen therapy significantly improves the cognitive performance.[23,38] Sex hormone deficiency in women is adequately treated with estrogen therapy, which improves their neurobehavioral and cognitive functions.

Cerebral salt wasting (CSW) occurs due to unregulated release of atrial natriuretic peptide.[40,43] Patients present with persistent hyponatraemia, hypernatriuresis with hyperosmolar urine. In CSW volume is depleted, hence volume is replaced with Na$^+$ containing fluid and hematocrit is to be restored. Infusion of saline, plasma and blood is necessary depending on the need. Fludrocortisone acetate is the specific treatment for CSW[9,40–43] which helps in sodium retention with fluid and correct hyponatremia.

CONCLUSIONS

Endocrinal abnormality related problems in head injury is a neglected aspect. Overall, 40% of severe head injuries to develop either short-term or long-term endocrinal problems. Basic reasons may be hypothalamic or pituitary damage, may be primary or even secondary to hypoxia or hypotension. Both anterior or posterior pituitary get involved. Pituitary stalk necrosis or avulsion can also occurs. Growth hormone deficiency, ADH secretion abnormalities and gonadotrophin insuffi-

ciency are more common problems. GH and gonadotrophin deficiency are also to some extent responsible for long-term behavioral and cognitive problems. Diabetes insipidus, inappropriate ADH secretion and CSW are quite frequent. All the endocrinal problem need proper evaluation and adequate short-term or long-term replacement to improve the overall outcome in patients with both severe and minor head injury.

REFERENCES

1. Bistritzer T, Theodor R, Inbar D, et al. Anterior hypopituitarism due to fracture sella turcica. Arne J Dis Child 1981;135:966–7.
2. Daniel PM, Prichard MML, Treip CS. Traumatic infarction of the anterior lobe of the pituitary gland. Lancet 1959;2:927–30.
3. Edwards OM, Clark JDA. Post-traumatic hypopituitarism. Six cases and review of the literature. Medicine 1981;65:281–90.
4. Halimi P, Sigal R, Doyon D, et al. Post-traumatic diabetes insipidus. MR demonstration of pituitary stalk rupture. J Comput Assist Tomogr 1988;12:135–7.
5. Miller WL, Kaplan SL, Grumbach MM. Child abuse as a cause of post-traumatic hypopituitarism. N Eng. J. Med 1980;302:724–8.
6. Ceballos R. Pituitary changes in head trauma (analysis of 102 consecutive cases of head injury) Albama J Med Sci 1966;3:185–98.
7. Daniel PM, Treip CS. The pathology of the pituitary gland in head injury. Mod Trends Endocrinol 1961;12:55–68.
8. Kornblum RN, Fisher RS. Pituitary lesions in craniocerebral injuries. Arch Patko 1969;188:242–8.
9. Ishikawa S, Saito T, Kaneko K, et al. Hyponatraemia response to fludrocortisone acetate in elderly patients with head trauma. Ann In Med 1987;16:707–11.
10. Agha A, Phillips J, Thompson CJ. Hypopituitarism following traumatic brain injury (TBI). Br J Neurosurg 2007;21:210–6.
11. Malik Zaben, Wessam El Ghoul, Antonio Belli Post-traumatic head injury pituitary dysfunction Perspectives in Rehabilitation, Disability and rehabilitation 2013;35:522–5.
12. Schneider HJ, Andermahr IK, Ghigo E, StallaGK, Agha A, MDHypothalamopituitary Dysfunction Following Traumatic Brain Injury and Aneury-

smal Subarachnoid HemorrhageA Systematic Review, JAMA 2007;298:1429–38.

13. Schneider HJ, Schneider M, Kreitschmann-Andermahr I, Tuschy U, Wallaschofski H, Fleck S, Faust M, Renner CI, Kopczak A, Saller B, Buchfelder M, Jordan M, Stalla GK. Structured assessment of hypopituitarism after traumatic brain injury and aneurysmal subarachnoid hemorrhage in 1242 patients: the German interdisciplinary database. J Neurotrauma 2011; 28:1693–8.

14. Justin Wagner, Joshua R. Dusick, David L. McArthur, Pejman Cohan, Christina Wang, Ronald Swerdloff, W. John Boscardin, Daniel F. Kelly, Acute Gonadotroph and Somatotroph Hormonal Suppression after Traumatic Brain Injury J Neurotrauma 2010;27:1007–19.

15. Kelly DF, Gonzalo 1TG, Cohan P, et al. Hypopituitarism following traumatic brain injury and aneurismal SAH: A preliminary report. J. Neurosurg 2000;93:743–52.

16. Eisenberg HM, Gary HE Jr, Aldrich EF, et al. Initial CT findings in 753 patients with severe head injury, a report from NIH traumatic coma Data Bank. J. Neurosurgery 1990;73:686–98.

17. Adams JR, Daniel PM, Prichard MML. Transection of the pituitary stalk in man. Anatomical changes in pituitary glands of 21 patients. J. Neurol Neurosurg Psychiat 1966;29:545–55.

18. Cohan P, Wang C, McArthur DL, Cook SW, Dusick JR, Armin B, Swerdloff R, Vespa P, Muizelaar JP, Cryer HG, Christenson PD, Kelly DF. Acute secondary adrenal insufficiency after traumatic brain injury: A prospective study. Crit. Care Med 2005;33:2358–66.

19. Halimi P, Sigal R, Doyon D, et al. Post-traumatic diabetes insipidus: MR demonstration of pituitary stalk rupture. J. Comput Asst Tomography 1988;12:135–7.

20. Massol J, Humbert P, Cattin F, et al. Post-traumatic diabetes insipidus and amenorrhoea-galactorrhoea syndrome after pituitary stalk rupture. Neuroradiology 1987;29:299–300.

21. Ziaber J, Chmielewski H, Laskowski A, et al. Profile of daily secretion of ACTH, beta endorphin and cortisol in patients with minor craniocerebral trauma. Wiado Nosci Leakarskie 1995;48:36–39.

22. Trivedi HS, Nolph 1C. Nephrogenic Diabetes Insipidus presenting after Trauma. Ame J. Nephrology 1994;14:145–7.

23. Steinbok P, Thompson GB. Metabolic disturbances after head injury: Abnormalities of sodium and water balance with specific reference to the effect of alcohol intoxication. Neurosurgery 1978;3:9–15.

24. Clark JD, Raggatt PR, Edwards DM. Hypothalamic hypogonadism following major head injury. Clinical Endocrinol 1988;29:153–65.

25. Woolf PD, Hamill RW, McDonald N, Lee LA, et al. Transient hypogonadiotrophic hypogonadism after head trauma: Effect on steroid precursors and correlation with sympathetic nervous system activity. Clinical Endocrinol 1986;25:265–74.

26. Hackl JM. Metabolic disorders in severe head injuries. Fortschritte der Medizm 1981;99:1562–6.

27. Shaul PW, Towbin RB, Chernausek SD. Precocious puberty following severe head trauma. Arne J Dischild 1985;139:647–69.

28. Dikmen SS, Ross BL, Machamer JE, et al. One year psychological outcome in head injury. J Int Neuropsychol Soc 1995;1:67–77.

29. Hellawell DJ, Taylor RT, Pentland B. Cognitive and psychosocial outcome following moderate or severe traumatic brain injury. Brain Inj 1999;13:489–504.

30. Levin HS, Gary HE, Eisenberg HM, et al. Neurobehavioural outcome one year after severe head injury. Experience of the traumatic data bank. J. Neurosurg 1990;73:699–709.

31. Saatman KE, Contreras PC, Smith DH, et al. Insulin like growth factor 1 (IGF1) improves both neurological motor and cognitive outcome following experimental brain injury. Exp. Neuro 1997;1(147):418–27.

32. Rollero A, Munaldo G, Fonzi S, et al. Relationship between cognitive function, growth hormone and insulin like growth factor I plasma level in aged subjects. Neuropsychobiology 1998;38:73–79.

33. Burman P, Broman JE, Helta J, et al. Quality of life in adults with growth hormone deficiency response to treatment with recombinant human GH in a placebo controlled 21 months trial. J. Clin Endocrinol Metab 1995;80:3585–90.

34. Deijen JB Vander Veen EA. The influence of growth hormone deficiency and GH replacement on quality of life in GH deficient patients. J Endocrinol Invest 1999;22 (Suppl. 5):127–36.

35. Sheldon WR Jr, De Bold CR, Evans WS, et al. Hypothalamic releasing hormones as combined anterior pituitary function test in normal subjects. J Clin Endocrinal Metab 1985;10:623–30.

36. NIH consensus Development Panel on Rehabilitation of persons with Traumatic Brain Injury: JAMA 1999;282:974–83.

37. Joete U, Endtz LJ. Traumatic disorders of pituitary hypothalamic function. Excretion of follicular stimulating hormone after closed head injury. A preliminary investigation. Applied Neurophysiology 1995;38:110–4.

38. Wang C, Alexander G, Berman N, et al. Testosterone replacement therapy improve mood in hypogonadal mena clinical research center study. J Clin Endocrinol Metab 1996;81:3578–83.

39. Wang C, Eyre DR, Clark R, et al. Sublingual testosterone replacement improves muscle mass and strength, decreases bone resoption and increases bone formation markers in hypogonadal men—a clinical research center study. J Clin Endocrinol Metab 1996;81:3654–66.

40. Amor M, Hasse J, Holmegard SN, et al. Cerebral salt wasting syndrome and syndrome of inappropriate antidiuretic hormone secretion in SAH caused by ruptured berry aneurysm. Pan Arb J Neurosurg 2000;4:25–31.

41. Weinand ME, Baynick PL, Goetz KL. A study of serum ADH and atrial natriuretic peptide level in a series of patients with intracranial disease and hyponatremia. Neurosurgery 1990;25:781–5.

42. Ganong CA, Kappy MS. Cerebral salt wasting in children. The need for recognition and treatment. Ame J Dis Child 1993;147:167–9.

43. Simma B, Burger R, Falk M, et al. A prospective randomized and controlled study of fluid electrolyte management in children with severe head injury: Lactated Ringers solution vs hypertonic saline. Crit Care Med 1998;26:1265–70.

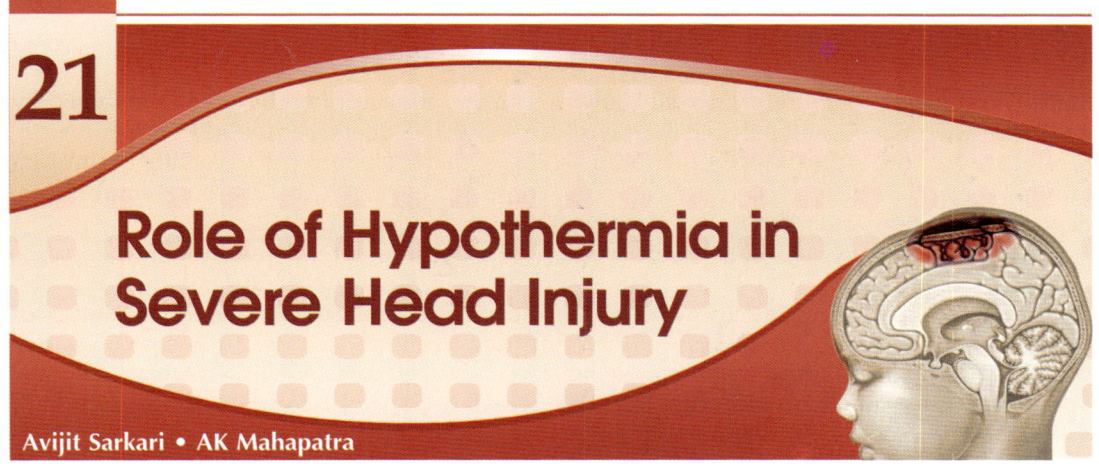

21

Role of Hypothermia in Severe Head Injury

Avijit Sarkari • AK Mahapatra

INTRODUCTION

Therapeutic hypothermia (TH) has been evaluated as a neuroprotective modality in cases of traumatic brain injury (TBI) by several researchers. From a historical perspective, the possibility that hypothermia provides neuroprotection in brain injury was first suggested in 1930s, when successful resuscitation following prolonged cold water asphyxia was reported.[1,2] Fay, in 1943, published the first report of using hypothermia as a treatment modality in patients with severe brain injury.[3] Since then, several authors have reported the potential therapeutic benefits of hypothermia in acute neurological injuries.[4-8]

Treatment of TBI has traditionally focussed on restoring and maintaining adequate brain perfusion, surgically evacuating large hematomas, whenever necessary, and preventing or promptly treating raised intracranial pressure (ICP).[9] The use of hypothermia in patients with TBI may have beneficial effects in both ICP reduction and possible neuroprotection.[10]

PATHOPHYSIOLOGY

TBI is a complex pathophysiological entity which can be described as two types pathologically: Primary and secondary brain injury. The primary brain injury is the physical damage to parenchyma (tissue, vessels) that occurs during traumatic event, resulting in shearing and compression of the surrounding brain tissue. The secondary brain injury is the result of a complex cascade of processes ensuing at the cellular level, beginning from minutes to hours after the primary injury and continuing for up to 72 hours or even longer. Thus, there may be a window of opportunity of several hours, or even days, during which injury can be lessened by various treatments, one of such is hypothermia.[9] Ischemia has a key role in all forms of brain injury and preventing ischemic or secondary injury is the basis of most neuroprotective strategies.[9] Results in animal studies have provided convincing evidence that if body or brain temperature is lowered during a brief period of transient cerebral ischemia, infarct size in brain is smaller as compared to that in normothermic or hyperthermic animals.[11-13]

The effects of systemic hypothermia (30 to 36°C) following fluid percussion brain injury in rats were first investigated by Clifton et al,[14] who showed that hypothermia of 33°C decreased mortality rates and reduced deficits in motor function and weight loss in experimental animals as compared with normothermia. Dietrich et al[15] demonstrated that post-traumatic hypothermia (30°C) initiated 5 minutes after fluid percussion brain injury reduced overall contusion volume and preserved survival of the overlying cortical neurons. Hence these studies concluded that hypothermia after a TBI provided histological/cellular protection, improved motor and cognitive function, and reduced mortality. Moderate hypothermia (30°C) initiated 5 minutes after TBI improved hippocampal-dependent learning and memory.[16] Traumatic axonal pathology, which is an important predictor of outcome in TBI patients, is attenuated with moderate hypothermia therapy.[17] Therefore, post-traumatic hypothermia modulates the major pathologies in TBI such as contusions, neuronal vulnerability, and traumatic axonal injury. As hypothermia modulates multiple pathways, it may have advantages over unipolar pharmacological attempts to provide neurological protection. The mechanisms through which this neuroprotection (Table 21.1) is achieved are elucidated below:

Effect on Blood–Brain Barrier

Alterations in blood–brain barrier (BBB) permeability after acute injury result in the crossing of water, electrolytes, blood-borne substances, and potential neurotoxic agents across the vascular system and into the brain parenchyma. Hypothermia has been found to significantly decrease the brain edema, after the focal cerebral ischemia.[18–20] One study demonstrated that mild hypothermia reduced extravasation of the protein tracer horseradish peroxidase.[21] Hypothermia may be attenuating BBB permeability by altering matrix metalloproteinases, (MMP, *refer* to Chapter 6), which are critical extracellular enzymes that can disrupt the BBB.[22] These modulating effects of hypothermia on BBB permeability are important in reducing the adverse post-injury outcomes.

Effect on Brain Metabolism

An important mechanism for the neuroprotective effect of hypothermia is a reduction or delay in metabolic demand during and after an acute CNS injury. Hypothermia lowers metabolic and energy demands, having potentially beneficial effects on cytoplasmic ATP and the maintenance of normal transmembrane ion and neurotransmitter gradients.

Oxygen consumption by brain is reduced by 5% per 1°C decrease in body temperature.[23] Slow metabolism reduces lactate accumulation. For every 1°C decrease in temperature, the pH increases by 0.016.[24]

Hypothermia has been shown to decrease need for glucose utilization compared with normothermia by using local measures of glucose metabolism with 2-deoxyglucose techniques,[25] and by using nuclear magnetic resonance spectroscopy.[26] The magnitude of preservation of ATP levels depends on both the temperature reduction and the severity of the injury.

Reduction in Inflammation and Edema

Hypothermia modulates the inflammatory response after TBI in a number of ways. It reduces leukocyte margination at the site of injury. It also reduces the endogenous inflammatory response of the central nervous system (CNS) by significantly decreasing the activation of both astrocytes and microglia.[27,28] **Hypothermia reduces tissue levels of reactive oxygen species such as superoxide, nitric oxide, and the hydroxyl radical.[29,30] Superoxide dismutase, the enzyme responsible for scavenging superoxide, is increased by hypothermia,[31] and nitric oxide synthase, the enzyme responsible for synthesizing nitric oxide, is reduced by hypothermia.[32]**

Effect on Neurotransmitters in Brain

Following TBI, the neurons become vulnerable to the excitotoxic effects of various neurotransmitters that are released (Table 21.1). Hypothermia reduces the levels of exicitatory neurotransmitters, thus decreasing seizure activity following head injury.[33] Globus et al[29] showed that intra-ischemic hypothermia (33°C and 30°C) attenuated the rise in extracellular levels of glutamate and dopamine after global cerebral ischemia. Lyeth et al[34] showed that hypothermia (30°C) reduced elevations in cerebrospinal levels of acetylcholine after TBI. Conversely, hypothermia delayed decreases in dopamine, norepinephrine, and serotonin after global cerebral ischemia.[35] Pharmaco-

Table 21.1: Mechanism of beneficial effects of hypothermia in brain injury

Secondary injury	Time after primary injury	Effect of hypothermia
• Release of excitatory neurotransmitters and kinase system activation	Minutes to hours	Reduces excitability and seizure activity
• Microthrombus formation	Minutes to days	Reduces thrombus formation
• Proinflammatory cytokines secretion	Minutes to days	Decreased proinflammatory mediators
• BBB disruption, capillary leakage	Hours to days	Decreased BBB permeability
• Free radical damage	Hours to days	Decreased
• Reperfusion injury	Hours to days	Decreased
• Mitochondrial dysfunction	Hours to days	Decreased
• Apoptosis	Days to weeks	Prevents apoptosis

logical treatments that reduce excitotoxicity further improve outcome in combination with hypothermia[36] and may be a promising strategy for future research. The glutamatergic receptors, AMPA (alpha-amino-3-hydroxyl-5-methyl-4-isoxazole-propionate) and NMDA (*N*-methyl-*D*-aspartate), are also modulated by hypothermia. Expression of hippocampal glutamate receptors is decreased after transient global ischemia and this is completely blocked by hypothermia.[37]

Cerebrovascular Effects

Cerebrovascular changes secondary to cooling the brain are important because changes in blood flow can have adverse effects on tissue survival and functional outcome. However, there are conflicting reports regarding the effects of hypothermia on cerebral blood flow. Rosomoff and Holaday[38] demonstrated that systemic hypothermia to 25°C significantly lowered cerebral blood flow. However, in a model of selective brain cooling (30°C), cortical blood flow measured by laser Doppler flowmetry had shown to increase above control levels.[39]

Effect on Intracellular Factors

There are marked changes in calcium-dependent intracellular signaling pathways after CNS injury. Temporary cerebral ischemia inhibits the activity of calcium/calmodulin-dependent protein kinase II (CaMK II), a key protein kinase that mediates synaptic strength.

This is attenuated by hypothermia.[40] Protein kinase C (PKC) translocates to the membrane after cerebral ischemia and undergoes inhibition; hypothermia reduces both translocation and inhibition of PKC.[41]

Hypothermia has also been found to alter transcription factors that participate in normal neuronal functioning. The immediate early gene *c-Fos*, which regulates key genetic responses of neurons, is activated by hypothermia after transient global ischemia.[42] These studies show that temperature changes can have profound effects on events associated with neuronal injury as well as the normal processing of neuronal signals throughout brain circuits.

Effect on Neuronal Cell Death

TBI is linked with not only neuronal necrosis but also apoptotic neuronal cell death. As with necrosis, this apoptotic cell death also seems amenable to prevention by the use of hypothermic strategies. Various genes are shown to be sensitive to post-injury temperature manipulations.[43] This may help in modulating both the acute and the more delayed genetic response to head injury.

Current Guidelines

Currently, the role of hypothermia after global cerebral ischemia associated with cardiac arrest is well established.[9,44] However its clinical efficacy for use in TBI remains speculative. One of the reasons is that because the diagnosis of TBI needs to be confirmed by CT scan, there is a delay in starting temperature reduction strategies. Hence, the results are not as convincing as in the experimental animal models wherein hypothermia commenced soon after injury has shown promising effects. Another reason is that most studies were conducted in severely injured patients only, and not in those with milder forms of head injury because of obvious ethical issues. Also, outcome is confounded by other important variables such as brain injury severity, age, gender, peripheral trauma, and a number of co-existing physiological responses (e.g. pupil size, intracranial pressure). At the time of admission, approximately 10% of patients presenting with TBI are hypothermic.[45] The International TBI data collaboration on modeling prognostic indicators of outcome after TBI (IMPACT)[46] was undertaken from 1982 to 1998. Univariate analysis of 26 predictors for outcome at 6 months was done in 8719 patients. Hypoxia, hypotension, and spontaneous hypothermia were significant prognostic markers of adverse outcome. However, the strength of the association between hypothermia on admission and adverse outcome after TBI was lessened after adjustment for other confounders such as age, GCS, motor score and pupil size and reactivity. Despite the large numbers of patients studied from the IMPACT database, there is still uncertainty about how best to manage body temperature after acute TBI. Guidelines for the best approach to temperature measurement do not exist. Currently the 2007 Brain Trauma Foundation (BTF) recommendations state that there is insufficient data to support the use of therapeutic hypothermia for management of traumatic TBI.[47] A review by Cochrane data group in 2009 made similar recommendations.

Prompted by the promising reports of the neuroprotective effects of hypothermia in brain injury, the Eurotherm3235Trial is being undertaken to provide precise evidence-based guidelines for the use of this modality in TBI.

Eurotherm3235Trial[10]

The Eurotherm3235Trial (European society of intensive care medicine study of therapeutic hypothermia (32–35°C) for intracranial pressure reduction after traumatic brain injury) is a multi-center, multinational, randomized controlled trial, examining the effects of hypothermia 32–35°C, titrated to reduce intracranial pressure < 20 mm Hg, on morbidity and mortality 6 months after TBI. The study aims to recruit 1800 patients over 41 months. The participants are randomized to either standard care or standard care with titrated therapeutic hypothermia. Hypothermia is initiated with 20–30 ml/kg of intravenous, refrigerated 0.9% saline and maintained using each centre's usual cooling techniques. There is a guideline for detection and treatment of shivering in the intervention group. Hypothermia is maintained for at least 48 hours in the treatment group and continued for as long as is necessary to maintain intracranial pressure < 20 mm Hg. The results of the trial are expected to provide a firm basis for the future guidelines for use of hypothermia in TBI.[10]

Methods of Hypothermia Induction

Currently, the optimal induction method is debatable. The ideal induction method is one which is safe, effective, with a sufficiently rapid cooling speed, easy implementation, widespread availability, and low cost. A combination of various modalities may be better suited than a single method alone.

A. *Pharmacological Cooling*

The use of anti-inflammatory drugs (i.e. ibuprofen) or antipyretic drugs (i.e. acetaminophen) for therapeutic hypothermia (TH) has been shown to cause only a modest reduction in temperature, and therefore, is insufficient alone to produce clinically significant hypothermia.

B. *Surface Cooling*

The various surface cooling techniques that have been studied are—water-circulating

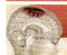
cooling blankets, ice-packs, water mattresses, ice-water and alcohol baths, whole body ice rubs, electric cooling fans, and/or forced air cooling. It is easy to implement, but induces severe shivering which may require heavy sedation and/or paralysis with neuromuscular blockade. In addition, it is difficult to maintain body temperature at a desired level. Overcooling can occur. However, an active surface cooling device with a feedback mechanism to actively regulate the body temperature has been developed. This device uses the Arctic Sun Temperature Management System (Medivance, Louisville, CO, USA), and was more effective than conventional surface cooling methods, for controlling fever in critically ill neurologic patients (Fig . 21.1).[48] The arctic sun has been explained as dry water immersion. It is a non-invasive method to induce hypothermia in comatose patients following sudden cardiac arrest (SCA) and patients at risk for brain damage. The arc sun uses gel pads, which stike to patients body using hydrogel (which adheses to the skin without removing hairs). Water circulates through there pads at a temperature between 4°–42°C. Cost of the disposable cooling pads is the main limitation of this device.

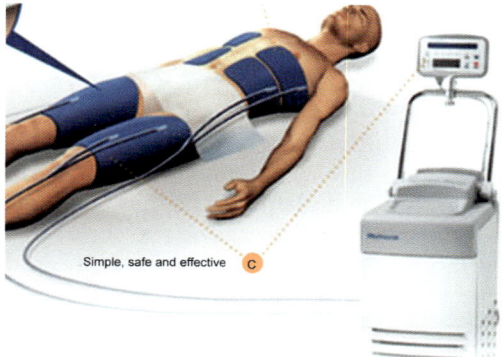

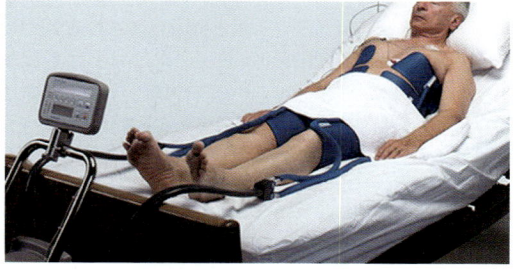

Fig. 21.1: Arctic sun pads, its application over body

C. Nasal Spray Coolant

Recently, a liquid coolant–oxygen mixture has been introduced to be used as a nasal spray. This rapidly evaporates with high-flow oxygen and results in significant cooling of the nasal passages and brain. However, some device-related adverse effects such as nasal whitening, epistaxis, and periorbital emphysema have been reported.[49]

D. Endovascular Cooling

This includes intravenous ice-cold saline infusion into peripheral or central veins, and active cooling catheters intra-arterially or intravenously. The average time to achieve the target temperature is much less with the use of intravenous cooling (~70 minutes) as compared to that with surface cooling (3–8 hours).[50] Another advantage is that since no surface equipment like cooling pads are required, surface counter-warming can be instituted which helps in attenuating the shivering response of the body, thus helping in a more efficient cooling of the core blood volume.

Being an invasive technique, the endovascular cooling carries the risks of infection and deep vein thrombosis (DVT). Patients may need close monitoring with duplex ultrasonography for DVT. Also, the technique requires greater technical skill.

E. Epidural Cooling

This is a novel technique that causes selective brain hypothermia. Studies suggest that with this technique, the target temperature is rapidly attained, easily controlled, and maintained for a long period of time, without altering the normal body temperature and hemodynamic stability.[51,52]

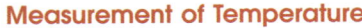

Measurement of Temperature

The accurate measurement of core temperature is of prime importance in treatment protocols using TH. Deep or 'core' body temperature[53] refers to that of the tissues deep within the skull or the thoracic and abdominal cavities. This is regulated mainly by the hypothalamus in the brain, which responds to input from thermoreceptors located centrally in the body core and peripherally in the skin. Various probes used to measure core temperature are as follows:[53,54]

I. Body Probes

The pulmonary artery is considered to be the 'gold standard' measurement site for core body temperature.[53] However, this site is rarely used due to practical considerations. Rectal temperature measurement is most commonly employed to assess core temperature. Others are bladder, esophageal and vaginal probes. Clinical infrared thermometers measuring temperature of tympanic membrane and temporal artery have also been used. The Deep Body Thermometer (DBT), first developed by Fox and Solman (1971),[54] is based on the 'zero heat flow' principle which states that if heat loss from the surface of the body is reduced to zero, the gradient between core and surface temperature will also tend towards zero. When equilibrium has been reached there should be a region of tissue below the surface which will be at a uniform temperature. The DBT achieves the zero heat flow condition by heating the skin surface such that outward heat flow from the core is matched by inward heat flow from the surface.

However, core body temperature does not always accurately predict brain temperature. Also, the body type sensors used to measure core temperature are susceptible to changes in their measurements caused by inadvertent position changes.[55]

II. Brain Probes

Various brain sensors are available which measure brain tissue temperature, directly and accurately, but they are invasive and expensive.[55]

III. Newer Non-invasive Methods

In recent years, newer non-invasive and accurate techniques to measure core temperature have been developed. One such technique is proton magnetic resonance spectroscopy that can be utilized for measuring absolute internal temperature.[56]

Early vs Delayed Cooling

Reaching the optimal level of cooling in the therapeutic window can have a significant impact on the outcome. It has been found that the best chance of neurological recovery is achieved when TH is induced within 15 minutes of ischemia initiation.[57] Early intra-ischemia cooling induction is supposed to modify ischemia-induced as well as post-reperfusion cellular abnormalities, but delayed TH induction is thought to target only the post-reperfusion cell death and inflammatory signaling pathways.[58] It has been suggested that ice-cold saline may be used for cooling before arriving at the hospital, where subsequently classical intravenous cooling can be started.[59]

Level of Hypothermia (Grading of Hypothermia)

Hypothermia can be classified based on the depth of cooling as follows:

- Normal body temperature = 37–38°C
- Mild hypothermia = 32–35°C
- Moderate hypothermia = 28–32°C
- Deep hypothermia < 28°C

Mild hypothermia seems to be sufficient enough for attaining the maximum neuroprotection possible while at the same time minimizing the side effects of TH. Studies have reported that there is no clinical benefit in cooling the patient below 35°C.[60,61]

Duration of Hypothermia

Cooling maintained for more than 48 hours, with gradual rewarming at a rate of 1°C per

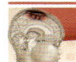

day, has been found to be associated with improved neurological outcome.[62]

Adverse Effects of TH (Table 21.2)

I. Shivering

This is the homeostatic mechanism which the body develops to counteract hypothermia. Shivering can lead to increased oxygen consumption of up to 40–100%, and can lead to detrimental effects in these patients. It can be controlled by sedatives, anaesthetic agents, opiates, and paralyzing agents. Since younger patients react to hypothermia earlier and with greater intensity of shivering, they require higher doses of these drugs to neutralize this counter-regulatory mechanism.[63]

II. Infection

Since leukocyte count and action decline due to hypothermia, there are increased risk of infection, the commonest being pneumonia. It occurs frequently in proportion to the duration and degree of hypothermia.[58]

III. Haemodynamic Instability

Bradycardia is the commonest cardiovascular effect, but is tolerated well. Hypotension and cardiac arrhythmias can occur. However, the risk of arrhythmias is substantial only when temperature is below 30°C.[64]

IV. Electrolyte Imbalance

Hypernatremia may be due to cold-induced diabetes insipidus (DI), or due to DI occurring as a direct effect of trauma. Hypokalemia, hypomagnesemia and hypophosphatemia can also occur and require appropriate monitoring and correction. The opposite imbalances can occur in rewarming.[58,65]

V. Thrombocytopenia

Though there is a tendency towards low platelet count, hypothermia in severe TBI did not show a significant difference in the coagulation parameters as compared to the normothermic patients.[65]

Table 21.2: Possible adverse effects of hypothermia

1. Infection
2. Electrolyte disturbances
3. Bradycardia
4. Hypotension
5. Cardiac arrhythmias
6. Decreased platelet count

Subsequent Rewarming

Most patients have a tendency to become hyperthermic with rebound rise in intracranial pressure in the rewarming phase.[58] Rewarming after hypothermia should be done slowly and in a controlled manner. During rewarming, the possiblility of mismatch between total body O_2 demand (VO_2) and oxygen delivery (DO_2) has been recognised. This rewarming shock is described as syndrome of acute acidosis characterised by decline in blood pH associated with respiratory inadequacy.[66] Hypotension and tachycardia are often present. Many alterations in cardiovascular system are completely reversed during rewarming.[66]

CONCLUSIONS

Hypothermia has a strong potential to become a valuable neuroprotective therapy in TBI. There is a need to determine the optimal parameters for its use in TBI. It is likely that a combination of various neuroprotective strategies, both invasive and non-invasive, will lead to a better outcome. Hence, TH induction to cool the deep brain structures appears to be a promising strategy to be used as a part of multimodal treatment strategies in the management of head injury.

REFERENCES

1. Gunn A, Thoresen M. Hypothermic neuro-protection. NeuroRx 2006;3:154–69.
2. Linares G, Mayer SA. Hypothermia for the treatment of ischemic and hemorrhagic stroke. Crit Care Med 2009;37(Suppl.):S243–9.
3. Fay T. Observations on generalized refrigeration in cases of severe cerebral trauma. Assoc Res Nerv Ment Dis Proc 1943;24:611–9.

4. Metz C, Holzschuh M, Bein T, Woertgen C, Frey A, Frey I, Taeger K, Brawanski A. Moderate hypothermia in patients with severe head injury: cerebral and extracerebral effects. J. Neurosurg 1996;85:533–41.

5. Krieger DW, DeGeorgia MA, Abou-Chebl A, Andrefsky JC, Sila CA, Katzan IL, Mayberg MR, Furlan AJ. Cooling for acute ischemic brain damage (coolaid): an open pilot study of induced hypothermia in acute ischemic stroke. Stroke 2001;32:1847–54.

6. Schwab S, Georgiadis D, Berrouschot J, Schellinger PD, Graffagnino C, Mayer SA. Feasibility and safety of moderate hypothermia after massive hemispheric infarction. Stroke 2001;32:2033–5.

7. Polderman KH. Keeping a cool head : how to induce and maintain hypothermia? Crit. Care Med 2004;32:2558–60.

8. Kollmar R, Schellinger PD, Steigleder T, Kohrmann M, Schwab S. Ice-cold saline for the induction of mild hypothermia in patients with acute ischemic stroke: a pilot study. Stroke 2009;40:1907–9.

9. Polderman KH: Induced hypothermia and fever control for prevention and treatment of neurological injuries. Lancet 2008;371:1955–69.

10. Sinclairs HL, Andrews PJD. Bench-to-bedside review: Hypothermia in traumatic brain injury. Crit Care 2010;14:204–13.

11. Busto R, Dietrich WD, Globus M, Scheinberg P, Ginsberg MD. Small differences in intraischemic brain temperature criti-cally determine the extent of ischaemic neuronal injury. J. Cereb. Blood Flow Metab 1987;7:729–38.

12. Kim Y, Busto R, Dietrich WD, Kraydieh S, Ginsberg MD. Delayed postischaemic hyper-thermia in awake rats worsens the histopatho-logical outcome of transient focal ischaemia. Stroke 1996;27:2274–81.

13. Yanamoto H, Nagata I, Nakahara I, Tohnai N, Zhang Z, Kikuchi H. Combination of intrais-chaemic and postischaemic hypothermia provides potent and persistent neuroprotection against temporary focal ischaemia in rats. Stroke 1999;30:2720–6.

14. Clifton GL, Jiang JY, Lyeth BG, Jenkins LW, Hamm RJ, Hayes RL. Marked protection by moderate hypothermia after experimental traumatic brain injury. J Cereb Blood Flow Metab 1991;11:114–21.

15. Dietrich WD, Alonso O, Busto R, Globus MY, Ginsberg MD. Post-traumatic brain hypothermia reduces histopathological damage following concussive brain injury in the rat. Acta Neuropathol 1994;87:250–8.

16. Bramlett HM, Green EJ, Dietrich WD, Busto R, Globus MY, Ginsberg MD. Posttraumatic brain hypothermia provides protection from sensorimotor and cognitive behavioral deficits. J Neurotrauma 1995;12:289–98.

17. Koizumi H, Fujisawa H, Ito H, Maekawa T, Di X, Bullock R. Effects of mild hypothermia on cerebral blood flow-independent changes in cortical extracellular levels of amino acids following contusion trauma in the rat. Brain Res 1997;747:304–12.

18. Kawai N, Nakamura T, Nagao S. Effects of brain hypothermia on brain edema formation after intracerebral hemorrhage in rats. Acta Neurochir Suppl 2002;81:233–5.

19. Mancuso A, Derugin N, Hara K, Sharp FR, Weinstein PR. Mild hypothermia decreases the incidence of transient ADC reduction detected with diffusion MRI and expression of c-fos and hsp70 mRNA during acute focal ischemia in rats. Brain Res 2000;887:34–45.

20. Park CK, Jun SS, Kim MC, Kang JK. Effects of systemic hypothermia and selective brain cooling on ischemic brain damage and swelling. Acta Neurochir Suppl 1998;71:225–8.

21. Dietrich WD, Busto R, Halley M, Valdes I. The importance of brain temperature in alterations of the blood–brain barrier following cerebral ischemia. J Neuropathol Exp Neurol 1990; 49:486–97.

22. Nagel S, Su Y, Horstmann S, Heiland S, Gardner H, Koziol J, Martinez-Torres FJ, Wagner S. Minocycline and hypothermia for reperfusion injury after focal cerebral ischemia in the rat: eff ects on BBB breakdown and MMP expression in the acute and subacute phase. Brain Res 2008;1188:198–206.

23. Faridar A, Bershad EM, Emiru T, Laizzo PA, Suarez JI, Divani AA. Therapeutic hypothermia in stroke and traumatic brain injury. Fron Neurol 2011;2:Art80.

24. Varon J, Acosta P. Therapeutic hypothermia: past, present, and future. Chest 2008;133:1267–74.

25. Tohyama Y, Sako K, Yonemasu Y. Hypothermia attenuates hyperglycolysis in the periphery of ischemic core in rat brain. Exp Brain Res 1998;122:333–8.

26. Lo EH, Steinberg GK, Panahian N, Maidment NT, Newcomb R. Profiles of extracellular amino

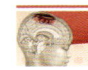
acid changes in focal cerebral ischaemia: effects of mild hypothermia. Neurol Res 1993;15:281–7.

27. Kinoshita K, Chatzipanteli K, Alonso OF, Howard M, Dietrich WD. The effect of brain temperature on hemoglobin extravasation after traumatic brain injury. J Neurosurg 2002;97:945–53.

28. Vitarbo EA, Chatzipanteli K, Kinoshita K, Truettner JS, Alonso OF, Dietrich WD. Tumor necrosis factor alpha expression and protein levels after fluid percussion injury in rats: the effect of injury severity and brain temperature. Neurosurgery 2004;55:416–24.

29. Globus MY, Alonso O, Dietrich WD, Busto R, Ginsberg MD. Glutamate release and free radical production following brain injury: eff ects of posttraumatic hypothermia. J Neurochem 1995;65:1704–11.

30. Sakamoto KI, Fujisawa H, Koizumi H, Tsuchida E, Ito H, Sadamitsu D, Maekawa T. Effects of mild hypothermia on nitric oxide synthesis following contusion trauma in the rat. J Neurotrauma 1997;14:349–53.

31. DeKosky ST, Abrahamson EE, Taff e KM, Dixon CE, Kochanek PM, Ikonomovic MD. Effects of post-injury hypothermia and nerve growth factor infusion on antioxidant enzyme activity in the rat: implications for clinical therapies. J Neurochem 2004;90:998–1004.

32. Van Hemelrijck A, Hachimi-Idrissi S, Sarre S, Ebinger G, Michotte Y. Post-ischaemic mild hypothermia inhibits apoptosis in the penumbral region by reducing neuronal nitric oxide synthase activity and thereby preventing endothelin-1-induced hydroxyl radical formation. Eur J Neurosci 2005;22:1327–37.

33. Mitani A, Kataoka K. Critical levels of extracellular glutamate mediating gerbil hippocampal delayed neuronal death during hypothermia: brain microdialysis study. Neuroscience 1991;42:661–70.

34. Lyeth BG, Jiang JY, Robinson SE, Guo H, Jenkins LW. Hypothermia blunts acetylcholine increase in CSF of traumatically brain injured rats. Mol Chem Neuropathol 1993;18:247–56.

35. Zhang H, Zhou M, Zhang J, Mei Y, Sun S, Tong E. Therapeutic effect of post-ischemic hypothermia duration on cerebral ischemic injury. Neurol Res 2008;30:332–6.

36. Zhu H, Meloni BP, Bojarski C, Knuckey MW, Knuckey NW. Post-ischemic modest hypothermia (35°C) combined with intravenous magnesium is more eff ective at reducing CA1 neuronal death than either treatment used alone following global cerebral ischemia in rats. Exp Neurol 2005;193:361–8.

37. Friedman LK, Ginsberg MD, Belayev L, Busto R, Alonso OF, Lin B, Globus MY. Intraischemic but not postischemic hypothermia prevents non-selective hippocampal downregulation of AMPA and NMDA receptor gene expression after global ischemia. Brain Res Mol Brain Res 2001;86:34–47.

38. Rosomoff HL, Holaday DA. Cerebral blood flow and cerebral oxygen consumption during hypothermia. Am J Physiol 1954;179:85–88.

39. Kuluz JW, Prado R, Chang J, Ginsberg MD, Schleien CL, Busto R. Selective brain cooling increases cortical cerebral blood flow in rats. Am J Physiol 1993;265:H824–7.

40. Hu BR, Kamme F, Wieloch T. Alterations of Ca^{2+}/calmodulin-dependent protein kinase II and its messenger RNA in the rat hippocampus following normo- and hypothermic ischemia. Neuroscience 1995;68:1003–16.

41. Shimohata T, Zhao H, Steinberg GK. Epsilon PKC may contribute to the protective effect of hypothermia in a rat focal cerebral ischemia model. Stroke 2007;38:375–80.

42. Akaji K, Suga S, Fujino T, Mayanagi K, Inamasu J, Horiguchi T, Sato S, Kawase T. Effect of intra-ischemic hypothermia on the expression of *c-Fos* and *c-Jun*, and DNA binding activity of AP-1 after focal cerebral ischemia in rat brain. Brain Res 2003;975:149–57.

43. Gressens P, Dingley J, Plaisant F, Porter H, Schwendimann L, Verney C, Tooley J, Thoresen M. Analysis of neuronal, glial, endothelial, axonal and apoptotic markers following moderate therapeutic hypothermia and anesthesia in the developing piglet brain. Brain Pathol 2008;18:10–20.

44. American Heart Association: Guidelines for CPR and ECC. Part 7.5 Post-resuscitation support. Circulation 2005;112 (24 Suppl) IV:84–88.

45. McHugh GS, Butcher I, Steyerberg EW, Lu J, Mushkudiani N, Marmarou A, Maas AIR, Murray GD. Statistical approaches to the univariate prognostic analysis of the IMPACT database on traumatic brain injury. J Neurotrauma 2007;24:251–8.

46. Maas AIR, Marmarou A, Murray GD, Teasdale TW, Steyerberg EW. Prognosis and clinical trial design in traumatic brain injury: the IMPACT study. J. Neurotrauma 2007;24:232–8.

47. Bullock RM, Povlishock JT. Guidelines for the management of severe traumatic brain injury. Brain trauma foundation guidelines. J. Neurotruma 2007; 24(Suppl. 1): S1–6.

48. Mayer SA, Kowalski RG, Presciutti M, Ostapkovich ND, McGann E, Fitzsimmons BF, Yavagal DR, Du YE, Naidech AM, Janjua NA, Claassen J, Kreiter KT, Parra A, Commichau C. Clinical trial of a novel surface cooling system for fever control in neurocritical care patients. Crit Care Med 2004;32:2508–15.

49. Castren M, Nordberg P, Svensson L, Taccone F, Vincent JL, Desruelles D, Eichwede F, Mols P, Schwab T, Vergnion M, Storm C, Pesenti A, PachlJ, Guérisse F, Elste T, Roessler M, Fritz H, Durnez P, Busch HJ, Inderbitzen B, Barbut D. Intra-arrest transnasal evaporative cooling : a randomized, prehospital, multicenter study (PRINCE: Pre-ROSC IntraNasal Cooling Effectiveness). Circulation 2010;122:729–36.

50. Keller E, Imhof HG, Gasser S, Terzic A, Yonekawa Y. Endovascular cooling with heat exchange catheters : a new method to induce and maintain hypothermia. Intensive Care Med 2003; 29:939–43.

51. Qiu W, Shen H, Zhang Y, Wang W, Liu W, Jiang Q, Luo M, Manou M. Noninvasive selective brain cooling by head and neck cooling is protective in severe traumatic brain injury. J. Clin. Neurosci 2006;13:995–1000.

52. Cheng H, Shi J, Zhang L, Zhang Q, Yin H, Wang L. Epidural cooling for selective brain hypothermia in porcine model. Acta Neuro-chirurgica 2006;148:559–64.

53. Fulbrook P. Core body temperature measurement: a comparison of axilla, tympanic membrane and pulmonary artery blood temperature. Intensive and Critical Care Nursing 1997;13:266–72.

54. Fox RH, Solman AJ, Isaacs R, Fry AJ, MacDonald IC.A new method for monitoring deep body temperature from the skin surface. Clin Sci 1973;44:81–86.

55. Childs C, Machin G. Reliability issues in human brain temperature measurement. Crit Care. 2009;13:R106 (doi:10.1186/cc7943).

56. Childs C, Hiltunen Y, Patankar T, Kauppinen R. Determination of regional brain temperature using proton magnetic resonance spectroscopy to determine brain-body temperature differences in healthy human subjects. Magn Reson Med 2007;57:59–66.

57. Kim F, Olsufka M, Nichol G, Copass MK, Cobb LA. The use of prehospital mild hypothermia after resuscitation from out of hospital cardiac arrest. J Neurotrauma 2009;26:359–63.

58. Lampe JW, Becker LB. State of the art in therapeutic hypothermia. Annu Rev Med 2011;62:79–93.

59. Clifton GL, Valadka A, Zygun D, Coffey CS, Drever P, Fourwinds S, Janis LS, Wilde E, Taylor P, Harshman K. Very early hypothermia induction in patients with severe brain injury (the National Acute Brain Injury Study: Hypothermia II): a randomised trial. Lancet Neurol 2011;10:131–9.

60. Shiozaki T, Nakajima Y, Taneda M, Tasaki O, Inoue Y, Ikegawa H, Matsushima A, Tanaka H, Shimazu T, Sugimoto H. Efficacy of moderate hypothermia in patients with severe head injury and intracranial hypertension refractory to mild hypothermia. J. Neurosurg 2003;99:47–51.

61. Tokutomi T, Miyagi T, Takeuchi Y, Karukaya T, Katsuki H, Shigemori M. Effect of 35% C hypothermia on intracranial pressure and clinical outcome in patients with severe traumatic brain injury. J Trauma 2009;66:166–8.

62. Peterson K, Carson S, Cairney N. Hypothermia treatment for traumatic brain injury: a systematic review and meta-analysis. J Neurotrauma 2008;25:62–65.

63. Polderman KH, Rijnsburger ER, Peerdeman SM, Girbes AR. Induction of hypothermia in patients with various types of neurologic injury with the use of large volumes of ice-cold intravenous fluid. Crit Care Med 2005;33:2744–51.

64. Wienberg AD. Hypothermia. Ann Emerg Med 1993;22:370–7.

65. Tokutomi T, Miyagi T, Morimoto K, Karukaya T, Shigemori, M. Effect of hypothermia on serum electrolyte, inflammation, coagulation and nutritional parameters in patients with severe traumatic brain injury. Neurocrit. Care 2004; 1:171–82.

66. Bigelow WC: Methods for inducing hypothermia and rewarming. Ann NY Acad Sci 1959;80:522–32.

22

Hypertonic Saline in Head Injury

Avijit Sarkari • AK Mahapatra

INTRODUCTION

Head injury is a complex clinical entity with a multifaceted pathophysiology, and its adequate management poses unique challenges to the neurointensive care unit specialists. The primary brain injury occurs at the time of the impact; however, this leads to the development of brain edema, increase in intracranial pressure (ICP), a decrease in cerebral perfusion pressure (CPP), cerebral hypoxia and secondary brain injury. Disruption of this vicious cycle of events is the basis of treatment in head injury. Osmotherapy has gained importance as a tool for decreasing cerebral edema and controlling intracranial hypertension, and contributes in improving the overall outcome after head injury. Among the treatment options available for the management of raised ICP, mannitol has been the traditional, predominant osmotherapeutic agent in use; however, researchers have explored other promising agents as substitutes for mannitol, the most promising of which is hypertonic saline (HTS).

Reflection Coefficient

The reflection coefficient of a substance is the osmotic gradient or tonicity that it creates. It depends upon its permeability across the blood–brain barrier (BBB). It can range from 0 for substances that can diffuse freely across the BBB, to 1.0 for those that cannot cross the BBB at all.[1,2]

Historical Perspective

Many osmotherapeutic substances have been tried and tested in head injury patients in the past. Some of them are—urea, glycerol, sorbitol, mannitol, hypertonic saline.

Urea was the first agent to be used clinically as an osmotic agent.[3–7] But its use was precluded by intolerable systemic side effects such as nausea, vomiting, diarrhea, hemoglobinuria, coagulopathies, and rebound intracranial hypertension. Also, it has a relative coefficient of only 0.59.[8]

Sorbitol and glycerol have only moderate efficacy as osmotherapeutic agents and cause significant hyperglycemia. Glycerol has a relative coefficient of only 0.48, making it a comparatively weak osmotic agent.[8]

Wise and Chater were the first to use osmotically active polyalcohol mannose called mannitol in 1962.[9] Since then, mannitol has been the traditional agent of choice for lowering intracranial hypertension. It is both safe and effective. It has a long duration of action (4–6 hours), and remains stable in solution form. Its use has been recommended by the Brain Trauma Foundation and the European Brain Injury Consortium as the osmotic drug of choice for head injury patients.[10,11] However, mannitol poses the dangers of severe dehydration and associated systemic hypotension and adverse renal effects, particularly in patients of hypovolemia.

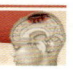

Accumulation of mannitol in brain tissue has been said to cause a rebound effect and raised ICP.

Hypertonic saline as an osmotic agent was first used in animal models by Weed and McKibben in 1919.[12] Shrinkage of brain tissue was found to occur with intravenous saline infusion. Almost 70 years later, Worthley et al in described its use in two patients of intracranial hypertension refractory to mannitol.[13] Since then, several authors have confirmed the therapeutic beneficial effects of HTS in managing intracranial hypertension in head injury.[14–30] The concentration of NaCl used in these reports is variable, ranging from 1.5 to 23.4%.

Mechanism of Action of HTS

The pathophysiology of cerebral edema from injury to the brain and the resultant intracranial hypertension involves a complex inter-relation between disruption of BBB volume of intracranial contents, and cerebral perfusion pressure. The magnitude of flow of fluid from cerebral capillaries into brain parenchyma is determined by the balance of Starling forces (the transcapillary hydrostatic pressure gradient counterbalanced by an osmotic pressure gradient).[31,32] In areas where the BBB is damaged, this balance is lost, facilitating flow of proteins and electrolytes across the membrane and causing vasogenic edema. In accordance with the Monro-Kellie doctrine (for details *refer* to Chapter 4), the consequences of focal or global cerebral edema can be lethal, as it leads to elevated ICP, and compromised cerebral perfusion and oxygenation. This results in ischemic and hypoxic damage to the brain, and causes compression of vital brain structures. HTS works by interrupting this cascade of events by a variety of mechanisms.

a. *Osmotic effect:* Classically, the mechanism of action of HTS has been attributed to the reduction of brain water content through its osmotic effects. HTS creates an osmotic gradient between the intravascular and interstitial compartments, thus causing shrinkage of brain in areas of intact BBB, and lowering ICP. Sodium has a reflection coefficient of 1.0 because of its high polarity and exclusion from the BBB[4,14,33] such that under normal circumstances, sodium needs to be actively transported across the BBB.[34,35] This makes sodium a potent osmotherapeutic agent.

However, this is not the only mechanism of action of HTS. Lescot et al[36] compared edema on CT scans done before and after HTS administration. They noticed that the fall in ICP was equal in those with no decrease in brain volume and in those with decreased brain volume. Also, a number of studies have reported a sustained decrease in ICP even after serum Na levels were such that the osmotic effect should not be active.[19,27] Based on these observations, several additional mechanisms through which HTS acts in head injury have been proposed. These are described below:

b. *Rheological effect:* HTS acts on blood rheology even before its osmotic effect on brain tissue begins. HTS reduces blood viscosity which improves CBF and cerebral oxygenation, causing autoregulatory vasoconstriction, thereby reducing ICP.[37] The measured volume expansion efficiency of HTS is ten times as compared to that of Ringer's lactate solution.[38] HTS also increases cardiac output and mean arterial pressure through both an increase in blood volume and a direct positive inotropic effect.[1,37]

c. *Improvement of blood circulation:* HTS is also thought to induce cerebrovascular endothelial cell shrinkage, causing an increase in vessel diameter and thereby an improvement in blood circulation.[19,25]

d. *Improve circulation:* HTS causes dehydration and reduction in size of erythrocytes, making them more capable of passing through capillaries, thus improving circulation.[39,40]

e. *CSF reduction:* HTS has been reported to cause reduction of CSF production.[41]

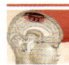

f. *Other functions:* Restoration of the neuronal membrane potential, maintenance of blood–brain barrier integrity, and an immunomodulatory effect whereby HTS attenuates the inflammatory response by decreasing adhesion of leukocytes to endothelium.[42,43]

HTS VS MANNITOL

The ideal osmotic agent is one which does not cross the blood–brain barrier, remains largely in the intravascular compartment and creates a strong osmotic gradient across the endothelium. It is inert and non-toxic, with negligible systemic side effects.[3,6] Out of all the osmotic agents that have been tested in head injury patients, mannitol and HTS are the closest to these properties of an ideal osmotic agent.

Mannitol, like HTS, has a biphasic action curve. Immediate reduction in ICP occurs through changes in blood fluid dynamics or *rheology*, leading to improved CPP and cerebral oxygenation.[44,45] The osmotic effect of mannitol takes around twenty minutes to develop after its administration.[46] Also, mannitol decreases CSF production by up to 50%, and this, in accordance with the Monro-Kellie's doctrine, can cause prolonged ICP decrease.[7]

Theoretically, HTS should be a more effective osmotic agent than mannitol. This is because mannitol has a reflection coefficient of 0.9, as compared to HTS which has a reflection coefficient of 1.0. This allows HTS to create a greater osmotic gradient.

Several clinical studies seem to confirm that HTS is possibly more effective than mannitol for the reduction of ICP.[14,29] Mortazir et al[30] review 36 articles, including ten RCTs (randomized control trials). A greater part of data suggested that HTS given as bolus or continuous infusion can be more effective than mannitol in reducing episodes of elevated ICP. Besides, there are several clinical reports where HTS has been successfully used to treat cases of raised ICP refractory to mannitol.[23,24]

The decline in ICP with HTS is sustained over a longer time period, as compared to mannitol.[25]

Neurological outcome: The results of various studies over this issue are not consistent. Ichai et al[18] showed in their RCT of 34 patients that 1 year GOS scores with HTS were better. In a retrospective study of 67 patients by Yildisdas et al,[26] the HTS group had a lower mortality rate and a lesser duration of comatose state than the mannitol group. However, in the 20 patient RCT by Vialet et al,[24] there was no difference in the mortality rate or the 90 day neurological outcome between the HTS group and the mannitol group.

Studies assessing the effect of mannitol and HTS on brain tissue oxygen tension are limited and inconclusive.[43,47,48]

Advantages of HTS over Mannitol

Adverse effect profile of HTS appears to be less than to that of mannitol.

1. Acute renal failure is a well-known, although rare complication of mannitol use. However, whether HTS is associated with renal failure or not is not clearly established. With mannitol use, a serum osmolality of greater than 320 mOsm/L is linked with renal failure, but an osmolality of up to 365 mOsm/L has been seen to be tolerated by head injury patients in case of HTS.[10,49] Mannitol cannot be used in patients with deranged renal function and renal failure.

2. Mannitol leads to delayed hypovolemia due to osmotic diuresis. This is potentially dangerous in patients of trauma who are commonly hypovolemic. On the other hand, HTS increases mean arterial pressure and blood circulatory volume, and has been found to double the survival of patients with hemorrhagic shock and traumatic brain injury.[50]

3. There are more chances of mannitol crossing the BBB (reflection coefficient 0.9), especially after prolonged use, and of subsequent development of rebound intracranial hypertension.

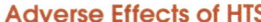
Adverse Effects of HTS

The use of hypertonic saline has been associated with a number of potential adverse effects which are elucidated below:

1. Sudden osmotic load by rapid HTS infusion causes a sudden decline in vascular resistance, leading to sudden hypotension. This is the most common side effect of HTS, and can be avoided by giving the saline solution slowly over 10 to 15 minutes.[51]

2. *Metabolic derangements:* Electrolyte abnormalities can occur during the use of hypertonic saline. When the kidney is presented with a heavy salt load, it responds by retaining bicarbonate and excreting calcium. Consequently, hypokalemia and hypocalcemia ensue, which are managed by appropriate repletion. HTS also causes a decrease in the plasma ion difference, leading to a non-anion gap metabolic acidosis and hyperkalemia. For this, addition of acetate is recommended. Acidosis does not pose a clinical threat except when it is severe and in presence of underlying co-morbid conditions.

3. *Acute renal failure:* The cut-off guideline for safe HTS serum osmolality given by neurotrauma guidelines is the same as that for mannitol, i.e. 320 mOsm/kg[10], although HTS seems to be safe up to an osmolality of 365 mOsm/L. In view of the paucity of nephrotoxicity data of HTS, renal insufficiency may be considered to be a relative contraindication for HTS use.

4. *Rebound intracranial hypertension:* Continuous osmotherapy leads to equalization of the osmotic gradient across the BBB. The total time window of effectiveness of the hyperosmolar agent depends upon the time taken to reach this equilibrium, and is inversely proportional to the degree of BBB damage. Withdrawal of the hyperosmolar agent after such an equilibrium is achieved leads to a reverse osmotic gradient, drawing water into the brain and causing rebound intracranial hypertension. Therefore, utmost care is needed while giving HTS to head injury patients with suspected extensive BBB damage. Some authors are of the view that continuous HTS infusions should be limited to 24–48 hours.[21] Others have suggested that it is even more critical to wean HS slowly, over a period of 24 to 48 hours.[29]

5. *Central pontine myelinosis or osmotic demyelination syndrome (ODS):* It is thought to result from sudden changes in osmotic gradient. There is evidence to suggest that for myelin injury to occur, the degree of rapid change in serum sodium level is much more for a normonatremic patient than a hypernatremic patient—to the order of 40 mEq/L.[6]

6. *Volume overload:* Volume overload and pulmonary edema are potentially dangerous complications that can occur with HTS administration, and in patients with poor cardiopulmonary reserve, it must be used cautiously.

7. *Herniation:* In patients with focal mass lesions, herniation can be precipitated with the use of HTS and mannitol. This is a potentially lethal, albeit understudied complication of HTS. This occurs because decrease in water content occurs more efficiently in the areas adjacent to the focal lesion rather than within the lesion itself, and the local ICP gradient increases, despite the overall fall in ICP.

8. *Phlebitis:* Phlebitis and local tissue damage can occur at the site of infusion of HTS. This can be avoided through proper nursing care. Solutions of greater than 2% saline should be infused through a central venous catheter.

Formulations

Different formulations of hypertonic saline solutions are used in clinical practice for the treatment of cerebral edema. Hypertonic saline solutions of 2, 3, or 7.5% contain equal amounts of sodium chloride and sodium acetate (50:50) to avoid hyperchloremic acidosis. Potassium supplementation (20–40 mEeq/L) is added to the solution as needed.

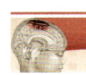
TREATMENT PROTOCOL

At present, there are no appropriate guidelines for HTS use. Indications for use, dosing and timing of use differ among institutions. There is no recommendation on the most optimal concentration, because all concentrations seem to have a favorable effect on ICP. It is logical to presume that it is the serum sodium that finally causes the osmotic effect on the brain. The target serum sodium concentration is 145 to 155 mEq/L (serum osmolality approximately 300–320 mOsm/L). A central venous catheter is used for continuous intravenous infusions at a variable rate to achieve euvolemia or slight hypervolemia (1–2 ml/kg/hr). In cases where a more rapid resuscitation is warranted, a 250 ml bolus of hypertonic saline can be administered carefully. This infusion is continued for 48 to 72 hours until there are signs of clinical improvement or there is a lack of response despite achieving the serum sodium target. Monitoring of serum sodium and potassium is done every 4 to 6 hours during both administration and withdrawal of therapy. Withdrawal of the saline solution infusion must be done with extreme caution to prevent any rebound intracranial hypertension. A careful watch for signs and symptoms of pulmonary edema from congestive heart failure is maintained. Chest radiographs are obtained daily for this purpose, especially in elderly patients with poor cardiovascular reserve.[8]

In cases, refractory to conventional therapies, intravenous bolus injections (30 ml) of 23.4% hypertonic saline have been used, with repetition as per need.[8]

Recommendations for Pediatric Head Injury

HTS has been proposed as an alternative to mannitol in the guidelines for management of pediatric head injury.[52] There are recommendations to use a 3% NaCl continuous infusion from 0.1 to 1.0 ml/kg/hr, given on a sliding scale, allowing a maximum serum osmolality of 365 mOsm/L.[53]

CONCLUSIONS

HTS is a safe and effective alternative to mannitol for use in head injury. In some situations it is even superior to mannitol such as hypovolemia and compromised renal function, which are worsened by mannitol. It has also proved useful for cases refractory to conventional therapy. If the benefits and safety profile of HTS are established by well-controlled trials in the future, it may as well become the first line therapy for raised ICP in head injury.

REFERENCES

1. Qureshi AI, Suarez JI. Use of hypertonic saline solutions in treatment of cerebral edema and intracranial hypertension. Crit Care Med 2000;28:3301–13.
2. Georgiadis AL, Suarez JI. Hypertonic saline for cerebral edema. Curr Neurol Neurosci Rep 2003; 3:524–30.
3. Bhardwaj A, Ulatowski JA. Cerebral edema: hypertonic saline solutions. Curr Treat Options. Neurol 1999;1:179–88.
4. Bhardwaj A, Ulatowski JA. Hypertonic saline solutions in brain injury. Curr Opin Crit Care 2004;10:126–31.
5. Fremont-Smith F, Forbes HS. Intravascular and intracranial pressure: an experimental study. Arch Neurol Psychiatr 1927;18:550–64.
6. Harukuni I, Kirsch J, Bhardwaj A. Cerebral resuscitation: role of osmotherapy. J Anesth 2002;16:229–37.
7. Paczynski RP. Osmotherapy—Basic concepts and controversies. Crit Care Clin 1997;13:105–29.
8. Raslan A, Bhardwaj A. Medical management of cerebral edema. Neurosurg Focus 2007;22 (5):E12.
9. Wise BL, Chater N. The value of hypertonic mannitol solution in decreasing brain mass and lowering cerebrospinal fluid pressure. J Neurosurg 1962;19:1038–43.
10. The Brain Trauma Foundation, The American Association of Neurological Surgeons, The Joint Section on Neurotrauma and Critical Care. Initial management. J Neurotrauma 2000;17:463–9.
11. Maas AI, Dearden M, Teasdale GM, et al. EBIC-guidelines for management of severe head injury

in adults: European Brain Injury Consortium. Acta Neurochir (Wien) 1997;139:286–94.

12. Weed LH, McKibben PS. Experimental alteration of brain bulk. Am J Physiol 1919;48:531–58.

13. Worthley LI, Cooper DJ, Jones N. Treatment of resistant intracranial hypertension with hypertonic saline. Report of two cases. J Neurosurg 1988;68:478–81.

14. Battison C, Andrews PJ, Graham C, Petty T. Randomized, controlled trial on the effect of a 20% mannitol solution and a 7.5% saline/6% dextran solution on increased intracranial pressure after brain injury. Crit Care Med 2005; 33:196–202, 257–8.

15. Berger S, Schwarz M, Huth R. Hypertonic saline solution and decompressive craniectomy for treatment of intracranial hypertension in pediatric severe traumatic brain injury. J Trauma 2002;53:558–63.

16. Einhaus SL, Croce MA, Watridge CB, Lowery R, Fabian TC. The use of hypertonic saline for the treatment of increased intracranial pressure. J Tenn Med Assoc 1996;89:81–82.

17. Harutjunyan L, Holz C, Rieger A, Menzel M, Grond S, Soukup J. Efficiency of 7.2% hypertonic saline hydroxyethyl starch 200/0.5 versus mannitol 15% in the treatment of increased intracranial pressure in neurosurgical patients— a randomized clinical trial [ISRCTN62699180]. Crit Care 2005; 9:R530–40.

18. Ichai C, Armando G, Orban JC, Berthier F, Rami L, Samat-Long C. Sodium lactate versus mannitol in the treatment of intracranial hypertensive episodes in severe traumatic brain-injured patients. Intensive Care Med 2009; 35:471–79.

19. Kerwin AJ, Schinco MA, Tepas JJ III, Renfro WH, Vitarbo EA, Muehlberger M. The use of 23.4% hypertonic saline for the management of elevated intracranial pressure in patients with severe traumatic brain injury: a pilot study. J Trauma 2009;67:277–82.

20. Oddo M, Levine JM, Frangos S, Carrera E, Maloney-Wilensky E, Pascual JL. Effect of mannitol and hypertonic saline on cerebral oxygenation in patients with severe traumatic brain injury and refractory intracranial hypertension. J Neurol Neurosurg Psychiatry 2009;80:916–20.

21. Qureshi AI, Suarez JI, Bhardwaj A. Malignant cerebral edema in patients with hypertensive intracerebral hemorrhage associated with hypertonic saline infusion: a rebound phenomenon? J Neurosurg Anesthesiol 1998;10: 188–92.

22. Saltarini M, Massarutti D, Baldassarre M, Nardi G, De Colle C, Fabris G. Determination of cerebral water content by magnetic resonance imaging after small volume infusion of 18% hypertonic saline solution in a patient with refractory intracranial hypertension. Eur J Emerg Med 2002;9:262–5.

23. Schwarz S, Schwab S, Bertram M, Aschoff A, Hacke W. Effects of hypertonic saline hydroxyethyl starch solution and mannitol in patients with increased intracranial pressure after stroke. Stroke 1998;29:1550–5.

24. Vialet R, Albanèse J, Thomachot L, Antonini F, Bourgouin A, Alliez B, et al. Isovolume hypertonic solutes (sodium chloride or mannitol) in the treatment of refractory posttraumatic intracranial hypertension: 2 ml/kg 7.5% saline is more effective than 2 ml/kg 20% mannitol. Crit Care Med 2003;31:1683–7.

25. Ware ML, Nemani VM, Meeker M, Lee C, Morabito DJ, Manley GT. Effects of 23.4% sodium chloride solution in reducing intracranial pressure in patients with traumatic brain injury: a preliminary study. Neurosurgery 2005;57:727–36.

26. Yildizdas D, Altunbasak S, Celik U, Herguner O. Hypertonic saline treatment in children with cerebral edema. Indian Pediatr 2006;43:771–9.

27. White H, Cook D, Venkatesh B. The use of hypertonic saline for treating intracranial hypertension after traumatic brain injury. Anesth Analg 2006;102:1836–46.

28. Rockswold GL, Solid CA, Paredes-Andrade E, Rockswald SB, Jancik JT, Quickel RR. Hypertonic saline and its effect on intracranial pressure, cerebral perfusion, and brain tissue oxygenation. Neurosurgery 2009;65:1035–41.

29. Ogden AT, Mayer SA, Connolly ES. Hyperosmolar agents in neurosurgical practice: the evolving role of hypertonic saline. Neurosurgery 2005;57:207–15.

30. Mortazavi MM, Romeo AK, Deep A, Griessenauer CJ, Shoja MM, Tubbs RS, Fisher W. Hypertonic saline for treating raised intracranial pressure: literature review with meta-analysis. J Neurosurg 2012;116:210–21.

31. Grande PO, Asgeirsson B, Nordstrom CH. Physiologic principles for volume regulation of a tissue enclosed in a rigid shell with application to the injured brain. J Trauma 1997;42:S23–31.

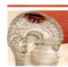

32. Nau R. Osmotherapy for elevated intracranial pressure: a critical reappraisal. Clin Pharmacokinet 2000;38:23–40.

33. Doyle JA, Davis DP, Hoyt DB. The use of hypertonic saline in the treatment of traumatic brain injury. J Trauma 2001;50:367–83.

34. Fishman RA. Blood brain barrier, in Fishman RA (ed): Cerebrospinal Fluid in Diseases of the Nervous System. Philadelphia, WB Saunders 1992;43–69.

35. Swanson PD: Neurological manifestations of hypernatremia, in Vinken PJ, Bruyn GW (eds): Handbook of Clinical Neurology: Metabolic and Deficiency Diseases of the Nervous System. Amsterdam, Elsevier/North-Holland 1976;28 part II:443–61.

36. Lescot T, Degos V, Zouaoui A, Préteux F, Coriat P, Puybasset L. Opposed effects of hypertonic saline on contusions and noncontused brain tissue in patients with severe traumatic brain injury. Crit Care Med 2006;34:3029–33.

37. Tseng MY, Al-Rawi PG, Pickard JD, Rasulo FA, Kirkpatrick PJ. Effect of hypertonic saline on cerebral blood flow in poor-grade patients with subarachnoid hemorrhage stroke 2003;34:1389–96.

38. Kramer GC. Hypertonic resuscitation: Physiologic mechanisms and recommendations for trauma care. J Trauma 2003;54:S89–99.

39. Kempski O, Behmanesh S. Endothelial cell swelling and brain perfusion. J Trauma 1997;42:S38–40.

40. Shackford SR, Schmoker JD, Zhuang J. The effect of hypertonic resuscitation on pial arteriolar tone after brain injury and shock. J Trauma 1994;37:899–908.

41. Forsyth LL, Liu-DeRyke X, Parker D Jr, Rhoney DH. Role of hypertonic saline for the management of intracranial hypertension after stroke and traumatic brain injury. Pharmacotherapy 2008;28:469–84.

42. Cross JS, Gruber DP, Gann S, et al. Hypertonic saline attenuates the hormonal response to injury. Ann Surg 1989;209:684–91; discussions 91–2.

43. Hartl R, Medary MB, Ruge M. Hypertonic/hyperoncotic saline attenuates microcirculatory disturbances after traumatic brain injury. J Trauma 1997;42:S41–7.

44. Burke AM, Quest DO, Chien S, Cerri C. The effects of mannitol on blood viscosity. J Neurosurg 1981;55:550–3.

45. Muizelaar JP, Lutz HA III, Becker DP. Effect of mannitol on ICP and CBF and correlation with pressure autoregulation in severely head-injured patients. J Neurosurg 1984;61:700–6.

46. Jafar JJ, Johns LM, Mullan SF. The effect of mannitol on cerebral blood flow. J Neurosurg 1986;64:754–9.

47. Sakowitz OW, Stover JF, Sarrafzadeh AS, Unterberg AW, Kiening KL. Effects of mannitol bolus administration on intracranial pressure, cerebral extracellular metabolites, and tissue oxygenation in severely head-injured patients. J Trauma 2007;62:292–8.

48. Pascual JL, Maloney-Wilenski E, Reilly PM, Sicoutris C, Keutmann MK, Stein SC, LeRoux PD, Gracias VH. Resuscitation of hypotensive head-injured patients: Is hypertonic saline the answer? Am Surg 2008;74:253–9.

49. Khanna S, Davis D, Peterson B. Use of hypertonic saline in the treatment of severe refractory posttraumatic intracranial hypertension in pediatric traumatic brain injury. Crit Care Med 2000;28:1144–51.

50. Wade CE, Grady JJ, Kramer GC, Younes RN, Gehlsen K, Holcroft JW. Individual patient cohort analysis of the efficacy of hypertonic saline/dextran in patients with traumatic brain injury and hypotension. J Trauma 1997;42 (Suppl 5):S61–65.

51. Wijdicks E, Zubkov AY. Principles of neurocritical care, in Yomans Neurological Surgery. 6th edition, Winn HR (ed), Philadelphia, Elsevier Saunders 2011; p. 435.

52. Carney NA, Chesnut R, Kochanek PM. Guidelines for the acute medical management of severe traumatic brain injury in infants, children, and adolescents. Pediatr Crit Care Med 2003;4:S1.

53. Adelson PD, Bratton SL, Carney NA. Guidelines for the acute medical management of severe traumatic brain injury in infants, children, and adolescents. Chapter 11. Use of hyperosmolar therapy in the management of severe pediatric traumatic brain injury. Pediatr Crit Care Med 2003;4:S40–4.

23

Prognosis after Traumatic Brain Injury

Sumit Sinha • Amandeep Jagdevan • AK Mahapatra

INTRODUCTION

Traumatic brain injury (TBI) is a major cause of death and disability worldwide. About 1.5 million people die every year and several millions affected receive emergency treatment. The prognosis of any medical condition can be defined as an opinion on its likely course, based on medical experience. The prognostication of the clinical course and outcome of patients with TBI is relevant for realistically informing the patient's relatives and friends about the future course of health of patient and for making diagnostic and therapeutic decisions. It can also be used to stratify patients with TBI, into prognostic groups for recruitment in clinical trials.

The estimates of prognosis after severe TBI are grossly ambiguous even today. The proposal of Glasgow Coma Scale (GCS) was the first step towards prognostication of TBI.[1,2] The GCS quantifies the level of consciousness. Though estimating the prognosis is relevant to making clinical decisions, not all clinicians treating TBI appreciate the role of prognosis in decision making. In a survey by Perel P et al, 80% of doctors treating TBI believed accurate prognostication to be important for decision making and only one-third believed that they were accurate in estimating prognosis.[3] The estimation of prognosis, based upon evidence-based analysis of data from a large number of patients, is likely to be more reliable than that derived from physician's own experience. With development of advanced statistical analysis, prognostic statistical models, which combine data from a large number of patients, have been developed, which are more accurate in estimating prognosis.[4] Prognostication cannot be done accurately keeping only one risk factor in mind. For this purpose, multiple risk factors have to be taken into account together and this can be done by using prognostic models.

In this chapter, we will discuss the prognosis of TBI and the various prognostic factors and prognostic models which determine the severity of TBI along with their application and limitations.

MEASURES OF OUTCOME AFTER TBI

The assessment of prognostic factors requires a clinically relevant end point like death or a measure of functional outcome. Death is often used as an endpoint in prognostic analysis; however, outcome measures like Glasgow Outcome Scale (GOS) are also used for this purpose.

Most of the studies on prognostication of TBI have used GOS or death as the end points. GOS was first introduced by Jannett and Bond in 1975.[2] It is an ordinal scale with five categories that assesses the overall outcome of patients (Table 23.1).

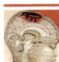

Table 23.1: Glasgow Outcome Scale (GOS)	
Scale	*GOS*
Poor	
1.	Dead
2.	Vegetative state
3.	Severe disability: Able to follow commands/ unable to live independently
Good	
4.	Moderate disability: Able to live independently; unable to return to work or school
5.	Good recovery: Able to return to work or school

The scale is often dichotomized to differentiate two groups with favorable and unfavorable outcome. Favorable outcome includes the categories 'moderate disability' and 'good recovery', while unfavorable outcome includes 'death', 'vegetative state' and 'severe disability'.

I. PROGNOSTIC FACTORS

A. Demographic Factors

1. *Age*

Increasing age is associated with worse outcome in patients with TBI. Several studies in the literature have documented age as an important and strong prognostic factor in patients with TBI.[5–10] The kind of association that patient age and outcome after TBI share remains unclear. In some studies, outcome has been mentioned as a continuous function of age.[10–12] However, there are studies in literature in which authors have reported threshold values of age.[5–7,13–15] Most of the studies have found that younger age is associated with better outcome.[16–19] The reason for poorer outcome in elderly population with TBI could be due to increased number of associated medical complications/ co-morbidities which leads to increased mortality and also because of the limited plasticity of elderly brain and limited regenerative capacity, which contribute to poor functional outcome in surviving patients.[20,21]

In a review of the literature addressing the issue of relationship between patient age and outcome following TBI, Chesnut et al[22] came to the conclusion that increasing age negatively affected outcome in a stepwise manner, with an age threshold of 60 years. Four class I studies have demonstrated that age > 60 years to be a threshold age in patients with severe TBI. The patients above this age have a mortality of more than 75%.[11,17,23,24] CRASH trial researchers reported that relation between age and log odds of death within 14 days showed no association until 40 years of age and a linear increase after 40 years.[25] The identification of different age thresholds by different authors[5–7,10,13–15] can be explained by difference in distribution of age of the patient population included in studies as well as by different statistical methods used in these studies.

Hukkelhoven et al,[26] in a review article analysing 5600 patients, concluded that age is an independent prognostic factor for poor outcome in patients with severe head injury and the association between age and outcome is continuous function while not supporting the existence of a threshold value for age.

So, one can conclude that, despite the controversy over existence of an age threshold that divides patients with severe head injury into good and poor prognostic groups, the role of age as an important and independent prognostic factor in patients with severe TBI has been clearly established.

2. *Gender*

Though males have higher risk of road traffic accidents and assaults leading to TBI, however, there is strong evidence in the literature that no relationship exists between gender and outcome after TBI.[27–32]

B. Clinical Factors

1. *Glasgow Coma Scale*

The Glasgow Coma Score (GCS) was initially developed by Teasdale and Janett[1] in 1974, and since then, it has been widely used in

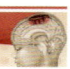

assessment of the severity of traumatic brain injury. In several studies GCS has been shown to have a good inter- and intra-rater reliability across the observers.[5,32] GCS has been shown to have a significant correlation with the outcome of patients with severe traumatic brain injury, both as a sum score[7,8] and including only the motor component.[8,25]

2. Pupillary Reactivity

Pupillary reactivity is an important clinical sign in patients with TBI. Abnormalities of pupillary reaction suggest brainstem compression and indicate poor outcome. Several studies have shown an association between abnormalities of pupillary reactivity and poor outcome.[17,31]

C. Laboratory Parameters

Abnormalities in the laboratory parameters are frequently encountered following TBI, however, the relationship between laboratory parameters and outcome following TBI has not been extensively investigated and laboratory parameters are not yet widely used as prognostic markers in TBI. A strong relationship has been shown by different studies between hyperglycemia, thrombocytopenia, anemia, coagulopathy and poor outcome. Van Beek et al[32] studied the relationship between lab parameters (glucose, sodium pH, Hb, platelet count and prothrombin time) and outcome following TBI from IMPACT database. They found a consistent and continuous relationship between these parameters and outcome. Hyperglycemia and low hemoglobin levels had strongest effect upon outcome. Similarly, hyponatremia was a predictor of poor outcome. However, the effects of treatment of these abnormal parameters on outcome are yet to be studied in detail.

D. Imaging Features

1. Marshall Grading

Marshall et al[33] proposed a CT based classification of TBI based upon the analysis of data from Traumatic Coma Data Bank. Marshall's CT-classification takes into consideration multiple CT characteristics including midline shift, status of basal cisterns, and presence of mass lesions. They identified six groups of patients based upon these features and broadly differentiated patients with mass lesions and diffuse injuries (Table 23.2). This CT-based classification has been widely used as a predictor of outcome in TBI.[22,30,34,35] However, there are certain drawbacks of Marshall's classification. It does not include traumatic subarachnoid hemorrhage and intraventricular hemorrhage into consideration, both of which have been shown to be predictors of outcome and mortality after TBI.[36–40] CT-classification also does not differentiate between different types of mass lesions, EDH has been shown to have a better prognosis than subdural hematoma and intracerebral hemorrhage.[22] Though, CT-classification is a strong predictor of outcome in TBI, individual parameters used in the classification can provide a greater discrimination in comparison to the classification itself.[41]

Table 23.2: CT based classification of TBI	
Category	*Definition*
Diffuse injury I	No visible intracranial pathology seen on CT scan
Diffuse injury II	Cisterns are present with midline shift-5 mm and/or
	• Lesion densities present
	• No high- or mixed-density lesion > 5 cc
	• May include bone fragments and foreign bodies
Diffuse injury III	Cisterns compressed or absent with midline shift –5 mm, no high- or mixed-density lesion > 5 cc
Diffuse injury IV	Midline shift > 5 mm, no high- or mixed-density lesion > 5 cc
Evacuated mass lesion	Any lesion surgically evacuated
Non-evacuated mass lesion	High- or mixed-density lesion > 5 cc, not surgically evacuated

2. Midline Shift

Midline shift has been shown to be a strong predictor of outcome after TBI.[27,41] Maas et al[41]

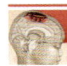

found that patients with midline shift </= 5 mm had better prognosis as compared with patients with midline shift > 5 mm.

3. Intracranial Hemorrhage

Subdural hematoma (SDH) is associated with poor outcome.[27,29] Prognosis in patients with EDH is better than SDH.[22] Traumatic subarachnoid hemorrhage is a strong predictor of outcome in TBI.[36–38,41] The evidence for prognostic value of intraventricular hemorrhage (IVH) in TBI is not very strong. There are studies[29] which report no relationship between IVH and outcome. Eisenberg et al[38] and Lee et al[40] reported the relationship between IVH and poor outcome in TBI to be caused by relation with other predictors. However, Maas et al[41] found IVH to be an independent predictor of poor outcome in patients with TBI.

4. Obliteration of Third Ventricle and Basal Cisterns

Obliteration of III ventricle and basal cisterns is associated with poor prognosis.[25,27,41] CRASH trial researchers[25] reported obliteration of III ventricle and basal cisterns to be worst predictor of 14 day mortality. Maas et al[41] also found the absence of basal cisterns to be the strongest predictor of six month mortality.

5. MR Spectroscopy (MRS)

Conventional neuroimaging techniques can detect macroscopic changes resulting from TBI. However, one commonly encounters severely disabled patients with normal neuroimaging.[38] After mechanical injury, multiple biochemical changes are initiated in addition to the structural changes, that are responsible for irreversible neuronal and axonal damage.[42,43] MRS is capable of detecting the neurochemical changes in the damaged brain despite normal neuroimaging.[44] NAA/Cho ratio has been shown to correlate with severity of injury in different studies.[44,45] However, the evidence for prognostic value of MRS in TBI is still inconclusive.

E. Electrophysiological Parameters

Somatosensory evoked potentials have been studied as prognostic markers in TBI.[46–50] Bilateral absence of cortical response has been shown to be a strong predictor of poor outcome, including death and vegetative state.[48] Pohlmann et al[46] reported that the reliability of SSEPs as a predictor of both good and poor outcome improved with serial recordings. Carter et al,[49] in a systematic review of studies addressing the role of SSEPs as predictors of outcome following TBI found that SSEPs had better sensitivity than GCS and CT scan and better specificity than pupillary response and CT scan in predicting favorable outcome. SSEPs had good sensitivity and specificity for prediction of unfavorable outcome as well. Similarly, in another review, Carrai et al[50] found a high predictive value (>90%) of SSEPs in predicting both favorable and unfavorable outcome in children with severe TBI. However, SSEPs have not found a wide acceptability as a practical prognostic factor in predicting theorist come after TBI.

II. PROGNOSTIC MODELS

From the previous discussion, it is clear that prognostication in TBI involves multiple factors. In a single patient with TBI, multiple factors play a role in determining the overall prognosis, some of these factors being favorable and others unfavourable. Therefore, a single prognostic factor cannot be relied upon as a sufficiently accurate predictor of the prognosis in a single patient. Prognostication in TBI, therefore, involves multivariate analysis of multiple factors. This can be done by combining the pertinent prognostic factors in a prognostic model.[51,52]

A prognostic model is a statistical model that predicts the prognosis of a patient by combining multiple factors. Prognostic models are more accurate in prognostication than expert clinicians.[4] Prognostic models can also be used to design the randomized controlled trials (RCTs) and to analyze the results of RCTs.[27] Many prognostic models are available in the literature but none of them is widely used clinically. For a prognostic model to be useful clinically, it should be validated clinically as well as methodologically.[51] Most of the models fail to fulfil these two requirements.

According to a review by Perel P et al,[3] more than 100 prognostic models have been described in the literature on TBI. They found that a total of 89 variables were used in these models. The mean number of variables included in each model was 5 (range: 2–12). The most commonly used variables were: GCS, age and pupillary reactivity. For multivariate analysis, in the development of the model, logistic regression, regression tree analysis and neural networks were used. Mortality and GOS were the main outcome measures used. Signorini et al[6] developed a prognostic model using clinical variables. The survival at 1 year was taken as outcome. This model was validated in 520 patients. Age, GCS, ISS, pupils reactivity and presence of hematoma on the CT scan were used as the prognostic factors. They reported a user-friendly normogram to predict probability of survival.

Hukkelhoven et al[35] also reported prognostic models. The outcomes measures used by them were: raised intracranial pressure (ICP), surgically removable lesions (SRL), un-favorable outcome (death, vegetative state or severe disability) and mortality at six months. The predictors for ICP were age, motor score, pupil size, pupillary reactivity, hypotension and ISS. For SRL, the predictors were the same as for ICP except motor score, and cause of injury was added. The predictor variables were age, gender, pupil reactivity, cause of injury, hypotension, hypoxia, CT classification and traumatic subarachnoid hemorrhage. They presented the model as a score chart to facilitate its use in clinical practice.

Recently, CRASH and IMPACT trials have come up with prognostic models. The Medical Research Council (MRC) CRASH (cortico-steroid randomization after significant head,

injury) trial is the largest clinical trial on TBI with a cohort of 10008 patients. Death and GOS were used as outcome measures. Age, sex, cause of injury, time from injury to randomization, Glasgow Coma Score at randomisation, pupillary reactivity, results of computed tomography, whether the patient had sustained a major extracranial injury, and level of income in country were used as prognostic variables. Analysis was done with multivariate logistic regression method. Both internal and external validation was done. The CRASH collaborators came up with two models: basic model and CT model.

a. Basic model–Four predictors were included in the basic model: age, GCS, pupillary reactivity, major extracranial injuries. GCS was the strongest predictor in low income countries and age was the strongest predictor in high income countries.

b. CT model–Following imaging features were included in this model: Petechial hemorrhages, obliteration of the third ventricle or basal cisterns, subarachnoid bleeding, midline shift, and non-evacuated hematoma. Obliteration of the third ventricle and midline shift were the strongest predictors of mortality at 14 days, and non-evacuated hematoma was the strongest predictor of unfavorable outcome at six months.

These models have shown an excellent discrimination. They have developed a web based calculator (www.crash2.lshtm.ac.uk/). The expected risk of death at 14 days and of death or severe disability at 6 months can be obtained by entering the values of the predictors.

CONCLUSIONS

Prognosis of severe head injury has improved significantly over the last 3 decades. Large number of factory influence the outcome. With the availability of multi-modal ICU monitoring and trained critical care personale outcome has further improved. However, in India till now proper ICU care in not available in many places. Hence, a lot needs to be done in India to improve the outcome of severe head injury. Recently, large number of studies are available dealing with biomarker in predicting the outcome. In future biomarkers will play a significant role in predicting the outcome of both severe and minor head injury.

REFERENCES

1. Teasdale G, Jennett B. Assessment of coma and impaired consciousness.A practical scale. Lancet 1974;2:81–84.

2. Jennett B, Bond M. Assessment of outcome after severe brain damage. Lancet 1975;1:480–4.

3. Perel P, Wasserberg J, Ravi RR, Shakur H, Edwards P, Roberts I. Prognosis following head injury: a survey of doctors from developing and developed countries. J Eval Clin Pract 2007;13: 464–5. CrossRefMedlineWeb of Science.

4. Lee KL, Pryor DB, Harrell FE Jr, Califf RM, Behar VS, Floyd WL, et al. Predicting outcome in coronary disease. Statistical models versus expert clinicians. Am J Med1986;80:553–60. CrossRefMedlineWeb of Science

5. Vollmer DG, Torner JC, Jane JA, et al. Age and outcome following traumatic coma:why do older patients fare worse? J Neurosurg 1991;75:S37–49.

6. Signorini D, Andrews P, Jones P, Wardlaw J, Miller J. Predicting survival using simple clinical variables:a case study in traumatic brain injury. J. NeurolNeurosurg Psychiatry 1999;66:20–25.

7. Gómez P, Lobato R, Boto G, De la Lama A, González P, de la Cruz J. Age and outcome after severe head injury. Acta Neurochir (Wien) 2000;142:373–81.

8. Braakman R, Gelpke GJ, Habbema JD, Maas AI, Minderhoud JM. Systematic selection of prognostic features in patients with severe head injury. Neurosurgery 1980;6:362–70.

9. Edna TH. Risk factors in traumatic head injury. ActaNeurochir (Wien) 1983;69(1–2):15–21.

10. Choi SC, Ward JD, Becker DP. Chart for outcome prediction in severe head injury. J Neurosurg 1983;59:294–7.

11. Narayan R, Greenberg R, Miller J, et al. Improved confidence of outcome prediction in severe head injury. J Neurosurg 1981;54:751–62.

12. Teasdale GM, Skene A, Parker L, Jennett B. Age and outcome of severe head injury. Acta Neurochir Suppl (Wien) 1979;28:140–3.

13. Overgaard J, Hvid-Hansen O, Land A, et al. Prognosis after head injury based on early clinical examination. Lancet 1973;2(7830): 631–5.

14. Piek J, Chesnut RM, Marshall LF, et al. Extracranial complications of severe head injury. J Neurosurg 1992;77:901–7.

15. Resnick DK, Marion DW, Carlier P. Outcome analysis of patients with severe head injuries and prolonged intracranial hypertension. J Trauma 1997;42:1108–11.

16. Bruce DA, Schut L, Bruno LA, Wood JH, Sutton LN. Outcome following severe head injuries in children. J Neurosurg 1978;48:679–88.

17. Berger MS, Pitts LH, Lovely M, Edwards MS, Bartkowski HM. Outcome from severe head injury in children and adolescents. J Neurosurg 1985;62:194–9.

18. Alberico AM, Ward JD, Choi SC, Marmarou A, Young HF. J. Outcome after severe head injury. Relationship to mass lesions, diffuse injury, and ICP course in pediatric and adult patients. Neurosurg 1987;67:648–56.

19. Andrews BT, Pitts LH. Functional recovery after traumatic transtentorial herniation. Neurosurgery 1991;29:227–31.

20. Peterson D. Stem cells in brain plasticity and repair. Curr Opin Pharmacol 2002;2:34–42.

21. Marshall LF. Head injury:past, present and future. J Neurosurgery 2000;47:546–61.

22. Chesnut R, Ghajar J, Maas AIR, et al. Management and prognosis of severe traumatic brain injury. Part 2: early indicators of prognosis in severe traumatic brain injury. J Neurotrauma 2000;17: 557–627.

23. Pazzagilla P, Frank G, Frank F, et al. Clinical course and prognosis of acute posttraumatic coma. J Neurol Neurosurg Psych 1975;38:149–54.

24. Lavati A, Farina ML, Vecchi G, et al. Prognosis of severe head injuries. J Neurosurg 1982;57;779–83.

25. CRASH Trial Collaborators. Final results of MRC CRASH, a randomised placebo-controlled trial of intravenous corticosteroid in adults with head injury—outcomes at 6 months. Lancet 2005;365: 1957–9.

26. Hukkelhoven CW, Steyerberg EW, Rampen AJ, Farace E, Habbema JD, Marshall LF, Murray GD, Maas AI. Patient age and outcome following severe traumatic brain injury: an analysis of 5600 patients. J Neurosurg 2003;99:666–73. Review.

27. Murray GD, Butcher I, McHugh GS, Lu J, Mushkudiani NA, Maas AI, et al. Multivariable prognostic analysis in traumatic brain injury: results from the IMPACT study. J Neurotrauma 2007;24:329–37.

28. Mushkudiani NA, Engel DC, Steyerberg EW, Butcher I, Lu J, Marmarou A, et al. Prognostic value of demographic characteristics in traumatic brain injury: results from the IMPACT study. J Neurotrauma 2007;24:259–69.

29. Wang JY, Bakhadirov K, Devous MD Sr, Abdi H, McColl R, Moore C, et al. Diffusion tensor tractography of traumatic diffuse axonal injury. Arch Neurol 2008;65:619–26.

30. F, Murray GD, Penny K, et al. The value of the "worst" computed tomographic scan in clinical studies of moderate and severe head injury. European Brain Injury Consortium. Neurosurgery 2000;46:70–5; discussion 75–7.

31. Marmarou A, Lu J, Butcher I, McHugh GS, Murray GD, Steyerberg EW, et al. Prognostic value of the Glasgow Coma Scale and pupil reactivity in traumatic brain injury assessed prehospital and on enrollment: an IMPACT analysis. J Neurotrauma 2007;24:270–80.

32. Van Beek JG, Mushkudiani NA, Steyerberg EW, Butcher I, McHugh GS, Lu J, Marmarou A, Murray GD, Maas AI. Prognostic value of admission laboratory parameters in traumatic brain injury: results from the IMPACT study. J Neurotrauma 2007;24:315–28.

33. Marshall LF, Marshall SB, Klauber MR, et al. A new classification of head injury based on computerized tomography. J Neurosurg 1991;75:S14–20.

34. RD, Gomez PA, Alday R, et al. Sequential computerized tomography changes and related final outcome in severe head injury patients. ActaNeurochir (Wien) 1997;139:385–91.

35. Hukkelhoven CW, Steyerberg EW, Habbema JD, Farace E, Marmarou A, Murray GD, Marshall LF, Maas AI. Predicting outcome after traumatic brain injury: development and validation of a prognostic score based on admission characteristics. J Neurotrauma Oct 2005;22:1025–39.

36. Greene KA, Marciano FF, Johnson BA, Jacobowitz R, Spetzler RF, Harrington TR. Impact of traumatic subarachnoid hemorrhage on outcome in nonpenetrating head injury. Part I: A proposed computerized tomography grading scale. J Neurosurg 1995;83:445–52.

37. Greene KA, Jacobowitz R, Marciano FF, Johnson BA, Spetzler RF, Harrington TR. Impact of traumatic subarachnoid hemorrhage on outcome in nonpenetrating head injury. Part II: Relationship to clinical course and outcome variables during acute hospitalization. J Trauma 1996;41:964–71.

38. Eisenberg HM, Gary HE, Jr, Aldrich EF, et al. Initial CT findings in 753 patients with severe head injury. A report from the NIH Traumatic Coma Data Bank. J Neurosurg 1990;73:688–98.

39. F, de la Fuente M, Lobato RD, et al. Intraventricular hemorrhage in severe head injury. J Neurosurg 1983;58:217–22.

40. Lee JP, Lui TN, Chang CN. Acute post-traumatic intraventricular hemorrhage analysis of 25 patients with emphasis on final outcome. Acta Neurol Scand 1991;84(2):85–90.

41. Maas AI, Hukkelhoven CW, Marshall LF, Steyerberg EW. Prediction of outcome in traumatic brain injury with computed tomographic characteristics: a comparison between the computed tomographic classification and combinations of computed tomographic predictors. Neurosurgery 2005;57:1173–82; discussion 1173–82.

42. Maxwell WL, Povlishock JT, Graham DL: A mechanistic analysis of nondisruptive axonal injury: a review. J Neurotrauma 1997;14:419–40.

43. TK, Smith DH, Meaney DF, Kotapka MJ, Gennarelli TA, Graham DI: Neuropathological sequelae of traumatic brain injury: relationship to neurochemical and biomechanical mechanisms. Lab Invest 1996;74:315–42.

44. S, Marmarou A, Aygok GA, Fatouros PP, Portella G, Bullock RM. Assessment of mitochondrial impairment in traumatic brain injury using high-resolution proton magnetic resonance spectroscopy. J Neurosurg 2008;108:42–52.

45. Garnett MR, Blamire AM, Rajagopalan B, Styles P, Cadoux-Hudson TA: Evidence for cellular damage in normal-appearing white matter correlates with injury severity in patients following traumatic brain injury: a magnetic resonance spectroscopy study. Brain 2000;123:1403–9.

46. Pohlmann-Eden B, Dingethal K, Bender HJ, Koelfen W. How reliable is the predictive value of SEP (somatosensory evoked potentials) patterns in severe brain damage with special regard to the bilateral loss of cortical responses? Intensive Care Med 1997;23:301–8.

47. Carter BG, Taylor A, Butt W. Severe brain injury in children: long-term outcome and its prediction using somatosensory evoked potentials (SEPs). Intensive Care Med 1999;25:722–8.

48. Lew HL, Dikmen S, Slimp J, Temkin N, Lee EH, Newell D, Robinson LR. Use of somatosensory-evoked potentials and cognitive event-related

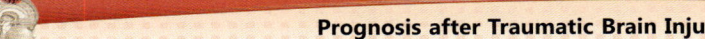

potentials in predicting outcomes of patients with severe traumatic brain injury. Am J Phys Med Rehabil 2003;82:53–61; quiz 62–4, 80.

49. Carter BG, Butt W. Are somatosensory evoked potentials the best predictor of outcome after severe brain injury? A systematic review. Intensive Care Med Jun 2005; 31(6):765–75. Epub 2005, Apr 22.

50. Carrai R, Grippo A, Lori S, Pinto F, Amantini A. Prognostic value of somatosensory evoked potentials in comatose children: a systematic literature review. Intensive Care Med 2010; 36:1112–26. Epub 2010, Apr 27.

51. Altman DG, Royston P: What do we mean by validating a prognostic model? Stat Med 2000; 19:453–73.

52. Pillai SV, Kolluri VR, Praharaj SS: Outcome prediction model for severe diffuse brain injuries: development and evaluation. Neurol India 2003;51:345–9.

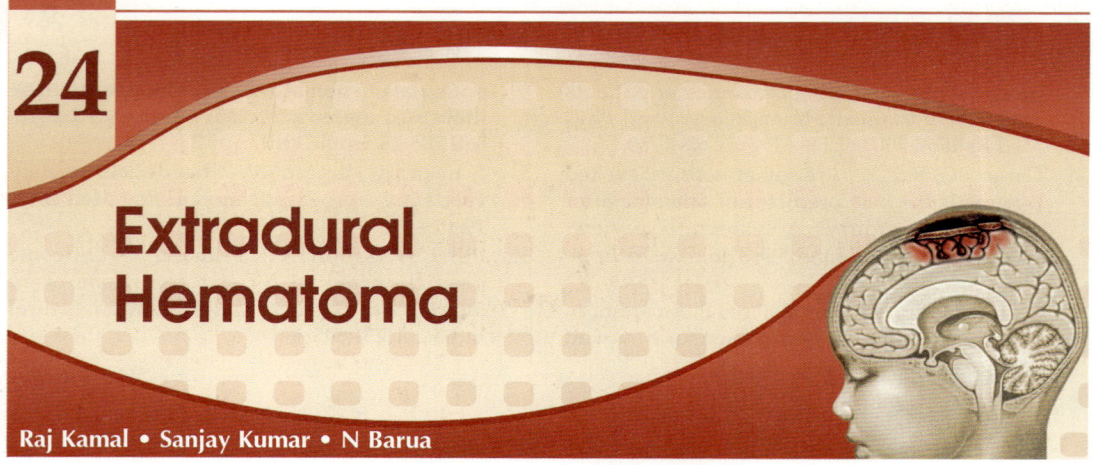

24

Extradural Hematoma

Raj Kamal • Sanjay Kumar • N Barua

INTRODUCTION

Epidural hematoma (EDH), also known as extradural hematoma, is a hemorrhage into the space between the dura and the overlying calvarium. It is almost exclusively caused by trauma. Incidence of extradural hematoma in patients admitted to the hospital for head injury ranges between 1 and 3%.[1,2] EDH is associated with diffuse axonal injury (DAI) in 5.8% of the patients. The latter explains the immediate coma (absence of lucid interval) and the grave prognosis.[3,4] In patients with GCS scores of 8 or less at admission the frequency of extradural hematoma can be as high as 9%.[5] Extradural hematomas commonly occur between the ages of 10 to 40 years.[6] Epidural hematomas are rare birth injuries, and spontaneous presentation is exceptional. EDH are rare over the age 60 years, because of close adherence of the dura to the inner table of the skull. It is commonly found in males (Male: Female ratio is 4:1). The morbidity and mortality result from mass effect on the brain as the hematoma grows and strips the dura away from the skull.

They usually develop from injury to the middle meningeal artery or one of its branches, and therefore, are usually temporo-parietal in location (Figs 24.1 and 24.2). A temporal bone fracture is often the cause, but is not essential. The expanding hematoma strips the dura from the skull; this attachment is quite strong such that the hematoma is confined, giving rise to its characteristic biconvex shape, with a well defined margin. It may present as primary depressed consciousness or following a lucid interval. The bleeding is usually acute and so of high attenuation. There is often significant mass effect with compression of the ipsilateral lateral ventricle and dilatation of the opposite lateral ventricle due to obstruction of the foramen of Munro. The basal cisterns may be effaced. The usual sites of occurrence for epidural hematomas (Fig. 24.3) are temporal (62–80%) and frontal (7–18%).[7] The other sites for EDH are middle fossa, parieto-occipital region, parasagittal region, and the posterior fossa.

The type of trauma that cause EDH are the same as those that cause other types of head injuries, i.e. falls, vehicular accidents, and assault.[8,9]

Pathogenesis

Following impact, the skull bends which can result in stripping of dura from the inner table of the skull. This bending of skull can also result in fracture of the skull. Skull bending, dural stripping and fractured skull are sufficient to cause vascular tears. The vascular tears cause bleeding into areas created by stripping of dura from the inner table of skull and the dura is further stripped by collecting

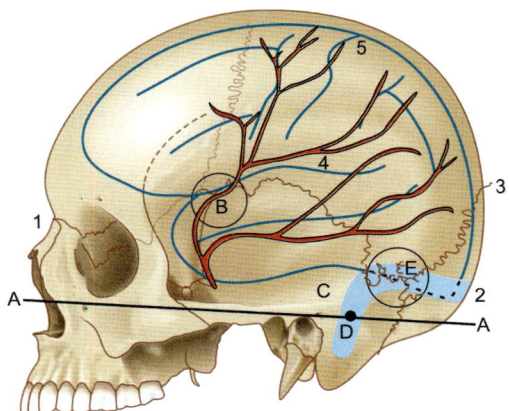

Fig. 24.1: Relations of the brain and middle meningeal artery to the surface of the skull. 1. Nasion, 2. Inion, 3. Lambda, 4. Lateral cerebral fissure, 5. Central sulcus. AA. Reid's base line, B. Point for trephining the anterior branch of the middle meningeal artery, C. Suprameatal triangle, D. Sigmoid bend of the transverse sinus, E. Point for trephining over the straight portion of the transverse sinus, exposing dura mater of both cerebrum and cerebellum. Outline of cerebral hemisphere indicated in blue; course of middle meningeal artery in red

extradural hematoma. Extradural hematomas are associated with **skull fractures** in more than 90% of patients.[7,10,11] In children, the incidence of associated fracture is lower owing to increased deformability of the skull in children.

The middle meningeal artery or vein is the commonest source of bleeding in patients with extradural hematoma, responsible in over 80% of patients, followed by torn dural venous sinuses or **diploic veins** (Fig. 24.1). The anterior division of the middle meningeal artery is most commonly involved. Foramen spinosum, located in the middle cranial fossa, transmits the middle meningeal artery from the infratemporal fossa into the cranial cavity (Fig. 24.2). The artery runs forward and laterally in a groove on upper surface of squamous part of temporal bone and the greater wing of sphenoid. After a short distance, the artery divides into anterior and posterior divisions. The anterior branch passes forward and upward to the anteroinferior angle of the parietal bone. Here the bone is deeply grooved by the artery for a short distance and is the site of damage after a blow. Artery then runs backwards and upwards on the parietal bone.

The hematomas are generally unilateral, and most are found in the temporal region (Fig. 24.3). Arterial or venous structures may

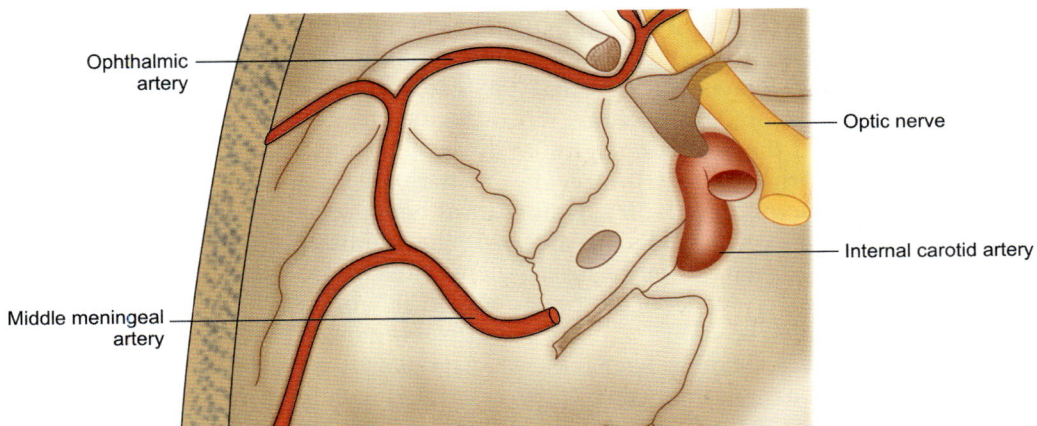

Fig. 24.2: Middle meningeal artery; after branching off the maxillary artery in the infratemporal fossa, it runs through the foramen spinosum to supply the dura mater. The anterior branch of the middle meningeal artery runs beneath the pterion. It is vulnerable to injury at this point, where the skull is thin. Rupture of the artery gives rise to an epidural hematoma

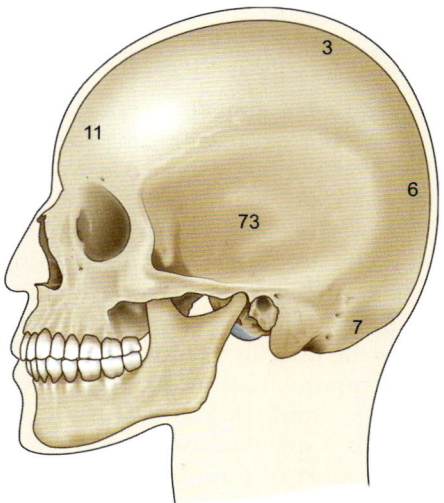

Fig. 24.3: Percentage distribution of site of epidural hematoma

be compromised, causing rapid expansion of the hematoma; however, chronic or delayed manifestations may occur when venous sources are involved. Extension of the hematoma usually is limited by suture lines owing to the tight attachment of the dura at these locations. Recent analyzs have revealed that epidural hematomas may actually traverse suture lines in a minority of cases.[12] The temporoparietal region and the middle meningeal artery are involved most commonly (66%), although the anterior ethmoidal artery may be involved in frontal injuries, the transverse or sigmoid sinus in occipital injuries, and the superior sagittal sinus in trauma to the vertex. Bilateral epidural hematomas account for 2–10% of all acute epidural hematomas in adults but are exceedingly rare in children. Posterior fossa epidural hematomas represent 5% of all cases of epidural hematomas (Fig. 24.3).

Bilateral extradural hematomas have been reported, chiefly after assault injuries.[10]

Associated injuries: Extradural hematomas are associated with other intracranial injuries in 10–15% of cases.[7,13] In presence of associated intracranial injuries the mortality increases.

Clinical Manifestations

Epidural hematoma should be suspected in any individual who sustains head trauma. Although classically associated with a lucid interval between the initial loss of consciousness at the time of impact and a delayed decline in mental status (10–33% of cases), alterations in the level of consciousness may have a variable presentation. Posterior fossa epidural hematoma may exhibit a rapid and delayed progression from minimal symptoms to even death within minutes.

Symptoms of epidural hematoma include the following:

The clinical course of presentation of a patient with an extradural hematoma can take one of five patterns[2,7]

1. Conscious throughout (8–24%).
2. Unconscious throughout (23–24%).
3. Initially unconscious and subsequently recovered (20–28%).
4. Initially conscious, followed by loss of consciousness (14–21%)[3,4]
5. Initially unconscious followed by recovery followed by a second loss of consciousness (12–34%).

Pattern 5 represents the classic **lucid interval** which occur in one-third or fewer patients with extradural hematomas.[10] The most important single sign of a developing extradural hematoma is clouding of consciousness or progressive depression of the level of consciousness.

There are no definite symptoms of extradural hematomas. The triad of head injury with lucid interval, mydriasis on the side of a hematoma and contralateral paresis occurs only in 18% of cases and mainly in temporoparietal region.

The dilated and non-reactive pupil can be associated with ipsilateral hemiplegia. This is due to indentation of the contralateral cerebral peduncle by the edge of the tentorium cerebelli (Kernohan's notch).

Initially pupil on the side of extradural hematoma contracts due to irritation of the

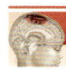

oculomotor nerve, the opposite pupil remains normal in size. In the next stage the ipsilateral pupil dilates due to paralysis of oculomotor nerve. Finally the pupils of both sides become dilated and fixed (Hutchinson's pupil). Paralysis of extraocular muscles supplied by oculomotor nerve occurs little after pupillary changes as pupillary fibers are more sensitive to pressure because of their peripheral arrangement in the oculomotor nerve. Poon et al[14] analyzed 73 patients with traumatic extradural hematoma (EDH) admitted to the neurosurgical unit and managed with surgical evacuation. Of these consecutive admissions, 22 patients (30%) with delayed EDH were reported. The overall mortality of traumatic EDH (5%; 4 of 73) was related to cases of delayed onset EDH. In addition to a high index of suspicion, early diagnosis of delayed EDH can be facilitated by liberal use of intracranial pressure monitoring and serial computed tomography.

Diagnosis of Acute Post-traumatic Extradural Hematoma

The operative mortality for EDH is directly related to the level of consciousness at the time of surgery.[15,16] Hooper had analyzed the mortality from epidural hematoma in patients who had optimal management with rapid diagnosis and early surgery and had concluded that a mortality of less then 10% should be reasonable. The mortality of EDH removal in awake, neurologically intact individual should be essentially zero regardless of hematoma size or location, but mortality dramatically increases to 40% if the patient is allowed to deteriorate to coma.[5]

EDH deserves a high index of suspicion in every patient with head injury of any type. Any patient with history of head injury and altered sensorium should undergo CT evaluation. Any patient with an abnormal neurological examination, clouding of consciousness by alcohol or drugs, or who may be lost to follow-up examination should undergo CT scan of head.

A CT head can safely and quickly rule out an EDH and identify associated intracranial lesions.

If a patient is admitted to a hospital without neurosurgeon or CT scanner then he should be immediately shifted to a hospital with these facilities.

Skull X-ray should be done in conscious patient, since the presence of skull fracture, increases the risk of an intracranial hematoma. **Mendelow et al[17] estimated that, for an alert patient without a skull fracture, the risk of developing an intracranial hematoma is about 1:6000, compared to 1:4 risk in a patient with an altered level of consciousness and a skull fracture.** A fracture seen on skull X-ray is an indication of CT scan.

CT APPEARANCE

The acute extradural hematoma is a relatively stereotyped lesion. Because the dura mater tends to adhere to the skull, the hematoma is seen on CT sections as a dense area immediately beneath the skull vault, convex towards both the brain and the vault.

Conventionally acute extradural hematomas are described as biconvex lens-shaped hyperdense lesion on CT scan. The temporo-parietal convexity is the most common site, in which the lesions are easily detected on axial sections (Fig. 24.4). Additional, coronal views may be necessary to identify the rare hematoma over the vertex. Large extradural hematoma may show significant mass effect with evidence of herniation.

A severe temporal lobe contusion may also obscure the EDH, although the temporal contusion or intracerebral hematoma may be of such size that operation would be performed regardless of the evidence of EDH. Delayed epidural hematomas are also known as 10–30% of head injury patients.[14] Early diagnosis of delayed EDH can be facilitated by liberal use of intracranial pressure monitoring and serial computed tomography.

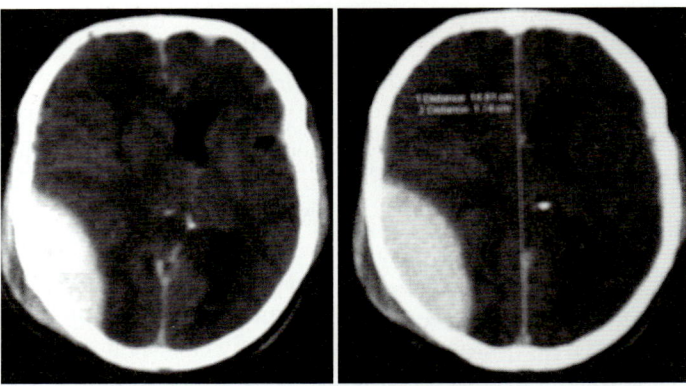

Fig. 24.4a: CT appearance of large, right temporoparietal hematoma with significant midline shift. Note the presence of biconvex extradural hematoma and compression of right lateral ventricle and midline shift towards left with dilatation of left lateral ventricle

TREATMENT OF ACUTE EXTRADURAL HEMATOMA

If a significant large epidural hematoma is diagnosed on CT scanning with evidence of herniation or rapid neurological deterioration, then the patient should be directly taken to operation theater for immediate removal of hematoma. With strong clinical diagnosis of epidural hematoma urgent exploratory burr hole exploration is mandatory when CT scan is not available or will be delayed significantly and the patient is deteriorating fast neurologically with evidence of transtentorial herniation. For the patient who can be scanned rapidly and taken directly to the operating room, CT scanning is preferred to the placement of burr holes.

Patients who are conscious with no neurological deficit and who is discovered to have an extradural hematoma, the necessity of surgical decompression can be questioned. Epidural hematoma may resolve on conservative treatment provided patient is under constant supervision with early detection of deterioration and operation. But this will result in prolonged stay in hospital. Such conservative approach should be avoided unless the hematoma is very small.

Bullock and Chestnut et al[18] recommended that an epidural hematoma (EDH) greater

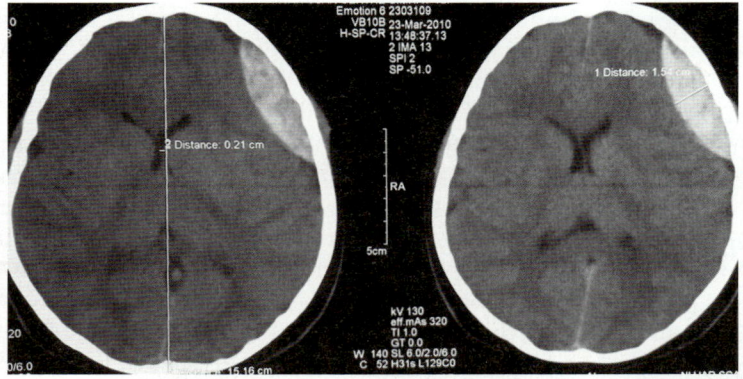

Fig. 24.4b: CT appearance of moderate sized left, frontal hematoma with minimal midline shift. Since the volume was more than 30 cc it was evacuated

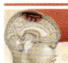
than 30 cu.cm (Figs 24.4a and b) should be surgically evacuated regardless of the patient's Glasgow Coma Scale (GCS) score. An EDH less than 30 cu.cm and with less than a 15 mm thickness and with less than a 5 mm midline shift (MLS) in patients with a GCS score greater than 8 without focal deficit can be managed nonoperatively with serial computed tomographic (CT) scanning and close neurological observation in a neurosurgical center. It was also strongly recommended that patients with an acute EDH in coma (GCS score < 9) with anisocoria undergo surgical evacuation as soon as possible. They recommended craniotomy as it provides a more complete evacuation of the hematoma.

Habibi et al[19] found 8 cases of acute epidural hematoma appearing isodense to brain parenchyma on computed tomography (CT), who had concomitant coagulopathy. These patients were managed by burr hole drainage for treatment of the liquefied EDH. A closed drainage system was then kept in the epidural space for 3 days. In all 8 patients, acute EDH was evacuated successfully via burr hole placement over the site of hematoma. The level of consciousness and other symptoms improved within the first day, and no patient required an additional routine craniotomy. For patients with slowly-developing EDH in the context of impaired coagulation, burr hole evacuation and drainage might be a less invasive method of treatment compared to conventional craniotomy.

Operative Technique

The classical epidural hematoma is due to the arterial bleeding from the middle meningeal artery and its branches. The patient should be placed on the operating table with the head positioned with the hematoma uppermost, and a skin and bone flap should be fashioned that encloses the area of hematoma as much as possible.

The vertical incision is placed one inch anterior to the external acoustic meatus, is

about 7 cm long, and reaches down to the zygomatic process. The incision should not go below the zygomatic process in order to prevent cutting the branches of the facial nerve which innervates the frontalis and orbicularis oculi muscles. The temporalis muscle and fascia are incised along their fibers and retracted by a self-retaining retractor. A **burr-hole is made and enlarged with a rongeur** (Figs 24.5 and 24.6). The craniectomy is carried down.

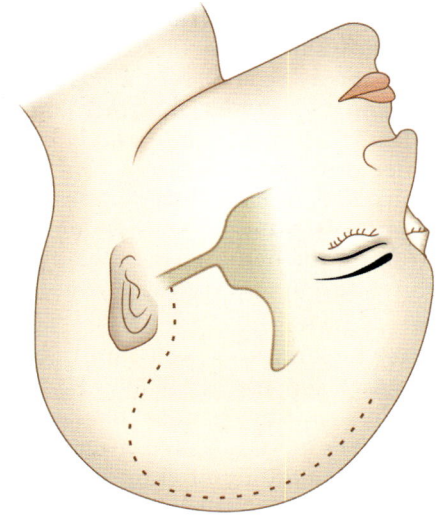

Fig. 24.5: Skin incision for removal of extradural hematoma

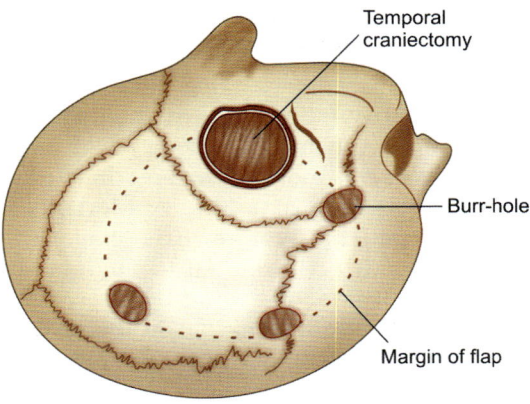

Fig. 24.6: Temporal craniectomy or bone flap

TEMPORAL CRANIECTOMY

Margin of bone flap to the floor of the temporal fossa and the hematoma is evacuated by suction. The burr hole should be made as quickly as possible so that extradural hematoma is decompressed rapidly. This reduces ICP quickly, hence improves the outcome.

The single burr hole can be converted into a craniotomy flap with craniotome or by making a trephine.

If the middle meningeal artery lies just over the fracture site, it may be coagulated at this point or it may be necessary to coagulate it at the foramen spinosum. In some patients the bleeding may originate directly from the foramen spinosum, with no visible artery available to coagulate. In these cases, foramen spinosum is plugged with bone wax for controlling the hemorrhage. Bleeding from fracture site will stop with application of bone wax.

After evacuation of clot and adequate hemostasis, a small incision in dura should be made to look acute subdural hematoma. The dura must be tacked securely around the perimeter of craniotomy or craniectomy (Hitch stitches). One dural stitch can be placed near the middle of exposed dura which passes through the corresponding holes near the center of craniotomy flap.

Outcome of Patients with Epidural Hematoma

The mortality from epidural hematomas should be less than 10%.[12] However, in large series, the overall mortality for epidural hematomas ranges from 20 to 40%.[20–22] Mortality is higher in patients over 40 years of age. The outcome is directly related to the level of consciousness at the time of operation. Patients who were conscious at the time of surgery had a mortality of 6.2% whereas in unconscious patients mortality may as high as 39%. Early evacuation of large acute epidural hematoma is highly recommended.

Seelig et al[3] found that in comatose patients suffering traumatic epidural hematoma after closed head injury overall mortality was 41%, with 4% remaining in the vegetative state. Fifty per cent of these patients, all of whom were in coma, also had an associated intracerebral contusion. There was no difference in outcome with regard to sex, mode of injury, or the presence or absence of contusion or shift on the computed tomographic (CT) scan. The motor score immediately before operation was the most powerful preoperative predictor of outcome. Sixty-seven per cent or two-thirds of the patients with a motor score of 4, 5, or 6 on the Glasgow Coma Scale had a satisfactory outcome at last follow-up examination. In contrast, in patients with a motor score of 3 or less, two-thirds either died or remained in a vegetative state. The acute traumatic epidural hematoma is often lethal in the comatose patient. They recommend early evacuation of epidural hematomas, i.e. when they are first noted on the CT scan, rather than waiting for clinical motor deterioration.

Some authors have reported zero mortality rate in non-comatosed patients. Mortality also varies significantly with modes of presentation as studied by McKissock et al.[7]

Table 24.1: Mode of presentation and mortality[5]	
Mode of presentation	*Mortality %*
1. Conscious throughout	0%
2. Unconscious throughout	57%
3. Initially unconscious and recovered	8%
4. Initially conscious, followed by loss of consciousness	29%
5. Initially unconscious, followed by recovery, followed by second loss of consciousness	57%

POSTERIOR FOSSA EXTRADURAL HEMATOMA (PFEDH)

Extradural hematoma in the posterior fossa is the most frequently encountered traumatic mass lesion in the posterior fossa.[19–20] It occurs in 3–13% of all post-traumatic extradural

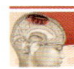

hematomas. It is not uncommon in young adults.

Sencer et al[23] found that traumatic posterior fossa epidural hematoma (PFEDH) is rare, but among children it may have a slightly higher incidence. Twenty-nine patients underwent surgery and 11 patients received conservative therapy and close follow-up. All patients fared well, and there was no surgical mortality or morbidity. They concluded that PFEDH in children can be treated in experienced centers with excellent outcome, and there is no need to avoid surgery when it is indicated.

Extradural hematoma of posterior fossa is almost always associated with a fracture of occipital bone which extends towards foramen magnum, and usually crosses the transverse sinus (Fig. 24.5).

Clinically, deterioration may be rapid, with respiratory depression occurring without any pupillary change or motor signs. Headache, nausea, vomiting and stiffness are the most common signs.[21,22] The clue to the diagnosis is an occipital injury, such as occipital bone fracture, scalp laceration in the occipital region.[11,24]

Patient may present with classic lucid interval, but in acute cases, patients more commonly present with signs of brainstem compression of rapid onset.[25]

Extradural clots in the posterior fossa may be recognized only when appropriate cuts are taken. Typical CT findings are those of a characteristic biconvex or lenticular area of increased density. These hematomas can extend above tentorium.

In these cases a transverse sinus laceration has to be considered.

Jang et al[26] analyzed 34 patients with regard to outcome and prognostic factors was carried out. The admission GCS score was the most valuable prognostic factor. Among the 28 patients with a GCS score of more than 9, 27 patients with GCS > 9 survived with good results; for the six patients with a GCS score of less than eight, two patients had good recovery and four patients had unfavorable outcome. The 15 patients that were conservatively treated and 14 out of the 19 patients surgically treated had a good recovery. Among the other surgically treated patients, two were moderately disabled, two remained in a vegetative state and one died (overall mortality 2.9%). An occipital fracture was present in 28 cases. Six patients with a diastatic fracture of the lambdoid suture had a more complicated venous sinus injury requiring early surgery compared to those with a simple linear fracture. The patients admitted with associated intracranial injuries, such as a contrecoup injury including subdural hemorrhage or traumatic subarachnoid hemorrhage had a poor outcome. The initial GCS score on admission and the presence of associated intracranial injuries were important factors associated with the patient prognosis. A diastatic fracture of the lambdoid suture was associated with complicated venous sinus injuries making surgery more difficult.

Management

Prompt diagnosis, rapid surgical evacuation are essential.

A suboccipital craniectomy for evacuation of posterior fossa extradural hematoma is done, but it may need to extend the craniectomy supratentorially if the hematoma has dissected above the level of transverse sinus (Fig. 24.6).

Operative Technique

The patient is placed in the prone position. The length of the skin incision is shown in Fig. 24.6. The trapezium muscle is cut 1 cm below its insertion and parallel to the superior nuchal line and scraped off the occipital bone with periosteal elevator. Two burr holes are made above and below the superior nuchal line. (The **superior nuchal line** corresponds to the transverse sinus). The burr holes are enlarged by a rongeur. The extradural hematoma is removed by suction and irrigation. Bleeding from sinus is usually controlled by placing surgicel and gelfoam. Dural sagging sutures are placed.

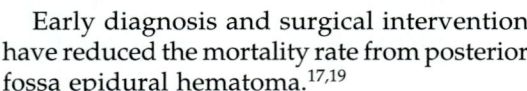

Early diagnosis and surgical intervention have reduced the mortality rate from posterior fossa epidural hematoma.[17,19]

CONCLUSIONS

Extradural hemorrhage is one of the most threatening lesions in patients with TBI, and early diagnosis is essential for its adequate treatment. It can be managed with excellent outcome with low GCS scores, abnormal pupillary reaction, and large hematoma size. However, these cases should be treated surgically without delay when necessary. EDH is more common in males between the ages of 10 and 40 years. It commonly occurs in temporal, frontal and basal middle fossa. Rarely EDH may be present in posterior fossa. The commonest source of extradural hematoma is middle meningeal artery. EDH should be suspected in patients with progressive deterioration in level of consciousness and patients with lucid interval. CT scan is the investigation of choice and shows biconvex lenticular hyperdense lesion on plain CT head. Early diagnosis and quick surgical evacuation is key to good result. Outcome depends on the level of consciousness at the time of operation, and associated brain and systemic injuries.

REFERENCES

1. Cordobes F, Lobata RD, et al. Observation on 82 patients with extradural haematoma. J Neurosurg 1981;54:179–86.

2. Jamieson KG, Yelland JDN. Extradural haematoma. Report of 167 cases. J Neurosurg 1968;28:13–23.

3. Eisenberg HM, Gary HE Jr, Aldrich EF, et al. Initial CT Finding in 753 patients with severe head injury. A report from NIH Traumatic Coma Bank. J Neuosurg 1990;73:88–98.

4. Gusmao SN, Pittella JE. Extradural haematoma and DA, in victims of fatal road traffic accidents. Br J Neurosurg 1998;12:123–6.

5. Seelig JM, Marshall LF, et al. Traumatic acute epidural-haematoma: Unrecognized high lethality in comatose patients. Neurosurgery 1984;15:617–20.

6. Heiskanen O. Epidural haematoma. Surg Neurol 1975;4:23–6.

7. McKissock W, Taylor JC, Bloom WH, et al. Extradural haematoma. Observations on 125 cases. Lancet 1960;1:167–72.

8. Cook RJ, Dorsch NWC, et al. Outcome prediction in extradural haematomas. Acta Neurochir (Wien) 1988;95:90–94.

9. Gutman MB, Moulton RJ, Sullivan I, et al. Risk factors predicting operable intracranial haematomas in head injury. J Neurosurg 1992;77:9–14.

10. Samudrala. S, Cooper P. Traumatic intracranial haematomas. In: Wilkins R, Rengachary S, eds. Neurosurgery, New York: McGraw-Hill 1997;2797–807.

11. Gupta PK, Mahapatra AK, Lad SD. Posterior fossa extradural haematoma. The Oman experience. Pan Arab J Neurosurgery 2001;5:1–7.

12. Huisman TA, Tschirch FT. Epidural hematoma in children: Do cranial sutures act as a barrier? J Neuroradiol. Aug 11 2008;[Medline].

13. Subramaniam MV, Rajendra Prasad G, Dibbala Rao B. Bilateral extradural haematoma. Br. J Surg 1975;62:5.

14. Poon WS, Rehman SU, Poon CYF, Li AKC, Traumatic extradural hematoma of delayed onset is not a rarity Neurosurgery May 1992; 30:681–6.

15. Gallaghar JP, Browder EJ. Extradural haematoma. Experience with 167 patients. J Neurosurg 1968;29:1.

16. Kvarnes T, Trumpy JH. Extradural haematoma. Report of 132 cases. Acta Neurochir (Wien) 1978;41:223–31.

17. Mendelow AD, Teasdale G, Jennett B, et al. Risks of intracranial haematoma in head injured adults. Br J Med 1983;287:1173–76.

18. Bullock MR, Chesnut R, Ghajar J, Gordon D, Hartl R, Newell DW, Servadei F, Walters BC, Wilberger JE; Surgical Management of Traumatic Brain Injury Author Group. Surgical management of acute epidural hematomas. Neurosurgery 2006;58:S7–15.

19. Habibi Z, Ali, Meybodi T, Seyed Mirsadegh MHi, Miri SM.Burr-Hole Drainage for the Treatment of Acute Epidural **Hematoma in Coagulopathic Patients: A Report of Eight Cases,** Journal of Neurotrauma 2012;2103–7.

20. Hooper RS. Extradural hemorrhages of the posterior fossa. Br. J Surg 1954;42:19–26.

21. Tsai FY, Teal JS, et al. Computed tomography of posterior fossa trauma. J Compute Assistant Tomogr 1980;4:291–305.

22. Stone JL, Schaffer L, et al. Epidural haematomas of the posterior fossa. Surg Neurol 1979;11:419–24.

23. Sencer A, Aras Y, Akcakaya MO, Goker B, Kiris T, Canbolat AT. Posterior fossa epidural hematomas in children: clinical experience with 40 cases. J Neurosurg Pediatr 2012;9(2):139–43.

24. Mahapatra AK, Bhatia R, Banerji AK. Posterior fossa extradural haematoma. A report of 5 cases. Neurology India 1982;30:239–44.

25. Gupta PK, Mahapatra AK, Lad SD. Limitation in management of extradural haematoma and their remedy. Oman Medical Journal 2001;18: 28–32.

26. Jang JW, Lee JK, Seo BR, Kim SH. Traumatic epidural haematoma of the posterior cranial fossa.Br J Neurosurg Feb 2011;25:55–61.

25

Posterior Fossa Extradural Hematoma

PK Gupta • AK Mahapatra • Raj Kamal

INTRODUCTION AND EPIDEMIOLOGY

Posterior fossa extradural hematoma (PFEDH) is an uncommon complication of head injury, which is sometimes associated with acute clinical deterioration (ACD) without significant warning symptoms and may results in death.[1] Traumatic space occupying lesions of the posterior fossa are uncommon, however, extradural hematoma is probably the commonest amongst them. It is seen in 0.1–0.3% of all head injury patients and 1.1–5.8% of all head injury patients requiring surgery.[2–5] Most of these cases are associated with calvarial fractures.

It accounts for up to 10% of extradural hematoma in our experience.[6] PFEDH is more common in males.[7] The GCS score at admission and the presence of hydrocephalus as detected by CT scan determines the outcome of the patients. The children have better outcomes than the adults.[7] Mostly younger individuals are affected in their most productive life and it is rare in extremes of age, less than 2 years and more than 60 years, due to the dense adherence of the dura to the overlying bone. Two-thirds of our patients were in pediatric age group, less than 16 years of age.[8]

Mode of Injury

RTA and fall from height are the usual modes of injuries causing PFEDH. Though extradural hematomas (EDH) are caused by trivial/minor injuries, slow traffic usually causes supratentorial EDH and PFEDH is less frequent due to protected location, smaller area and excessive bony reinforcement by stresses. High-speed traffic and severe impact is more often associated with PFEDH. In a pediatric series by Berker, out of 16 cases of PFEDH,15 had fall and traffic accident in one case.[9] Assault is yet another but uncommon mode of injury causing PFEDH.

PATHOGENESIS

PFEDH, which is reported to constitute 0.1%–0.3% of all cranial traumatic conditions, is of venous origin in 85% of the cases and develops as a result of injury to the transverse or sigmoid sinuses secondary to occipital fracture.[7–9] Since most of the PFEDHs are of venous origin and expand slowly, it takes longer for the clinical picture to develop in PFEDH and it is of vital importance to use imaging methods for early diagnosis. Currently, CT has replaced the skull series that were used in order to detect calvarial fractures in patients with posterior fossa trauma. Hematoma usually evolves slowly and takes 18 hours to few days to manifest. Hyperacute EDH in the posterior is unusual as the, bleeding in not arterial in most of the cases. Usual source of bleeding is venous, i.e. dural sinuses or one of the draining veins and fracture hematoma. At some stage, bleeding

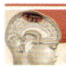

stop due to the tamponade effect of the cerebellum. Hence, the patients take some time to accumulate enough PFEDH to become symptomatic. Exceptionally, the source of bleeding is arterial. The occipital branch of the vertebral artery and distal branches of middle meningeal artery are usual blood vessel involved.[9–11] Source of bleeding is, identifiable in 60–65% of the patients only.[12,13]

Epidural hematoma of nonarterial origin should be suspected if preoperative CT shows a hematoma overlying a dural venous sinus or in the posterior fossa and convexity. The sinus-origin group had a high frequency of fractures which crossed the sinuses, and this might be diagnostically and surgically useful in such cases.[14]

Once a significant volume gets accumulated, then the clinical course is rapid and catastrophic in most of the cases. Almost 50–60% of the cases presents within 18–24 hours (acute) following trauma. Remaining patients may present as subacute or even chronic (after 7 days). Hematoma may be confined to posterior fossa unilaterally or may extend to both the sides or may sometimes even extend into supratentorial compartment.[6] Bilateral separate PFEDH has been very infrequently reported.[15] Pediatric PFEDH is more often confined to posterior fossa where as the PFEDH in adults tend to extend supratentorial.[16] Up to 40% of cases have associated intracranial pathology.[2,6,17]

Clinical Profile

Early symptoms and signs of PFEDHs are uncertain and unpredictable. Patient can remain unconscious or conscious throughout, may have single or double lucid interval[18] or may remain conscious initially to lapse into unconsciousness later. A conscious patient may complain of persistent and severe occipital pain and persistent vomiting. Large numbers of patients have external evidence of occipital trauma. Battles sign may also indicate presence of ongoing PFEDH collection but it is not a common sign and has

been reported in less than 5% of the cases.[6] Neurological examination of these patients may reveal papilloedema as early as 6–8 hours due to acute hydrocephalus that may be missed in an unconscious patient unless specifically looked for. In chronic cases, the patient may present with classical symptoms and signs of cerebellar mass lesion. Rarely a patient may present with torticollis. In subacute cases, the clinical picture will be indistinct and only a thoughtful/fastidious clinician will be able to pick up the subtle signs and reach the diagnosis. Initial assessment has no bearing on the diagnosis, hence it is important to closely and continuously observe such patients. Evolution of localizing signs, failure to improve completely, persistent altered state of consciousness and persistent headache and vomiting are indications to further investigate such patients. Clinical deterioration once sets in, is usually rapid and even an asymptomatic significant PFEDH will not give time to act. Only prompt decompression can save the life and limit of the morbidity. However, small and insignificant PFEDH with no mass effect can still be treated conservatively and expectantly under close observation. High index of suspicion is essential to identify such cases in time.

Investigations

In centres, where CT scanning is not a routine norm in the initial evaluation of head injury patients, X-ray of the skull (including the townes view) is a good screening investigation for radiological evaluation of such patient. Occipital fracture is noted in 55–60% of the cases when Towne's view is also included in the initial radiological assessment of the patient in best centers.[2] A CT scan should evaluate a patient with occipital fracture, even though only 6–8% of occipital fractures are associated with PFEDH, irrespective of clinical status of the patient. CT scan is the most valuable investigation. CT scan helps in early diagnosis, as it is reliable and predictive and also shows associated intracranial pathologies in almost one-third of the cases (Fig. 25.1). CT scan shows biconvex hyper or mixed density lesion besides compression of the cerebellum, shift of the IVth ventricle, compression of the brainstem and obstructive hydrocephalus involving both lateral and III ventricle and fracture of the occipital bone in bone windows. Compared to supratentorial EDH, PFEDH are usually less dense on CT scanning, more so in younger age group.[16] CT scan done soon after injury (within 6 hours of trauma), small EDH and a fracture overlying a vascular marking stands high chances of delayed deterioration due to hematoma enlargement and even if asymptomatic, CT scan should be repeated in them before expiry of 24 hours.[20] Rapidly evolving hydrocephalus and direct compression over the brainstem are the usual causes of mortality whereas associated intra and extracranial lesions are primarily responsible for morbidity.[21]

On MR imaging, acute epidural hematoma is seen as a localized extra-axial collection between the dura and the inner table.[14] Imaging of the dura as a line with very low signal between the hematoma and the brain parenchyma is pathognomonic for epidural hematoma. While it is not always possible to differentiate small epidural hematomas that have not formed a biconvex shape yet due to small volume, demonstration of dura between the parenchyma and the hematoma is diagnostic on MR imaging. Also, MR imaging is more sensitive in the detection of associated parenchymal conditions or dural venous sinus thromboses possibly associated with PFEDH.[22,23] In recent studies, it has been reported that with diffusion weighted MR images with very short acquisition times, dural venous sinus thrombus and early ischemic changes could easily be demonstrated, but no additional benefit from the diffusion-weighted imaging has been defined in the evaluation of acute epidural hematoma.[14,24] Since obtaining an MR imaging study is difficult in unstable trauma patients, the initial imaging of choice and the most commonly used method is still unenhanced CT. In a study by Dirim,[14] of the 49 patients with a traumatic posterior fossa condition, 59% had only occipital fracture. When this group of patients is excluded from the study, the rate of epidural hematoma in the group with traumatic pathology associated with occipital fracture is found to be 35%.

Treatment/Surgery

PFEDH more than 15 mm in thickness, compressing and obliterating IV ventricle causing obstructive hydrocephalus, poor visualization of the posterior fossa cisterns and compression of brainstem irrespective of GCS/neurological status should be promptly evacuated to achieve good result.[25] Hematoma less than 15 mm in thickness, less than 10 ml in volume with a maximum of 5 mm shift of midline structures and no associated

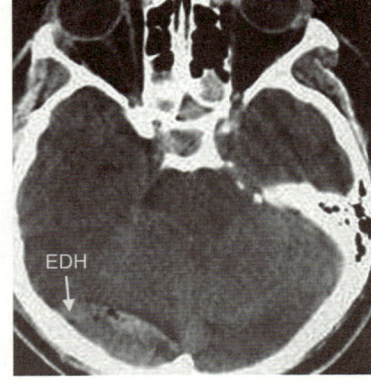

Figs 25.1a and b: CT scan showing PFEDH

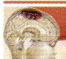

intracranial pathologies can still be observed but even mild deterioration in such situation warrants immediate evacuation of PFEDH.[19] Posterior fossa craniectomy (Figs 25.2 and 25.3) with or without supratentorial craniotomy is necessary to evacuate a solid acute or subacute clot, however, a chronic PFEDH with liquid blood requires only a burrhole to drain out the fluid hematoma.

Outcome

Outcome is good provided the condition is identified and treated in time, before any catastrophic deterioration occurs. Poor outcome is associated with delayed or missed diagnosis, poor primary neurological status, associated intra- and extracranial injuries and

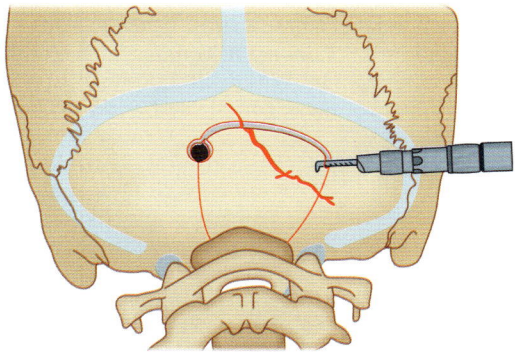

Fig. 25.2: Posterior fossa craniotomy through burr hole and craniotome

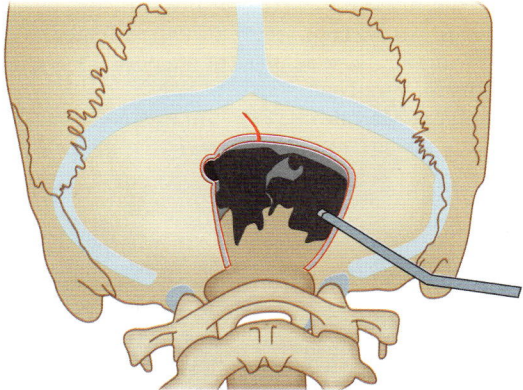

Fig. 25.3: Posterior fossa craniotomy and removal of extradural hematoma using a suction device

unstable cardiopulmonary functions.[6,21,26,27] Compared to supratentorial EDH, PFEDH has a poorer outcome. Early diagnosis and urgent surgical intervention may give the patient a chance of total recovery and craniotomy with hematoma evacuation is an appropriate surgical technique as in the case of supratentorial extradural hematoma.[9,27] Non-invasive imaging techniques like CT and MR scanning has tremendously changed the prognosis in such patients, as they are identified well in time and treated, to an extent that now zero-mortality has been obtained in these patients[5] at the cost of increasing morbidity due to associated lesions or poor primary neurological status.

CONCLUSIONS

Posterior fossa EDH is a rare condition and constitutes less than 10% of cranial EDH. Clinical presentation is varied, however, diagnosis must be kept in mind in patients having impact over occipital or sub-occipital region or in patients having radiological evidence of occipital fracture. A patient with an acute PFEDH is an acute neurosurgical emergency and if treated in time, can result in good outcome. CT scan has significantly facilitated early, prompt and appropriate diagnosis. Associated brain pathology, presence of an acute hematoma and acute hydrocephalus are a few prognosticating factors. High index of suspicion, early diagnosis and prompt evacuation are the essential components of good outcome.

REFERENCES

1. Hayashi T, Kameyama M, Imaizumi S, Kamii H, Onuma T. Acute epidural hematoma of the posterior fossa—cases of acute clinical deterioration. Am J Emerg Med 2007; 25(9):989–95.
2. Mahajan RK, Sharma BS, Khosla VK, Tewari MK, Mathuriya SN, Pathak A, Kak VK. Posterior fossa extradural haematoma. Annals Academy of Medicine 1993;22:410–413.
3. Mahapatra AK, Bhatia R, Banerji AK. Posterior fossa extradural haematoma. Report of 5 cases Neurology India 1982;30:239–44.

4. Sadik AR, Epstein FJ, Ransohoff J. Epidural haematoma of posterior fossa. NY State J Med 1978,78:801–3.

5. Thomas LM, Gurdjian ES. Intracranial haematomas of traumatic origin. In: Youmans JR, ed Neurological Surgery vol 2 Philadelphia: WB Saunders 1973:960–8.

6. Gupta PK, Mahapatra AK, Lad SD. Posterior fossa extradural haematoma an Oman experience. Pan Arab J Neurosurg 2001;5:1–7.

7. Malik NK, Makhdoomi R, Indira B, Shankar S, Sastry K. Posterior fossa extradural hematoma: our experience and review of the literature. Surg Neurol 2007;68(2):155–8; discussion 158.

8. Gupta PK, Mahapatra AK, Lad SD. Pediatric posterior fossa extradural haematoma. Ind J Pediatrics 2002;69(6):489–94.

9. Berker M, Cataltepe O, Ozcan OE. Traumatic epidural haematoma of the posterior fossa in childhood: 16 new cases and a review of the literature.Br J Neurosurg 2003;17(3):226–9.

10. Jamieson KG. Angiographic demonstration of bleeding points in posterior fossa extradural haematoma. J Neurosurg 1972;36:644–5.

11. Perot P, Ethier R, Wong A. An arterial posterior fossa extradural haematoma demonstrated by vertebral angiography. J Neurosurg 1967; 26:255–60.

12. Koc RK, Pasaoglu A, Menku A, Oktem S, Meral M. Extradural haematomas of the posterior fossa. Neurosurg Rev 1998;21:52–7.

13. Holzschuh M, Schuknecht B. Traumatic epidural haematomas of the posterior fossa: 20 new cases and a review of the literature since 1961. Br J Neurosurg 1989;3:171–80.

14. Dirim BV, Orük C, Erdoðan N, Gelal F, Uluç E.Traumatic posterior fossa hematomas. Diagn Interv Radiol 2005;11(1):14–8.

15. Gelabert M, Prieto A, Allut AG. Acute bilateral extradural haematomas of the posterior cranial fossa. Br J Neurosurg 1997;11:573–5.

16. Suyama Y, Kajikawa H, Yamamura K, Sumioka S, Kajikawa M. Acute epidural haematoma of posterior fossa: comparative analysis between 20 cases in adults and 10 cases in children. No Shinkei Geka 1996;24:621–4.

17. Roda JM, Gimenez D, Perez-Higueras A, Blazquez MG, Perez-Alvarez M. Posterior fossa epidural haematomas: a review and synthesis. Surg Neurol 1983;19:419–24.

18. Parkinson D, Hunt B, Shields C. Double lucid interval in patients with extradural haematoma of the posterior fossa. J Neurosurg 1971;34:534–6.

19. Knuckey NW, Gelbard S, Epstein MH. The management of asymptomatic epidural haematomas. A prospective study 1989;70:392–6.

20. Wong CW. The CT criterion for conservative treatment but under close clinical observation of posterior fossa epidural haematoma. Acta Neurochir (Wien) 1994;126:124–7.

21. Kawakami Y, Tamiya T, Tanimoto, Shimamura Y, Hattori S, Ueda T, Ishida T. Non-surgical treatment of posterior fossa epidural haematoma. Pediatr Neurol 1990;6:112–8.

22. Samudrala S, Cooper PR. Traumatic Intracranial Hematomas. In: Wilkins RH, Rengachary SS, eds. Neurosurgery. 2nd ed. New York: McGraw-Hill 1996;2797–807.

23. Osborn AG. Craniocerebral Trauma. In: Diagnostic Neuroradiology. St. Louis: Mosby 1994;204–205.

24. Lovblad KO, Bassetti C, Schneider J, Guzman R, El-Koussy M, Remonda L, Schroth G. Diffusion-weighted MR in cerebral venous thrombosis. Cerebrovasc Dis 2001;11:169–76.

25. Otsuka S, Nakatsu S, Matsumoto S, Sato S, Motozaki T, Ban S, Yamamoto T. Study on cases with posterior fossa epidural haematoma - clinical features and indications for operation. Neurol Med Chir (Tokyo) 1990;30:24–8.

26. Pozzati E, Tognetti F, Cavallo M, Acciarri. Extradural haematomas of the posterior cranial fossa. Surg Neurol 1989;32:300–3.

27. Garza-Mercado R. Extradural haematomas of the posterior cranial fossa. J Neurosurg 1983; 59:664–72.

26

Acute Subdural Hematomas

Raj Kamal • D Gupta

INTRODUCTION

An acute subdural hematoma is a collection of fresh blood under the dura, which may compress the brain.[1] Subdural hematomas (SDHs) can be classified into:

1. Acute subdural hematoma presents within 48 to 72 hours of injury.
2. Subacute subdural hematoma between 3 and 20 days.
3. Chronic subdural hematoma presents from 3 weeks to several months.

The source of acute subdural blood is bridging cortical vein near sagittal sinus, veins from Sylvian fissure to sphenoparietal sinus, the inferior cerebral veins draining into the transverse and the superior petrosal sinuses. Traumatic acute subdural hematoma remains one of the most lethal of all head injuries.[1] Since 1981, it has been strongly held that the critical factor in overall outcome from acute subdural hematoma is timing of operative intervention for clot removal; those operated on within 4 hours of injury may have mortality rates as low as 30% with functional survival rates as high as 65%. Wilberger et al[2] found that the extent of primary underlying brain injury is more important than the subdural clot itself in dictating outcome; therefore, the ability to control ICP is more critical to outcome than the absolute timing of subdural blood removal.

Leitgeb et al[3] in an Austrian study reported that out of the 738 patients with severe TBI, 360 (49%) had acute SDH. Of these, 168 (46.7%) died in the hospital, 67 (18.6%) survived with unfavorable outcome, and 116 (32.2%) survived with favorable outcome. They concluded that age, severity of TBI, and neurological status were the main factors influencing outcomes after severe TBI due to acute SDH. Nonoperative management was associated with significantly higher mortality.

Epidemiology

Acute SDH occurs in approximately 10–30% of patients with severe head injury.[4–6] Males are much more likely to present with acute subdural hematomas than females. In 80% of acute SDH it is the extent of the underlying brain injury which determines the outcome.[7] The reported male to female ratio varies from 3:1 to 6:1.[5] Falls and assaults are the most frequent mechanisms of injury associated with acute subdural hematomas. Older people have a greater risk of developing acute SDH, and the average age of patient with acute subdural hematoma is greater than other types of head injury.[1] Subdural hematomas account for 50 to 60% of acute traumatic intracranial hematomas, and they are more likely to occur after falls or assaults than after motor vehicle accidents.[8,9] They can also occur with increased frequency in patients with coagulopathy (iatrogenic or pathological). Annual incidence of patients with closed head injury admitted to hospitals in the US is estimated at 200 per 100,000 people.[10] In a 2006 University of California Los Angeles study evaluating all patients undergoing cranial CT scanning for suspected blunt head trauma, 8.7% had significant acute traumatic brain injury.[11] Older studies suggest the overall incidence of head injury to be 0.3%, with a peak at age 10 to 29 years.[12] Subdural hematomas have also been linked to chronic renal dialysis. A study from the Northern US found that the incidence of subdural hematoma in 2002 was 58 cases per 100,000 in the general population compared with 191 per 100,000 among dialysis recipients.[13]

Pathogenesis

Acute subdural hematomas are caused by rupture of parasagittal or Sylvian bridging veins draining into dural venous sinuses. Acute SDH result entirely from inertial forces. The parasagittal veins are susceptible to damage during short duration angular acceleration of the head as they are superficially located.[14] Rarely, acute SDH can be due to rupture of cortical artery.[15] Matsuyama et al[15] in 1997 reported a series of 19 cases of SDH due to arterial rupture.

Acute subdural hematomas typically result from torsional or shear forces causing disruption of bridging cortical veins emptying into the dural venous sinuses. This causes subdural hematomas along the convexity.[14,16] Direct force to the skull and brain may cause contusions or lacerations, and typically results in bleeding from a subdural vessel near the temporal pole.[14,16] In some cases, arterial injury may occur, resulting in rapid neurological decline and poor chances for recovery.[16] When the head strikes a broad, hard surface (as in fall), the impact energy causes brain to accelerate within the skull. The strain that occurs during these conditions is confined to the surface, if the acceleration is present for a brief period of time. The types of injury that can be produced in these circumstances are those at the brain surface and those to vascular tissue (bridging veins). If the duration of acceleration is prolonged the strains penetrate deeper into brain and cause **diffuse axonal injury** (DAI). Hence acute SDHs and DAI often coexist. This diffuse brain injury can have a greater influence on the patients outcome and prognosis than the presence of a hematoma in the subdural space.[17]

Another source of bleeding that can result in subdural hematoma is laceration or rupture of small cortical arteries and veins associated with cerebral contusion or injury. Subdural hematomas are usually located over cerebral convexities. The most common site of cerebral contusion associated with a subdural hematoma is the temporal pole, followed by frontal pole and cerebral convexity. Subdural hematoma extend to nearest dural reflection. It may extend along the tentorium. Subdural hematomas may occur medially between falx and medial surface of cerebral hemisphere. Acute SDHs at this site occur due to rupture of veins bridging the medial aspect of the hemisphere and superior sagittal sinus. This is commonly called as parafalcine subdural hematoma, which is clinically characterized by contralateral hemiparesis in which the lower extremity is weaker than the upper extremity (Falx syndrome).

Injuries Associated with Acute Subdural Hematoma

Acute subdural hematomas are commonly associated with contrecoup injuries, including contusions and lacerations of frontal and temporal poles (Fig. 26.1). If an acute SDH is associated with an extensive area of lobar contusion and intracerebral hemorrhage, this combination is often referred to as burst lobe.

The contusions frontal poles and temporal poles are common because brain sustains an impact against irregular bony prominences at the time of injury. Other associated injuries are epidural hematomas, posterior fossa lesions, and contralateral subdural hematomas.[4]

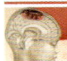

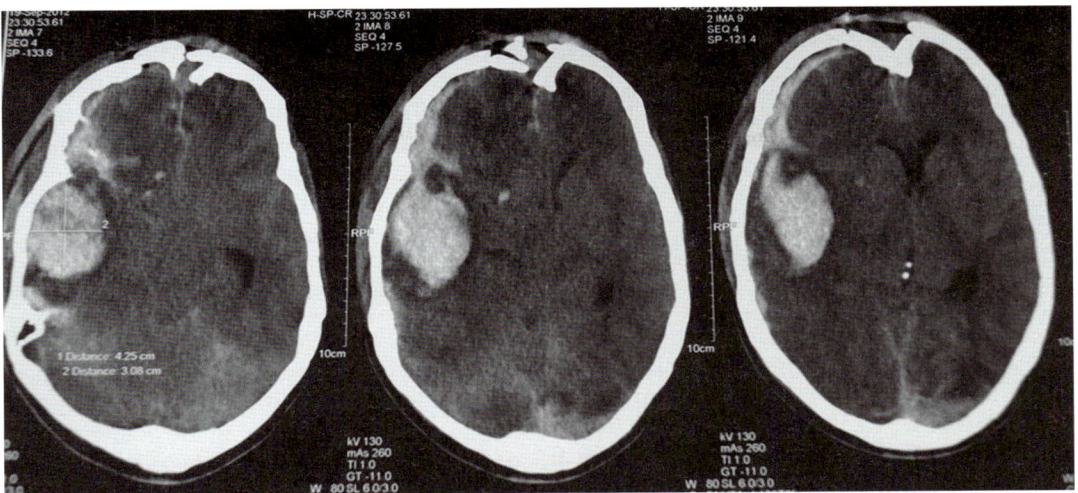

Fig. 26.1: NCCT head showing acute subdural hematoma with large temporal contusion with frontal bone fracture. Please note significant mass effect with developing right PCA infarct

As already stated, diffuse axonal injuries of the brain are commonly associated with acute SDH. This finding may explain the high morbidity and mortality rates in patients with acute SDHs, despite appropriate management of these hematomas.

Clinical Findings

The clinical finding in patients with acute subdural hematoma are related to an acute raised intracranial pressure and the severity of diffuse injury to the brain (Table 26.1). The evolution of symptoms may be rapid and thus simulate the picture of an acute extradural hemorrhage.[18]

It is too early for papilloedema to develop in a patient with an acute subdural hematoma, though an occasional case is seen where severe papilloedema with or without retinal hemorrhages may be seen within a day or two of the injury.[19,20] Patients who sustain severe injuries, become unconscious with decerebrating posture since the time of injury or decerebrate rapidly may be assumed to have sustained diffuse cerebral injury.

In patients with less severe injuries, the deteriorating level of consciousness is deter-

mined by the severity of brain injury at the time of impact and the rate of growth of hematoma. Transtentorial herniation is indicated by the bradycardia associated with hypertension (Cushing's response).

Patients with minor head injuries may lose consciousness initially because of concussion and later on become unconscious due to collecting hematoma (lucid interval).

Lateralizing Findings (Localizing Signs)

It includes ipsilateral pupillary dilatation with impaired reaction and motor deficit. Usually the pupillary dilatation will be ipsilateral and motor deficit (hemiparesis or hemiplegia) will be contralateral to the site of subdural hematoma (Table 26.2).

Table 26.1: Clinical symptoms and signs in patient with acute supratentorial subdural hematoma

Symptoms and signs	McKissock et al[21]	Jamieson[16] et al
Pupillary abnormalities	57	43
Hemiparesis	44	40
Seizures	6	11
Aphasia	6.1	7.5
Decerebrate posturing	—	16

Table 26.2: True and false localizing signs
True localizing signs
1. Ipsilateral pupillary dilatation with nonreaction
2. Contralateral motor weakness
False localizing signs
1. Contralateral pupillary dilatation (cause—optic or oculomotor nerve injury)
2. Ipsilateral motor weakness (Kernohan's notch)

False localizing signs may also occur such as contralateral pupillary dilatation due to opposite optic nerve injury or oculomotor nerve injury. Another false localizing sign would be motor weakness of same side due to compression of the contralateral cerebral peduncle against tentorial edge (Kernohan's notch).[22]

Diagnosis

In the presence of lateralizing signs the diagnosis between epidural and subdural hematoma is usually impossible. Early onset disturbances of consciousness are indicative of SDH.

The role of skull X-ray in evaluating patient of an intracranial mass lesion is controversial. The skull X-ray provides little information that will help the neurosurgeons to make therapeutic decisions. However, the risk of an intracranial hematoma is increased 50 times when a skull fracture is present.[23] Therefore, CT scanning is essential in any patient with an abnormal skull film.

CT SCAN BRAIN

On CT scan (Figs 26.2a and b) an acute subdural hematoma appears as a hyperdense extra-axial collection which are usually crescent shaped.[24]

The concavity of the crescent follows the brain surface. The inner surface of the hematoma outline the contours of the brain and therefore a characteristic saw tooth appearance in the region of Sylvian fissure.

The subdural hematomas do not cross the falx or tentorium. Rarely, acute SDH can be present in interhemispheric fissure (Fig. 26.3)

There may be mass effect on brain in the form of compression of ipsilateral ventricle, midline shift and obliteration of basal cisterns.

A typical CT findings include mixed density subdural hematomas with varying degree of hypodensity within the high density clot due to CSF within the subdural space or due to clot retraction.

MAGNETIC RESONANCE IMAGING

Magnetic resonance imaging (MRI) is superior at identifying subacute or chronic traumatic lesions, including intracerebral or extra-axial hematomas, particularly in the posterior fossa or brainstem. However, MRI is not as sensitive as CT scan in diagnosing acute hemorrhage because fresh blood is not well delineated; MRI takes longer time. In sick patients on monitors/ventilators MRI scanning is often not possible.

Management

Generally, the most important criteria for determining management of acute subdural hematomas are neurological signs/symptoms and radiographic appearance. Subacute hematomas can be treated in the same way as chronic hematomas; acute-on-chronic hematomas are usually treated in the same way as acute subdural hematomas. Many patients with severe head injury present with coagulopathy and require normalization of their coagulation profile. Correcting coagulopathy is imperative in all patients with subdural hematoma. All patients on anticoagulation must have their antiplatelet or anticoagulant agent stopped and/or reversed.[25,26] All patients require serial prothrombin time (PT), partial thromboplastin time (PTT), INR, and platelet and fibrinogen levels followed.

Management of Raised Intracranial Pressure

In patients with increased intracranial pressure (ICP), a standard protocol is used for management. It is important to follow traditional traumatic brain injury principles,

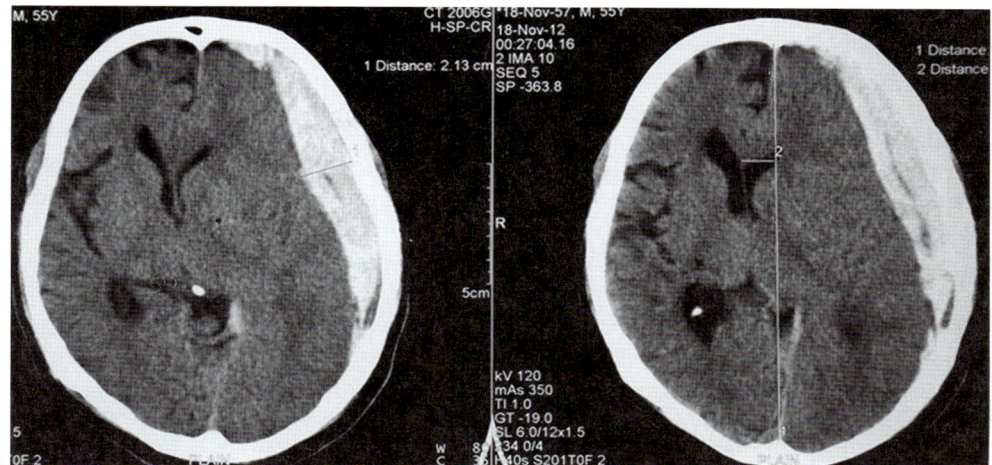

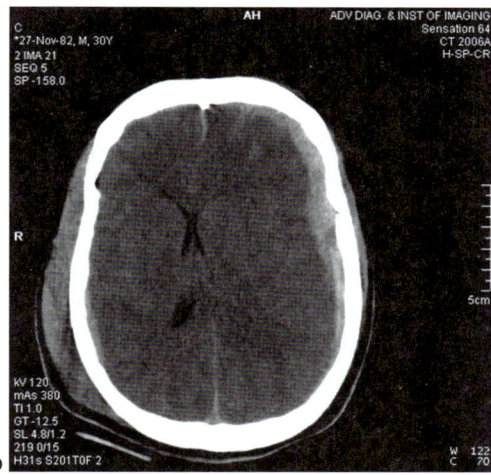

Figs 26.2a and b: NCCT head (a and b) showing acute subdural hematoma with mass effect exhibited by effacement of sulci and midline shift with subfalcine herniation

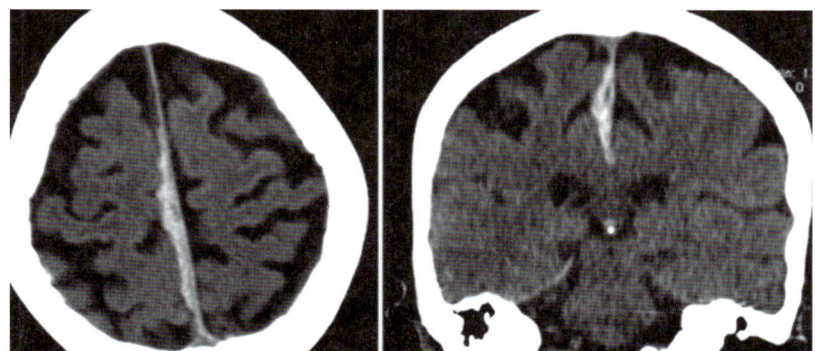

Fig. 26.3: Interhemispheric acute SDH

including maintaining a cerebral perfusion pressure of 60 to 70 mm Hg and ICP < 20 mm Hg (in adults). While surgical evacuation would be considered in many patients with an acute subdural hematoma and signs of increased ICP, there is a subset of patients with small acute subdural hematomas whose neurological symptoms are due to other injuries, such as intraparenchymal contusions or diffuse axonal injury. In these patients, surgical evacuation would not be a first-line therapy.

Primary options that can be used to lower ICP include raising the head of the bed to 30°, using the reverse Trendelenburg position if spinal instability or injury is present. Analgesics and sedation can be useful, as pain and agitation can increase the ICP. Using paralytics in intubated patients can help to attenuate the effects of suctioning. Hyperventilation to a goal pCO$_2$ of 30 to 35 mm Hg (monitored with serial ABGs) can be beneficial.

Secondary treatment options to lower ICP include osmotic therapy with 3% hypertonic saline, with a dosing limit based on an upper serum sodium limit of 155 mmol/L. Some studies have shown 7.2% hypertonic saline to be very effective in lowering ICP without reducing cerebral blood flow. Osmotic diuretics such as mannitol can be used, but should be avoided if serum osmolality is > 320 mOsm/kg.

Other treatment options include maintaining the patient in a pentobarbital coma (requires continuous EEG monitoring), inducing hypothermia by intravascular cooling or topical cooling blankets, and decompressive hemicraniectomy.

Small subdural hematomas may be associated with other intracranial hematomas requiring either management of raised ICP or surgical evacuation. Occasionally, small subdural hematomas may cause significant cerebral edema and neurological deterioration. Management should, therefore, be based on size and on clinical symptoms/signs. All patients with Glasgow Coma Scale (GCS) score < 9 need to have ICP monitoring with ventriculostomy, subarachnoid bolt, or intraparenchymal monitor. Other functions can be monitored with a pressure of brain tissue oxygen monitor for partial pressures of oxygen in brain tissue in areas of interest; jugular bulb monitoring for global cerebral oxygenation.

The initial management of acute **subdural hematoma** includes maintenance of airway, maintenance of blood pressure and measures to lower intracranial pressure (ICP). The aim of decreasing ICP and maintaining BP is to maintain cerebral perfusion pressure (CPP).

The treatment for a subdural hematoma causing increased intracranial pressure, significant midline shift and signs of brainstem compression is surgical evacuation. In general, all SDHs that are more than 5 mm thick with midline shift are considered for surgical evacuation.

At the other extreme, patients with absent brainstem reflexes after resuscitation will almost certainly have a poor result and are rarely operative candidates.[27,28] Patients with good Glasgow Coma Scale (GCS) with small subdural hematoma may not need surgery.

An acute subdural hematoma should be removed by wide craniotomy centered over maximum width of hematoma. Adequate exposure will allow to remove complete removal of subdural clot with visualization and control of the source of hemorrhage. Removal and debridement of underlying contusion or intracerebral hemorrhage may be accomplished at the time of evacuation of the subdural hematoma.

Surgical Technique
(Figs 26.4a to d and 26.5a to d)

The mechanism of injury responsible for producing acute SDH also leads to high incidence of temporal and frontal contusions and tearing of midline **bridging veins.** To achieve all the surgical objectives, the operative exposure must provide access to the frontal and temporal lobes.

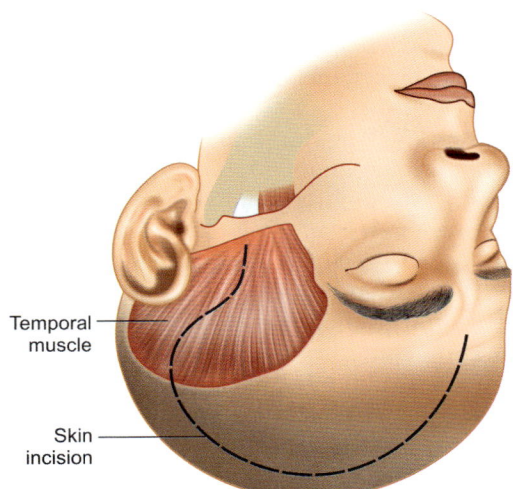

Fig. 26.4a: Skin incision for craniotomy

Skin incision: A large frontotemporo-parietal skin flap is made by using a question mark incision. The incision starts 1 cm anterior to the tragus at the level of the zygomatic arch and turns posterosuperiorly and then curved anteriorly towards frontal region as shown in Fig. 26.3.

Incision over the temporal region should be made first, because in patients who are deteriorating rapidly quick decompression can be achieved by making a burr hole craniectomy followed by cruciate dural incision. This cruciate dural incision allows rapid surgical decompression and may be crucial for the patient.

Bone flap is made as shown in Fig. 26.4.

Dural opening and evacuation of hematoma: Dura is opened in C shaped manner. The dura is opened by gently curving the incision anteriorly. Care should be taken not to injure the cortical vessels particularly in Sylvian fissure.

After dura is opened, the clot is removed gently from the cortical surface with the help of suction catheter and irrigation. Frontal lobe or temporal lobe contusions, if present, are evacuated. Hemostasis should be meticulously done with bipolar.

Closure: Dura should be closed in all cases with or without dural graft. Bone flap is replaced and fixed. Multiple tack up sutures **(Hitch sutures)** should be used to prevent

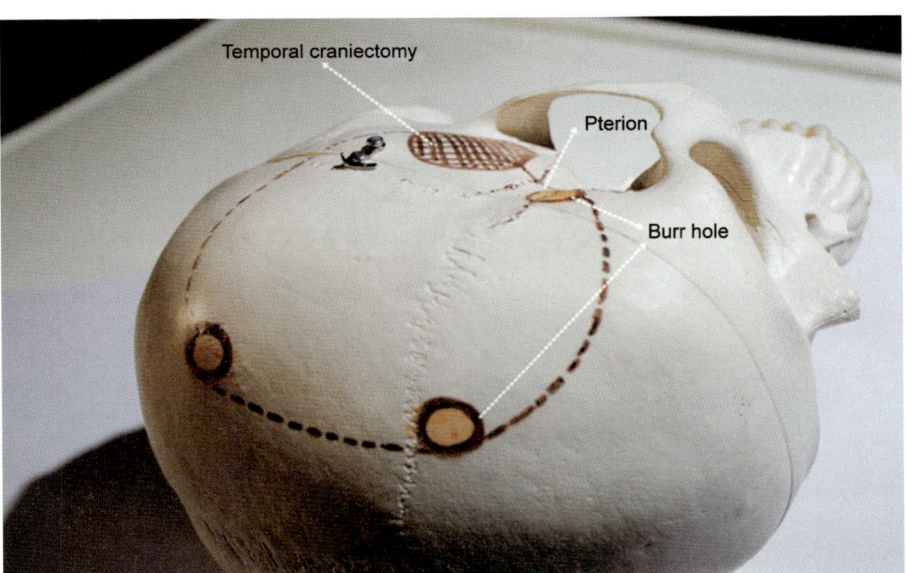

Fig. 26.4b: Burr hole placement for standard trauma craniotomy. Also note temporal craniotomy for initial decompression

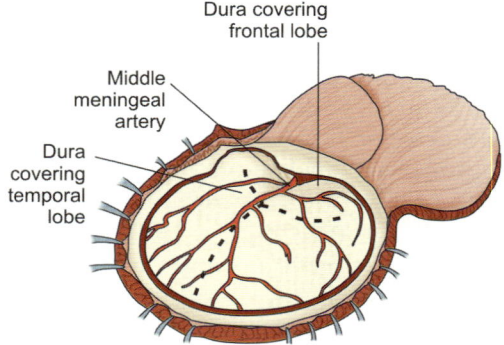

Fig. 26.4c: Dural incision for evacuation of acute SDH

postoperative extradural hematoma. If possible, intracranial pressure (ICP) should be done in all cases postoperatively.

Following problems are frequently encountered during evacuation of acute post-traumatic subdural hematoma.

1. Intraoperative brain swelling.
2. Intraoperative bleeding.

1. *Intraoperative brain swelling:* This is not an uncommon problem. Immediately after opening the dura and evacuation of SDH, the brain starts swelling up into the incision. If this happens, the endotracheal tube and position of patient should be checked.

Causes of intraoperative swelling

a. Cerebral vascular engorgement.
b. Epidural hematoma on opposite side.
c. Intracerebral contusion hematoma.
d. Residual hematoma.

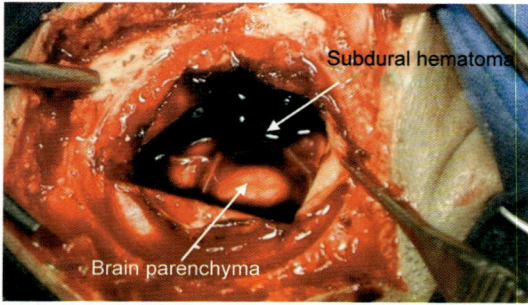

Fig. 26.4d: Acute SDH after opening dura

Intraoperatively mannitol should be administered or a bolus of phenobarbitone (10 mg/kg) may be beneficial, provided patient is not hypotensive.

Brain swelling can result from cerebral vascular engorgement following failure of cerebral **autoregulation.** Practical problem of massive brain swelling is closure of dura and whether to replace bone flap or not. It is recommended that dural should be closed with dural grafts. Some authors advocates that the dura should not be closed and the bone flap should be left out. However, this will usually lead to infarction of herniated brain. Aldrich and Eisenberg[29] strongly recommend replacement of bone flap.

2. *Intraoperative bleeding:* Venous hemorrhage is an important cause of acute subdural hematoma.

Important veins from which bleeding can occur

a. Bridging veins along the sagittal and transverse sinus.
b. Vein at the anterior aspect of the Sylvian fissure.
c. Inferior cerebral veins and dural sinuses.

These veins may continue to bleed as the subdural hematoma is removed because of release of tamponade effect. Sinus bleeding can be controlled by packing with surgical or gelfoam.

Bleeding from cortical arteries are not uncommon.

In a few cases of acute SDH, surgery may not be necessary, because of the reason that SDH is thin and not producing man effect, patient may be in good GCS or patients may be unfit for surgery. Thus conservative management can be used in selected cases.[31] Rarely, acute SDH can disappear rapidly in 12–24 hours.

Outcome of Patients with Acute Post-traumatic Subdural Hematomas

Acute subdural hematomas are associated with high mortality ranging from 36 to 90% (Table 26.3) of various factors attributing to

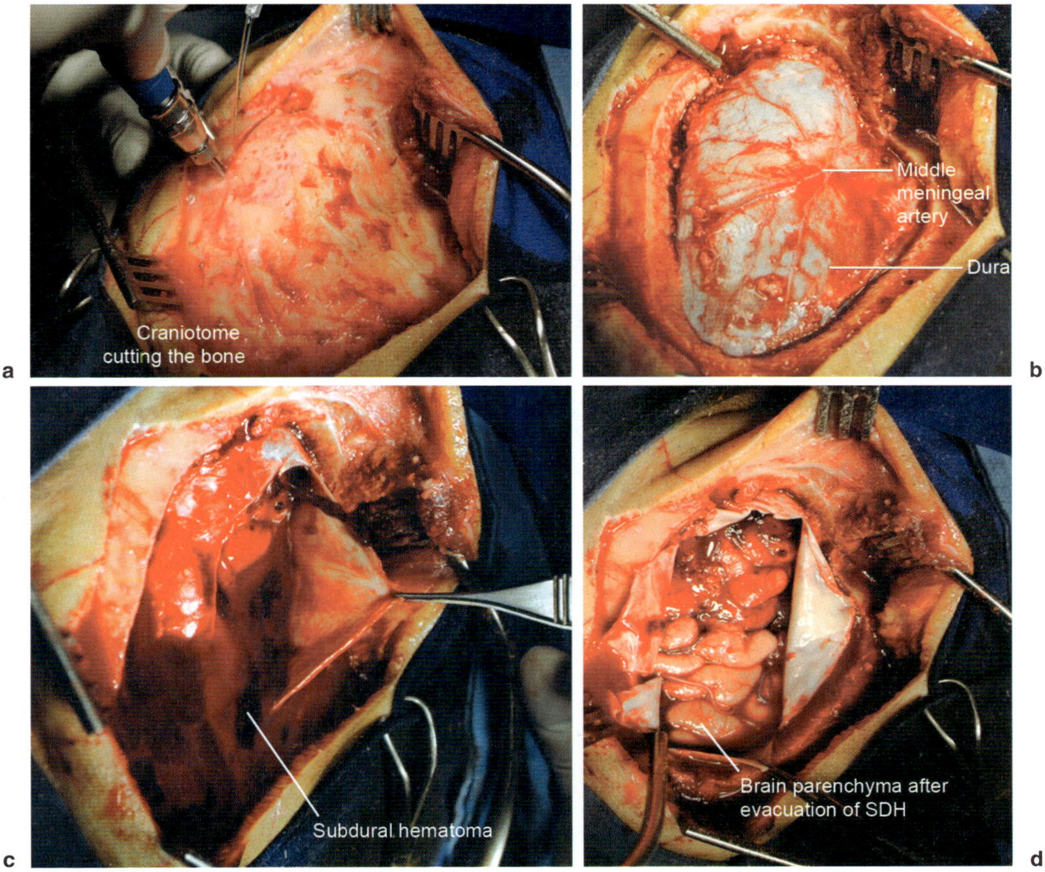

Figs 26.5a to d: Evacuation of acute SDH steps (a) making a bone flap; (b) exposure of dura; (c) cutting the dura in C shaped manner; (d) lax brain after removal of SDH

Table 26.3: Outcomes from acute subdural hematoma		
Source	*Mortality*	*Severe disability*
Gennarelli et al[14]	74 (GCS 3–5)	16
	36 (GCS 6–7)	
Stone et al[30]	59	14
Wilberger et al[2]	66	15
Marshall et al[9]	50	36

mortality, the level of consciousness at the time of presentation and at the time of operation is highly predictive of outcome. In the series of Gennarelli et al mortality correlated directly with **Glasgow Coma Scale** (GCS) score; patients with a GCS score of 3 to 5 and an acute subdural hematoma had a mortality of 76%, while patients with a GCS score of 6 to 8 had a mortality rate of 36%.[9]

Mortality and morbidity are lower in patients who are conscious when the decision to operate is made compared with those who have lucid intervals with subsequent deterioration to unconsciousness or who are unconscious throughout.

Patients who present with pupillary dilatation is strongly predictive of high mortality and morbidity.[32] Unilateral pupillary abnormality have mortality of ranging from 41 to 74%, while bilateral pupillary abnormalities ranges from 82 to 98%. Hatashita et al[33] analyzed sixty patients with acute subdural hematoma were between 1981 and 1989 and found that overall mortality was 55% and the functional recovery rate 30%. Thirteen (93%) of 14 patients with a Glasgow Coma Scale (GCS) score of 3 died, while all eight patients with a GCS score of 7 or more achieved functional recovery. The mortality of patients with GCS scores of 4–6 ranged from 45 to 67%. Patients with GCS scores of 4–6 over 65 years old had a mortality of 82%, compared to 50% mortality for those aged 19–40 years. The mortality for patients with GCS scores of 4–6 operated on within 4 hours of injury was 62% in contrast to 33% for those operated on from 4 to 10 hours. Patients with GCS scores of 4–6 who underwent craniotomy with evacuation of the hematoma achieved significantly better recovery than those treated by burr holes. Four patients with GCS scores of 4–6 died in spite of decompressive craniectomy or craniotomy with duroplasty. The mortality is only influenced by age and type of surgical intervention among patients with GCS scores of 4–6. Shorter time from injury to surgical evacuation does not affect mortality within 10 hours of injury.

Young patients have a better outcome than older patients with acute subdural hematoma.[34]

In one series, mortality increased from 39% in patients at or under 40 years of age to 70% in those older than 40 years.

Poor Prognostic Factors

1. Patients older than 40 years
2. Glasgow Coma Scale < 8
3. Pupillary abnormalities
4. Postoperatively raised intracranial pressure.
5. Delay in diagnosis and operation.

CONCLUSIONS

Acute subdural hematoma is a collection of blood under dura which results from rupture of parasagittal and Sylvian bridging veins following angular acceleration injuries to brain. Acute SDH is commonly associated contrecoup injuries and DAI. The clinical presentation in patients with acute subdural hematoma are related to increased ICP and the severity of diffuse injury to the brain. In severe injuries patient may become unconscious since the time of injury. CT scan is the investigation of choice. Acute SDH appears as a hyperdense, crescenteric extra-axial collection with or without mass effect. Surgical intervention is required in patients with thick subdural hematomas with midline shift. Intraoperative brain swelling is a common problem, which results due to vascular engorgement, EDH on opposite side and increase in intracerebral contusion/hematoma. Acute subdural hematomas have high mortality rate ranging from 36 to 90%. In selected cases patients can be managed conservatively.

REFERENCES

1. Gutman MB, Moulton RJ, et al. Risk factors predicting operable intracranial hematomas in head injury. J Neurosurg 1992;77:9–14.
2. Wilberger JE, Harris M, Diamond DL. Acute subdural hematoma: morbidity, mortality, and operative timing. Journal of Neurosurgery 1991;74(2):212–8.
3. Leitgeb J, Mauritz W, Brazinova A, Janciak I, Majdan M, Wilbacher I, Rusnak M. Outcome after severe brain trauma due to acute subdural hematoma. Journal of Neurosurgery 2012;117(2): 324–33.
4. Fell DA, Fitzgerald S, Moid RH, Caram P. Acute subdural hematomas. Review of 144 cases. J Neurosurg 1975 Jan;42(1):37–42.
5. Sosin DM, Sniezek JE, Waxweiler RJ. Trends in death associated with traumatic brain injury, 1979 through 1992: Success and failure. JAMA 1995;273:1778–80.
6. AL Hani Q, Gupta PK, Mahapatra AK, Lad SD. Development of chronic subdural hematoma. A reminder for its pathogenes Oman Medical Journal 2001;17:20–4.
7. Seelig JM, Becker DP, et al. Traumatic acute subdural hematoma: major mortality reduction in comatose patients treated within four hours. N Eng. J Med 1981;304;1511–8.

8. Zwienenberg-Lee M, Muizelaar JP. Clinical pathophysiology of traumatic brain injury. In: Winn HR, Youmans JR (eds): Youmans Neurological Surgery. Philadelphia, PA: WB Saunders 2004;5039–64.

9. Marshall L, Gautille T, Klauber M. The outcome of severe closed head injury. J Neurosurg 1991;75:S28–36.

10. Narayan RK, Michel ME, Ansell B, et al. Clinical trials in head injury. J Neurotrauma 2002;19:503–57.

11. Holmes JF, Hendey GW, Oman JA, et al. Epidemiology of blunt head injury victims undergoing ED cranial computed tomographic scanning. Am J Emerg Med 2006;24:167–73.

12. Klauber MR, Barrett-Connor E, Marshall LF, et al. The epidemiology of head injury: a prospective study of an entire community—San Diego County, California, 1978. Am J Epidemiol. 1981;113:500–9.

13. Sood P, Sinson GP, Cohen EP. Subdural hematomas in chronic dialysis patients significant and increasing. Clin J Am Soc Nephrol 2007;2:956–9.

14. Gennarelli T, Jhibault L. Biomechanics of acute subdural hematoma. J Trauma 1982;22:680–86.

15. Matsuyama T, Shimomura T, Okumura Y, et al. Acute subdural hematoma due to rupture of cortical arteries: a study of the points of rupture in 19 cases. Surg Neurol 1997;47(5):423–7.

16. Jamieson KG, Yelland JDN. Surgically treated traumatic subdural hematomas. J Neurosurg 1972;37:137–49.

17. Marshall LF, Gautile T, et al. The outcome of severe head injury. J Neurosurg 75 (Suppl) 1991;28–36.

18. Balasubramaniam V, Ramamurthi B. Subdural hematoma. J Ind Med Assn 1961;36:1.

19. Kalyanraman S, Ramamurthi B, et al. Subdural hematoma. Neurol (India) 1970;18:18.

20. Kalyanraman S. Traumatic Intracranial Hemorrhage. In:Ramamurthi B, Tandon PN (eds). Textbook of Neurosurgery, 2nd edn. BI Churchill Livingstone 1996;307–14.

21. McKissock W, Richardson A, et al. Subdural hematoma. A review of 389 cases. Lancet 1960;1:1365–69.

22. Kernohan JW, Woltman HW. Incisura of the cinus due to contralateral brain tumour. Arch Neurol Psychiatry 1929;27:274–87.

23. Mendelow AD, Teasdale G, Jennett B, et al. risks of intracranial hematoma in head injured adults. BMJ 1983;287:1173–6.

24. Samudrala S, Cooper PR: Traumatic Intracranial hematomas. In Wilkin RH, Rengachary SS (Eds): Neurosurgery McGraw-Hill, 1996:2797–807.

25. Cortiana M, Zagara G, Fava S, et al. Coagulation abnormalities in patients with head injury. J Neurosurg Sci 1986;30:133–8.

26. Goodnight SH, Kenoyer G, Rapaport SI, et al. Defibrination after brain-tissue destruction: A serious complication of head injury. N Engl J Med 1974;290:1043–47.

27. Obana WG, Pitts LH. Extracerebral Lesions. Neurosurg Clin N Am 1991;2:351–72.

28. Meyer SH, Chesnut RM: Post-traumatic Extra-axial Mass Lesions: Subdural and extradural hematoma. In Tindall GT, Cooper PR, Barrow DL (eds): The Practice of Neurosurgery, Williams and Wilkins 1996;1461–72.

29. Aldrich EF, Eisenberg HW: Acute Subdural hematoma. In Apuzzo MLZ (ed) Brain Surgery complication Avoidance and Management, Churchill Livingstone 1993;1283–98.

30. Stone JL, Lowe RJ, et al. Acute subdural hematoma: direct admission to a trauma centre yields improved results. J Trauma 1986;26:445–50.

31. Croce MA, Dent DL, Menke PG, et al. Acute Subdural hematoma: nonsurgical management of selected patients J. Trauma 1994;36:820–26.

32. Me Laurin RL, Tutor FT. Acute subdural hematoma. Review of ninety cases. J Neurosurg 1961;18:61–7.

33. Hatashita S, Koga N, Hosaka Y, Takagi S. Acute subdural hematoma: severity of injury, surgical intervention, and mortality. Neurol Med Chir (Tokyo) 1993;33(1):13–8.

34. Jennett B, Bond M. Assessment of outcome after severe brain damage: a practical scale. Lancet 1975;1:480–84.

27

Cerebral Contusion and Intracerebral Hematoma

Raj Kamal

INTRODUCTION

A cortical contusion is a bruise of the brain's parenchyma. Contusio cerebri, a form of traumatic brain injury, is a bruise of the brain tissue.[1] A cerebral laceration is a similar injury except that, according to their respective definitions, the pia-arachnoid membranes are torn over the site of injury in laceration and are not torn in contusion.[2,3] Cerebral contusions are similar to other bruises in tissues and can be associated with multiple microhemorrhages, small blood vessel leaks into brain tissue. It consists of heterogeneous areas of hemorrhage, brain necrosis and infarction.[4] A cerebral contusion is distinctive of mechanical injury. Contusions formed at the site of cranial impact are **coup contusions** and those opposite the cranial impact are **contrecoup contusions**. Herniation contusions occur in the margins of brain hernias located most frequently along the margin of the falx cerebri, tentorium or foramen magnum.[5] In several series of head-injured patients, the occurrence of cerebral contusion has varied from 20 to 40%.[6–9]

Traumatic parenchymal hematoma may result from the coalescence of the hemorrhages within contusion. The pathogenesis of production of intracerebral hematomas are similar to pathogenesis of contusions.

Pathology and Pathogenesis

Coup contusions are due to direct injury to the brain tissue and its surface vessels by fracture fragments. The direct injury causes highly localised compressive strains. Coup contusions result from high negative pressure, that develop when an area of inbent skull rapidly snaps back into place (*see* Chapter 3 on biomechanics of head injury). This results in high tensile strains causing rupture of pial vessels, cortical vessels and cause brain tissue damage.[10]

Contrecoup contusions result from translational or angular head motion. Angular head motion produces high tensile strains throughout the brain. According to Gennarelli and Meaney[10] if these tensile strains exceeds the vascular tolerance in a given region, contusion results. These tensile strains are concentrated in certain regions of the brain due to geometric effects. **These areas are adjacent to the bony structures with considerable irregularity to the surface of the frontal lobe and the temporal lobes. In clinical practice, contusions of frontal and temporal lobe are very common.**[11,12] Contusion of the occipital lobe is rare because it is surrounded by the falx cerebri and the tentorium on two sides and on the third side by the smooth, curving skull adjacent to the occipital lobe.

Frosch et al[13] concluded that as with any other organ, a blow to the surface of the brain,

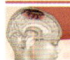

transmitted through the skull, leads to rapid tissue displacement, disruption of vascular channels, and subsequent hemorrhage, tissue injury, and edema. The crests of gyri are most susceptible, since this is where the direct force is greatest. The most common locations for contusions correspond to the most frequent sites of direct impact and to regions of the brain that overlie a rough and irregular inner skull surface, such as the frontal lobes along the orbital ridges and the temporal lobes. Contusions are less frequent over the occipital lobes, brainstem, and cerebellum unless these sites are adjacent to a skull fracture (fracture contusions) (Fig. 27.1). When seen on cross-section, contusions are wedge shaped, with the broad base lying along the surface, deep to the point of impact. The histologic appearance of contusions is independent of the type of trauma. In the earliest stages, there is edema and hemorrhage, which is often pericapillary. During the next few hours, the extravasation of blood extends throughout the involved tissue, across the width of the cerebral cortex, and into the white matter and subarachnoid space. Morphologic evidence of neuronal injury (pyknosis of the nucleus, eosinophilia

of the cytoplasm, and disintegration of the cell) takes about 24 hours to appear, although functional deficits may occur earlier. Axonal swellings develop in the vicinity of damaged neurons or at great distances away. The inflammatory response to the injured tissue follows its usual course, with the appearance of neutrophils followed by macrophages.[13]

Contusions involve gyral crests, are wedge shaped extending through the cortex to the white matter. According to definition if the pia is torn then the injury becomes cerebral laceration.

Lindenberg and Freytag[14] described gliding contusion as areas of focal hemorrhages along superior medial margins of cerebral hemispheres. These are deep parenchymal injuries that may or may not be comparable to surface contusion.[5,14]

Pathogenesis of intracerebral hematoma is similar to cerebral contusion. The mechanisms of coup and contrecoup injury described for cerebral contusion also apply for intracerebral hematoma.[15] Intracerebral hematomas frequently occur in frontal and/or temporal lobes. Hematomas can be adjacent to contusion. Traumatic intracerebral hematoma

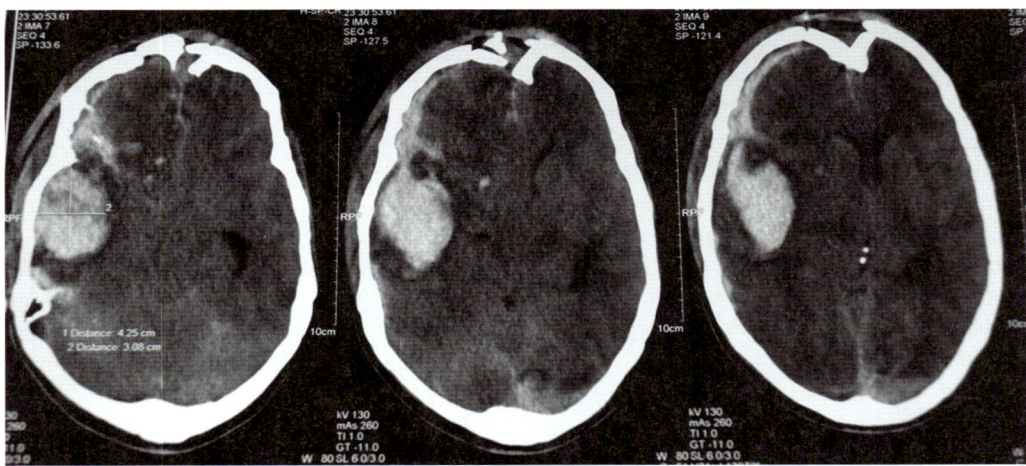

Fig. 27.1: Axial CT scan shows right temporal contusion hematoma with acute subdural hematoma and frontal depressed fracture. There is associated right frontal contusion. This lesion is causing significant mass effect as evident by compressed-ipsilateral frontal horn, and obliterated basal cisterns. Dilated contralateral temporal horn indicates brain herniation

can be present without cerebral contusion. In 20% case hematomas are multiple and in 30 to 60% are associated with extracerebral hematomas.[16–18]

Certain factors such as loss of autoregulation and post-traumatic coagulopathies can lead to delayed formation and increase in size of intracerebral hematoma.[19–21] Delayed post-traumatic hematoma have been noted following surgical removal of cerebral contusions. This most probably occurs because of loss of initial tamponade effects of mass lesion.[22,23]

Clinical Features

There is no specific clinical picture that suggests cortical contusion. The symptoms associated with cerebral contusion vary widely depending on patient factors, other coexistent traumatic injuries and the size and severity of the contusion. Frequently, significant contusion is associated with other traumatic brain injury and thus the clinical presentation of the patient is the result of multiple pathologies. If a contusion is big enough, it can cause significant swelling and resultant increase in intracranial pressure causing different degree of depression of their level of consciousness.

It is progressive neurological deterioration following head injury that makes contusions and intracerebral hematoma likely especially if there has been progressive deterioration of consciousness with localizing signs.[16] Signs of brainstem compression and transtentorial herniation are more common in temporal contusion and hematoma. Traumatic temporal contusion and hematomas produce brainstem compression because of their location in the middle fossa with bone on their inferior, lateral, and anterior side. The path of least resistance would appear to be towards the brainstem.[16,24]

Bifrontal contusions can produce delayed neurological deterioration in the patient. The shift in bifrontal contusion may be more in anteroposterior direction than in lateral direction.[15,24] Temporal contusions and

hematomas can be dangerous because they can produce brainstem compression in presence of normal or slightly raised ICP.

Delayed intracerebral hematoma is diagnosed by serial CT scans. The indication for repeat CT scan are:

i. Development of focal neurological deficit.
ii. Failure to improve.
iii. Neurological deterioration.

Gudeman et al[21] found the incidence of delayed intracerebral hematoma to be 8% among 162 consecutive severe closed head injuries. In 90% cases the diagnosis of delayed traumatic intracerebral hematoma by CT was within 48 hours.

Cerebellar hematoma following head injury are uncommon and results from coup injury. They are associated with occipital bone fracture and cerebellar contusion. They can cause brainstem compression and obstructive hydrocephalus.[25–27]

CT Scan Findings

On CT scan, contusions appear as lesions of mixed density, with areas of high density blood surrounded by low density areas of edema and tissue necrosis with or without mass effect (Figs 27.1 and 27.2). They may be entirely of low density after 24 to 48 hours due to resorption of blood.[28,29]

On CT scan, traumatic intracerebral hematoma is visualized as a focal, well defined rounded areas of abnormal density in the brain (Fig. 27.1). Early CT findings include patchy, ill-defined low density lesions that may be mixed with smaller hyperdense foci of petechial hemorrhage (Figs 27.2a, 27.3a and b). In 20% of cases delayed hemorrhages develop in what previously appeared as non-hemorrhagic low density areas. Traumatic parenchymal hematomas may result from the coalescence of the hemorrhages within contusion. Normal, fresh whole blood is hyperdense (50 to 60 Houns-field units [HU] relative to normal brain (20 to 35 HU). This density is accounted for almost entirely by the globin (protein) moiety of hemoglobin. CT

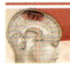

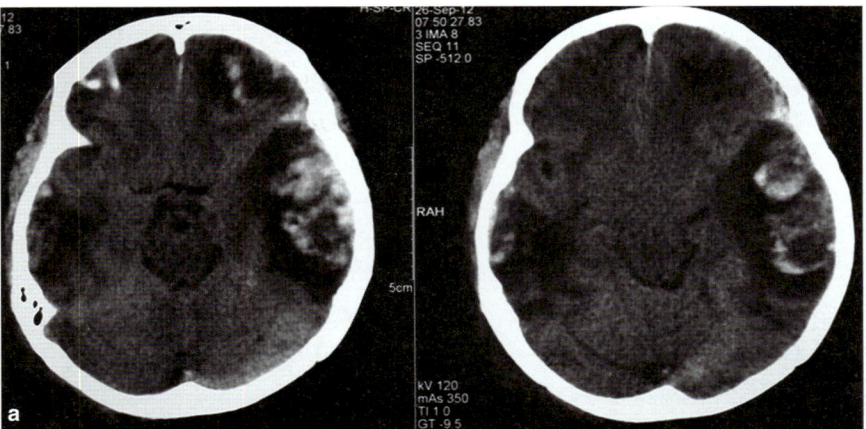

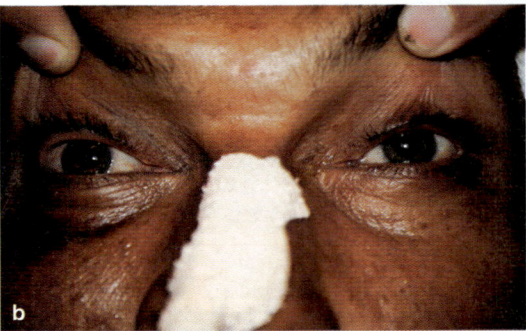

Figs 27.2a and b: (a) CT scan brain showing large left temporal contusion with small right temporal and left frontal contusion; (b) patient (CT scan in Fig. 27.2a) showing dilated left pupil indicating that early surgical decompression is required

scan may fail to show non hemorrhagic contusion or small contusion in brainstem, which can be well visualised by MR scan. MR is much more sensitive than CT Scan in visualizing contusions and the demarcation is much clear and distinct (Figs 27.4a and b). Multiple superficial areas of hyperintense signal abnormalities are seen on T_2-weighted images.[30,31]

Management

The optimal management of cerebral contusion and hematoma is variable. Management depends upon clinical condition of the patient, size of contusion and intracranial pressure. Patients with small, deep, lesions are managed conservatively.[27] Patients with large intra-cerebral hematoma and/or contusion with mass effect, altered sensorium should be surgically evacuated. Prompt surgical removal of significant SDH and EDH is well established and is widely accepted procedure. Surgical practice in the treatment of traumatic ICH differ widely around the world. The aim of surgery in traumatic ICH removal is to prevent secondary brain damage. To determine role of surgery in TICH, STITCH (surgical trial in traumatic intracerebral hemorrhage) trial[35] is going on (*refer* to Chapter 18).

Patients whose hematomas are small (irrespective of neurological deficit) and patients with hemorrhages involving the deep

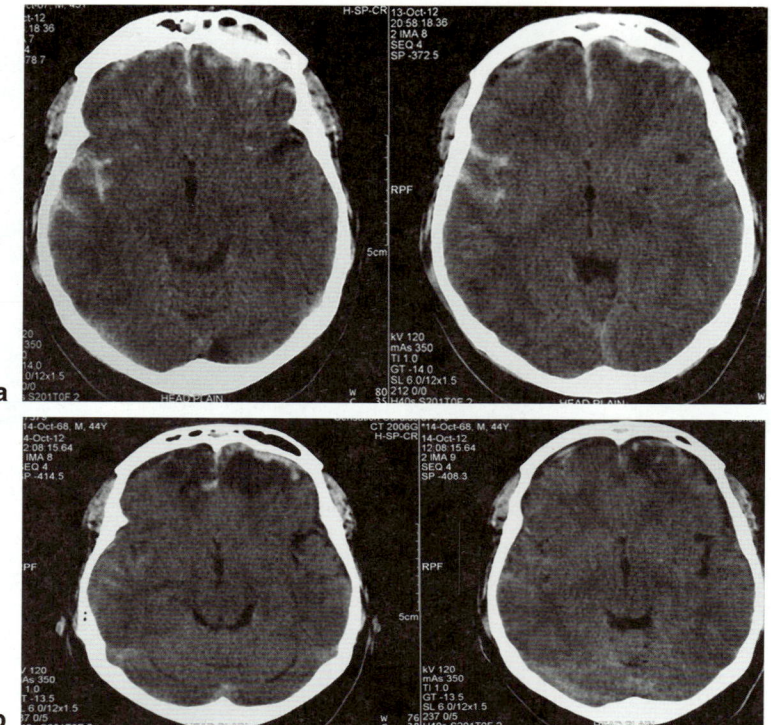

Figs 27.3a and b: Axial CT scan in a patient with severe closed head injury. Immediately after head injury showing bifrontal and right temporal contusion with traumatic SAH in right Sylvian fissure (a). CT scan after 24 hours showing resolution of SAH and contusions with hypodensity in left frontal region (b)

white matter, basal ganglia or in brainstem usually do not require surgery.[4]

Intracranial pressure monitoring should be done in all severe head injury patients with intracerebral hematoma and/or contusion. Intracranial hypertensive unresponsive to medical treatment, midline shift on CT on deteriorating neurological condition are indications for surgical removal of contusion/hematoma.

Intracranial pressure of over 20 mm Hg sustained for more than 5 minutes should be treated. In patients with temporal lobe or deep frontal lobe lesions, in whom the risk of uncal herniation is greater, and ICP of over 15 mm Hg should be treated.[25,33]

Measures to control intracranial hypertension includes normothermia, head elevation, sedation, hyperventilation ventricular drainage, Mannitol and barbiturate coma. These measures are described in detail elsewhere.

If the ICP is not controlled by above means then repeat CT scan should be done to rule out new or increasing intracerebral hematoma. Phenytoin should be given postoperatively for prophylaxis against post-traumatic seizures.

Post-traumatic Cerebellar Hematoma

larger than 30 cc and/or greater than 3 cm should be evacuated through suboccipital craniectomy. Cerebellar hematomas cause direct brainstem compression and needs urgent attention.

Outcome

Outcome in intracerebral hematomas and cerebral contusions vary widely. Mortality

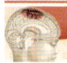

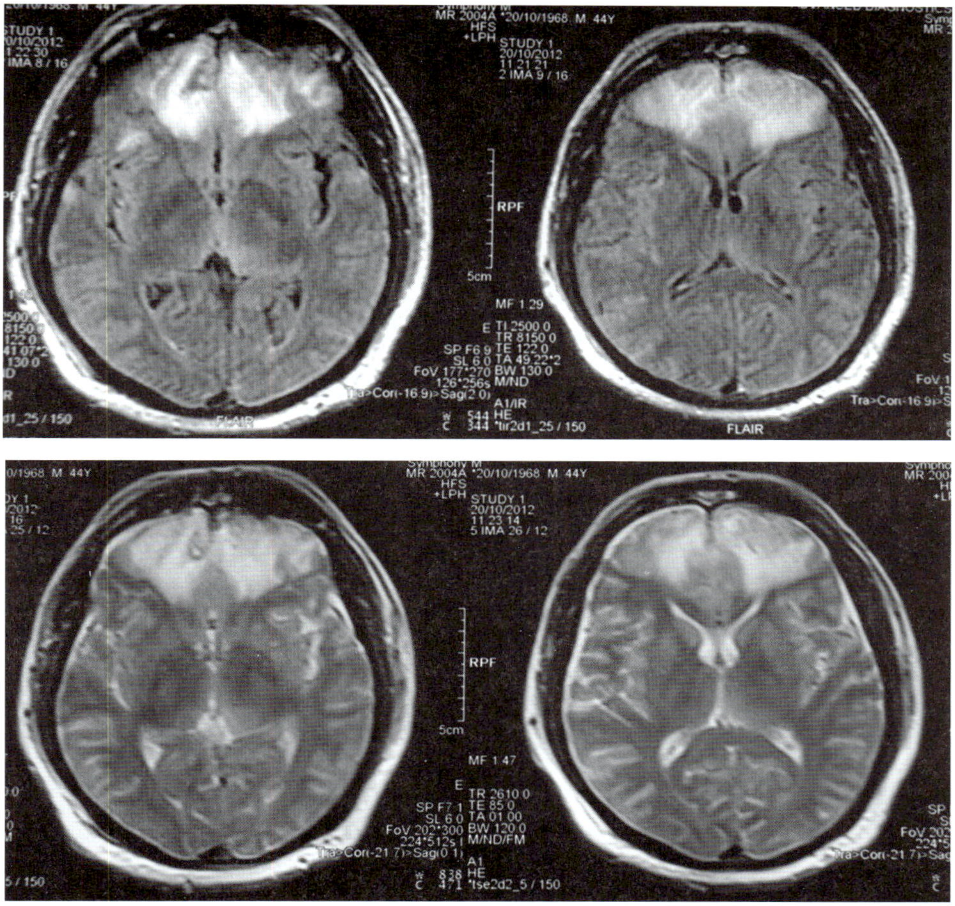

Figs 27.4a and b: MRI brain of patient on 7th day after head injury. Axial T_1- and T_2-weighted images show hyperintense bifrontal contusions

and morbidity depends on the neurological status at the time of operation.

Associated intracranial lesions, as well as the severity of the primary brain injury itself markedly influences the prognosis.

Intracerebral hematomas: Mortality rate varies from 25 to 72%.[29,34]

Contusion: Mortality rate varies from 25 to 60%. For delayed intracerebral hematomas mortality reported is more than 50%.[19]

CONCLUSIONS

Contusion and post-traumatic intracerebral hematomas are relatively frequent in head injury. The pathogenesis traumatic intracerebral hematoma is similar to cerebral contusion. Cerebral contusion and traumatic intracerebral hematoma occur due to coup and contrecoup injuries. These frequently occur in frontal and temporal lobes because of bony irregularities and high tensile strains in these areas of brain. Clinical symptoms and signs vary with location and size of the intracerebral hematoma. Larger contusions produce significant neurological deterioration in the patient. Temporal lobe contusion and hematoma can present with deteriorating level of consciousness, oculomotor nerve

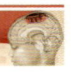

palsy or an uncal herniation syndrome. Large bifrontal contusions result in delayed, abrupt clinical deterioration. Traumatic intracerebral hematoma and contusions can be diagnosed easily by CT scan. Contusions and hematomas producing mass effect should be evacuated surgically. Small contusion with no mass effect should be managed conservatively.

REFERENCES

1. Hardman JM, Manoukian A. "Pathology of Head Trauma". Neuroimaging Clinics of North America 2002;12(2):175–87.
2. Granacher RP. Traumatic Brain Injury: Methods for Clinical and Forensic Neuropsychiatric Assessment, Second Edition. Boca Raton: CRC 2007;26.
3. Gennarelli GA, Graham DI. "Neuropathology". In Silver JM, McAllister TW, Yudofsky SC. Textbook of Traumatic Brain Injury. Washington, DC: American Psychiatric Association 2005:29.
4. Samudrala S, Cooper PR. Traumatic Intracranial hematomas. In Wilkins RH, Rengachary SS (Eds.), Neurosurgery Second, (eds.) McGraw-Hill 1996;2797–2807.
5. Hardman JM. Cerebrospinal trauma. In Davis RL, Robertson DM (eds). Textbook of Neuropathology, 3rd edn Williams and Wilkins 1997; 1179–232.
6. Khoshyomn S, Tranmer BI. "Diagnosis and management of pediatric closed head injury". Seminars in Pediatric Surgery 2004;13(2):80–6.
7. Dublin AB, French BN, Rennick JM. Computed tomography in head trauma. Radiology 1977;122:365–9.
8. French BN, Dublin AB. The value of computerised tomography in the management of 1000 consecutive head injuries. Surg Neurol 1977;7:171–83.
9. McPherson BCM, McPherson P, Jennett B. CT evidence of intracranial contusion and hematoma in relation to the presence, site and type of skull fracture. Clin Radiol 1990;42:321–26.
10. Gennarelli TA, Meaney DF. Cranial trauma, In Wilkins RH, Rengachary SS (eds). Neurosurgery (2nd edn), McGraw-Hill 1996;2611–21.
11. Hirsh LF. Delayed traumatic intracerebral hematomas after surgical decompression. Neurosurgery 1979;5(6):653–5.
12. Stender A, Schulze A. The surgical treatment of space occupying contusions and intracerebral hematoma after blunt cerebral trauma. Excepta Med-Intern Congress Series 1966;110:231–5.
13. Frosch MP, Anthony DC, Girolami UD, The Central Nervous System, In Kumar, Abbas, Fausto, Aster (eds); Robbins and Cotran Pathologic Basis of Disease, 8th edn, Elsevier 2010; 1279–1344.
14. Lindenberg R and Freytag E. A mechanism of cerebral contusions: A pathologic-anatomic study. Arch Pathol 1960;69:440–69.
15. Gaylan L. Rockswod. Post-traumatic intra-axial mass lesions: hematomas, contusions, edema. In Tindall GT, Cooper PR, Barrow DL. The practice of Neurogery, 1st edn. Williams and Wilkins 1995;1461–72.
16. Browder J, Turney MF. Intracerebral hemorrhage of traumatic origin: Its surgical treatment. NY State J Med 1942;42:2230–35.
17. Solonick D, Pitts LH, et al. Traumatic intracerebral hematomas: Timing of appearance and indications for operative removal. J. Trauma. Rockswold GL. Post-traumatic intra-axial mass lesions 1986;26:787–94.
18. Fukamachi A, Kohnok, Nagaseki Y, et al. The incidence of delayed traumatic intracerebral hematoma with extradural hemorrhage. J. Trauma 1985;25:145–9.
19. Diaz FG, Yock DH, Larson D, et al. Early diagnosis of delayed post-traumatic intracerebral hematomas. J Neurosurg 1979;50:217–23.
20. Evans JP, Scheinker IM. Histological studies of the brain following head trauma II. Post-traumatic petechial and massive intracerebral hemorrhage. J Neurosurg 1946;3:101–13.
21. Gudeman SK, Kishore PRS, et al. The genesis and significance of delayed traumatic intracerebral hematoma. Neurosurgery 1979;5:309–13.
22. Gupta PK, Mahapatra AK, Lad SD. Delayed hematoma in head injury. Pan Arab J Neurosurg 2003;7:40–5.
23. Hirsh LF. Delayed traumatic intracerebral hematomas after surgical decompression. Neurosurgery 1979;5(6):653–5.
24. Statham PF, Johnston RA, McPherson P. Delayed deterioration in patients with traumatic frontal contusions. J Neurol Neurosurg Psychiatry 1989;52:351–4.
25. Kelly DF, Mebride DQ, Becker DP. Surgical Management of Severe closed Head Injury in Adults. In: Schmidek HH, Sweet WH (eds). Operative Neurosurgical Techniques. Indications, Methods and Results, 3rd edn. WB Saunders company 1995;47–67.

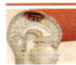 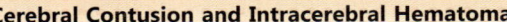

26. Firsching R, Frowein R, Thun F. Intracerebellar hematoma: eleven traumatic and non-traumatic cases and a review of literature. Neurochirurgia, 1987;30:182–5.

27. Nagata K, Ishikawa T, et al. Delayed traumatic intracerebellar hematoma: Correlation between the location of the hematoma and the pre-existing cerebellar contusion. Neurol Med Chir (Tokyo) 1991;31:792–6.

28. Jamieson KG, Yelland JDNR. Traumatic intracerebral hematoma: report of 63 surgically treated cases. J Neurosurg 1972;37:528–32.

29. Jay a Kumar PN, Sastry KVR, et al. Prognosis in contrecoup intracranial hematoma—a clinical and radiological study of 63 patients. Acta Neurochir (Wien) 1991;108:30–3.

30. Osborne AG, In diagnostic Neuroradiology, Mosby, Craniocerebral trauma 1994;199–244.

31. Lane B, Stevens JM, Moseley IF. Cranial and intracranial pathology. In Grainger RG, Allison DJ (eds), Grainger and Allison's Diagnostic Radiology, A Textbook of Medical Imaging, Churchill Livingstone 1997:2127–48.

32. Soloniuk D, Pitts LH, Lovely M, et al. Traumatic intracerebral hematomas: timing of appearance and indications for operative removal; J. Trauma 1986;26:787–94.

33. Chestnut RM, Marshall LF, Marshall SB. Medical Management of intracranial pressure, in Cooper PR (ed.): Head Injury, 3rd edn. Baltimore, Williams and Wilkins 1993; 225–46.

34. Bullock R, Golek J, Blake G. Traumatic intracerebral hematoma—which patient should undergo surgical evacuation? CT scan features and ICP monitoring as a basis for decision-making. Surg Neurol 1989;32:181–7.

35. Gregson BA, Rowan EN, Patrick M Mitchell, Unterverg A, et al. Surgical trial in traumatic intracerebral hemorrhage [STITCH (trauma)]: study protocol for randomised controlled trial; Trials 2012;13:193.

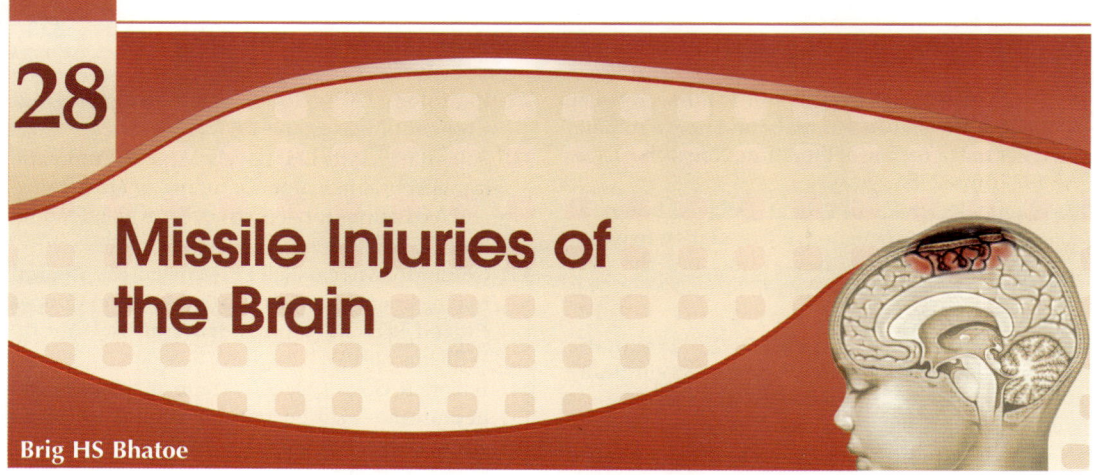

28

Missile Injuries of the Brain

Brig HS Bhatoe

INTRODUCTION

Missile injuries of the brain have traditionally viewed with pessimism due to their supposedly poor outcome. While their incidence is rising all over the world due to rise in ethnic armed struggle, militancy and terrorist related violence, civilian injuries are also showing a rise due to easy availability of firearms.[25] There has been improved understanding of these injuries due to pioneering works of Horsley, Cushing and more recently by experience in the Korean and Vietnam wars. Missile ballistics is now understood better and CT has revolutionized the evaluation and prognostication of these injuries. Multi- and univariate analysis of various factors influencing the likely outcome has been attempted, and the Glasgow Coma Scale score has remained the most reliable predictor of the outcome. Surgical techniques have been standardized and postoperative monitoring is better. Outcome of such injuries, both during war or war-like situations and in civilian gunshot wounds has shown improvement and there has been rethinking on the problem of retained intracranial fragments. A better understanding of pathology and adherence to basic neurosurgical principles of definitive surgical management will ensure saving of more lives and improved neurological preservation. Nevertheless, mortality due to these injuries remains high, a fact to be borne in mind by all those who attend to victims of craniocerebral missile injuries.

HISTORICAL PERSPECTIVE

Penetrating wounds of the head have challenged physicians since medieval ages. Within a few hundred years of the Mongols' bringing gunpowder to Europe from China in the fourteenth century, a firearm (Spanish musket) was invented which could propel a projectile at 1000 feet/sec and could inflict previously unimaginable wounds.[53] There was little attempt to treat these injuries over the next three centuries, and until the turn of the twentieth century, missile injuries of the brain were almost universally fatal. Modern management of these injuries began with the experimental studies of Sir Victor Horsley,[30] in which he described the hydrodynamic nature of CMIs, and cessation of respiration with rise in intracranial pressure. This was followed by application of antiseptic techniques to combat neurosurgery in the Anglo-Boer war (1899–1902). Management was further advanced and standardized by Harvey Cushing during his wartime service in France during the First World War, which resulted in a decrease in mortality from 54 to 28%.[18]

The literature on missile wounds sustained during war is more extensive than that deals with such injuries incurred in peacetime. Each war has furthered experience in this regard.

World War I proved the efficacy of definitive surgical intervention. The Spanish Civil War showed that the blast effect was a significant component of craniofacial injury. During World War II, initial dural repair and antibiotic medication showed distinct improvement in outcome.[37] The Korean War confirmed the effectiveness of prompt evacuation of the patient to a neurosurgical centre, often by helicopters from the battle site, followed by definitive neurosurgical intervention. This resulted in improved survival and reduced infection.[38] The civil disturbances in Belfast took place close to the neurosurgical center and the natural history of penetrating injury could be studied from the moment of injury.[10,41] During the Israeli expedition into Lebanon, all the victims of head injuries were brought to a single institution and for the first time, the place of CT scan in combat neurosurgery was established and a less aggressive debridement could be followed.[9] Finally, after the Vietnam conflict, the Vietnam Head Injury Study (VHIS) involving the US Army, Navy, Air Force and American Red Cross followed up the head injury survivors of war for 18 years and elicited valuable data.[40] Significantly, during the Gulf War (1991), there were only two cases of missile injuries of the brain among the American troops.[11] From India, Bajpayee[4] reported on missile injuries of the brain sustained during the 1971 Indo-Pak war. Experiences with civilian gunshot wounds too have been reported.[14,19,39,43] Experiences in management of low velocity missile injuries (LVMIs) to the brain during low intensity military conflicts and antimilitancy operations have recently been analyzed.[8,20] Experiences with CMIs during OP VIJAY (Kargil) have been analyzed and the role of conservative debridement and meticulous dural closure has been firmly established.[49] The management principles have been successfully extrapolated to the management of civilian casualties.

Applied Ballistics the Missiles

Projectiles travelling at less than 2000 feet/sec fall into the category of low velocity missiles, while those traveling above this speed are high velocity missiles. There is a distinct difference in the pattern of injury and outcome of low velocity missile injuries (LVMIs) and high velocity missile injuries (HVMIs). Most handguns and revolvers use heavy bullets weighing about 0.5 oz and have muzzle velocities ranging from 550 to 900 ft/sec. In contrast, most rifles and small arms (rifles, stenguns, machine-guns, etc.) used in war use light bullets having muzzle velocities averaging 3000 ft/sec. High velocity missiles as they reach the limit of their range become low velocity (*spent bullet*) and may inflict less severe wounds as compared to that within their effective range. The handgun ammunition can achieve muzzle velocity of 1200 ft/sec effective over a short distance. Pieces of shrapnel from exploding devices may have a velocity of 600 ft/sec; unlike rifled bullets however, they rapidly lose energy due to their irregular shape and non-aerodynamic nature. The commonly observed CNS missile injuries are inflicted by one of the following missiles:

1. *The 7.62 mm bullet:* This can be fired by AK-47 assault rifle (Kalashnikov), self loading rifle (SLR), light machine gun or medium machine gun (LMG/MMG). The bullet weighs 150 grams and has a muzzle velocity of more than 2000 ft/sec.

2. The 5.56 mm bullet fired from Indian Small Arms System (INSAS), M-16 rifle. The bullet weighs 55 grams and has a muzzle velocity of more than 3000 ft/sec.

3. Low velocity missiles fired from a variety of firearms, viz. revolvers, shotguns, handguns, 12 bore single/double barrel guns, country made weapons (*katta, tamancha*, etc. as prevalent in parts of Bihar and Uttar Pradesh).

4. *Fragments of exploding devices:* The variety of exploding devices reflects the ingenuity of the minds that assemble them, often in innocuous looking forms. They may be made to look like toys, transistors, CD players, etc. which are often detonated by handling or by remote access. A domestic

LPG cylinder placed on its top often makes an innocuous looking but deadly combination for explosion. Other familiar sources of missiles are the HE 36 mm grenade, rockets, and exploding artillery/mortar shells. Fragments of exploding devices initially travel at high speeds of over 3000 ft/sec, and then rapidly lose speed because their volume, weight, irregular shape and become low velocity at distances of 10 metres or more.

5. Glass fragments, nails, etc. may rarely act as missiles.[42, 55]

Energy Transfer

A bullet is stable in its flight through the atmosphere, but becomes less stable on entering the tissues, when it tends to yaw, deform, tumble due to resistance offered by the tissues, thus releasing kinetic energy (KE). Injury to the tissues by a missile is a function of energy release over time, and of the volume and location of tissue disruption. The amount of kinetic energy contained in the missile is defined by the formula $E = -1/2mv^2$, where m is the mass of the missile and v its velocity. Since energy contained in the missile varies directly with the square of its velocity, the latter is relatively more important in determining the energy transfer by the missile than the mass. The amount of tissue damage caused by a missile may be correlated with the amount of energy deposited within the tissues by the missile. The energy transferred can be expressed by the equation:

$$E_t = E_{en} - E_{ex}$$

where E_t = missile energy transferred, E_{en} = energy of entry at the time of impact, and E_{ex} = energy contained in the missile at the time of its exit from the tissues.

If the missile exits, only part of its kinetic energy will be deposited within the tissues. The same amount of energy may be deposited by a missile of a smaller mass with a high velocity, or a greater mass missile with low velocity. The amount of energy transfer to the brain is the difference of the energies of the missiles at entry into and exit from the skull. If the missile does not exit from the skull, the energy transferred is the energy contained in the missile at the moment of impact. Thus, lower the residual velocity, greater the energy liberated.[29]

The extent and degree of damage in wounds are proportional to the amount of KE of the missile dissipated in the wound. The injury produced by the missile is increased by factors causing it to give up more of its energy intracranially. A missile that yaws will give up more of its energy. Similarly, a hollow point bullet that shatters upon impact will tend to give up more KE to the brain, is more destructive than bullets that do not shatter. Likewise, shotgun injuries caused by multiple pellets at close range, each with relatively small amount of KE are extremely destructive; each of these pellets acts as an independent missile invested with KE according to its mass and velocity. Other factors that determine KE transfer by a missile are the resistance offered by the tissues and the tendency of the bullet to deform and increase the area with which it impacts the brain with a consequent increase energy transfer to the tissues. Bullets with a flat front and expansion on impact (*dumdum bullets*) present a large surface area to the tissues to transfer energy. A rifled bullet fired at low velocity, spinning with its ling axis parallel to the trajectory may pass cleanly through the tissue and exit retaining much of its KE it had on impact. A high velocity rifle bullet of the same caliber will more likely strike with its long axis at a slight angle to its trajectory,[6] and as a consequence of this and its great velocity, deform and may even disintegrate in the tissues. The much greater tissue resistance to this high velocity deformed and 'tilted' missile and its fragments leads to release of an enormous amount of KE. The tissue damage is proportionately greater. Transfer of energy is greatest in dense tissues with a high water content. Thus, wounds of brain (and those of liver, kidney, muscle and bone) are more destructive than wounds of less dense tissue such as lung or fat.

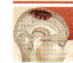

Physical Effects of Missile Wounding[23]

Missile wounding can be understood in terms of physical interactions between the missile and the tissues through which it passes. The primary destructive effects of a missile interacting with tissues is caused by two mechanisms:

1. *Crushing action of the missile:* There is fracture of the skull, laceration and fragmentation of brain tissue and injury to vascular structures.

2. *Pressure waves and cavitation* (Fig. 28.1): Besides the direct crushing action, a missile moving in water or tissue medium generates distinctive types of pressures waves within the medium it transits:

    a. *Juxta-missile pressure:* Extremely high pressures (thousands of atmospheres) are generated immediately infront of and at right angles to a moving missile, owing to flow of medium (through which the missile is travelling) around the missile.

    b. *Longitudinal shock wave:* When a missile strikes animal tissues, a high pressure compression front or shock wave is formed which moves spherically away from the point of impact. It is doubtful whether these shock waves result in any energy transfer to cause tissue damage.[28]

    c. *Pressure waves from KE transfer (Cavitation):* Cavitation (Fig. 28.1) was first recognized as a pathological phenomenon in missile injuries by Woodruff.[54] At the same time, Sir Victor Horsley[30] demonstrated experimentally the cavitation in missile injuries of the brain by firing into clay models of brain. When a high velocity missile passes through tissues, KE is transferred to adjacent tissue elements, which are propelled radially, creating, creating a large sub-atmospheric temporary cavity directly behind the missile. When the elastic limit of this outwardly displaced tissue is reached, it falls inward whence it was displaced. This cycle may be repeated several times before the deranged tissue comes to rest around the permanent track created by the missile. The oscillatory, outward and inward rush of tissue created a long lasting (milliseconds) lower amplitude (20 to 30 atmospheres) pressure wave which propagates throughout the medium. It has been considered that these lower amplitude, longer lasting pressure waves are the cause of damage to the tissues at a distance from the site of actual missile injury. Kinetic energy deposited by a missile is partitioned between that which directly crushes tissues in its path and that which displaces tissues adjacent to the missile track. The latter is less destructive than the former owing to the elastic properties of the displaced tissue which may be

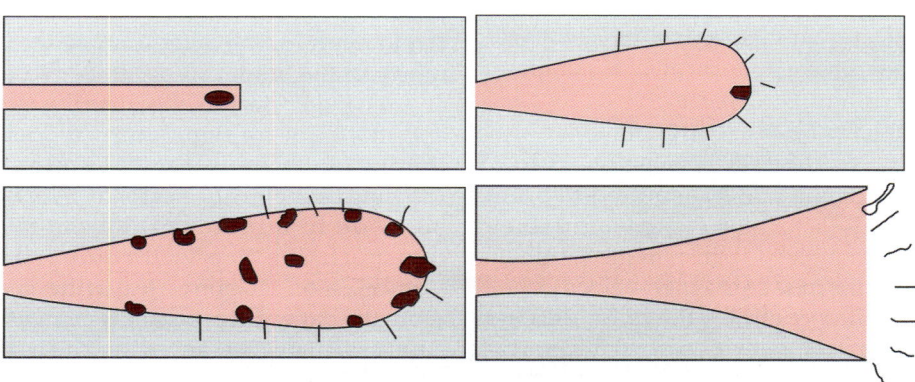

Fig. 28.1: Passage of high- and low-velocity missiles through the animal tissues

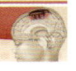

deformed without being irrevocably destroyed.[12,16]

Pathophysiology

Pathophysiology of CMI remains a complicated and poorly understood aspect of neurotrauma although some deductions arrived at from head injury management can be applied to it. Absence of specific data, and scant literature on experimental studies (unlike that seen in closed head injuries) are major limiting factors in further understanding of pathophysiology of CMI.

Effect on ICP and cerebral perfusion: Experimental studies have revealed an instantaneous rise in ICP immediately after tissue penetration, due to shock waves lasting 15–25 microseconds; the magnitude of rise is determined by the amount of KE of the missile and can reach up to 80 kg/cm^2.[2,29] Such a rise in ICP may produce instant brainstem compression, internal brain herniations resulting in death or decerebration while there may be no demonstrable significant mass effect.[32] Such acutely raised ICP may be the cause of instant death in humans following CMI. Experimental studies have demonstrated a second rise in ICP 60–100 mm Hg within two to five minutes of injury, and a rapid rise in mean arterial blood pressure (MABP); MABP shows a subsequent fall, and a low MABP with persistently raised ICP results in poor cerebral perfusion, decerebration and higher mortality.[12,17,34] Transcranial Doppler studies in patients with CMI have shown vasospasm in 37% cases; these patients have poor survival as compared to those without vasospasm.[33]

Mechanism of brain injury: Immediate rise of ICP due to shock wave lasting 15 to 25 microseconds may be transmitted to brainstem, and this factor along with internal brain herniations may lead to instantaneous death, especially if the missile is a high-velocity one.[32] As the missile penetrates the brain, cerebral parenchyma in its path is crushed and spread apart, creating a permanent cavity that is slightly larger than the diameter of the missile.[23] Formation of a temporary cavity, which may be 30 times the diameter of the missile (depending on the KE of the missile) stretches and tears the brain parenchyma. KE transfer to the brain may be cumulative with injuries from multiple pellets, secondary missiles or from internal ricochet, and injuries remote to the observed missile track are quite common.

Contusion and hemorrhage may occur in areas distant from the missile track. Laceration of major vessels may produce large parenchymal hematomas, extending considerable distances from the site of the track. Patients who have no intracranial missile penetration may develop neurological deficit as a result of blast wave. They may suffer fracture of the skull as well. White matter edema has been observed in experimental CMI in primates,[3] with widespread swelling of perivascular astrocytes within 30 minutes of injury.[2] Edema has been observed in minutes in patients with CMI, who died subsequently.

Experimental studies on cats have shown the early stage changes in the cerebral microcirculation after a craniocerebral missile wound. The blood flow in the microvessels may increase progressively in the areas of concussion, contusion and laceration, induce reperfusion injury following ischemia and hypoxia of the brain tissue resulting from microcirculation disorder caused by the wound.[34, 35, 52]

Evaluation and Initial Management

Rapid neurological deterioration after missile injury to the brain can occur due to primary and secondary factors. Because the morbidity and mortality are significantly influenced by the patient's neurological status before reaching the neurosurgical care, efforts should be made to minimize the time taken for transportation to a well-equipped neurosurgical center.[31] Upon arrival in the emergency room the patient is completely evaluated after ensuring an adequate airway and hemodynamic stability. All external bleeding should be controlled and search for abdominal, thoracic

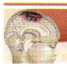

and extremity injury is made, and their appropriate treatment is planned. Complete head is shaven and extruded brain matter or CSF leak, boggy scalp swelling, eye injury (indicating oculocerebral injury), bleeding or CSF leak from nose or ears, subcutaneous emphysema over the face and neck and pulsations in the carotids in the neck are carefully looked for. The mouth and oropharynx are cleared by suction and examined for bone fragments, splinters and brain matter.

A detailed neurological evaluation, as practical in the prevailing circumstances, is carried out, which will be the baseline for all subsequent evaluations. Rapid examination of sensorium by Glasgow Coma Scale (GCS) is done, pupils and visual status, ocular movements are noted and facial paresis, focal motor deficit, etc. are looked for. An enlarging intracranial mass lesion should be suspected when there is progressive loss of brainstem function in a pattern consistent with herniation, or if the brainstem examination is dramatically better than the overall GCS score.[25]

Imaging

Skull radiograph (Fig. 28.2): Skull radiographs are done routinely in all the patients. The commonest finding is the presence of intracranial radio-opaque foreign bodies. Their

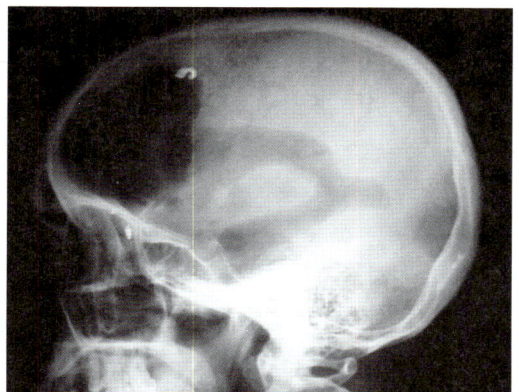

Fig. 28.2: Skull radiograph (lateral view) showing intracranial metallic Shrapnell and pneumoventriculogram

location and distribution can give an idea about the direction of the missile track and the structures likely to have been injured. Comminuted fractures, depressed fractures, stellate and linear fractures can be appreciated. Skull radiographs are superior to CT in delineating certain fractures, such as horizontal linear fractures and fractures in the same plane as axial CT slices that can be missed on CT. Another important finding is the presence of pneumocephalus, and, rarely an air ventriculogram if the ventricle has been entered. Other findings that may be present are sinus opacification and contralateral shift of calcified midline structures.

Skull radiographs may also be done after CT, when trying to locate a single intracranial foreign body which is suspected to have changed its position, and in patients with postoperative neurological deterioration, when it may show a treatable lesion like pneumocephalus (Fig. 28.1).

Computed tomography (Figs 28.3 to 28.5): CT is the imaging procedure of choice for evaluation of these injuries, which can diagnose as well as prognosticate the injuries. Usually, a depressed comminuted fracture with indriven fragments are seen in LVMIs. On the other hand, HVMIs may result in extensive skull fracturing remote from the impact site. The parenchymal laceration is seen as a conical track with base of the cone at entrance site. Hemorrhage into the track outlines it as a high attenuating track. However, the shape of the track is variable according to the missile yaw and energy transfer to the tissues (Figs 28.3 and 28.4). CT will also show the ricocheted missile tract, intracranial hemorrhage, indriven radioopaque material, pneumocephalus, cerebral edema, brain contusion. Besides being the most important diagnostic imaging modality, CT is also valuable in prognostication of CMIs. Patients with multilobar injury, subarachnoid hemorrhage, cerebral infarction carry a worse prognosis, as compared to those with localized damage.

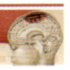

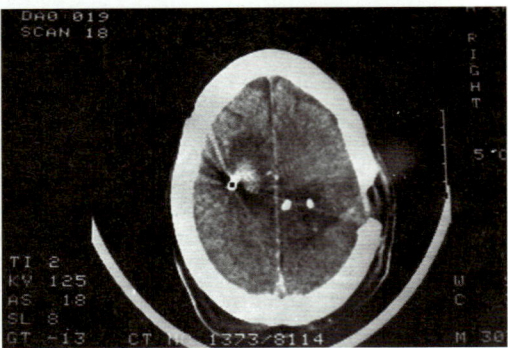

Fig. 28.3: CT brain showing skull fracture with missile track

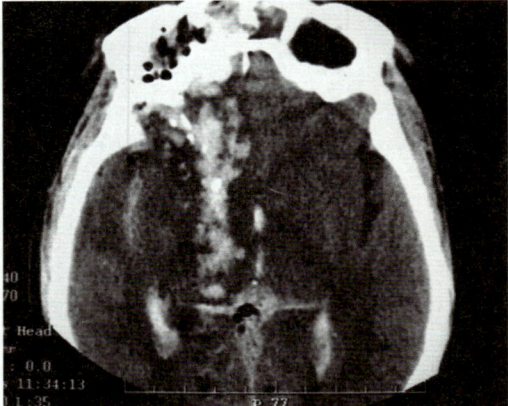

Fig. 28.4: CT brain showing extensive brain injury due to high velocity missile injury

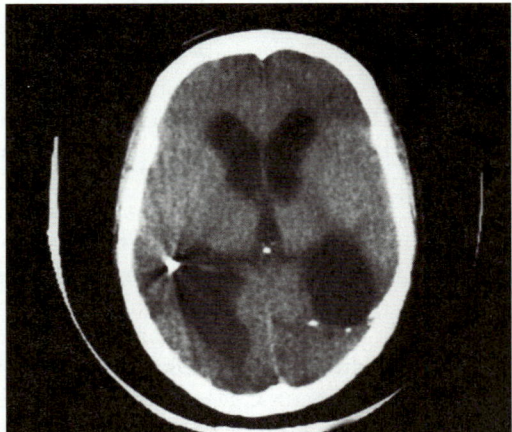

Fig 28.5: CT showing retained intraventricular Shrapnell with hydrocephalus

CT is also valuable in serial evaluation of CMI patients, especially in the presence of neurological deterioration.

Carotid angiography: Evaluation of CMI with carotid angiography in the acute phase is given up. Angiography is however valuable in evaluation of certain sequelae of CMI like traumatic aneurysms, arteriovenous fistulae, etc.

OPERATIVE MANAGEMENT

The aim of surgical management in missile injuries of the brain is to increase the incidence and quality of survival by reducing raised the intracranial pressure and prevention of infection. The principles of surgery enunciated by various authors are:

a. The mass lesion consisting of intracranial hematoma and non-viable brain tissue along the path of missile must be evacuated.

b. The missile and bone fragments wherever feasible must be removed, but without enhancing the pre-existing neurological deficit. The brain is usually swollen and retraction can be hazardous. Therefore, one should avoid digging into the brain to retrieve the elusive missile.

c. Dura and scalp must be closed over the brain in a watertight fashion.

d. Postoperative elevations of intracranial pressure should be minimized and adjunctive therapy (vide infra) should be instituted aggressively.

Availability of adequate anesthesia support during and after surgery, good fiberoptic illumination, suction, bipolar cautery, etc. are mandatory prerequisites for optimum management.

The choice of approach is between debridement via small craniectomies[27] and large bone flaps centered over the wound of entrance.[26] The latter allows greater control of hemorrhage and better decompression,[4] and lower infection rate.[44,45] Craniectomy should be wide enough to allow access to normal dura from all sides. Recent military data[9,21,50] indicate that aggressive approach is not necessary and efforts should be made to preserve as much neural tissue as possible. After debridement, missile and bone fragments should be retrieved only if they are accessible without producing any further neurological damage. Exit wounds if present are also debrided and dura is closed with pericranial graft, temporalis fascia or fascia lata.

Orbitocranial injuries and fronto-orbito-maxillary injuries are usually associated with compound fracture of the skull base resulting in profuse CSF rhinorrhea and orbitorrhea. Such injuries may not be accompanied by alteration in sensorium but are potentially dangerous due to their communication with the oral cavity or air sinuses. These injuries have to be recognized and repair of dural defect (usually by bifrontal craniotomy) to stop the CSF leak should be carried out at the earliest. Pericranial flaps, mashed muscle and fascia lata are extremely useful in dealing with these CSF leaks.

Gunshot wounds of the paranasal sinuses and orbit are uncommon. Their severity depends on the missile track in the tissues. Such injuries can involve the brain from below. Endoscopic sinus surgery is appropriate technique for removing projectiles.[5] Penetrating orbitocranial non-missile injuries (e.g. stab injuries) caused by metallic foreign bodies are very rare among civil population. After careful radiological evaluation of the shape and position of the foreign object, a combined frontal craniotomy and orbitotomy is performed, in order to remove achieve the safe removal of the metallic bar.[41] Neuronavigation techniques have been utilized for secondary removal of retained missile fragments.[47]

PROBLEM OF RETAINED INTRACRANIAL FRAGMENTS

It may not be possible to extricate all the metallic fragments lodged within the brain, due to the unpredictable trajectory of the missile and accompanying factors like brain swelling. Attempts to aggressively remove these missiles may aggravate neurological injury due to retraction, hemorrhage, etc. The problems to be kept in mind while dealing with retained fragments are:

A. Infection

In the past, military neurosurgeons believed that it was imperative to remove all the bone and metallic pieces. Reoperation was advocated if retained fragments were evident after initial debridement.[27,36] Retained fragments were believed to be fraught with intracranial suppurative complications.[38] Martin and Campbell[35] recorded infection rate of 16% based on their World War II experience. Over 40% of their patients with retained fragments became infected. Reoperation in such patients was associated with increased neurological deficit.

Recent reports have advocated a more conservative approach. Brandvold et al[9] while treating Israeli soldiers during their expedition into Lebanon reported 60% survivors had retained fragments, and none of them developed suppurative complications. In the wartime experience of Bajpayee,[4] 22 patients out of 63 treated for missile brain injuries had retained intracranial missiles; 2 of these 22 developed brain abscess and 2 developed recurrent meningitis. In a recent series of patients with retained intracranial splinters in low intensity military conflicts,[7,8] there were suppurative complications in 4 out of 37 cases with retained fragments; all 4 had either orbitocranial injury or breach of paranasal sinuses. They had recurrent episodes of pyogenic meningitis; 2 of these developed brain abscesses and 2 developed hydrocephalus requiring ventriculoperitoneal shunt. Intraventricular fragments may be associated with meningitis and ventriculitis (Fig. 28.5). Metallic foreign body in the cavernous sinus causing delayed formation of brain abscess after missile injury has been reported.[48] It is now evident that the extent of brain damage as evident on initial CT is of greater prognostic value than the fragment

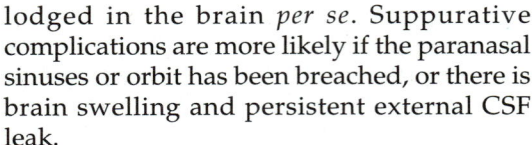

lodged in the brain *per se*. Suppurative complications are more likely if the paranasal sinuses or orbit has been breached, or there is brain swelling and persistent external CSF leak.

B. *Epilepsy*

The epileptogenic effects of retained fragments especially those containing copper have been mentioned.[15] However, the true incidence is difficult to assess since these patients are routinely put on antiepileptic drugs.

C. *Migration*

Migration of retained intracranial fragments has been of considerable interest. Migration possibly occurs due to creation of paths wider than the diameter of the missile itself, the weight of the missile and pulsation of the brain. Migration can occur across the midline[19] and into the cervical canal.[56] Migration can lead to fresh neurological deficits, hydrocephalus and traumatic aneurysm.[26] Migration of a bullet from the cranium to the lower end of spinal canal may occur months after the injury.

ADJUNCTS TO OPERATIVE MANAGEMENT

Anticonvulsants

The exact role of prophylactic anticonvulsants in CMI is not yet settled, although what is clear is that there is higher incidence of post-traumatic epilepsy after CMI as compared to that seen after closed head injury. Although anticonvulsants were used in Korean and Vietnam conflicts, the incidence of PTE following CMI was same as in earlier wars where these were not used.[13,15] In the VHIS, one-half of the patients with early seizures had late epilepsy.[13, 46] During the Iran-Iraq War, 32% patients developed PTE after CMI.[1] Thus, it would be reasonable to assume that approximately one-third of patients with combat CMIs develop seizures.[13] There are a few series that document the incidence of PTE after civilian CMIs. Crockard[17] reported a seizure incidence of 35%, and Gordon,[24] an incidence of 40–50%. Thus, it would be reasonable to believe that all penetrating brain injuries must have anticonvulsant prophylaxis since the true incidence of epilepsy in such injuries may be as high as 35%.[51]

Management of Raised Intracranial Pressure

Management of CMI is a source of trepidation because a few of the therapies aimed at ICP reduction and maintenance of CPP are physiologically benign. While head elevation by 30° in euvolemic patients can significantly reduce ICP without altering CPP,[22] some of the other therapeutic measures used in routine management of head trauma, such as hyperventilation and diuresis risk converting relatively uncomplicated neurologic injuries into complicated multisystem injuries. Hyperventilation can result in alkalosis which contributes to hypokalemia, and diuresis can provoke hypotension, hypovolemia and hypokalemia. Hence the therapy for lowering raised ICP has to be carefully monitored, so that electrolyte disturbances are avoided or promptly recognized and treated, and CPP is maintained. Current concepts in the management of missile injuries to the brain emphasize the frequent occurrence of raised ICP in the postoperative period. To a large extent, judicious debridement of injured cerebral tissue and evacuation of intraparenchymal and extra-axial hematomas can minimize ICP elevations. Medical management of raised ICP consists of proper positioning, ensuring adequate oxygenation, and administration of osmotic and loop diuretics. Hyperventilation can be valuable in selected patients. ICP monitoring is a valuable adjunct in the postoperative management.

Antibiotics

Antibiotics that cross into the CSF should be administered in antimeningitic dosages for 4 to 6 weeks. Previously, a combination of chloramphenicol and penicillin was widely used; at present, one of the third generation cephalosporins (cefotaxime, ceftazidime, ceftriaxome) along with an aminoglycoside (netilmicin, amikacin) are favored. Metronidazole may be added especially in the presence of extensive soft tissue injury.

CONCLUSIONS

Initial GCS is the single most important prognostic factor in predicting outcome in missile injuries of the brain. Rapid evacuation of these patients to a neurosurgical center, aggressive resuscitation in both field and during transit and prompt correction of physiologic abnormalities are of paramount importance to clinical outcome. CT is the cornerstone in the diagnostic evaluation of these patients. The surgical principles of aggressive treatment of mass lesions, limited brain debridement, watertight dural closure and tension free scalp closure should be applied to all situations. Postoperative management of raised ICP, administration of antibiotics and anticonvulsants are required for optimizing the outcome of victims of missile brain injuries.

Acknowledgments

To the publishers (Jaypee) and the editors of the textbook: Ramamurthi and Tandon's Textbook of Neurosurgery, 2011.

REFERENCES

1. Aarabi B, Taghipour M, Haghnegahdar A, Farokhi M, Mobley L. Prognostic factors in the occurrence of post-traumatic epilepsy after penetrating head injury suffered during military service. Neurosurg Focus 2000;8(1)Article 1.
2. Allen IV, Kirk J, Maynard RI, et al. An ultrastructural study of experimental high velocity penetrating head injuries. *Acta* Neuropathol (Berl) 1983;59:277–82.
3. Allen IV, Scott R, Tauner JA. Experimental high velocity missile injury. Injury 1982;14:183–93.
4. Bajpayee C P. Penetrating head injuries. *Medical* Journal Armed Forces India 1976;32:490–4.
5. Balseris S, Einoriene D, Martinkenas JL, et al. Sinoorbital gunshot injuries. Endoscopic diagnostics and management. Medicina (Kaunas) 2008;44:308–12.
6. Berlin RH, Janzon B, Liden E, et al. Wound ballistics of Swedish 5.56 mm assault rifle AK 56 J Trauma 28 (suppl): 1988;76–83.
7. Bhatoe HS. Retained intracranial splinters: A follow-up study in survivors of low intensity military conflicts. Neurol India 2001;49:29–32.
8. Bhatoe HS, Garg A, Kapoor S, et al. Experiences in the management of splinter injuries of brain in low intensity military conflicts. Asian Archives of Critical Care Medicine XLVI 1997;(2):63–8.
9. Brandvold B, Levi L, Feinsod M, et al. Penetrating craniocerebral injuries in the Israeli involvement in the Lebanese conflict, 1982–1985; Analysis of a less aggressive surgical approach. Journal of Neurosurgery 1990;72:15–21.
10. Byrnes DP, Crockard HA, Gordon DG. Penetrating craniocerebral missile injuries in the civil disturbances in Northern Ireland. British Journal of Surgery 1971;61:169–76.
11. Carey ME. Analysis of wounds incurred by US Army Seventh Corps personnel treated in Corps Hospitals during Operation Desert Storm, Feb 20–Mar 10, 1991. Journal of Trauma 1996;40(3):165–9.
12. Carey ME, Sarna GS, Farrell JB, et al. Experimental missile wound to brain. J Neurosurg 1989;71:754–764.
13. Caveness WF. Onset and cessation of fits following craniocerebral trauma. Journal of Neurosurgery 1963;20:570–83.
14. Cooper PR. Gunshot wounds of the brain. In, Cooper PR (Ed). Head Injury. 3rd ed. Baltimore, Williams and Wilkins 1993;355–71.
15. Caveness WF, Meirowsky AM, Rish BL, et al. The nature of post-traumatic epilepsy. J Neurosurg 1979;50:545–53.
16. Crockard HA, Brown FD, Johns LM, Mullan S. Physiological consequences of experimental cerebral missile injuryand use of data analysis to predict survival. J Neurosurg 1977;46:784–94.
17. Crockard HA. Bullet injuries to the brain. *Ann Roy Coll Surg Engl* 1974;55:111–23.
18. Cushing H. A study of a series of wounds involving the brain and its enveloping structures. British Journal of Surgery 1918;5:558–684.
19. Laxman Das, Karamchand, Premsagar I C, et al. Missile injuries of the head. Neurology India 1995; 43:174–5.
20. DeMuth WE. Bullet velocity as applied to military rifle wounding capacity. Journal of Trauma 1969;9:27–38.

21. Fackler M L. Wound Ballistics: The management of assault rifle injuries. Military Medicine 1990;155:222–5.

22. Feldman Z, Kanter MJ, Robertson CS, et al. Effect of head elevation on intracranial pressure, cerebral perfusion pressure, and cerebral blood flow in head-injured patients. J Neurosurg 1992;76:207–11.

23. Freytag E. Autopsy findings in head injuries from firearms. Statistical evaluation in 254 cases. Archives of Pathology 1963;76:215–25.

24. Gordon DS. Missile wounds of the head and spine. Br Med J 1975;1:614–6.

25. Grahm TW, Williams FC Jr., Harrington T, et al. Civilian gunshot wounds to the head: A prospective study. Neurosurgery 1990;27:696–700.

26. Haddad FS. Nature and management of penetrating head injuries during Civil war in Lebanon. Canadian Journal of Neurosurgery 1978;21:233–40.

27. Hammon WM. Analysis of 2187 consecutive penetrating wounds of the brain from Vietnam. Journal of Neurosurgery 1971;34:127–31.

28. Harvey EN, McMillen JH. An experimental study of shock waves resulting from the impact of high velocity missiles on animal tissues. J Exp Med 1947;85:321–8.

29. Hopkinson DAW, Marshall TK. Firearm injuries. British Journal of Surgery 1967;54:344–53.

30. Horsley V. A clinical lecture on penetrating wounds of the central nervous system. The Clinical Journal 1898;12:261–7.

31. Kaufman HH, Makela ME, Lee KF, et al. Gunshot wounds to the head: A perspective. Neurosurgery 1986;18:689–95.

32. Kirkpatrick JB, DiMaio V. Civilian gunshot wounds of the brain. Journal of Neurosurgery 1978;49:185–98.

33. Kordestani RK, Neil AM, McBride DQ. Cerebral hemodynamic disturbances following penetrating craniocerebral injury and their influence on outcome. Neurosurg Clin N Amer 1995;6:657–67.

34. Lindegaard KF, Nornes H, Bakke SJ, et al. Cerebral vasospasm after subarachnoid hemorrhage investigated by means of transcranial Doppler ultrasound. Acta Neurochir 42(suppl): 1988;81–4.

35. Martin J, Campbell EH. Early complications following penetrating wounds of the skull. Journal of Neurosurgery 1946;3:239–49.

36. Mathews WE. The early treatment of cranio-cerebral missile injuries: Experience with 92 cases. Journal of Trauma 1972;12:939–54.

37. Matson DD. The treatment of craniocerebral injuries due to missiles. Springfield, III, Charles C Thomas, 1948.

38. Meirowsky AM. The retention of bone fragments in brain wounds. Military Medicine 1968;133: 887–90.

39. Mohanty S, Asthana S, Shankar V, et al. Gunshot injuries of the head in civilian practice in India. Neurology India 1991;39:141–5.

40. Myers PW, Brophy J, Salazar AM, et al. Retained bone fragments after penetrating brain wounds: Long term follow up in Vietnam Veterans. Journal of Neurosurgery 1989;70:319–23.

41. Pascual JM, Navas M, Carrasco R. Penetrating vballistic-like frontal brain injury caused by a metallic rod. Acta Neurochir (Wien) 2009;151: 689–91.

42. Rahimizadeh A, Shakeri M, Amirdjamshidi. Unusual craniocerebral injury by glass fragments. Neurosurgery 1987;21:427–8.

43. Ramesh Chandra. Missile wounds of the head. In, Ramamurthi B, Tandon P N (Eds). Textbook of Neurosurgery Vol I, 2nd edn, New Delhi. B I Churchill Livingstone 1996:383–92.

44. Rish BL, Dillon JD, Weiss GH. Mortality following penetrating craniocerebral injuries. An analysis of deaths in the Vietnam Head Injury Registry population. Journal of Neurosurgery 1983;59: 775–80.

45. Rosenberg WS, Harsh GR. Penetrating wounds of the head. In, Wilkins RH, Rengachary SS (Eds). Neurosurgery Vol II, 2nd edn. New York, McGraw-Hill 1996:2813–20.

46. Salazar AM, Jabbari B, Vance SC, et al. Epilepsy after penetrating head injury I. Clinical Correlates: A report from Vietnam Head Injury Study. Neurology 1985;35:1406–14.

47. Schulz C, WoernerU, Luelsdorf P. Image-guided neurosurgery for secondary operative removal of projectiles after missile injury of the brain. Surg Neurol 2008;69(4):364–8.

48. Shurbaji A, Rosahl SK, Feigl GC, et al. Metallic foreign body in the cavernous sinus causing delayed formation of brain abscess after missile injury. J Trauma 2006;60:1135–7.

49. Singh Prakash. Missile injuries of the brain. Results of less aggressive surgery. Neurology India 2003;51:215–9.

50. Taha JM, Saba ML, Brown JA. Missile injuries to the brain treated by simple wound closure:

results of a protocol during Lebanese conflict. Neurosurgery 1991;29:380–4.

51. Temkin NR, Dikman SS, Winn HR. Management of head injury: Post-traumatic seizures. Neurosurgical Clinics of North America 1991;2:425–35.

52. Wang F, Chen CC, Mao BY, et al. Early stage changes of calibre and blood flow of cat pial microvessels following craniocerebral missile wound. Di Wi Jun Yi Da Xyu Xyu Bao 2004;24:889–91 (Chinese).

53. West CGH. A short history of the management of penetrating missile injuries of the head. Surgical Neurology 1981;16:145–9.

54. Woodruff CE. The causes of explosive effect of modern small caliber bullets. NY Med J 1898; 67:593–601.

55. Wu JJ, Shih CJ. Unusual penetrating injury of the superior sagittal sinus. Surg Neurol 1982;17:43–6.

56. Young WF Jr, Katz MR, Rosenwasser R H. Spontaneous migration of an intracranial bullet into the spinal canal. South Medical Journal 1993;86:557–9.

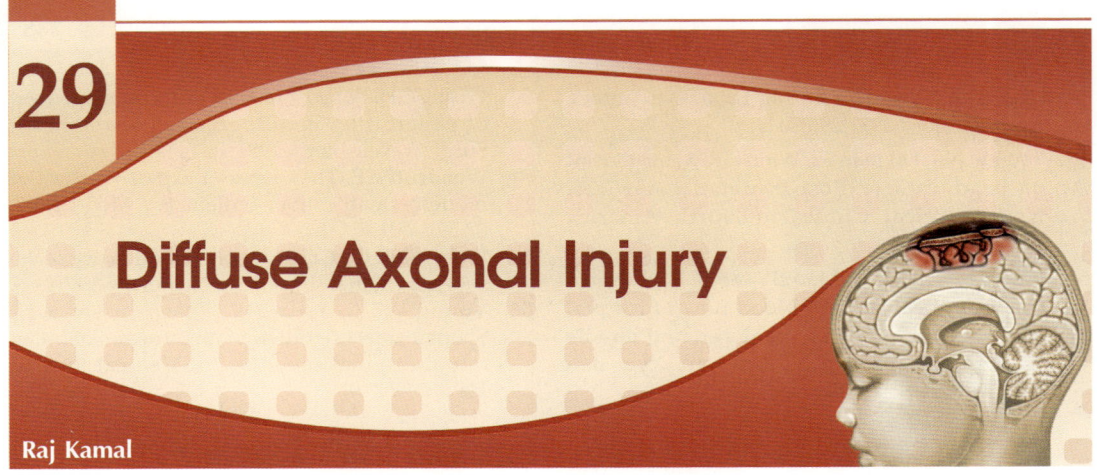

29

Diffuse Axonal Injury

Raj Kamal

Diffuse brain injury is defined as the pathology of comatose patients who are unconscious from the moment of impact and do not experience a lucid interval without evidence of space occupying intracranial lesions on computed tomography (CT) scan or magnetic resonance imaging (MRI). The two subgroups of diffuse brain injury are traumatic diffuse axonal injury (DAI) and diffuse brain swelling.

Traumatic diffuse axonal injury (DAI) was first described by Strich[1] as "diffuse degeneration of white matter following severe head injury". Since then, a number of terms have been used to describe DAI and include "shearing injury/"diffuse white matter shearing injury" and "inner cerebral trauma."

The new definition includes severely head-injured patients with normal scans, tissue tear hemorrhages, traumatic subarachnoid and intraventricular hemorrhages, diffuse brain swelling and unilateral swelling with midline shifts.

In diffuse axonal injury case, the brain may appear surprisingly normal when viewed with the naked eye. However, distinctive gross and microscopic features characterize severe DAI. **Axonal swelling (retraction balls)** are the microscopic hallmark of DAI. Widely distributed lesions contain reactive axonal swellings in the cerebral white matter, corpus callosum and upper brainstem. **Diffuse axonal injury (DAI) is a frequent result of traumatic acceleration/deceleration or rotational injuries and a frequent cause of persistent vegetative state in patients.** In fact, DAI represents approximately one half of all intra-axial traumatic lesions.[2] This lesion is the most significant cause of morbidity in patients with traumatic brain injuries, which most commonly result from high-speed motor vehicle accidents. Any patient with a closed head injury who experiences extensive loss of consciousness and neurological deficits warrants neuroimaging.[3] DAI typically consists of several focal white-matter lesions measuring 1–15 mm in a characteristic distribution.

Diffuse brain swelling occurred approximately twice as often in children (aged 16 years or younger) as in adults. A high mortality rate (53%) was found in these children, which was three times that of the children without diffuse brain swelling (16%). Adults with diffuse brain swelling had a mortality rate (46%) similar to that of children, but only slightly higher than that for adults without diffuse brain swelling (39%).[4] DAI has been considered a primary-type injury, with damage occurring at the time of the accident. Secondary injury is thought to result in retraction balls.

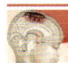
The degree of microscopic injury usually is considered to be greater than that seen on diagnostic imaging and the clinical findings reflect this point. DAI is suggested in any patient who demonstrates clinical symptoms disproportionate to his or her CT-scan findings. DAI results in instantaneous loss of consciousness and most patients (> 90%) remain in a persistent vegetative state, since brainstem function typically remains unaffected. DAI rarely causes death.

The frequency of DAI in head injury varies according to the degree of severity of injury, but patients that survive with any degree of DAI will always show sequelae, whether psychological or neurological. More severe injuries ending up in vegetative state.[5]

PATHOGENESIS OF DAI

It is caused by angular or rotational acceleration and deceleration inertial effects and not by contact phenomena. The severity of axonal damage is related to the magnitude, duration and onset rate of the **angular acceleration.**[6]

The direction of impact plays an important role. **Sagittal** movement is the best tolerated by the brain whereas lateral and horizontal movements are not well tolerated. The **angular acceleration** results in shearing and tensile strains on axons, typically at the gray, white matter interphases.[6] In response to a lateral head motion, small centers of rotation occurs in temporal and superior frontal lobes. Xiao-Sheng et al,[7] 2000, had demonstrated diffuse axonal injury in rats due to lateral head rotation. The regions shown in the figure indicate the areas where the brain is the most prone to axonal damage due to high level of strain at the site.

By only using angular acceleration in monkeys, Gennarelli et al[6] produced injury patterns seen in humans. Such injuries result from shear and/or tensile strains on axons in the cerebral white matter, corpus callosum, and brainstem. The severity of axonal injury was proportional to the rapidity of angular acceleration of head. These findings suggest

that minute injuries sometimes found after concussion may also be the result of angular acceleration.

Remaining surviving axons may be vulnerable because of secondary events leading to hypoxia, ischemia and subsequent release of excitatory amino acids and free radicals. The ultimate event in the neuronal death appears to be the influx of calcium ions.[8] Buki et al[9, 10] had demonstrated calpain mediated spedin proteolysis in pathogenesis of traumatically induced axonal injury. In another study they reported cytochrome C release and caspase activation in DAI.

Pathology of Traumatic Diffuse Axonal Injury

Diffuse axonal injury is one of the most important types of brain damage that can occur as a result of non-missile head injury, and it may be very difficult to diagnose post mortem unless the pathologist knows precisely what he is looking for. Increasing experience with fatal non-missile head injury in man has allowed the identification of three grades of diffuse axonal injury. **Three grades of DAI** have been described by Adams et al[11] based on their neuropathological studies (Table 29.1): Grade 1 DAI denotes widespread, microscopic axonal damage in any location; in Grade 2 DAI there are additional focal abnormalities in the corpus callosum; and in Grade 3 DAI, focal lesions in the rostral brainstem are also found. From these early studies, DAI was noted in one-third of all fatal cases. However, using newer techniques to visualize the axonal damage, DAI has been almost universally demonstrated in fatal TBI.[12] Diffuse axonal injury was identified in 122 of a series of 434 fatal non-missile head injuries–10 grade 1, 29 grade 2 and 83 grade 3. In 24 of these cases the diagnosis could not have been

Table 29.1: Grading of DAI[11]	
Grade 1	Widespread damage in any location
Grade 2	Grade 1 + focal abnormalities in corpus callosum
Grade 3	Grade 2 + lesion in rostral brainstem

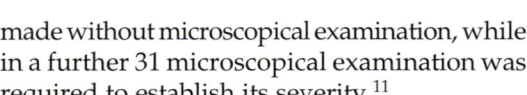
made without microscopical examination, while in a further 31 microscopical examination was required to establish its severity.[11]

Three "classic" lesions, characterize severe DAI.[13]

i. Reactive axonal "retraction" balls.

ii. Hemorrhagic necrosis in the dorsolateral quadrant of the rostral brainstem.

iii. Hemorrhagic necrosis in the corpus callosum.

The axonal swellings are the microscopic hallmark of DAI. They become apparent within hours after injury and may persist for a year or more. Shearing injury can lead to tearing of the axon and death of the neuron. Axonal transport continues up to injured site, but no further, leading to a buildup of transport products and local swelling at that point.[14, 15] When it becomes large enough, swelling can tear the axon at the site of the break in the cytoskeleton, causing it to draw back toward the cell body and form a bulb.[6] This bulb is called a retraction ball, the hallmark of diffuse axonal injury.[15] Microglial stars develop in these damaged sites and may eventually replace the swollen axons. Degeneration of long tracts will evolve and ventricular dilation will follow.[16]

The lesion in the dorsolateral quadrant of the rostral brainstem are usually hemorrhagic and involve dorsolateral-lateral part of midbrain and the rostral pons, almost always involving the superior cerebellar peduncle.

The lesions in corpus callosum usually lie lateral to the midline, affect the inferior and posterior part of corpus callosum. These lesion may extend over several centimeters. The callosal injury may be focal, may be segmental, or may extend from the genu to the splenium.

DAI appears to be a distinct entity which may develop after mild concussion up to and including persistant coma. The finding of occasional clusters of microglia in patients dying soon after head injury suggested that axonal injury has occurred. More recently antibody against p-amyloid precursor protein has been demonstrated in patients who died

from unrelated causes after sustaining a minor head injury.[17, 18]

Recently evidence from animal experiments[19] and observations in humans[20] have shown that the initial axonal injury is in continuity. The disruption of axon occurs only later, as a result of a so-called secondary or delayed axotomy.

Accumulation of precursor protein of amyloid within 2 or 3 hours of injury indicates beginning of delayed axotomy. This process may continue for 24 hours or more.[20–22] The exact mechanisms causing secondary axotomy are not yet known. But proposed mechanisms include increased permeability to Ca^{++} in the region of Ranvier's node or, alternatively, within the internal cytoskeleton itself.[23] This leads to disorganization of microtubules and neurofilaments hence block in axonal transport resulting in axonal focal swelling. Later on classical axonal bulb appears. Any measure which prevents or minimize secondary axotomy can improve clinical outcome. Till now no such specific measure is available for use in human beings.

Incidence of DAI

The incidence of DAI will be higher at autopsy than would be obvious on radiographic (CT, MRI) examination.

Adams et al.[24, 25] found DAI in 28% of non-missile head injuries histologically at autopsy. In 20% of these cases, the diagnosis of DAI could not have been made without microscopic examination. The CT incidence of DAI in various series varies from 2.4 to 15.5%.[26, 27]

Clinical Presentation

DAI occurs most commonly in patient injured in high velocity traffic accidents. The hallmarks of severe diffuse brain injury are coma from the onset of trauma, with the majority of severely injured patients showing a combination of generalised extensor posture or flexion. Classically these patients become unconscious immediately upon impact. About one-third of DAI patients may recover sufficiently from the initial head injury to talk before lapsing into coma.

Diagnostic Studies

1. Computed Tomography (CT)

The classic CT appearance of DAI is small focal punctate tissue tear hemorrhages in the cerebral white matter, basal ganglia, corpus callosum or dorsal part of the brainstem. **The three most common locations for the hemorrhages are the lobar white matter, corpus callosum and the dorsolateral quadrant of rostral brainstem in the region of superior cerebral peduncle** (Fig. 29.l).

Tissue tear hemorrhages characteristically appear as small, discreet areas without mass effect or other associated abnormalities. The size of these lesions vary from 0.5 to 2.5 cm. They may not be evident in early CT scans. Patients eventually proven to have DAI, 50–80% demonstrate a normal CT scan upon presentation. Delayed CT scanning may be helpful in demonstrating edema or atrophy, which are later findings. For this reason, when CT-scan findings are negative and DAI is suggested clinically, MRI may be performed, as MRI modality can demonstrate lesions not observed through CT scanning. However, although MRI is more sensitive in the detection of subtle soft-tissue abnormalities, CT scanning is more available and practical in the current medical environment and is therefore, according to teasdale, the "mainstay of acute investigation of head injury."[28]

2. MRI

MRI is superior to CT in depicting non-hemorrhagic contusions, which appear as high intensity areas on T_2-weighted images and as iso-intense or hypointense areas on T_1-weighted images (Figs 29.2a and b). Magnetic resonance imaging of DAI has shown hemorrhagic and nonhemorrhagic lesions in the white matter in the hemispheres, corpus callosum and rostral brainstem, compatible with the neuropathological characteristics of this type of injury[29] and a modified staging has been used in imaging studies. Stage 1 represents a pattern of traumatic lesions confined to lobar white matter, whereas in Stages 2 and 3, lesions are depicted in the corpus callosum and brainstem, respectively.[30, 31] MRI sequences which are recommended include T_1-weighted, T_2-weighted, T_2-gradient-echo, proton density-weighted and diffusion-weighted images.[32] The degree of confidence is high, as abnormal signal in the characteristic locations, discovered in the clinical setting of recent trauma, leaves little doubt about the diagnosis of DAI. In a prospective cohort study, Skandsen et al examined MRI scans from patients in the early phase of moderate to severe head injury and determined the prognosis was better in patients with DAI whose lesions were confined to the lobar white matter or who had callosal lesions than it was in patients with DAI who had lesions in the dorsolateral brainstem.[31]

T_1-weighted images are helpful for anatomic localization;[33] however, nonhemorrhagic lesions may be isointense to surrounding tissue. Hemorrhagic lesions appear hyperintense on T_1-weighted images. However, on T_2-weighted sequences, nonhemorrhagic lesions appear hyperintense. Diffusion-weighted sequences can reveal hyperintensities in areas of axonal injury.

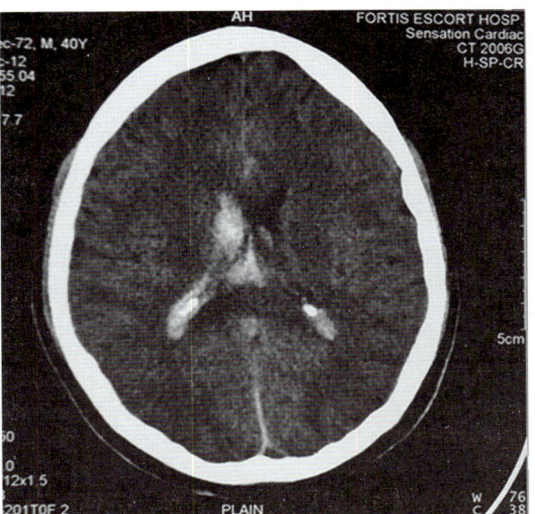

Fig. 29.1: CT scan showing corpus callosum contusion with intraventricular hemorrhage suggestive of DAI

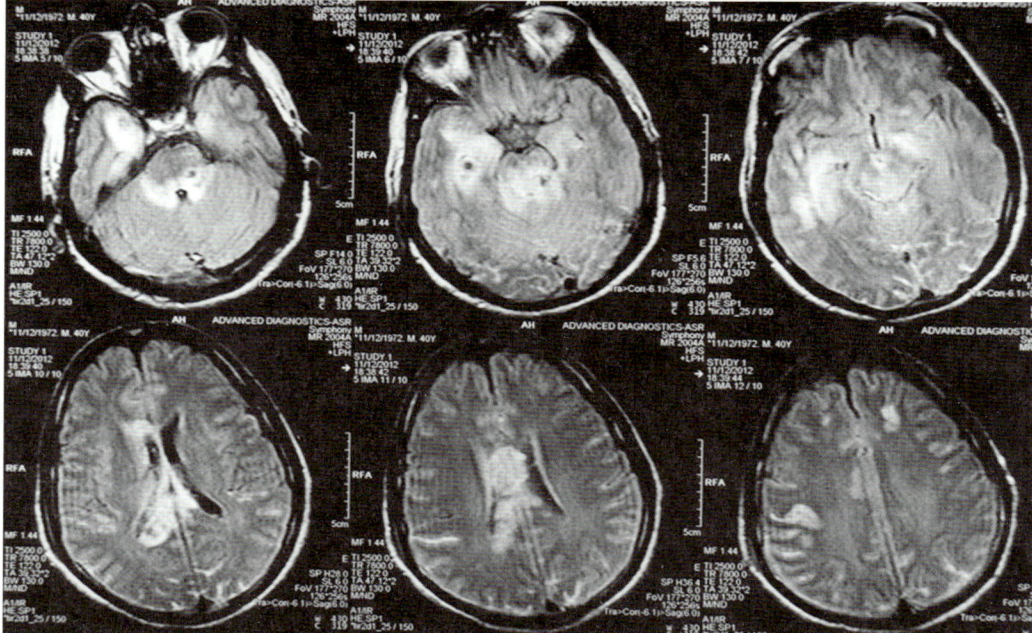

a

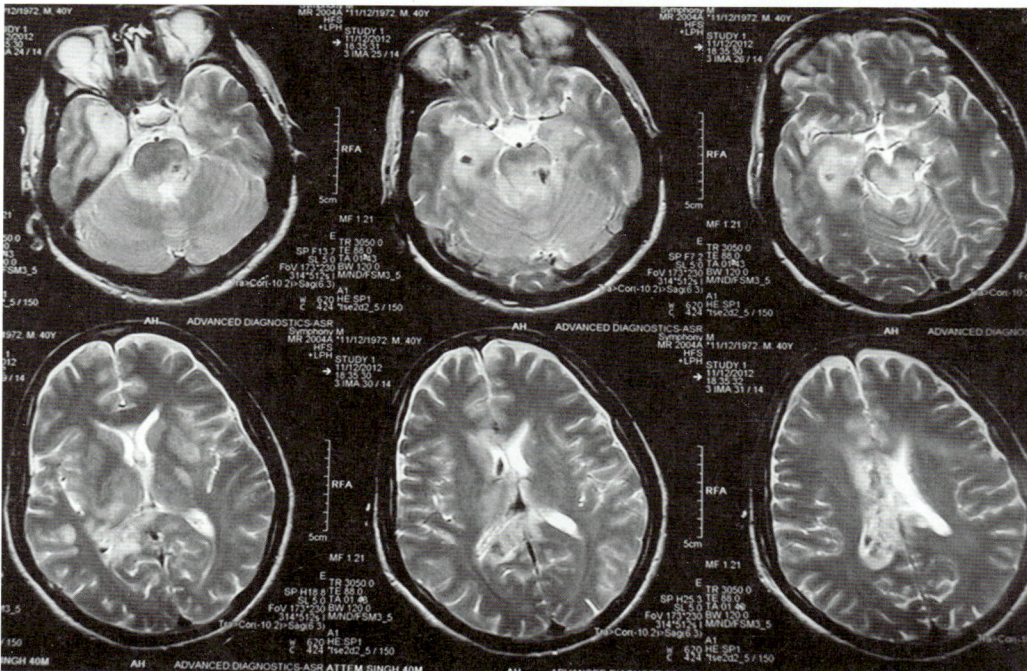

b

Figs 29.2a and b: (a) T$_1$-weighted image and (b) MRI brain of same patient showing the presence of multifocal areas of abnormal signal (bright on T$_2$-weighted images) at the white matter in the temporal or parietal corticomedullary junction or in the splenium of the corpus callosum. Other areas that frequently are abnormal include the dorsolateral rostral midbrain and the corona radiata

As demonstrated in the image below, gradient-echo sequences are particularly useful in revealing the paramagnetic effects of petechial hemorrhages. Gradient-echo imaging can often shows signal abnormality in areas that appear normal in T_1- and T_2-weighted spin-echo sequences. For this reason, gradient-echo imaging has become a mainstay of MRI exams for patients with suggested shearing-type injuries. The abnormal signal on gradient-echo images can persist for many years after the injury.

The most common MRI finding of DAI, as seen in the image (Fig. 29.2), is the presence of multifocal areas of abnormal signal (bright on T_2-weighted images) at the white matter in the temporal or parietal corticomedullary junction or in the splenium of the corpus callosum. Other areas that frequently are abnormal include the dorsolateral rostral midbrain and the corona radiata. Eventually, nonspecific atrophic changes are observed.

Patient with Diffuse Axonal Injury

Diffusion-weighted imaging (DWI) and the corresponding apparent diffusion coefficient (ADC) differentiate between lesions with increased and decreased diffusion based on the net movement of water molecules. Traditionally, DWI has been used for the diagnosis of acute stroke, given its high sensitivity for acute ischemia; however, DWI has been shown to be sensitive for other cerebral disease processes, including DAI.[34] Characteristic imaging findings on DWI/ADC can be broken down into 3 types: (1) Lesions that are hyperintense on DWI and ADC, (2) lesions that are hyperintense on DWI and hypointense on ADC and (3) hemorrhagic lesions that are hypointense on DWI and ADC but are surrounded by a hyperintense signal on DWI and ADC.[35]

One area of research has been magnetization transfer imaging. Studies have reported that the magnetic transfer ratio has shown promise in identifying areas of injury not visible on the above MRI pulse sequences. This may allow the radiologist to appreciate a truer representation of the degree of microscopic injury. Studies have also indicated that MRI can play a role in predicting the length of coma in DAI patients. The volume of white matter lesions has been correlated to the degree of injury, as measured by MRI.[36] MRI has also been used to quantify cerebral blood flow in damaged areas of the brain, thus predicting injury severity.

Multiple biomarkers are used to quantify the severity of traumatic brain injury (TBI) and to predict outcome. CT and conventional MR imaging underestimate injury and correlate poorly with outcome.[37] New MR imaging techniques, including diffusion tensor imaging (Figs 29.3 and 29.4), can provide information about brain ultrastructure by quantifying isotropic and anisotropic water diffusion. Our objective was to determine if changes in anisotropic diffusion in TBI correlate with acute Glasgow Coma Scale (GCS) and/or Rankin scores at discharge. Apparent diffusion coefficients (ADCs) and fractional anisotropy (FA) values were measured at multiple locations and correlated with clinical scores. ADC and FA values were significantly reduced within the splenium. DTI reveals changes in the white matter may be a valuable biomarker for the severity of tissue injury and a predictor for outcome.[37]

Sugiyama et al[38] evaluated clinical usefulness of diffusion tensor imaging (DTI) and found significantly more brain regions with decreased fractional anisotropy (FA) were found on the DTI scans of patients with DAI than on those of control subjects. In addition, DTI revealed more brain lesions than did conventional MRI. Moreover, fiber tractography-based analysis revealed that DAI patients with memory disorders exhibited an interruption of fibers within the fornix. This study concluded that DTI is an effective modality for detecting lesions and examining cognitive disorders in patients with DAI.[38]

MRI is more sensitive than CT scan in detecting tissue tear hemorrhages. A com-

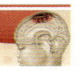
parison between T_2-weighted MRI and CT scanning showed that non-hemorrhagic lesions were identified in 90% of the cases diagnosed with MRI, but in only 20% on CT scan. However, small hemorrhagic lesions were seen with approximately the same frequency on both CT scans and MRI studies.

Treatment of Traumatic Diffuse Axonal Injury

Following basic principles are applicable for managing patients with diffuse axonal injuries:

1. Immediate establishment of ventilation and circulation at the accident site.
2. Aggressive monitoring and control of intracranial pressure.
3. Intensive care to achieve neuronal recovery.

The patency of the respiratory tract must be maintained or established and restoration of an adequate ventilation should have top priority. **Endotracheal intubation** is often necessary to protect the airway and maintain ventilation.

Cerebral perfusion pressure (CPP) is defined as **mean arterial pressure (MAP) minus intracranial pressure.** CPP = MAP – ICP. The initial approach to maintain MAP (hence CPP) is to establishment and maintenance of circulatory volume by administering adequate volumes of crystalloids, colloid, or blood products, as appropriate.

It is important to identify the patient who are at risk of developing increased intracranial pressure. Risk factors, which can predict intracranial hypertension are:

1. Subarachnoid hemorrhage
2. Midline shift
3. Abnormal mesencephalic cistern.

Patients with subarachnoid hemorrhage are twice likely to develop increased ICP and presence of abnormal mesencephalic cistern are almost three times prone to develop increased ICP. More the midline shift more is the chance of developing raised ICP.

Severe head injured patients with a normal CT scan have 10–15% chance of developing intracranial hypertension after 72 hours, hence serial follow-up CT scans are necessary. Most investigators report improved outcome with treatment at levels from 15 to 20 mm Hg. ICP may be measured from intraventricular, intraparenchymal, subdural and extradural sites. At our center, we are using subdural bolt for measuring ICP. A bolt utilizes the technology of fluid filled systems with an external transducer that is consistently referred to a point on the patients head as the zero level (external auditory meatus).

Various medical methods for controlling an increased intracranial pressure are:

1. *Hyperventilation:* Hyperventilation induces **hypocapnia** which rapidly lowers the ICP by the mechanism of metabolic autoregulation. There is vasoconstriction which decreases the cerebral blood volume. $PaCO_2$ is usually kept around 30–33 mm Hg using sedation, analgesia and full neuromuscular blockage.

2. *Position of the patient's head:* Elevating the head of the bed in the range of 15 to 30° from horizontal decreases ICP by improving venous outflow.

3. *Osmotherapy and diuretics:* Mannitol is the drug of choice to reduce ICP. It increases osmotic gradient across the blood–brain barrier (BBB) leading to water movement from area of edema across area of BBB. Mannitol also increases erythrocyte membrane flexibility which decreases blood viscosity and results in reflex vasoconstriction and decreased cerebrovascular volume. These effects are pronounced if mannitol is administered in bolus.

Barbiturates: It effectively reduces increased ICP by sedation, vasoconstriction, reducing $CMRO_2$ and by inhibiting free radical-induced lipid peroxidation. Important side effects of barbiturate are hypotension and myocardial depression.

Dosage: Loading dose (10 mg/kg) of thiopental given during 30 min.

Maintenance: 1 mg/kg/hr infusion loading dose should be given in well-equipped ICU under supervision.

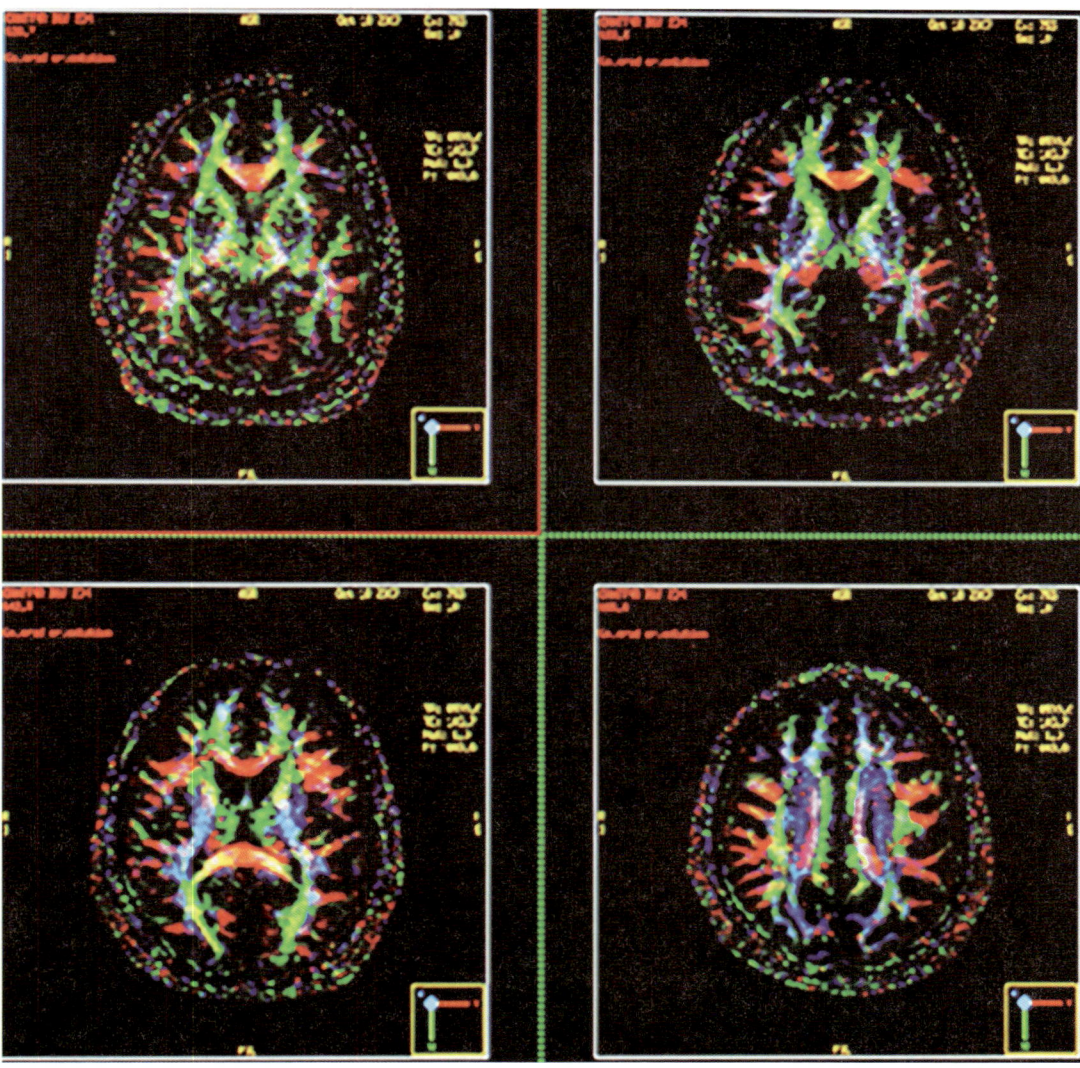

←→ Left-right

↕ Anterior-posterior

X Superior-inferior

Fig. 29.3: Normal diffusion tensor imaging (DTI): Axial tractographic image demonstrates white matter tracts in the brain in the left-right (red), anterior-posterior (green), and superior-inferior (blue) directions

Treatment of barbiturate induced hypotension.

Intravascular volume should be increased and dopamine/dobutamine to be started.

Cerebrospinal fluid drainage: It is an effective means of reducing ICP. Complications are infection and hemorrhage.

Prognosis: In diffuse axonal injuries little can be done about the primary axonal injury.

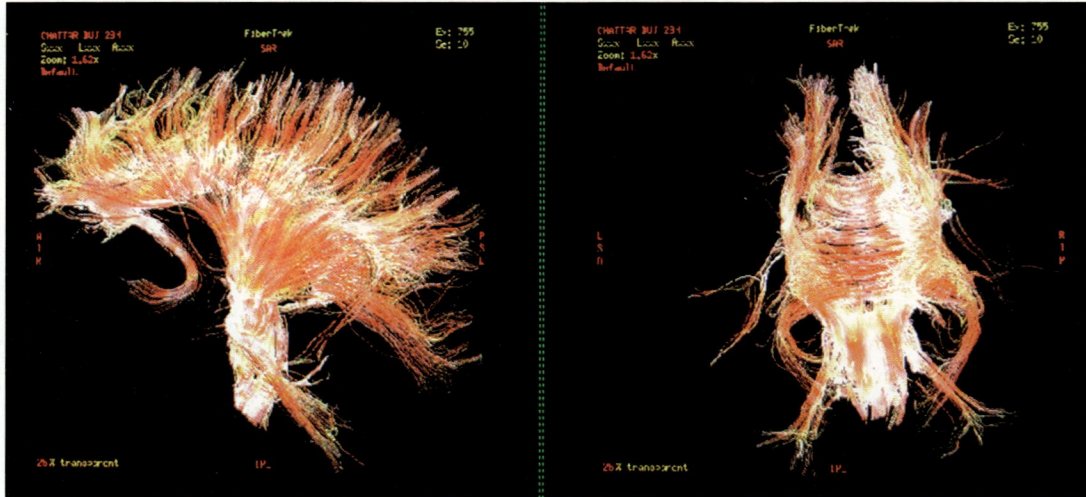

Fig. 29.4: Normal tractography demonstrating normal corona radiata fibers and corpus callosal fibers which are clearly damaged or reduced in DAI

Measures to reduce intracranial pressure and **measures to prevent or reverse the secondary insults** (such as edema, ischemia and secondary neuronal death) should be taken aggressively as it may improve the mortality and morbidity in diffuse axonal injuries.

Wilberger et al[27] found a correlation between the admission GCS scores and the eventual outcomes of patient with diffuse axonal injury.

In severe head injury 42% of the patients either died or were severely disabled or vegetative at discharge. Mild and moderate head injuries did well; no patient was severely disabled or **vegetative** at discharge, and no patient died. In patients with brainstem or corpus callosum tissue tear hemorrhages, the outcome were especially poor.[27] Paterakis et al[39] in 2000 had reported outcome in patients of DAI and highlighted prognostic role of MRI.

CONCLUSIONS

Traumatic diffuse axonal injury is characterized by reactive axonal retraction balls, hemorrhagic necrosis in dorsolateral quadrant of brainstem, hemorrhagic necrosis in the corpus callosum. Diffuse axonal injury is caused by angular acceleration or rotational acceleration, the extent of axonal damage depends upon magnitude, duration and rate of angular acceleration. Classically these patients become unconscious immediately upon impact. CT shows small focal punctate hemorrhages in the cerebral white matter, basal ganglia, corpus callosum or dorsal part of the brainstem. MRI is superior to CT scan in demonstrating non-hemorrhagic contusions. Recently, prognostic role of biomarkers like DTI has gained importance. Maintenance of cerebral perfusion pressure and aggressive monitoring and control of intracranial pressure are mainstay of medical management.

REFERENCES

1. Strich SJ. Diffuse degeneration of the cerebral white matter in severe dementia following head injury. 3 Neurol Neurosurg Psychiatry 1956;19: 163–85.

2. Thomas M, Dufour L. Challenges of diffuse axonal injury diagnosis. Rehabil Nurs Sep–Oct 2009;34(5):179–80.

3. Kinoshita T, Moritani T, Hiwatashi A, et al. Conspicuity of diffuse axonal injury lesions on

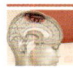

diffusion-weighted MR imaging. Eur J Radiol 2005;56(1):5–11.

4. Aldrich EF, Eisenberg HM, Saydjari C, Luerssen TG, Foulkes MA, Jane JA, Marshall LF, Marmarou A, Young HF. Diffuse brain swelling in severely head-injured children; Journal of Neurosurgery 1992 ;76(3):450–4.

5. Crooks DA, Berry CL: The pathological concept of diffuse axonal injury; its pathogenesis and the assessment of severity The Journal of Pathology Sep 1991;165(1):5–10.

6. Gennarelli TA, Thibault LE, Adam JH, et al. Diffuse axonal injury and traumatic coma in the primate. Ann Neurol 1982;12:564–74.

7. Xiao-Sheng H, Sheng YuY, Xiang Z, et al. Diffuse axonal injury due to lateral head rotation in rat model. J. Neurosurg 2000;93:626–33.

8. Aldrich EF, Eisenberg HM. Diffuse Brain Injury. In Tindal GT, Cooper PR, Barrow DL (eds). The Practice of Neurosurgery, Williams and Wilkins 1996;1490–1501.

9. Buki A, Povlishock JT. Evidence for calpain mediated spectin proteolysis in the pathogenesis of traumatically induced axonal injury. J. Neuropathol Exp Neurol 1999;58:365–75.

10. Buki A, Okonkwo DO, Wang KKW, et al. Cytochrome C release and caspase activation in traumatic axonal injury. J Neurosci 2000; 20:2825–34.

11. Adams JH, Doyle D, Ford I, Gennarelli TA, Graham DI, McLellan DR. Diffuse axonal injury in head injury: definition, diagnosis and grading. Histopathology 1989;15:49–59. Cross Ref, Medline.

12. Gentleman SM, Roberts GW, Gennarelli TA, Maxwell WL, Adams JH, Kerr S. Axonal injury: A universal consequence of fatal closed head injury? Acta Neuropathol 1995;89:537–43. Cross Ref, Medline.

13. McCormick WE. Pathology of closed head injury. In Wilkins RH, Rengachary SS (eds). Neurosurgery McGraw-Hill 1997:2639–66.

14. Staal JA, Dickson TC, Chung RS, Vickers JC. Cyclosporin-A treatment attenuates delayed cytoskeletal alterations and secondary axotomy following mild axonal stretch injury. Dev Neurobiol 1995;67(14):1831–42.

15. Gultekin SH, Smith TW.Diffuse axonal injury in craniocerebral trauma. A comparative histologic and immunohistochemical study. Arch pathol Lab Med 1994;118(2):168–71.

16. Hardman JM, Cerebrospinal trauma. In Davis RL, Robertson DM (Eds). Textbook of neuropathology. Williams and Wilkins 1997;1179–232.

17. Blumbergs PC, Scott G, et al. Staining of amyloid precursor protein to study axonal damage in mild head injury. Lancet 1994;344:1055.

18. Grady MS, Me Laughin MR, et al. The use of antibodies targetted against the neurofilament subunits for the detection of diffuse axonal injuries in humans. J Neuropathol Exp Neurol 1993;52:143.

19. Povlishock JT, Jenkins LW. Are the pathobiological changes evoked by traumatic brain injury immediate and irreversible? Brain pathol 1995;5:415–26.

20. McKenzie KJ, Me Lellan DR, Gentleman SM, et al. Is p-APP, a marker of axonal damage in short surviving head injury? Actaneuropathol (Berl) 1996;92:608–13.

21. Sherriff FE, Bridges LR, et al. Markers of axonal injury in postmortem human brain. Actaneuropathol (Berl) 1994;88:433–9.

22. Park E, Bell JD, Baker AJ, Traumatic Brain Injury: Can the consequences be stopped? Can Med Assoc J 2008;17:137–52.

23. Teasdale GM, Graham GI. Craniocerebral Trauma: Protection and retrieval of neuronal population after injury. Neurosurgery 1998;43: 723–38.

24. Adam JH, Doyle D, et al. Diffuse axonal injury definition, diagnosis and grading. Histopathology 1989;15:49–59.

25. Adam JH, Dajle D, et al. Microscopic diffuse axonal injury in cases of head injury. Med Sci Law 1985;25:265–9.

26. Lindenberg R, Fisher R, et al. Lesions of corpus callosum following blunt mechanical trauma to the head. Am J Pathol 1955;31:297–317.

27. Wilberger JE, Rothfus WE, et al. Acute tissue tear hemorrhages of the brain: Computed tomography and clinicopathological correlations. Neurosurgery 1990;27:208–13.

28. Teasdale GM. Head injury. J Neurol Neurosurg Psychiatry May 1995;58(5):526–39.

29. Grados MA, Slomine BS, Gerring JP, Vasa R, Bryan N, Denckla MB: Depth of lesion model in children and adolescents with moderate to severe traumatic brain injury: use of SPGR MRI to predict severity and outcome. J Neurol Neurosurg Psychiatry 2001;70:350–8. Cross ref.

30. Gentry LR, Godersky JC, Thompson B: MR imaging of head trauma: review of the distribution and radiopathologic features of traumatic lesions. AJR Am J Roentgenol 1988; 150:663–72.

31. Skandsen T, Kvistad KA, Solheim O, et al. Prevalence and impact of diffuse axonal injury

in patients with moderate and severe head injury: a cohort study of early magnetic resonance imaging findings and a 1-year outcome J Neurosurg, 2009.

32. Schrader H, Mickeviciene D, Gleizniene R, et al. Magnetic resonance imaging after most common form of concussion. BMC Med Imaging 2009;9:11.

33. Gentry LR, Godersky JC, Thompson B. MR imaging of head trauma: review of the distribution and radiopathologic features of traumatic lesion. AJR Am J Roentgenol 1988; 150(3):663–72.

34. Schefer PW, Grant PE, Gonzalez RG. Diffusion-weighted MR imaging of the brain. Radiology Nov 2000;217(2):331–45.

35. Hergan K, Schefer PW, Sorensen AG, Gonzalez RG, Huisman TA. Diffusion-weighted MRI in diffuse axonal injury of the brain. Eur Radiol Oct 2002;12(10):2536–41.

36. De la Plata CM, Ardelean A, Koovakkattu D, et al. Magnetic resonance imaging of diffuse axonal injury: quantitative assessment of white matter lesion volume. J Neurotrauma 2007;24(4):591–8.

37. Huisman TA, Schwamm LH, Schefer PW, Koroshetz WJ, Shetty-Alva N, Ozsunar Y, Wu O, Sorensen AG. Diffusion tensor imaging as potential biomarker of white matter injury in diffuse axonal injury. AJNR Am J Neuroradiol. 2004;25(3):370–6.

38. Sugiyama K, Kondo T, Oouchida Y, et al. Clinical utility of diffusion tensor imaging for evaluating patients with diffuse axonal injury and cognitive disorders in the chronic stage. J Neurotrauma 2009;26(11):1879–90.

39. Paterakis K, Karantanas AH, Komnos A, et al. Outcome of patients with diffuse axonal injury: the significance and prognostic value of MRI in the acute phase. J Trauma 2000;49:1071–5.

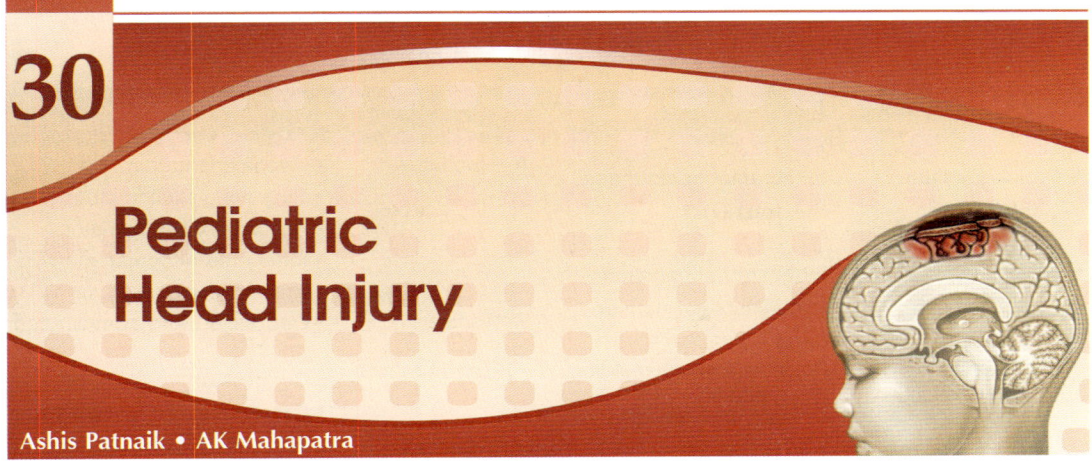

30

Pediatric Head Injury

Ashis Patnaik • AK Mahapatra

INTRODUCTION

Head trauma leading to brain injury is an important cause of morbidity and mortality both in adults and children. Although head injuries in children and adults have several similarities, pediatric patients have a more susceptible cranial vault due to thinner bones, large head-to-torso ratio, late development of air sinuses and differences in the immune system and in their capability of maintaining body temperature.[1] It is almost 30 years Prof. McLaurin, a famous Pediatric neurosurgeon said, "Child is not a small adult". When he said that, he tried to emphasize that the management protocol being used in adult cannot be applicable to children, especially so, if the children are less than 5 years of age. The vast majority of head trauma in pediatric patients suffer from mild injury, require no specific therapy and may not develop any sequelae but, it is important to identify individuals at risk of significant injury.[2] Severe head trauma in children is less frequent than in young adults, and the mortality rate is also lower due to different pathomechanisms and response of the pediatric brain to trauma.[3] This along with different mode of management and specific problems in pediatric age group, makes these an entirely different management problem compared to the adult population.

INCIDENCE

In India, pediatric age population below the age of 16 years, constitute around 40% of total population and 30% of head injury patients are in fact children. Considering the total number of head injury patients in India of about 1,000,000–1,200,000 per annum, there occurs near about 300,000 to 400,000 pediatric head injury cases each year, which is a huge burden to our society.[3] More than half of the patients of head injuries who come to emergency department in US are children.[4] Schutzman et al,[5] reported cranial injury in 84.3% of their 2100 children, below 13 years, who were admitted for trauma. Out of 161 mortality, 145 cases were accounted by head injury. Fall from a height is the most common cause of head injury in children, followed by motor-vehicle-related accidents.[6]

MECHANISMS OF INJURY

Most common mechanism of head injury depends upon the age of the child. Pediatric population can be divided into four groups:

1. *Neonates and infants:* Below 1 year of age— Birth trauma is the most common type causing head injuries in this age group. This is induced by various conditions like prolonged labor, cephalopelvic disproportion and difficult labor (Table 30.1). Use of forceps or vacuum for difficult labor is also

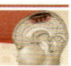

Table 30.1: Causes of neonatal head injury

Causes	Type of lesions
a. Prolonged labor	a. Intracranial hemorrhage
b. Cephalopelvic disproportion	Subarachnoid
c. Difficult labor	Intracerebral hematoma
d. Use of forceps and vacuum extractors	Intraventricular hemorrhage
	Posterior fossa hematoma
e. Fall from height	b. Brain edema

Table 30.2: Common intracranial lesions in children due to head injury

A. Neonates	• Cephalohematoma
	• Ping-pong skull fracture
	• Acute subdural hematoma
	• Intracerebral hematoma
	• Brain swelling
B. Toddlers	• Depressed and comminuted fracture
	• Concussion
	• Extradural and subdural hematoma
	• Contusion
	• Laceration
	• Brain swellings
	• Combination of the above pathologies
C. Older children	• Extradural hematoma
	• Subdural hematoma
	• Cerebral contusion/ laceration
	• Intracerebral hemorrhage
	• Ischemic hypoxic injury
	• Brain swelling

responsible for causing damage to head. Normally, there occurs moulding of parietal bones over each other and of the frontal and occipital bones over the parietals. However, during obstructed and difficult labors, this normal moulding process gets exaggerated, leading to damage to the underlying brain. Such complications can be avoided by elective cesarean section in high risk patients.

2. *Between 1 and 5 years of age:* Falls from height or object falling on the head of child, constitute around 80% of head injuries in this group. Falling of coconut and causing head injury is an occasional and typical mechanism in children below 16 years. In the Western literature, child abuse has been mentioned as one of the important causes head injury in young children.[7,8]

3. Between 5 and 10 years of age.

4. Above 10 years.

Both fall and sports related injury are important cause of head injury.

Pathology

Similar to those in adults, pathological changes in brain following head injury can be:

1. *Primary:* It includes all types of hematomas, contusions, and lacerations (Table 30.2).

2. *Secondary:* It includes changes induced by the primary pathology such as brain edema, hypoxia and ischemic changes.

Specific Injuries in Newborns and Neonates

Normally, during moulding at the time birth, some amount of edema of scalp in form of serosanguinous, subcutaneous, extraperiosteal fluid collection with poorly defined margins occurs and is known as **caput succedaneum**. This is caused by the pressure of the presenting part of the scalp against the dilating cervix during delivery. It is often treated by pediatricians and usually does not require neurosurgical consultation. **Subgaleal hematoma** is a blood collection between periosteum and galea aponeurotica, and passes the suture lines. It is usually related to vacuum extraction, trauma and rarely in coagulation disorders.[9] It is usually develops gradually. Prompt diagnosis is of paramount importance since patient may present with shock. Similarly **cephalohematoma**, a larger blood collection, which do not cross the suture lines can give rise to hypovolemic shock and needs blood transfusion. Exaggerated

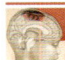

moulding of skull bones during labor or rough use of forceps can lead to intracranial hemorrhage in neonates. Extradural hematomas are rare in neonates and very small children as the dura is densely adherent to skull bone. Acute subdural hematomas are not uncommon in newborns. About 20–25% of neonatal deaths are due to intracranial hemorrhage.[10]

Fractures in neonatal period are rare due to the elasticity of the bone. More commonly a typical **ping-pong** fracture (Fig. 30.1) occurs which is may depressed or fissured type. As the dura is densely adherent to the overlying bone, any fracture is liable to damage the dura and when unrepaired, can lead to **growing skull fractures**. This type of fractures are common up to the age of 5. Due to non-pneumatization of paranasal sinuses, fracture through the anterior cranial fossa is also common and can lead to CSF rhinorrhea.

Head Injuries in Toddlers and Older Children

Children between 5 and 16 years are prone to sustain head injuries due to fall from height due to lack of parent supervision or during kite flying. Small children are susceptible to head injury when allowed to travel standing or sitting unharnessed, and the moving car is suddenly brought to a halt. Head of the baby gets squashed between mother and dashboard ("Baby Dashboard syndrome").

Fracture Skull

There are four major types of skull fractures in children: linear, depressed, diastatic and of skull base. Linear fractures are most common and usually are parietal in location (Fig. 30.2). Although not significant, they give rise to extradural hematoma, especially if they cross a major vessel. In younger children, the fracture may look like a dimple or "gutta-percha doll's head" due to pliability of skull bone. Comminuted fractures in children tend to associated with dural tears, laceration and are often compound and depressed in nature (Fig. 30.3). All diastatic fractures should be followed up to timely identify the presence of a growing fracture. Skull base fractures are rare in children. They can be suspected in the presence of specific signs such as periorbital ecchymosis (Raccoon's eyes), mastoid ecchymosis (Battle's sign), otorrhagia and epistaxis. The most common physical findings are hemotympanum and bleeding in the ear canals.

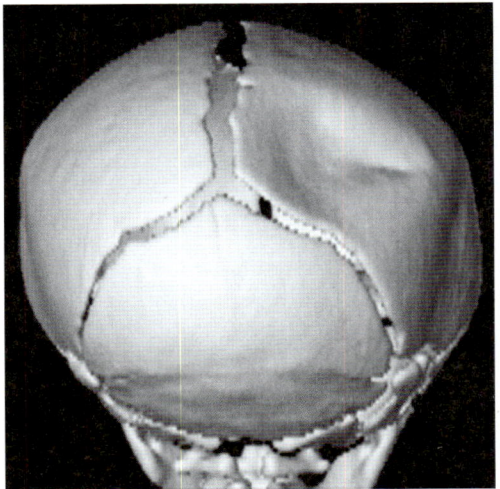

Fig. 30.1: 3D CT scan showing a ping-pong fracture without any break in outer or inner table of the skull

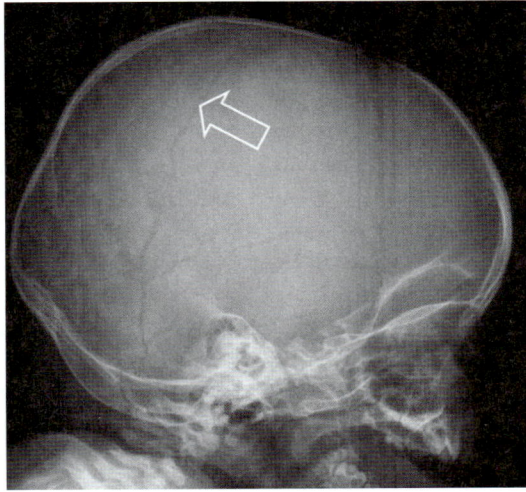

Fig. 30.2: Vertical linear fracture involving parietal and occipital bones

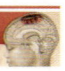

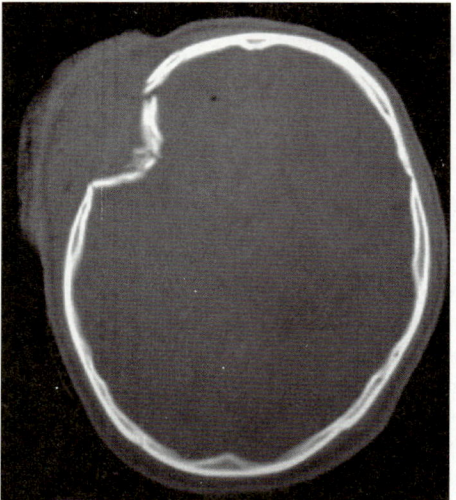

Fig. 30.3: CT bone window showing comminuted depressed fracture in a child

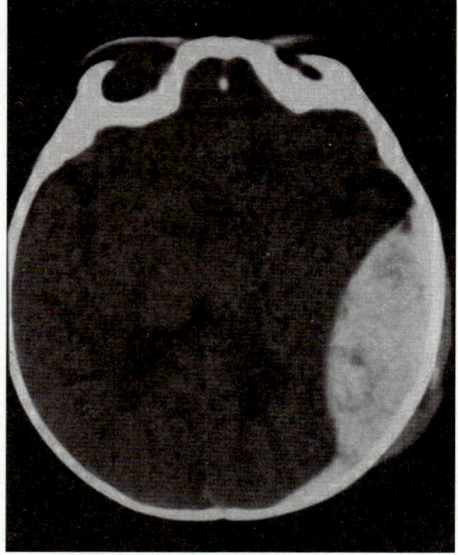

Fig. 30.4a: Extradural hematoma appearing hyperdense in left parietal region

Concussion

Concussion means reversible neurologic dysfunction. It is associated with transient loss of consciousness, memory loss (both retrograde and post-traumatic amnesia). Etiology of concussion is the injury in the occipital area and shearing strain at the brainstem level. Children recover faster from concussion injuries than the adults.

Extradural Hematoma

Most of the extradural hematomas in older children are frontal or temporal in location (Figs 30.4a and b). Rarely posterior fossa hematomas have been reported. Ammirati and Tomita[11] reviewed 36 cases of posterior fossa extradural hematomas in children. These hematomas can extend above the tentorium.[12] The lucid period may be absent; and in children, only in one-third of the cases the clinical presentation is typical.

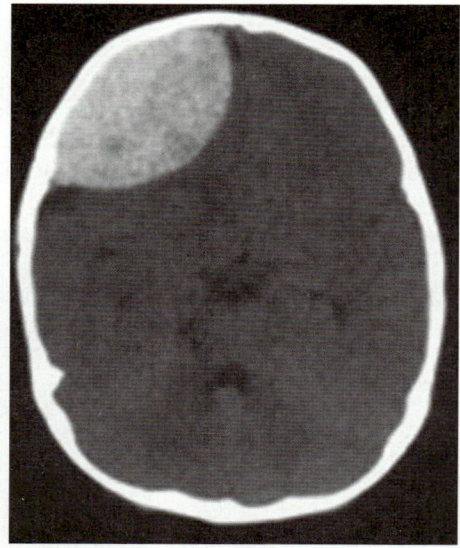

Fig. 30.4b: CT scan head: Large EDH with mass effect

Acute Subdural Hematoma

Acute subdural hematomas (Fig. 30.5) are common in children with two peak ages, one at the infancy, and the other in older children. Usually it results due to severe injuries like fall from height, only rarely it may be due to minor injury. When the fontanelle is open in small children, the expanding hematoma can present as tense anterior fontanelle which may wrongly be diagnosed as a case of hydrocephalus.

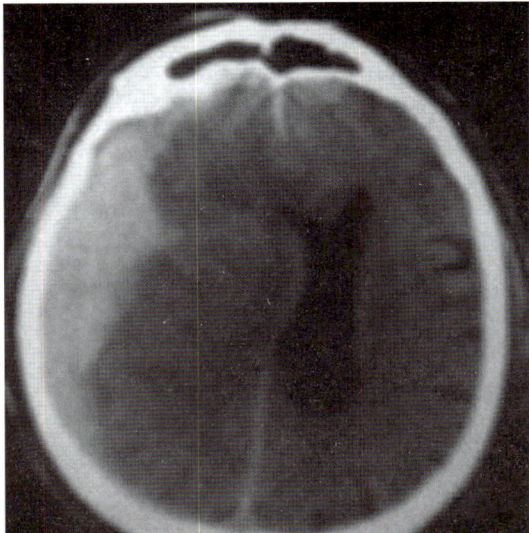

Contusions/Laceration and Intracerebral Hematoma

Contusions (Fig. 30.6) and intracerebral hematomas are unusual in children and may be the result of focal brain injury or penetrating trauma. Most often they involve the temporal and frontal lobes. Many intracerebral hematomas can be treated conservatively. Those with significant mass effect or shift may require evacuation if clinically indicated.

Chronic Subdural Hygroma/Effusion

Majority of these are seen in infants, predominantly male, with 93% occurring below the age of three.[13] Head injury due to birth trauma can cause such pathology (Fig. 30.7). Children present with seizure, macrocrania, bulging fontanelle, irritability, anemia, cranial nerve palsy. Various modalities of treatment like burr hole drainage, repeated tapping, membranectomy, superior sagittal sinus reconstruction have been instituted with subdural-peritoneal shunting of collection being the most accepted one.

Penetrating Head Trauma

Penetrating head injuries are rare in children but belong to the class of most severe traumatic brain injuries. In these cases,

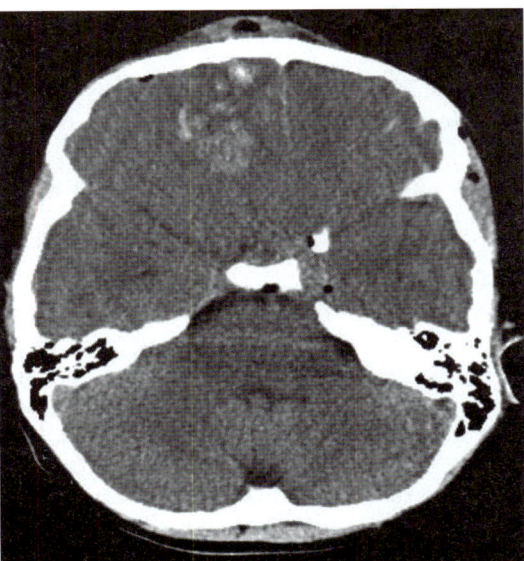

Fig. 30.6: Right side basifrontal region contusion

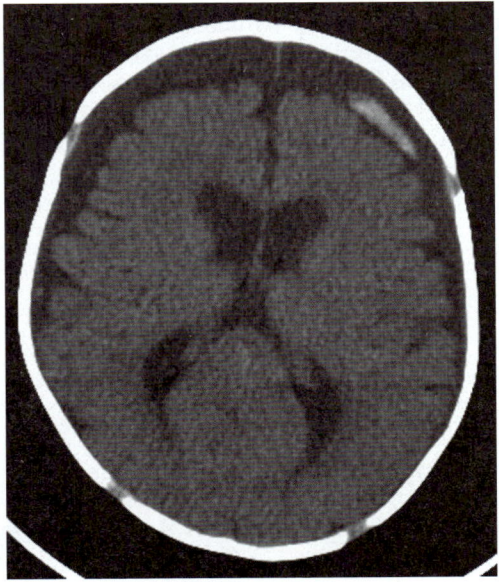

Fig. 30.7: Bilateral frontal subdural hematoma due to birth trauma

communication arises between the intra-cranial cavity and surrounding environment. Gunshot head injuries,[14] injuries from knife, nails, pencils, chopsticks and scissors are some of the examples of this injury.[15–18]

Brain Edema

Although the situation of brain edema are common in both adults and children, different pathomechanisms account for them (Table 30.3). In adults, the edema is due to increased water content and is known vasogenic edema. Venous congestion and stasis accounts for the intractable brain swelling in children, termed as malignant brain edema. Brain injuries release excitatory neurotransmitters and these can cause breakdown of blood–brain barrier (BBB). This leads to disturbance of autoregulation and leakage of fluid into extravascular spaces causing brain edema.

Traumatic Ischemic Damage

It has been established that the ischemia plays an important role in secondary brain injury. Studies have shown that the incidence of ischemic damage is 85–90% in fatal head injuries[19,20] (Fig. 30.8). This ischemia can be focal or diffuse due to microcirculatory failure. Ischemic damage to brain after injury in children is not uncommon as fine vasculature in children and sludging effect of blood in capillaries due to increased viscosity predisposes to microcirculatory failure.

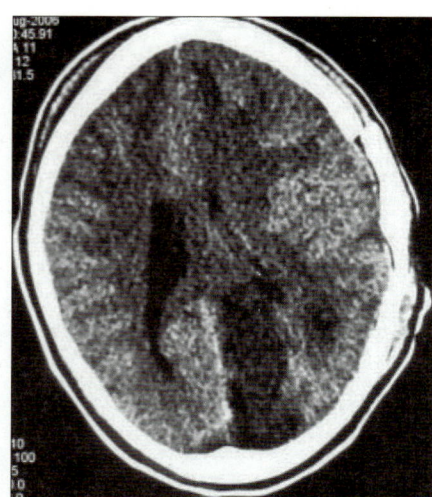

Fig. 30.8: Gross brain edema on left hemisphere with left PCA infarct following trauma in a child

CLINICAL ASSESSMENT

1. Breathing

Similar to adults, quick evaluation of breathing is of utmost importance. But, the children tolerate hypoxia poorly as:
- Children have high oxygen demand compared to adults (double that of adults).
- Air passage is narrower and the adenoids and tonsils are larger further compromising the airway.
- Soft tracheal rings result in easy obstruction of trachea on flexion.
- Delicate vocal cords and larynx get easily damaged by repeated suction and attempt to intubate.
- To intubate a child is more difficult than adult.

All the above factors can facilitate the irreversible brain damage during hypoxia.

Breathing can be assessed by noting the chest movement. Noisy breathing suggest a partial obstruction to the air passage. Chest injury should be ruled out as children are sensitive to pain arising out of fractured ribs and lead to inadequate chest movement and inadequate respiration. Children have a tendency to swallow air which pushes

Table 30.3: Mechanism of brain edema formation
Head trauma
↓
Disturbance in autoregulation
↓
Deranged microcirculation

• Opening of tight junction	• Release of vasoactive neurotransmitters
• Breakdown of BBB	• Release of free radicals
• Exudation of fluid	• Opening of calcium channel
• Edema	• Development of edema

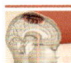

Table 30.4: Pediatric Glasgow Coma Scale					
Eye opening		*Best verbal response*		*Best motor response*	
Spontaneous	4	Coos, babbles	5	Normal spontaneous movement	6
To speech	3	Irritable, cries	4	Withdraws to touch	5
To pain	2	Cries to pain	3	Withdraws to pain	4
None	1	Moans to pain	2	Abnormal flexion	3
		None	1	Abnormal extension	2
				None	1

diaphragm upwards, thereby worsening the breathing.

2. Assessment of Blood Pressure

In adults, head injury usually produce shock. But the children can develop hypotension due to scalp hematoma or bleeding from lacerated wound, as children have poor response to blood loss and only 10–15% of blood loss can be tolerated, as compared to adults, who can stand up to 35–40%.

3. Systemic Examination

Thorough examination of the limbs for fracture, chest, abdomen for an occult abdominal, pelvic or retroperitoneal injury is important. Evacuation of distended urinary bladder should be done to reduce abdominal pressure as well as the agitation of the patient and intracranial pressure.

4. Neurological Assessment

While assessment of children above the age of 10 years is easier, same in neonates and very young children is quite difficult due to lack of co-operation. Similar to adults, it consists of:

a. *Level of consciousness:* The implementation of Glasgow Coma Scale (GCS), which has been universally accepted method to evaluate the neurological status of adult patients, has limitations in very small children. Pediatric Glasgow Coma Scale has been devised to be used in this conditions[21] (Table 30.4).

Head trauma is classified according to GCS as follows

• *GCS 13 to 15:* Minor head trauma

• *GCS 9 to 13:* Moderate head trauma
• *GCS ≤ 8:* Severe head trauma.

Pediatric Coma Score

It considers six factors:
1. Size.
2. Respiratory status.
3. Sytolic blood pressure.
4. CNS status.
5. Open wound.
6. Fractures.

Each factor graded according to the abnormality: +2 for minor abnormality, +1 for major abnormality and –1 for severe and life-threatening abnormality. Therefore, the total score has range of –6 which signifies 100% mortality to +12 score which indicates excellent outcome.

Pediatric Rapid Score (Table 30.5)

It is a simple and rapid scoring system modified from original GCS. However, it does not considers the systemic factors.

b. *Focal neurological deficit:* Presence of hemiparesis, monoparesis or plegia signifies focal brain damage. Cranial nerve palsies particularly 3rd cranial nerve involvement is considered to be the most significant finding in head injury similar to that in adults. Upper motor facial palsy can

Table 30.5: Pediatric rapid score (AVPU system)
A—Alert and fully conscious
B—Responds to verbal command
P—Responds to pain
U—Unresponsive

occur as part of hemiparesis. Lower motor facial palsy is usually associated with fracture of petrous temporal bone and ecchymoses of retroauricular and mastoid areas (Battle's sign), CSF otorrhea, etc. Cerebellar signs are rarely present in head injuries in children and are suggestive of posterior fossa lesions. In neonates, acute subdural hematomas can present as irritability, hypotonia, lethargy, tense fontanelle and opisthotonus posture.

INVESTIGATIONS

1. X-ray Skull

Use of X-ray skull after the widespread availability of CT scan has grossly reduced due to:

- Difficult to get a good quality X-ray in children due to movement.
- Significant intracranial pathology can exist without a single skull fracture.
- Provides no informations about the brain parenchyma damage, hematomas.

However, X-ray skull can provide important informations in comminuted fractures such as position and displacement of the fragments, in PNS opacity and in foreign bodies such as metallic fragments and bullets.

2. CT Scan

CT scan is the investigation of choice, for all the types of head injury (Figs 30.3 to 30.6), as it is widely available, rapidly obtained, more informative and can be easily repeated. It clearly delineates the intracranial pathology including hematomas, parenchymal injury,

edema and infarction. Bone window shows the associated skull bone fractures both simple and comminuted, thereby decreasing the need for X-ray skull. CT scans are also used to long-term follow-up of a head injury patient.

Although routine CT scan is desirable in moderate and severe head injuries, there is still an uncertainty over which children with minor head trauma require CT, as fewer than 10% of these children suffer from a traumatic brain injury.[22] CT scan is also associated radiation exposure[23] which may impair the cognition development in children. Rice et al[24] reported that there may 1 case of lethal cancer for every 1000 CT scans performed in a young child. Therefore, identification of children having low risk after head trauma is of paramount importance. Atabaki et al[25] in their series of 1000 pediatric patients with minor head trauma, 65 patients had a CT scan with intracranial pathology and only 6 out of 65, required neurosurgical intervention.[16] Kuppermann et al[26] in a prospective study of 42, 412 children with minor head trauma, obtained CT scans on 14969 (35.3%) children and only 60 (0.1%) underwent surgery. They developed prediction rules which help in the identification of children in whom CT can be omitted (Table 30.6).

Members of the Pediatric Emergency Research, Canada, Head Injury Study Group led by Osmond et al[27] derived the Canadian Assessment of Tomography for Childhood Head Injury (CATCH) rule (Table 30.7), by means of a prospective cohort study involving 3886 children presenting with symptomatic

Table 30.6: Low risk of harboring clinically important traumatic brain injury[26]	
< 2 years of age	**> or = 2 years of age**
a. Normal mental status	a. Normal mental status
b. No scalp hematoma except frontal	b. No loss of consciousness
c. No loss of consciousness or loss of consciousness for less than 5 sec	c. No vomiting
d. Non-severe injury mechanism	d. Non-severe injury mechanism
e. No palpable skull fracture	e. No signs of basilar skull fracture
f. Acting normally according to the parents	f. No severe headache

Table 30.7: CT reqirement criteria in mild head injury in children (catch rule)[27]

High risk:
1. GCS score < 15 at 2 hours after injury
2. Suspicion of open skull fracture
3. Worsening headache
4. Irritability on examination

Moderate risk:
1. Large scalp hematoma
2. Signs of skull base fracture
3. Dangerous injury mechanism

minor head trauma to 10 Canadian pediatric teaching institutions.

MRI

Although MRI can provide all the details given by CT scan except skull fractures and subarachnoid hemorrhage, it has the following limitations in comparison to CT:

- High cost.
- Not widely available in emergency situations.
- Long scanning time which is not possible in neonates and small children.
- Claustrophobia.

However, MRI gives better resolution of parenchymal injuries (Fig. 30.9) and posterior fossa and is the most sensitive neuroimaging study available for brain injury (Fig. 30.10). Cerebral blood flow (CBF), cerebral blood volume (CBV) can be measured by MRI. MRI spectroscopy can show the location of ongoing ischemia, frequency of vasogenic edema and the presence of intracellular edema.

Diffusion-weighted imaging: Images on DWI are sensitive to differences in the diffusion rate of water molecules and can detect vasogenic and cytotoxic edema.[28] Increased diffusion is thought to occur with vasogenic edema due to increased water in the extracellular space where there is increased mobility, while restricted diffusion due to decreased water movement in the intracellular space is thought to be due to cytotoxic edema.[29, 31] DWI also can quantify water mobility by determining apparent diffusion coefficient (ADC) values, a measure of random water motion limited by cellular composition. ADC measurements are useful in detecting diffuse axonal injury (DAI) in pediatric TBI patients.

While there are numerous studies of DWI and ADC (apparent diffusion coefficient) for lesion detection and outcome following TBI in adults, less is known about DWI and ADC in pediatric TBI. In one recent study, ADC values (obtained within 7 days of injury) in the peripheral white matter tracts were signi-

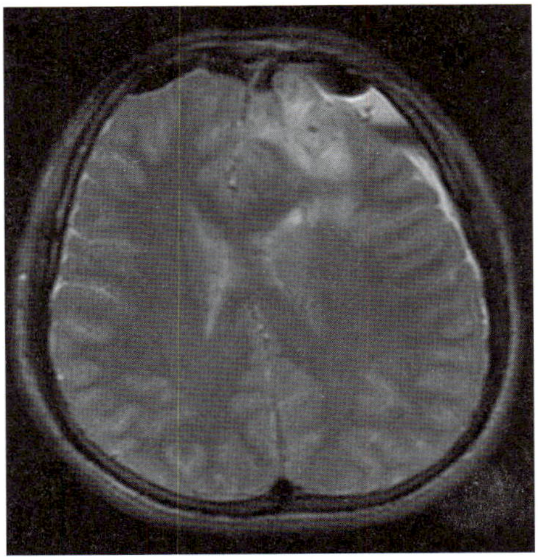

Fig. 30.9: MRI; T_2-weighted image showing small left frontal contusion

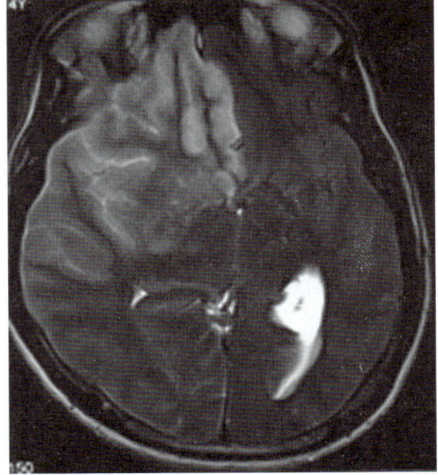

Fig. 30.10: MRI brain showing post-traumatic ischemic changes on T_2-weighted image

ficantly reduced in children with severe TBI that had poor outcomes compared to children with severe TBI that had good outcomes at 6–12 months after trauma.[30] Furthermore, acute ADC values in the peripheral white and gray matter regions following pediatric TBI were inversely correlated with long-term (1–4 years) neurocognitive outcomes.[63] DWI has also been shown to allow earlier detection of acute cerebral ischemia (Fig. 30.11) than conventional CT or MRI as processes associated with ischemic injury result in greater diffusion restriction.[31,32]

Susceptibility weighted imaging (SWI): In pediatric TBI, hemorrhagic shearing lesions associated with DAI are a very common pathologic entity.[33,34] Unlike the large hemorrhages seen in contusions, epidural and subdural hematomas, conventional CT or MRI will usually not pick up these small shearing hemorrhagic lesions. Susceptibility weighted imaging (SWI) is a form of MRI that utilizes the paramagnetic properties of blood products (intravascular and extravascular deoxyhemoglobin, methemoglobin, and hemosiderin) based on their magnetic susceptibility effects in order to increase the visibility of microscopic hemorrhages.[34,35] SWI has been shown to be superior in detecting hemorrhagic DAI after TBI in children compared to conventional MRI.[36,37]

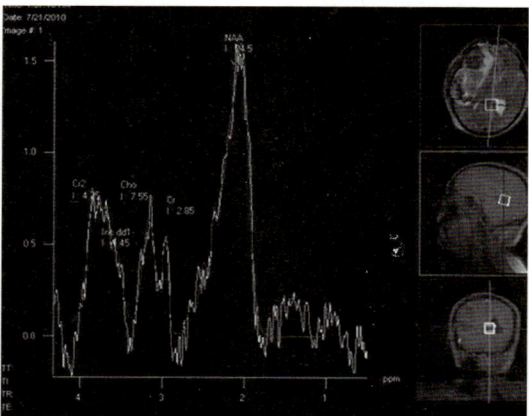

Fig. 30.11: MR spectroscopy showing NAA peak

Diffusion tensor imaging (DTI): Diffusion tensor imaging (DTI), which is a more complex form of DWI. DTI takes advantage of the directionality of water diffusion in the human brain and allows analysis of the white matter tracts.[38,39] Water diffusion is considered isotropic when motion is free and equal in all directions. In the normal brain tissue, there are physical boundaries that restrict water diffusion in the white matter tracts, with greater water mobility parallel to the axons and restriction of mobility perpendicular to the axons. This diffusion restriction is termed fractional anisotropy (FA) or the ratio of anisotropy to isotropy;[40] FA ranges from 0 to 1, where values closer to 0 represent isotropy or increased diffusion, for example, as a result of injury.[41] In contrast, values closer to 1 represent water diffusion more parallel to the white matter tracts in normal brain tissue.

Pediatric DTI studies done within weeks to years after TBI generally reveal reduced FA.[42,43] Another study revealed reduced FA and increased ADC in the white matter tracts of the TBI group compared to controls[44,45] and correlated with cognitive and global outcome.

Magnetic resonance spectroscopy (MRS): MRI uses signals from the proton nuclei of water to reconstruct anatomical images, MRS uses the protons located on neurochemicals within brain tissues (Fig. 30.11). Several key brain metabolites measured by MRS include N-acetylaspartate (NAA), an amino acid synthesized in the mitochondria, that is a neuronal and axonal marker that decreases with neuronal dysfunction or loss.[46] Total Creatine (Cr) composed of phosphocreatine and its precursor Cr are markers of intact brain energy metabolism. Total choline (Cho) which predominantly consists of phosphoryl and glycerophosphoryl Cho is a marker for membrane repair or synthesis, demyelination, or inflammation. Lactate is a result of anaerobic glycolysis and/or may be a response to release of glutamate.[47] Glutamate and glutamine are excitatory amino acid neurotransmitters that are released after TBI and may play a major role in neuronal death. Myoinositol is an organic osmolyte in astrocytes and increases with glial proliferation.[48]

MANAGEMENT

Although management of head injuries should start from the time of accidents, most of the time, interventions cannot be done till the patient reaches the casualty. This initial 1 hour following trauma is the golden hour for both adult and pediatric head injury patients as the events occurring in this period indicate the long-term outcome.

Similar to any trauma patient, pediatric head injury patients should be assessed in the order of (Table 30.8):

1. Airway
2. Breathing
3. Circulation (to detect any hypotension early and correct it)
4. Disability

Respiratory obstruction and hypotension are the two important killers in pediatric age group followed by intracranial hematomas. Therefore, adequate oxygenation is the important step. Sometimes the patient may need endotracheal intubation and ventillatory support. As pediatric patients are more prone to shock, proper intravenous fluid replacement should be started if there are signs of dehydration and hypotension. Patients with raised ICP or intracranial hematoma need mannitol 0.5–1.0 gm per kg body weight. Hypoglycemia should be prevented by giving glucose containing fluid.

Anticonvulsants should be administered in cases of brain parenchyma injuries including contusions, lacerations, compound fractures with in-driven bony fragments into the brain substance. Proper antibiotics in case of wounds, indwelling catheter to prevent bladder distension should be given.

ICU Care of Pediatric Head Injury

Pediatric head injuries account for 10% of total ICU admissions and 10% of total ICU days by

Table 30.8: Initial assessment in pediatric head injury and stabilization procedure[49]

Airway (A)
Consider possible injury to the cervical spine
Maintain head and neck in a neutral position
Immobilization: Sandbags, intravenous solution bags, towel rolls (younger patients)
Age-appropriate rigid cervical collar or manual in-line immobilization (older patients)
Orotracheal intubation if cannot maintain airway adequately with positioning and after suctioning

Breathing (B)
Intubation if unable to maintain adequate oxygenation and ventilation, despite provision of supplemental oxygen
Use rapid-sequence induction technique
Maintain cervical spine precautions

Circulation (C)
Hemodynamic instability unlikely to be caused by intracranial injury alone (exception: Significant intracranial or scalp bleeding in a young infant)
If present:
• Investigate extracranial lesions causing hemorrhagic or hypovolemic shock
• Insert two large-bore intravenous catheters; fluid bolus of 20 ml/kg of normal saline
• Repeat until vital signs improve

Disability (D)
Perform rapid assessment, including:
Glasgow Coma Scale score adapted to age
Pupil size and reactivity to light
Tone, reflex and movement of all four limbs
Fontanelle (infants)
Signs of basal skull fracture: Periorbital ecchymosis ('Raccoon eyes'), ecchymosis over the mastoid bone (Battle's sign), obvious leakage of CSF from the nose or ears, hemotympanum. If one or more of these signs is present, no tube should be placed by the nasal route

Table 30.9: Indications for admission into ICU

1. Severe head injury with patient in intubated state
2. Children with proven or suspected raised ICP
3. Multiple episodes of seizure
4. Impending or sudden deterioration of neurological status from a stable condition
5. Postoperative status
6. Polytrauma patients

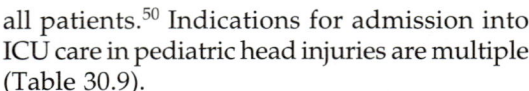

all patients.[50] Indications for admission into ICU care in pediatric head injuries are multiple (Table 30.9).

Management in ICU can broadly be:

a. Monitoring of hemodynamic parameters like blood pressure, central venous pressure, fluid and electrolyte, end tidal carbon dioxide (ETCO$_2$) in ventilated patients.

b. Maintenance of proper nutrition through enteral (preferable) or parenteral route.

c. *Monitoring of ICP:* To prevent any sudden deterioration. However, it has not been considered as a part of standard care in pediatric head injuries.[51]

d. Monitoring cerebral metabolism and cerebral blood flow.

e. General measures to keep the ICP low like elevated head position, sedation and paralysis, mannitol and diuretic therapy to lower the ICP.

Role of Surgery

Surgery should be done in cases of:

• Compound injury with brain herniation.

• Large hematoma with raised ICP.

• Depressed fracture when the bone fragment is depressed deeper than the adjacent inner table (with or without seizure).

Postoperatively, the children can be electively ventilated till they have good spontaneous respiration maintaining the normal oxygen saturation. If a patient needs long-term ventilation, then an elective tracheostomy is necessary. As children have little glycogen or fat reserve, nasogastric feeding should be started as soon as possible.

Outcome

Initial neurological status such as pediatric coma score is the most important predictor of outcome. Patients with post-trauma low GCS score or systolic BP of less than 135 mm of Hg have a poor prognosis. Neonates have a strong correlation with high mortality. Similarly a bulging fontanelle, bilateral 3rd nerve palsy, irregular respiration and persistent unrespon-siveness have a positive correlation with the severity of brain injury. Coagulopathy and development of early post-traumatic seizures are also associated with a worse outcome.

The overall mortality in severe head injury is around 40–60%. Mortality is multifactorial and depends upon large number of factors (Table 30.10).

BRAIN DAMAGE MARKERS

Various markers have been evaluated for possible use in the diagnosis and prognosis of brain damage in children. S100 calcium-binding protein B, or S100 β is usually elevated in children after traumatic brain injury.[52–55] It has been extensively studied as a diagnostic tool[53, 54] and selection of patients for CT.[55] Neuron specific enolase (NSE)[54,56–58] coagulo-pathy[59,60] hyperglycemia[61,62] are the other markers which have been reported to be associated with poor outcome in pediatric head injuries.

CONCLUSIONS

Head injury is common in pediatric age group and accounts for 25–30% of all head injuries. Causes are heterogeneous and depend on the actual age of the patient. Birth trauma is a more frequent cause in neonate, while falls are overall major cause of head injuries in pediatric age group. All kinds of intracranial pathology similar to that seen in adults, can occur in pediatric patients. However, children are more prone for malignant brain swellings and ischemic brain damage. Children withstand the hypotension and hypoxia poorly. Head injuries in children, in general

Table 30.10: Factors influencing outcome
a. Coma score
b. Associated injury
c. Age of the patient
d. Hypotension
e. Fixed dilated pupils
f. Decerebrate rigidity or decortication
g. Cold caloric response

have to be managed more aggressively than the adults as they have less reserve. Surgery in pediatric head injury patients requires experienced surgeons and anesthetists. Overall mortality ranges from 40 to 50%.

REFERENCES

1. Alexiou GA, Sfakianos G, Prodromou N. Pediatric head trauma. J Emerg Trauma Shock 2011;4:403–8.

2. Farrell CA. Management of the pediatric patient with acute head trauma. Peditr Child Health 2013;18:253–8.

3. Kumar R, Mahapatra AK. The changing "epidemiology" of pediatric head injury and its impact on the daily clinical practice. Childs Nerv Syst 2009;25:813–23.

4. Duhaime AC. Closed head injury without fractures. In: Albright LA, Pollack IF and Adelson PD (Eds). Principles and Practice of Pediatric Neurosurgery. Thieme 1999;799.

5. Schutzman SA, Barnes P, Duhaime AC, Greenes D, Homer C, Jaffe D, et al. Evaluation and management of children younger than two years old with apparently minor head trauma: proposed guidelines. Pediatrics 2001;107:983–93.

6. Adirim TA, Wright JL, Lee E, Lomax TA, Chamberlain JM. Injury surveillance in a pediatric emergency department. Am J Emerg Med 1999;17:499–503.

7. Canadian Pediatric Society, Child and Youth Maltreatment Section, Guidelines Working Group. Multidisciplinary Guidelines on the Identification, Investigation and Management of Suspected Abusive Head Trauma. Ottawa: Canadian Pediatric Society, 2007.

8. King WJ, McKay M, Simick A. Canadian Shaken Baby Study Group. Shaken baby syndrome in Canada: Clinical characteristics and outcomes of hospital cases. CMAJ 2003;168:155–9.

9. Kirkpatrick JS, Gower DJ, Chauvenet A, Kelly DL Jr. Subgaleal hematoma in a child, without skull fracture. Dev Med Child Neurol 1986;28:511–4.

10. Bagchi AK. Head injury in neonates. In an introduction to head injury. Chapter 11, AK Bagchi (ed), Oxford University Press, Calcutta 1980;77–80.

11. Ammirati M, Tomita T. Posterior fossa epidural hematoma during childhood. Neurosurgery 1984;14:541–4.

12. Mahapatra AK. Posterior fossa extradural haematoma. Indian Pediatrics 1990;27:989–92.

13. White JR, Farukhi Z, Bull C, Christensen J, Gordon T, Paidas C, Nichols DG. Predictors of outcome in severely head-injured children. Crit Care Med 2001;29:534–40.

14. Irfan FB, Hassan RU, Kumar R, Bhutta ZA, Bari E. Craniocerebral gunshot injuries in pre-schoolers. Childs Nerv Syst 2010;26:61–6.

15. Pascual-Castroviejo I, Pascual-Pascual SI, Viaño J. Diplegia due to transcranial knife-blade injury in a 20-month-old child. J Child Neurol 2006;21:340–1.

16. Karim T, Topno M. An unusual case of penetrating head injury in a child. J Emerg Trauma Shock 2011;3:197–8.

17. van As AB, van Dijk J, Numanoglu A, Millar AJ. Assaults with a sharp object in small children: A 16-year review. Pediatr Surg Int 2008;24:1037–40.

18. Mackerle Z, Gal P. Unusual penetrating head injury in children: Personal experience and review of the literature. Childs Nerv Syst. 2009;25:909–13.

19. Graham DI. Pathology of hypoxic brain damage in man. J Clin Pathol Suppl (R Coll Pathol) 1977;11:170–80.

20. Graham DI, Adama JH, Doyle O. Ischemic brain damage in fatal non-missile head injuries. J Neurol Sciences 1976;39:213–34.

21. Holmes JF, Palchak MJ, McFarlane T, Kuppermann N. Performance of the Pediatric Glasgow Coma Scale in children with blunt head trauma. Acad Emerg Med 2005;12:814–9.

22. Halley MK, Silva PD, Foley J, Rodarte A. Loss of consciousness: When to perform computed tomography? Pediatr Crit Care Med 2004;5:230–3.

23. King MA, Kanal KM, Relyea-Chew A, Bittles M, Vavilala MS, Hollingworth W. Radiation exposure from pediatric head CT: A bi-institutional study. Pediatr Radiol 2009;39:1059–65.

24. Rice HE, Frush DP, Farmer D, Waldhausen JH. APSA Education Committee. Review of radiation risks from computed tomography: Essentials for the pediatric surgeon. J Pediatr Surg 2007;42:603–7.

25. Atabaki SM, Stiell IG, Bazarian JJ, Sadow KE, Vu TT, Camarca MA, et al. A clinical decision rule for cranial computed tomography in minor pediatric head trauma. Arch PediatrAdolesc Med 2008;162:439–45.

26. Kuppermann N, Holmes JF, Dayan PS, Hoyle JD Jr, Atabaki SM, Holubkov R, et al. Identification

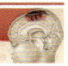

of children at very low risk of clinically-important brain injuries after head trauma: A prospective cohort study. Lancet 2009;374:1160–70.

27. Osmond MH, Klassen TP, Wells GA, Correll R, Jarvis A, Joubert G, et al. CATCH: A clinical decision rule for the use of computed tomography in children with minor head injury. CMAJ 2010;182:341–8.

28. Schaefer PW, Grant E, Gonzalez G. Diffuse weighted MR Imaging of the brain. Radiology 2000;217:331–45.

29. Friess SH, Kilbaugh TJ, Huh JW, Advanced Neuromonitoring and Imaging in Pediatric Traumatic Brain Injury. Critical Care Research and Practice.Volume 2012 (2012), Article ID 361310, 11 p.

30. Galloway NR, Tong KA, Ashwal S, Oyoyo U, and Obenaus A. "Diffusion-weighted imaging improves outcome prediction in pediatric traumatic brain injury" Journal of Neurotrauma, 2008;25:1153–62.

31. Hergan K, Schaefer PW, Sorensen AG, Gonzalez RG, and Huisman TA. "Diffusion-weighted MRI in diffuse axonal injury of the brain," European Radiology 2002;12:2536–41. View at Scopus.

32. Huisman TA. "Diffusion-weighted imaging: basic concepts and application in cerebral stroke and head trauma," European Radiology, 2003;13:2283–97.

33. EM Haacke, NY Cheng, MJ House, et al. "Imaging iron stores in the brain using magnetic resonance imaging," Magnetic Resonance Imaging 2005;23:1–25.

34. Sehgal V, Delproposto Z, Haacke EM, et al. "Clinical applications of neuroimaging with susceptibility-weighted imaging," Journal of Magnetic Resonance Imaging 2005;22:439–50.

35. Tong KA, Ashwal S, Holshouser BA, et al. "Hemorrhagic shearing lesions in children and adolescents with post-traumatic diffuse axonal injury: improved detection and initial results," Radiology 2003;227:332–9.

36. Beauchamp MH, Ditchfield M, Babl FE et al. "Detecting traumatic brain lesions in children: CT versus MRI versus susceptibility weighted imaging (SWI)," Journal of Neurotrauma, 2011;28:915–27.

37. Tong KA, Ashwal S, Holshouser BA et al. "Diffuse axonal injury in children: clinical correlation with hemorrhagic lesions," Annals of Neurology, 2004;56:36–50.

38. Mori S, Crain BJ, Chacko VP, van Zijl PC. "Three-dimensional tracking of axonal projections in the brain by magnetic resonance imaging," Annals of Neurology, 1999;45:265–9.

39. McGraw P, Liang L, and Provenzale JM. "Evaluation of normal age-related changes in anisotropy during infancy and childhood as shown by diffusion tensor imaging," American Journal of Roentgenology 2002;179:1515–22.

40. Suskauer SJ, Huisman TA. "Neuroimaging in pediatric traumatic brain injury: current and future predictors of functional outcome," Developmental Disabilities Research Reviews, 2009;15:117–23.

41. Sundgren PC, Dong Q, Gómez-Hassan D, Mukherji SK, Maly P, Welsh R. "Diffusion tensor imaging of the brain: review of clinical applications," Neuroradiology, 2004;46:339–50.

42. Akpinar E, Koroglu M, Ptak T. "Diffusion tensor MR imaging in pediatric head trauma," Journal of Computer Assisted Tomography, 2007;31:657–661.

43. Wu TC, Wilde EA, Bigler ED, et al. "Longitudinal changes in the corpus callosum following pediatric traumatic brain injury," Developmental Neuroscience, 2011;32:361–73.

44. Levin HS, Wilde EA, Chu Z, et al. "Diffusion tensor imaging in relation to cognitive and functional outcome of traumatic brain injury in children," Journal of Head Trauma Rehabilitation, 2008;23:197–208.

45. Wilde EA, Chu Z, Bigler ED, et al. "Diffusion tensor imaging in the corpus callosum in children after moderate to severe traumatic brain injury," Journal of Neurotrauma 2006;23:1412–26.

46. Alessandri B, Al-Samsam R, Corwin F, Fatouros P, Young HF, Bullock RM. "Acute and late changes in N-acetyl-aspartate following diffuse axonal injury in rats: an MRI spectroscopy and microdialysis study," Neurological Research 2000;22:705–12.

47. Bullock R, Zauner A, Woodward JJ, et al. "Factors affecting excitatory amino acid release following severe human head injury," Journal of Neuro-surgery, 1998;89:507–18.

48. Parry L, Shores A, Rae C, et al. "An investigation of neuronal integrity in severe pediatric traumatic brain injury," Child Neuropsychology, 2004;10:248–61.

49. American College of Surgeons Committee on Trauma, (eds). Advanced Trauma Life Support

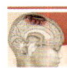
for Doctors Manual, 8th edition. Chicago: American College of Surgeons, 2008.

50. Duhamie AC, O'Rourke M. Intesive care manangement of children with head injuries. In: Andrews BT and Hammer GB (eds). Pediatric Neurosurgical Intensive Care. American Association of Neurological Surgeons 1997;125.

51. Adelson DP. Pediatric trauma made simple. Clinical Neurosurgery. Lippincott, Williams and Wilkins 2000;319–35.

52. Berger RP, Pierce MC, Wisniewski SR, Adelson PD, Kochanek PM. Serum S100 β concentrations are increased after closed head injury in children: A preliminary study. J Neurotrauma 2002;19:1405–9.

53. Hallén M, Karlsson M, Carlhed R, Hallgren T, Bergenheim M. S100 β in serum and urine after traumatic head injury in children. J Trauma. 2010;69:284–9.

54. Geyer C, Ulrich A, Gräfe G, Stach B, Till H. Diagnostic value of S100 β and neuron-specific enolase in mild pediatric traumatic brain injury. J Neurosurg Pediatr 2009;4:339–44.

55. Müller K, Townend W, Biasca N, Undén J, Waterloo K, Romner B, et al. S100 β serum level predicts computed tomography findings after minor head injury. J Trauma 2007;62:1452–6.

56. Fridriksson T, Kini N, Walsh-Kelly C, Hennes H. Serum neuron-specific enolase as a predictor of intracranial lesions in children with head trauma: A pilot study. Acad Emerg Med 2000;7:816–20.

57. Bandyopadhyay S, Hennes H, Gorelick MH, Wells RG, Walsh-Kelly CM. Serum neuron-specific enolase as a predictor of short-term outcome in children with closed traumatic brain injury. Acad Emerg Med 2005;12:732–8.

58. Kövesdi E, Lückl J, Bukovics P, Farkas O, Pál J, Czeiter E, et al. Update on protein biomarkers in traumatic brain injury with emphasis on clinical use in adults and pediatrics. Acta Neurochir (Wien) 2010;152:1–17.

59. Keller MS, Fendya DG, Weber TR. Glasgow Coma Scale predicts coagulopathy in pediatric trauma patients. Semin Pediatr Surg 2001;10:12–6.

60. Swanson CA, Burns JC, Peterson BM. Low plasma D-dimer concentration predicts the absence of traumatic brain injury in children. J Trauma 2010;68:1072–7.

61. Cochran A, Scaife ER, Hansen KW, Downey EC. Hyperglycemia and outcomes from pediatric traumatic brain injury. J Trauma 2003;55:1035–8.

62. Melo JR, Di Rocco F, Blanot S, Laurent-Vannier A, Reis RC, Baugnon T, et al. Acute hyperglycemia is a reliable outcome predictor in children with severe traumatic brain injury. Acta Neurochir (Wien) 2010;152:1559–65.

31

Traumatic Brain Injury in Elderly

Sumit Sinha • Kanwaljeet Garg • AK Mahapatra

INTRODUCTION

The elderly population is defined as age greater than 65 years. They constitute rapidly growing population in the US and other developed nations.[1-4] Between 1900 and 1990, the number of people aged 65 and over in the US has increased by tenfold, from 3.1 to 31.1 million.[5] As the population continues to age, knowledge about TBI as an etiologic factor in cognitive impairment will become increasingly important. It remains unclear how the association between patients age and outcome after closed TBI can be described. However, in some studies researchers have treated outcome as a continuous function of age,[5] whereas others have identified age threshold values between 30 and 60 years.[3,6]

In a recent study dealing with geriatric patients with a mild head injury, 14% of patients had evidence of lesion on CT scans which required intervention in 20% of the patients.[7-9] Because research was unable to pinpoint useful clinical predictors of lesion formation, head CT scans are now recommended for all patients aged 65 and older presenting with neurological symptoms and signs or history of head trauma.[9] The financial and human costs of treating TBI in older adults are extensive. Various studies have reported higher mortality rates in range of 30–80% in elderly population compared to young patients.[10-12] Mortality rates in adults with severe TBI aged 55 and older range from 30 to 80%,[10] significantly higher than those reported in younger patients. One study[13] reported greater mortality rates from TBI beginning at age of 31 years, but the likelihood of death was maximal after 70 years of age. In a meta-analysis evaluating, the association between age and outcomes, another study[14] reported an optimal change point for mortality at age 60. Majority of elderly population having associated co-morbidities is high, which influence the outcome after TBI.[13,14]

In the United States, 48% of community-dwelling adults aged 65 and older have arthritis, 36% have hypertension, 27% have coronary disease, 10% have diabetes mellitus, and 6% have a cerebrovascular accidents.[15,16] One study[17] found that 73% of elderly TBI patients had medical conditions before injury, compared with 28% of younger adults. This significant increase in comorbidity may be important in primary and secondary prevention efforts. The relative risk of fall in older adults with diabetes mellitus is 1.97, compared with those without diabetes mellitus.[18] Because falls are the primary mechanism of injury in TBI in older adults, this population may be appropriate target for primary prevention strategies.

Incidence

Traumatic brain injury (TBI) is a major health and socioeconomic problem throughout the

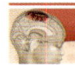

world and is a leading cause of death and disability. Traumatic brain injury is most common among younger age group and much of the literature on TBI has focused on this age group. However, the elderly are also at increased risk. Following a period of relatively, low risk in the middle adult year risk for TBI increases substantially in 6–7th decade with unintentional falls being a common cause.[1] According to the Ontario Trauma Registry Report, for 1996/1997[2], 41% of all hospital injury admissions occurred in the > 65 years age group, with 86% of these due to unintentional falls. Among these patients, head injury was 3rd most common type of injury. Motor vehicle accidents are another particularly common cause of this injury in this age group. Dementia and cognitive decline in the elderly age group may be important predisposing factors to both falls[3] and motor vehicle accidents.[4] Conversely, there are data suggesting that TBI in elderly is associated with adverse cognitive sequelae, including dementia.

Factors for High Incidence

The elderly population pose some inherent factors which place them at risk for greater incidence of poor outcome after TBI. First, in elderly the dura is more adherent to the skull. Second, as part of routine management of chronic cardiovascular and cerebrovascular conditions, majority of older adults receive aspirin and other anticoagulant therapies. Thus, the mechanisms of injury most likely to be seen in elderly persons (e.g. fall, motor vehicle accident) increase the risk for poor outcome after TBI. Other normal aging changes include cerebrovascular, atherosclerosis and decreased free radical clearance.[19] The former could increase the risk of injury or cause a secondary insult, and the latter may increase oxidative damage after a TBI.[20] Moderate cerebral atrophy may be present in some older adults, which can cause occult findings to be present on head computed tomography (CT), despite of an initial intact neurological examination.[19]

PATHOPHYSIOLOGY

It is still not very clear whether the current published guidelines for the management of TBI are adequate for older adults with TBI and in elderly with comorbid health conditions. No study has yet identified whether the current cerebral perfusion pressure (CPP) guidelines are appropriate for management of the older adult with a TBI. Current guidelines recommend maintaining CPP at a minimum of 60 mm Hg.[21] CPP is defined as mean arterial blood pressure minus intracranial pressure. After severe TBI, cerebral autoregulation is altered. However, little is known about the response of older brain to injury. A single study completed in healthy middle-aged and older adults (mean age 54 ± 8) found no change in dynamic cerebral autoregulation, under the normal conditions.[22] In older adults, the several age-specific factors contribute to making cerebral autoregulation CPP in TBI a complex issue, that requires further investigation, within this population. First, there is a high incidence of comorbid conditions, including hypertension and diabetes mellitus, which could affect the responsiveness and perfusion needs of the cerebral vasculature. Secondly, because of the normal systemic changes attributable to aging, the ability of the cardiovascular system to respond to shock is impaired in older adults.[20] Lastly, this ability may be further compromised by medicines taken by many elderly patients, such as beta blockers and antiplatelet agents, which could affect cerebrovascular response to injury.

Clinical Features

Older age has long been recognized as an independent predictor of worse outcome from TBI.[23–25] The mechanism by which this occurs remains unknown. Although a single study has reported that adults aged 60 and older who suffered mild TBI had significantly better functioning ($p < .05$) at 1 month postinjury on the Glasgow Outcome Scale (GOS) than younger persons with mild TBI, significance was not maintained when employment status was controlled for.[26] In studies those have examined disability after TBI, there is evidence to suggest that elderly adult TBI survivors have greater dependence than younger survivors, using global outcome measures, including the GOS[26, 27] and the functional independence measure (FIM).[11] In addition, older adults with TBI have longer lengths of stay[26] and are more likely to have delayed neurological decline.[28, 29] As a result of the longer hospital stays, the cost of their care is significantly greater. These longer stays occur despite lower injury severity scores and higher mean GCS scores than those of their younger counterparts. Once admitted to inpatient rehabilitation facilities. Older patients with TBI require longer hospital stay, resulting in greater costs.[30, 31] Additional understanding of the outcomes in older patients with TBI has been gleaned from the trauma literature. For any given injury, older trauma patients required more medical and subspecialty consultations and had more complications than their younger injured counterparts while hospitalized.[31] Various currently available outcome studies, in elderly population with TBI, focus on early outcome time points (e.g. discharge). However, since the elderly demonstrate slower rates of functional improvement during recovery from TBI,[30] hence this factor should be an important consideration in future interventions and study designs.

Outcome

With regards to global outcome post-TBI, the results of studies looking at the effect of age are inconclusive. Some studies have shown that recovery is worse for older patient compared to younger counterpart as measured by the Glasgow Outcome Scale (GOS) [32] both at discharge from hospital[33–35] and several months post-injury.[36–38] Reeder et al[39], however, found that amount of improvement during in-patient rehabilitation was not associated with age when controlling for injury severity, injury etiology and demographic variables. More recently, Mosenthal et

al[17] found no difference in acute care discharge GOS between young and elderly patients with isolated TBI. Rapoport[26] found that elderly patients with mild TBI showed better GOS scores compared to younger patients and that they reported less psychosocial impairment, less psychological distress and less physical symptoms than younger patients 1 month post-trauma. More consistent results are found in studies comparing functional outcome in younger and older patients with TBI. Some studies have shown that scores on the Rancho Los Amigos Scale (RLAS)[40] were significantly higher upon discharge from rehabilitation for younger patients with TBI.[41] The FIMTM[42] rating and the Disability Rating Scale (DRS) score upon admission to and discharge from rehabilitation were also found to be significantly higher for the younger patients in a study using data from the TBI Model Systems (TBIMS).[30] Other researchers have also shown a statistically significant difference favoring younger patients compared to older on a modified FIMTM measure including scores for locomotion, feeding and expression upon discharge from acute care[11,17] and 6 months post-trauma.[17]

In the area of cognitive outcome, it has been clearly shown in several studies that the elderly present decreased cognitive functioning following mild and moderate TBI.[6,43,44] Moreover, Aharon-Peretz et al[45] found poorer cognitive functioning in a group of elderly patients with TBI compared to a normal control group from the community but no significant difference between patients with TBI and orthopedic control patients. Very little information, however, is found in the literature comparing cognitive functioning between the young and elderly patients with TBI. One study found poorer cognitive functioning in older subjects having suffered mild-to-moderate TBI, when compared to a younger group and community age-matched controls, but the time post-injury was very broad, ranging from 2 to 63 years.[46]

Studies comparing the elderly and the young on length of stay (LOS) in the hospital and the services required after TBI have also been reported in the literature. Some earlier studies have shown an increased length of hospitalization for the older patient with TBI.[47] More recent research, however, showed no difference in acute care stay for older patients[17,30] but significantly longer LOS in rehabilitation for the elderly compared to those younger than age 55.[30,42,45] It has also been shown that significantly more elderly patients are more likely to require increased family involvement and use of community support services[48] or require a change of domicile[47,48] including need for a nursing home.[33] Moreover, Testa et al[48] found that patients over the age of 50 years are less likely to return to work post-TBI compared to those subjects younger than 50. An initial study from rehabilitation centers found no significant difference in the number of younger and older patients with TBI discharged to the community post-rehabilitation.[42] A recent follow-up to this research, which included a larger number of subjects showed that significantly more patients' older than 55 years were discharged to a skilled nursing facility or another hospital compared to younger group post-rehabilitation.

The review of the literature reveals that most studies on outcome in the elderly patients with TBI have been carried out post-rehabilitation. However, some data are available on global outcome at the time of discharge but very little information exists regarding the effect of age on functional outcome upon discharge from acute care and according to severity of TBI. Furthermore, studies of differences in functional and cognitive performance between younger and older patients with TBI are lacking. This is extremely important from a clinical point of view, as this information help to guide the treating team in determining the prognosis and in order to better respond to elderly population's particular needs for early rehabilitation programming as well as rehabilitation and placement services post-acute care.

CONCLUSIONS

Head injury in elderly is important because of various factors. Lack of cerebral compliance, defective cerebral autoregulation, and co-morbid factors add to the problems and further reduce the chance of good or functional outcome. These patients need careful monitoring and meticulous care. The hospital stay is longer and overall outcome is much poorer than younger adults. Proper and planned cognitive and physical rehabilitation can help in early and satisfactory recovery.

REFERENCES

1. Fields RB, Coffey CE. Traumatic brain injury. In: CE coffey and JL. cumming (eds). Textbook of Geriatric Neuropsychiatry (Washington, DC: American Psychiatric Press) 1994;479–508.
2. Canadian Institute For Health Information: Ontario Trauma Registry Report. Hospital injury admissions 1996/97 (Ottawa, Ontario), 1998.
3. Tinetti ME, Doucette JT, Claus EB. The contribution of predisposing and situational risk factors to serious fall injuries. J Am Geriatr Soc 1995;43:1207–13.
4. O'neill D, Neubauer K, Boyle M. et al. Dementia and driving. JR Soc. Med. 1992;85:199–202.
5. Tauber C: Sixty-five plus in America. US Bureau of the Census, Current Population Reports, Special Studies (Washington, DC, US Government Printing Office), 1992;23–178.
6. Goldstein FC, Levin HS, Goldman, et al. Cognitive and behavioral sequelae of closed head injury in older adults according to their significant others. J Neuropsychiatry Clin Neurosci 1999;11:38–44.
7. Agency for Healthcare Quality and Research [on-line]. H-CUPnet, Healthcare cost and utilization project. [May 1, 2006]. Available at www.ahrq.gov/HCUPnet.
8. Shinoda-Tagawa T, Clark DE. Trends in hospitalization after injury: Older women are displacing young men. Inj Prev 2003;9:214–19.
9. Mack LR, Chan SB, Silva JC, Hogan TM. The use of head computed tomography in elderly patients sustaining minor head trauma. J Emerg Med 2003;24:157–62.
10. Rozzelle CJ, Wofford JL, Branch CL. Predictors of hospital mortality in older patients with subduralhematoma. J Am Geriatr Soc 1995;43: 240–4.

11. Susman M, DiRusso SM, Sullivan T, et al. Traumatic brain injury in the elderly: Increased mortality and worse functional outcome at discharge despite lower injury severity. J Trauma 2002;53:219–23.

12. Kotwica Z, Jakubowski JK. Acute head injuries in the elderly.An analysis of 136 consecutive patients. Acta Neurochir (Wien) 1992;118:98–102.

13. Harris C, DiRusso S, Sullivan T, Benzil DL. Mortality risk after head injury increases at 30 years. J Am Coll Surg 2003;197:711–6.

14. Hukkelhoven CW, Steyerberg EW, Rampen AJ, et al. Patient age and outcome following severe traumatic brain injury: An analysis of 5,600 patients. J Neurosurg 2003;99:666–73.

15. Hoffman C, Rice D, Sung HY. Persons with chronic conditions.Their prevalence and costs. JAMA 1996;276:1473–9.

16. Adams PF, Hendershot GE, Marano MA. Current estimates from the National Health Interview Survey, 1996. Vital Health Stat 10 1999;1–203.

17. Mosenthal AC, Livingston DH, Lavery RF, et al. The effect of age on functional outcome in mild traumatic brain injury: 6-month report of a prospective multicenter trial. J Trauma 2004;56:1042–8.

18. Kennedy RL, Henry J, Chapman AJ, et al. Accidents in patients with insulin-treated diabetes: Increased risk of low-impact falls but not motor vehicle crashes—a prospective register-based study. J Trauma 2002;52:660–6.

19. Timiras P. The nervous system: Structural and biochemical changes. In: Timiras P, (ed). Physiological Basis of Aging and Geriatrics. 3rd edn. CRC Press; Boca Raton, FL: 2003;99–118.

20. Thompson HJ, Bourbonniere M. Elderly trauma from head to toe. Crit Care Nurs Clin North Am. 2006;18:419–31.

21. Guidelines for the Management of Severe Brain Injury: Guidelines for the management of severe traumatic brain injury. Brain Trauma Foundation, American Association of Neurological Surgeons, Congress of Neurological Surgeons. J Neurotrauma 2007; 24 Suppl 1:S1–106.

22. Yam AT, Lang EW, Lagopoulos J, et al. Cerebral autoregulation and ageing. J Clin Neurosci 2005; 12:643–6.

23. Hukkelhoven CW, Steyerberg EW, Rampen AJ, et al. Patient age and outcome following severe traumatic brain injury: An analysis of 5,600 patients. J Neurosurg 2003;99:666–73.

24. Coronado VG, Thomas KE, Sattin RW, et al. The CDC traumatic brain injury surveillance system: Characteristics of persons aged 65 years and older hospitalized with a TBI. J Head Trauma Rehabil 2005;20:215–28.

25. Czosnyka M, Balestreri M, Steiner L, et al. Age, intracranial pressure, autoregulation, and outcome after brain trauma. J Neurosurg 2005;102:450–4.

26. Rapoport MJ, Feinstein A. Age and functioning after mild traumatic brain injury: The acute picture. Brain Inj 2001;15:857–64.

27. Miller JD, Pentland B. Head injuries in elderly patients. Neurosurg Rev 1989;1 (Suppl 12): 441–5.

28. Pennings JL, Bachulis BL, Simons CT, et al. Survival after severe brain injury in the aged. Arch Surg1993;128:787–93.

29. Luukinen H, Viramo P, Koski K, et al. Head injuries and cognitive decline among older adults: A population-based study. Neurology 1999;52:557–62.

30. Frankel JE, Marwitz JH, Cifu DX, et al. A follow-up study of older adults with traumatic brain injury: Taking into account decreasing length of stay. Arch Phys Med Rehabil 2006;87:57–62.

31. Mc Kevitt EC, Calvert E, Ng A, et al. Geriatric trauma: Resource use and patient outcomes. Can J Surg 2003;46:211–5.

32. Jennett B, Bond M. Assessment of outcome after severe brain damage, a practical scale. Lancet 1975;1(7905):480–4.

33. Mosenthal AC, Lavery RF, Addis M, Kaul S, Ross S, Marburger R, Deitch DA, Livingston DH. Isolated traumatic brain injury: Age is an independent predictor of mortality and early outcome. J Trauma 2002;52:907–11.

34. Vollmer DG, Torner J, Jane JA, Eisenberg HM, Foulkes MA, Marmarou A, Marshall LF. Age and outcome following traumatic coma: Why do older patients fare worse? J Neurosurg 1991;75: S37–49.

35. Hukkelhoven CWPM, Steyerberg EW, Rampen AJJ, Farace E, Habbema JDF, Marshall LF, Murray GD, Maas AIR. Patient age and outcome following severe traumatic brain injury: An analysis of 5600 patients. J Neurosurg 2003;99: 66–73.

36. Gan BK, Lim JH, Ng IH. Outcome of moderate and severe traumatic brain injury amongst the elderly in Singapore. Ann Acad Med, Singapore 2004;33:63–7.

37. Rothweiler B, Temkin NR, Dikmen SS. Aging effect on psychosocial outcome in traumatic brain injury. Arch Phys Med Rehabil 1998;79:881–7.

38. Kilaru S, Garb J, Emhoff T, Fiallo V, Simon B, Swiencicki T, Lee KF. Long-term functional status and mortality of elderly patients with severe closed head injuries. J Trauma 1996;41:957–63.

39. Reeder KP, Rosenthal M, Lichtenberg P, Wood D. Impact of age on functional outcome following traumatic brain injury. J Head Trauma Rehabil 1996;11:22–31.

40. Malkmus D, Booth BJ, Kodimer C. Rehabilitation of the Head Injured Adult: Comprehensive Cognitive Management. Downey CA: Professional Staff Association of Rancho Los Amigos Hospital, Inc., 1989.

41. Cifu DX, Kreutzer JS, Marwitz JH, Rosenthal M, Englander J, High W. Functional outcomes of older adults with traumatic brain injury: A prospective multicentre analysis. Arch Phys Med Rehabil 1996;77:883–8.

42. Granger CV, Cotter AC, Hamilton BB, Fielder RC. Functional assessment scales: A study of persons with multiple sclerosis. Arch Phys Med Rehabil 1990;71:870–5.

43. Goldstein FC, Levin HS, Presley JS, Colohan ART, Eisenberg HM, Jann B, Bertolino-Kusnerik L. Neurobehavioural consequences of closed head injury in older adults. J Neurol Neurosurg Psychiatry 1994;57:961–6.

44. Aharon-Peretz J, Kliot D, Amyel-Zvi E, Tomer R, Rakier A, Feinsod M. Neurobehavioural consequences of closed head injury in the elderly. Brain Inj 1997;11:871–5.

45. Klein M, Houx PJ, Jolles J. Long-term persisting cognitive sequelae of traumatic brain injury and the effect of age. J Nerv Ment Dis 1996;184:459–67.

46. Roy CW, Pentland B, Douglas Miller J. The causes and consequences of minor head injury in the elderly. Injury 1986;17:220–3.

47. Wilson JA, Pentland B, Currie C, Douglas Miller J. The functional effects of head injury in the elderly. Brain Inj 1987;1:183–8.

48. Testa JA, Malec JF, Moessner AM, Brown AW. Outcome after traumatic brain injury: Effects of aging on recovery. Archives of Physical Medicine and Rehabilitation 2005;86:1815–23.

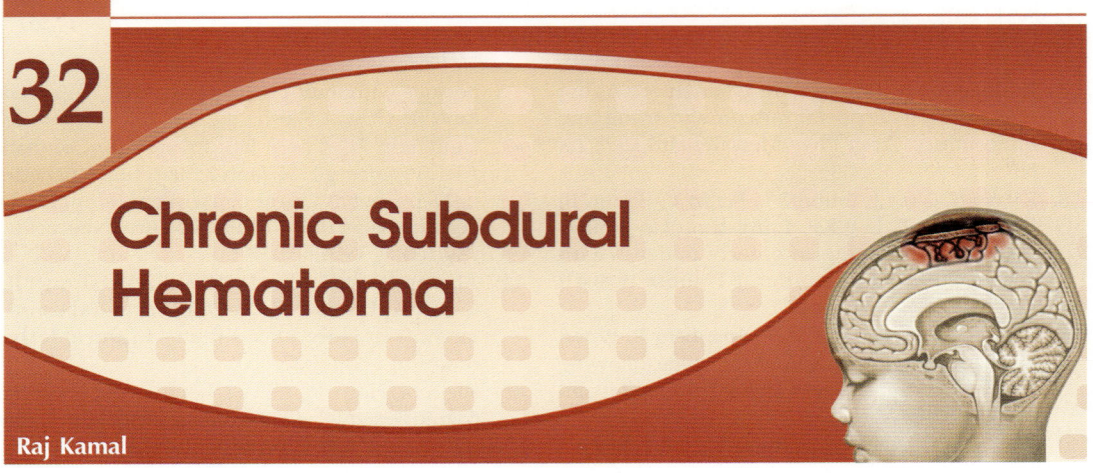

32

Chronic Subdural Hematoma

Raj Kamal

INTRODUCTION

A subdural hematoma (SDH) is a collection of blood below the inner layer of the dura but external to the brain and arachnoid membrane. **Chronic subdural hematomas** are usually 3 week or older and are hypodense compared with the brain. However, subdural hematomas may be mixed in nature, such as when acute bleeding has occurred into a chronic subdural hematoma. Subdural hematoma develops when the tiny veins that run between the dura and surface of the brain (bridging veins) tear and leak blood. This is usually the result of a mild head injury.

A subdural hematoma is more common in the elderly because of normal brain shrinkage that occurs with aging. This shrinkage stretches and weakens the bridging veins. These veins are more likely to break in the elderly, even after a minor head injury. Most of the times family members may not remember any injury that could explain it.

According to the time of onset of symptoms after the injury the subdural hematoma is classified into 3 types: **Acute, subacute and chronic.**

Acute   : within 48 to 72 hours.
Subacute : 3 to 20 days.
Chronic   : >3 weeks to several months.

Into last group are placed the cases in which either no history of trauma or the trauma described is of such trivial nature that its relationship to trauma is doubtful. About 20 to 30% of cases have no history of trauma. The incidence of chronic subdural hematoma is 1 to 2 per 100,000 people per year.[1] Most patients are 50 years of age or older.

PATHOGENESIS AND PATHOLOGY

Chronic subdural hematoma is seen in elderly patients in whom **cerebral atrophy causes widening of the subdural space thus exposing the bridging veins to a greater risk of rupture when subjected to angular shearing forces.**[2,3]

Oozing of blood is usually gradual and spreads over a large area of the surface of the brain and may extend in the interhemispheric fissure along the falx cerebri. Several hundred milliliters of blood may accumulate gradually in this space without causing symptoms. **Subdural hematomas evoke a peculiar reaction largely derived from the inner surface of the dura and results in granulation tissue, referred to as "neomembrane,"** that encircle the hematoma.[4] The neomembrane facing the dura is called outer membrane and that facing the surface of brain is called inner membrane. **The outer membrane is thick and highly vascular whereas inner membrane is thin, relatively avascular and sometimes adherent to the arachnoid.** Formation of outer membrane begins as thin membrane and by 4 weeks it becomes thick and vascular.

According to Yamashima[5] (Fig. 32.1a), there is a dura-arachnoid interface layer, which is structurally the weakest throughout the meninges. An extravasation of blood within the dural border layer splits it, leaving a few tiers of dural border cells over the arachnoid. These cells cover the internal surface of the hematoma, proliferate and later on, form the inner membrane. The outer membrane is related to hematoma enlargement because of the repetitive hemorrhages whereas the inner membrane is related to liquefaction of the subdural hematoma. As the inner membrane plays a pivotal role in the pathophysiogenesis and determination of the location of chronic subdural hematoma, histologic, ultrastructural and clinical analyses were performed with correlations to the dura-arachnoid interface and the so-called "subdural space."

When the veins that bridge the subdural space are excessively stretched, they rupture, and venous blood escapes into the subdural space. Yamashima and Friede[7] examined cerebral bridging veins by electron microscopy and emphasized their fragility in their subdural portions. Some authorities deny that such a space exists and propose instead a space opened within the dural border cell layer.[6,7]

Although some subdural clots reabsorb spontaneously, the encapsulated fluid may slowly increase in volume, creating a chronic subdural hematoma. The lack of counter-pressure in predisposed patients may permit growth of a small hematoma that might otherwise resolve spontaneously.[8–10]

Another mechanism for subdural hematoma growth is recurrent bleeding from the hematoma capsule.[11] Chronic subdural hematomas are a local inflammatory process that causes the formation of a granulation tissue often referred to as the external or outer membrane.[5, 6, 12] This membrane has abnormally permeable macrocapillaries. Exudation from

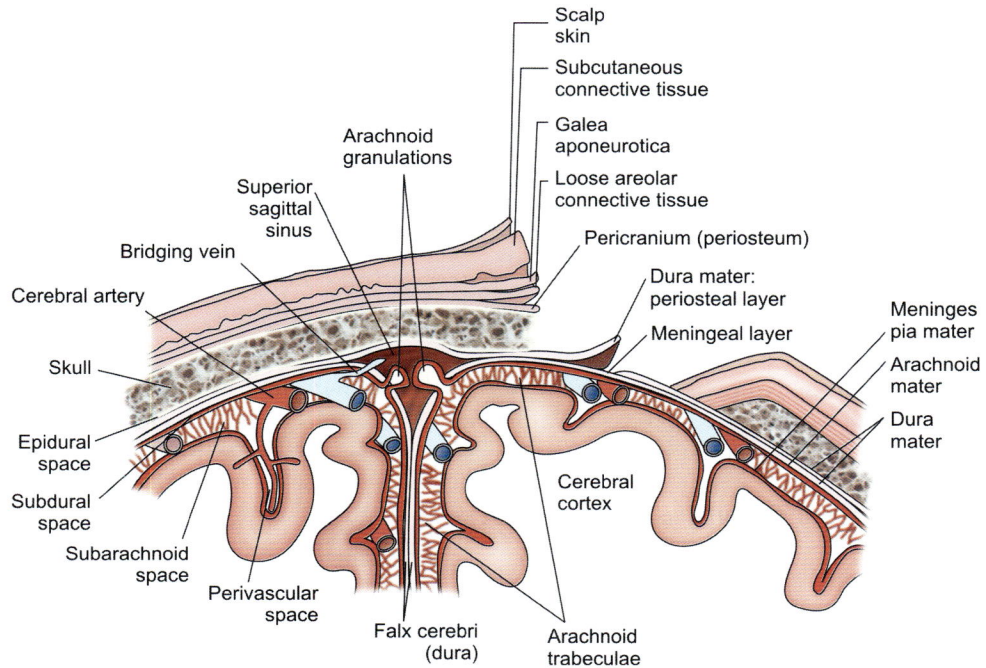

Fig. 32.1a: Anatomy of subdural space

the macrocapillaries in the outer membrane plays an important role in the enlargement of hematoma.[13]

Initially a fibrin layer forms around the periphery of the clot on the dural but not the arachnoid side, this is invaded by fibroblasts and blood vessels. The outer membrane, which looks more like pigmented dura with the passage of time, is continuous with the much thinner inner membrane in which a thin layer of fibroblasts appears, presumably by migration from the edges of the outer layer.

The subdural blood clot liquefies in the center with passage of time and is resorbed. The capillaries of the neomembrane are abnormal and friable.[5,6]

Progressive enlargement of hematoma occurs due to repeated microhemorrhages from the friable capillaries of the neomembranes[2, 14]

Repeated microhemorrhages cause the enlargement of the chronic subdural hematoma by directly increasing the volume of the clot and resupplying substrates for coagulation and fibrinolysis.[15–17] Another postulation for the enlargement of a chronic SDH is that the outer and inner membrane acts as an osmotic membrane, imbibing cerebrospinal fluid into the hematoma thus increasing its volume.[18] Sometimes the loculated fluid is totally absorbed and the two membranes fuse.

Bilateral subdural hematomas, more common in children, may impede the free flow of CSF in the subarachnoid space and can cause hydrocephalus and dementia.[2]

Sources of non-traumatic, so-called spontaneous chronic subdural hematomas are convexity angiomas, aneurysms and other cerebral vascular disorders such as inflammations, thrombosis and hemorrhagic diasthesis.

Factors which can predispose to chronic subdural hematomas
1. Low intracranial pressure
2. Cerebral atrophy
3. All coagulopathies
4. Anticoagulants.

Low intracranial pressure can occur following overdrainage of CSF following VP shunt, dehydration and spinal anesthesia. Due to decrease in cerebral volume, tangential movements occur easily, predisposing rupture of bridging veins. Also because of reduced pressure hemorrhages are not immediately stopped.

Alcoholics are also more prone to develop chronic subdural hematoma due to higher rate of accident than general population, secondary coagulation disturbances and/or generalized vascular fragility as a result of avitaminosis.

Clinical Manifestations

The most frequent presenting symptoms are **headache, drowsiness, gait abnormalities and hemiparesis.** Headache occurs in 30–90% of patients.[19, 20] At times, the headache is described as mild and generalized. Altered mental status is a frequent complaint. Although this may manifest as mild confusion or dementia, the changes may be more profound and the patient may have a markedly decreased level of consciousness or may even be obtunded. Mental status changes are probably responsible for the labeling of many patients with chronic subdural hematomas as suffering from psychiatric disease. Hemiparesis is also a common presenting complaint and the neurologic dysfunction is usually contralateral to the hematoma.

Chronic subdural hematoma patients may have suffered a significant head injury. However, in approximately one-third of patients there is no definite history of preceding head injury.

The incidence of chronic subdural hematoma increases steadily and more rapidly approaching the 60–70 age group. Chronic SDH shows male predominence. The symptoms and signs are given in Table 32.1.[19]

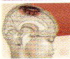

Table 32.1: Manifestations of chronic subdural hematoma in 194 patients [Luxon and Harrison][19]

	Initial symptom		Symptom present	
	N	%	N	%
Headache	125	64	149	77
Mental change	23	12	97	50
Limb symptoms	11	6	69	36
Loss of consciousness or epilepsy	11	6	33	17
Drowsiness	8	4	102	53
Fluctuation in symptoms	–	–	21	11
Vomiting	–	–	68	35
Hemiparesis	–	–	113	58
Papilledema	–	–	66	34
Neck stiffness	–	–	27	14
Hemianopsia	–	–	21	11
Dysphasia	–	–	38	20

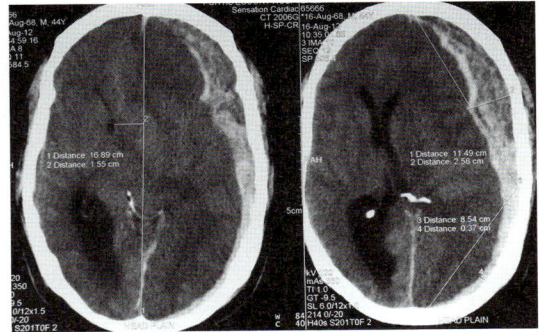

Fig. 32.1b: Chronic subdural hematoma. CT scan showing hyperdense cellular component occupying the dependent part and significant midline shift with contralateral dilated ventricles

INVESTIGATION

CT is the investigation of choice for evaluation of chronic subdural hematoma. A chronic subdural hematoma is hyperdense in first week after injury. It becomes isodense in about ten days to 2 weeks and thus could be overlooked on the CT scan examination. After 3 weeks, chronic subdural hematoma usually appears hypodense or relatively hyperdense on CT (Fig. 32.1b). It is often difficult to distinguish isodense chronic SDH from cerebral parenchyma. Isodense subdural hematoma displaces surface sulci of the brain away from inner table. They have been often misdiagnosed as cerebral swelling or tumor. Chances of missing bilateral isodense subdural hematoma is still higher.

Large chronic subdural hematomas resulting in subfalcine and transtentorial herniations. Associated subfalcine and transtentorial herniation can be diagnosed very well on CT scan (Figs 32.1b) and MRI (Fig. 32.4).

Subacute subdural hematoma (1–2 weeks) have high signal on both T_1- and T_2-weighted images due to presence of extracellular methemoglobin.

Chronic subdural hematomas may be hyperintense relative to brain and CSF in both short TR and long TR images due to presence of extracellular methemoglobin.

MRI can also demonstrate acute hemorrhage within chronic SDH. **MRI is more sensitive than CT in identifying isodense SDH.** Subacute subdural hematomas are bright on T_1-weighted images (hyperintense) and relatively dark (hypointense) on T_2-weighted images (Figs 32.2, 32.3a and b). MRI is often the most informative and precise study.[21] MRI signal intensity may vary with time, but chronic subdural hematomas are generally hyperintense on both T_1- and T_2-weighted scans. Rarely, a chronic subdural hematoma is isointense on T1 images due to methemoglobin, which is related to the age of the extravasated blood. Often, on either CT or MRI, one sees a subdural hematoma that is heterogeneous or with layering of blood; these types are secondary to mixing of fresh blood (from intermittent hemorrhages from the external membrane) with the chronic subdural fluid. On T_2-weighted MRI scans, a black band is frequently observed on the inner membrane of symptomatic chronic subdural hematomas.[22]

Treatment. Chronic subdural hematomas have been evacuated by craniotomies, burr holes and twist-drill craniotomies, each procedure having its advocates. Surgical

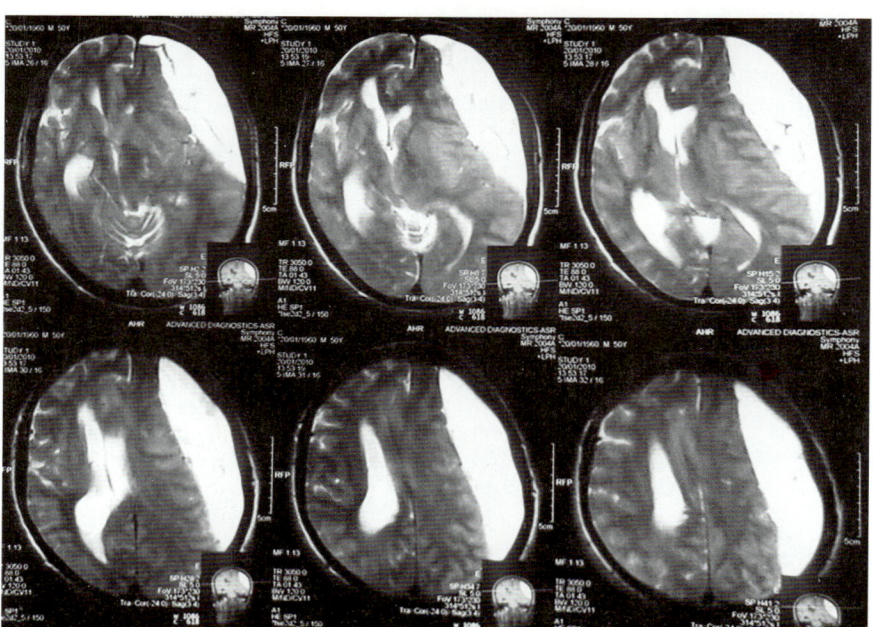

Fig. 32.2: Chronic subdural hematoma: MRI showing bright signal on T_2-weighted images

intervention causes decreased fibrinolytic and increased coagulant activity in the hematoma fluid.[23] The role of corticosteroids in the management of chronic subdural hematomas is not well defined. Current evidence neither supports nor refutes the use of corticosteroids. A randomized controlled trial is warranted.[24] Recent data suggested that in surgical treatment of chronic subdural hematoma with burr hole craniostomy, extended preoperative corticosteroid administration is associated with a lower recurrence rate.[25]

Hematoma drainage and irrigation through multiple burr holes, is usually effective in reducing their size and in speeding their reabsorption. Burr hole location is guided by hematoma size and shape. The patient is positioned on the operating table with the affected side up (for bilateral hematomas, both sides of the head are draped and the larger hematoma drained first). Two burr holes suffice in most cases; frontal and parietal placement at the anterior and posterior margins of the collection usually works well.

The dura over the anterior burr hole is opened first to prevent premature collapse of the subdural space. On opening the dura, a thick outer hematoma membrane is encountered. The composition of the hematoma varies with the age of the blood, from fresh clot to thin xanthochromic fluid.

The following treatment modalities are available for chronic subdural hematoma.
1. **Medical management—bedrest,** osmotic diuretics, corticosteroids.
2. **Surgical management**
   a. Twist drill craniostomy
   b. Burr holes
   c. Craniotomy.

1. Medical Management

Suzuki and Takakua[26] treated 23 chronic subdural hematoma patients with 20% mannitol, 500–1000 ml daily. The average duration of treatment was 31 days. Most of their patients became asymptomatic within 1–2 months from the beginning of treatment.

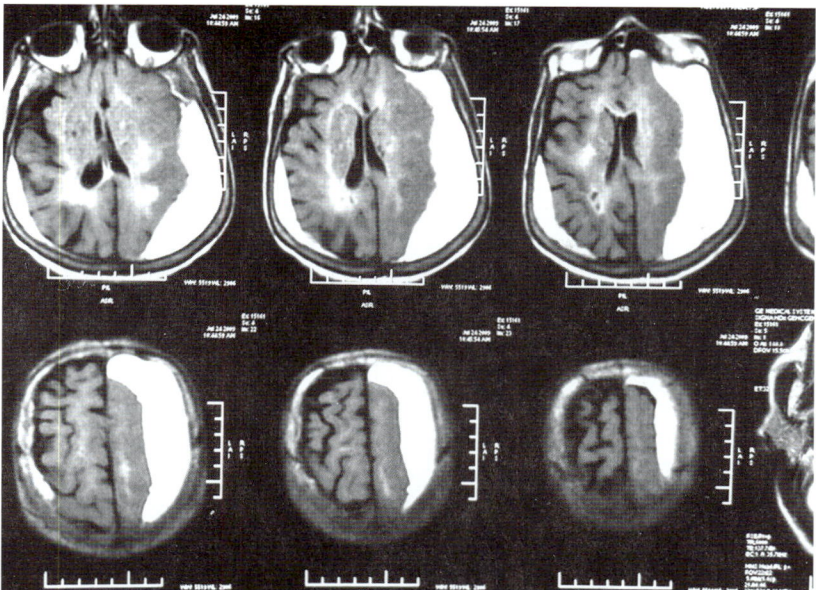

Fig. 32.3a: Chronic subdural hematoma: MRI showing bright signal on T_1-weighted images

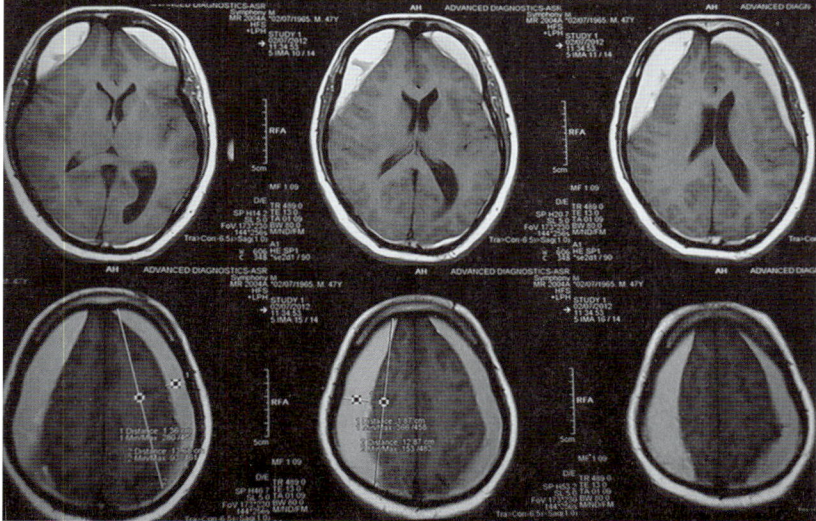

Fig. 32.3b: MRI showing bilateral chronic subdural hematoma, hyperintense on T_1-weighted images

Unfortunately, these good results could not be verified in a control series by Gjerris and Schmidt[27] in which mannitol regime failed in first seven patients and the study has to be abandoned.

Conservative treatment may be tried in patients with minimal neurological signs and small chronic subdural hematoma found incidently or those who refuse surgery. In these cases, ultimately surgery may be

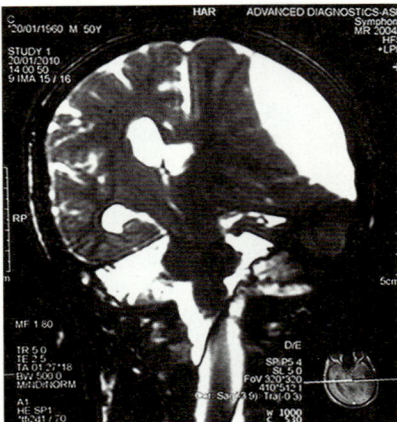

Fig. 32.4: MRI brain (coronal) T$_2$-weighted image showing large left chronic SDH with transtentorial herniation

required. Conservative treatment alone either is not effective or requires very long hospitalization.

Twist Drill/Burr Hole Craniotomy

This procedure is performed under local anesthesia. Complete head shaving is mandatory for twist drill aspiration. Head is prepared meticulously with povidone iodine after cleaning with savlon. About 1 cm long incision is placed 3 cm away from midline and anterior to coronal suture or should be placed adjacent to the thickest part of subdural hematoma as determined by the CT scan. The twist drill hole should be placed accordingly. The direction of twist should be posteriorly and inferiorly usually making an angle of 45° to the perpendicular.

The drainage of chronic subdural hematoma should be slow and controlled otherwise intracerebral hemorrhage may occur following rapid decompression. A catheter may be passed into subdural space and connected to closed sterile drainage system.

Burr holes: Two burr holes (Fig. 32.5) are usually placed under local anesthesia after preparing the head as described for twist drill aspiration. If the collection extends down into the temporal fossa, a third burr hole is also advisable.

Burr holes are guided by the site and size of chronic SDH on CT scan. Posterior burr hole is placed just posterior to the thickest portion of hematoma, which is parietal eminence in most cases. The anterior frontal burr hole is placed anterior to the coronal suture 3 cm lateral to the midline (Fig. 32.5).

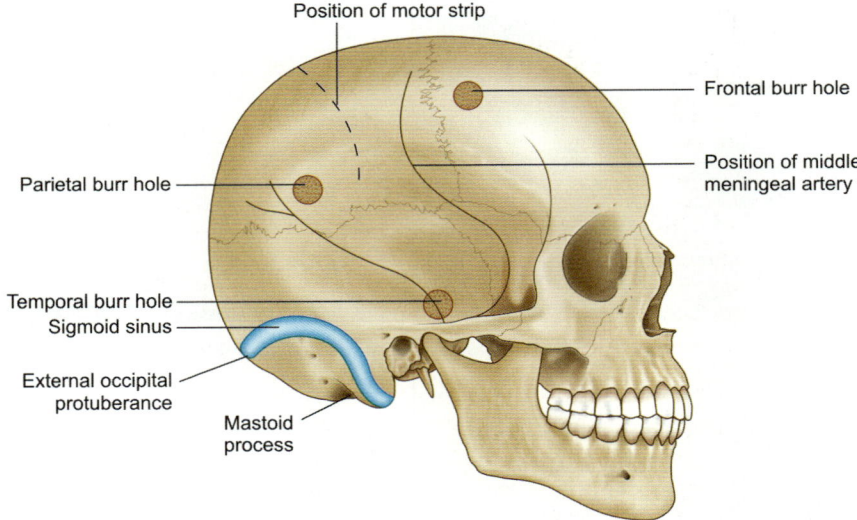

Fig. 32.5: Burr hole position in relation to middle meningeal artery

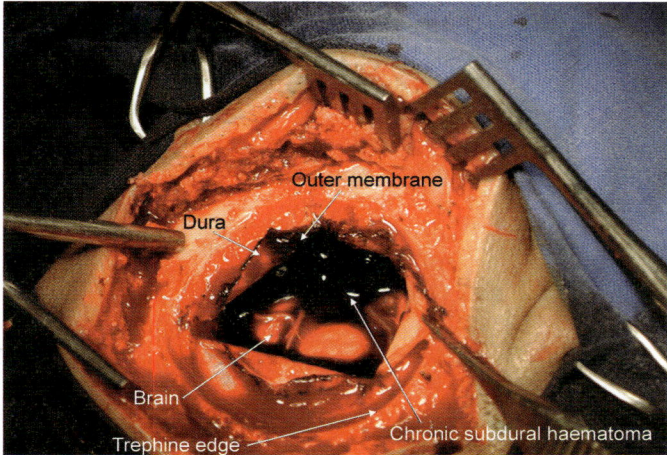

Fig. 32.6: Peroperative photograph of draining chronic SDH through trephine

The dura over the anterior burr hole is opened first to prevent premature collapse of the subdural space. On opening the dura, a thick outer hematoma membrane is encountered (Fig. 32.6). The composition of the hematoma varies with the age of the blood, from fresh clot to thin xanthochromic fluid. In most cases the hematoma has an intermediate appearance and has been described as resembling crankcase oil. If intracranial pressure is high, considerable fluid leakage will occur, and the brain often re-expands. Irrigation is recommended for the residual fluid; catheters with multiple fenestrations are gently threaded into the subdural spaces and irrigated by gravity until the return is clear. Failure of the irrigating solution to communicate between burr holes suggests interposed solid clot or fibrous septations. Dura is incised in cruciate manner identifying outer membrane (Fig. 32.6). Outer membrane is incised separately with slow and controlled drainage of hematoma. The second burr hole is made to facilitate irrigation with isotonic saline. A drain can be placed in the subdural space postoperatively for 24–48 hours for drainage of residual hematoma. Care should be taken while inserting pediatic feeding tube inside subdural space, drain-tip should be soft and directed over the convexity of the brain.

The proximal end of drain should be taken out from separate incision. Drain is not necessary if the brain expands adequately after the drainage of subdural hematoma. If brain fails to expand following evacuation of chronic subdural hematoma then measures recommended by various authors are:

Lumbar puncture and intrathecal infusion of 40–300 ml isotonic or ringer lactate solution. Favorable results saline shown by La Londe and Gardner,[28] Cameron,[29] Grisoli et al.[30]

Craniotomies for chronic subdural hematoma evacuation and removal (stripping) of the subdural membranes were advocated to prevent hematoma recurrence.[35] However, the effectiveness of this technique has been challenged; it is sometimes used as a primary surgical therapy but is reserved for recurrences or cases with considerable fresh clot or multiple loculations.[36, 37]

Complications

1. *Recurrence:* Twist drill 5–24%

   Burr hole 0–26%

2. Subdural empyema occurs in < 2%[29,30] of burr hole evacuation of chronic subdural hematoma

3. Intracerebral hemorrhage is 1–5%.[31, 32]

CONCLUSIONS

Chronic subdural hematoma is a common neurosurgical problem which produces symptoms from three weeks to several months after injury. Subacute subdural hematoma, produces symptoms, from 3 to 20 days. Most patients are over 50 years of age. History of trauma is absent in 25–50% of cases. Chronic alcoholism, brain atrophy, epilepsy, and coagulopathies are important precipitating factors.

Headache, altered sensorium are most common presenting symptoms. For evaluation, CT scan is investigation of choice. After three weeks, the vast majority of SDH will be **hypodense** and will assume lenticular appearance but because of recurrent bleeding from hematoma membranes, chronic SDH can also appear **hypo-** and **hyperdense.**

Isodense SDH on CT scan are easily diagnosed by MRI. For symptomatic chronic subdural hematoma treatment should be in favour of operation. Recurrence in chronic subdural hematoma is not uncommon.

REFERENCES

1. Fogdholm R, Waltimo O. Epidemiology of chronic subdural haematoma. Acta Neurochir (Wien) 1975;32:247–50.

2. Giuffre R. Physiopathogenesis of chronic subdural hematomas: A new look to an old problem. Riv Neurol 1987;5:298.

3. Yamashima T, Friede RL: Why do bridging veins rupture into the virtual subdural space? J Neurol neurosurg psychiatry 1984;47:121.

4. Powers JM, Horoupian. Central Nervous System. In Damjanov I, Linder J (eds.). Anderson's Pathology ed. 10 Mosby 1996;2693–793.

5. Yamashima T, Yamamoto S. How do vessels proliferate in the capsule of a chronic subdural hematoma? Neurosurgery 1984;15:672.

6. Yamashima T, Yamamoto S, Friede RL. The role of endothelial gap junctions in the enlargement of chronic subdural hematomas. J Neurosurg 1983;59:298.

7. Yamashima T. The inner membrane of chronic subdural hematomas: pathology and pathophysiology Neurosurg Clin N Am 2000;11(3):413–24.

8. Maurice-Williams RS. Chronic subdural hematoma: an everyday problem for the neurosurgeon. Br J Neurosurg 1999;13:547–9.

9. Lee KS, Bae WK, Doh JW, Bae HG, Yun IG. Origin of chronic subdural hematoma and relation to traumatic subdural lesions. Brain Inj 1998;12:901–10.

10. Lee KS, Bae WK, Park YT, Yun IG. The pathogenesis and fate of traumatic subdural hygroma. Br J Neurosurg 1994;8(5):551–8.

11. Ito H, Yamamoto S, Saito K, Ikeda K, Hisada K. Quantitative estimation of hemorrhage in chronic subdural hematoma using the 51Cr erythrocyte labeling method. J Neurosurg 1987;66:862–4.

12. Sato S, Suzuki J. Ultrastructural observations of the capsule of chronic subdural hematoma in various clinical stages. J Neurosurg 1977;47:311–5.

13. Tokmak M, Iplikcioglu AC, Bek S, Gokduman CA, Erdal M. The role of exudation in chronic subdural hematomas. J Neurosurg 2007;107(2):290–5.

14. Kawakami Y, Chikama M, et al. Coagulation and fibrinolysis in chronic subdural hematoma. Neurosurgery 1989;25:25.

15. Markwalder TM, Reulen HJ. Influence of neomembraneous organization, cortical expansion and subdural pressure on the postoperative course of chronic subdural hematoma, an analysis of 201 cases. Acta Neurochir (Wien) 1986;79:100.

16. Weir B. Oncotic pressure of subdural fluids. J Neurosurg 1980;53:512.

17. Ito H, Komai T, Yamamoto S. Fibrinolytic enzymes in the lining walls of chronic subdural hematoma. J Neurosurg 1980;48:197–200.

18. Zollinger R, Gross RE. Traumatic subdural hematoma: An explanation of the late onset of pressure symptoms. JAMA 1934;103:245–9.

19. Luxon LM, Harrison MJ. Chronic subdural hematoma. Q J Med 1979;48(189):43–53.

20. Mc Kissock W, Richardson A, Bloom WH. Subdural hematoma: A review of 389 cases. Lancet 1960;1:1365.

21. Williams VL, Hogg JP. Magnetic resonance imaging of chronic subdural hematoma. Neurosurg Clin N Am 2000;11:491–8.

22. Imaizumi T, Horita Y, Honma T, Niwa J. Association between a black band on the inner membrane of a chronic subdural hematoma on T_2-weighted magnetic resonance images and enlargement of the hematoma. J Neurosurg 2003;99(5):824–30.

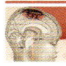

23. Matsumoto M, Sakata Y, Yamazaki T, Endo G, Ohishi H, Takasu N. Local coagulofibrinolysis in the postsurgical recovery of patients with chronic subdural hematoma. Acta Neurochir (Wien) 1999;141:177–81.

24. Zarkou S, Aguilar MI, Patel NP, et al. The role of corticosteroids in the management of chronic subdural hematomas: a critically appraised topic. Neurologist 2009;15(5):299–302.

25. Berghauser Pont LM, Dammers R, Schouten JW, et al. Clinical factors associated with outcome in chronic subdural hematoma: a retrospective cohort study of patients on pre-operative corticosteroid therapy. Neurosurgery 2012; 70(4):873–80.

26. Suzuki J, Takakua A. Non-surgical treatment of chronic subdural hematoma. J Neurosurg 1970;33:548.

27. Gjerris F, Schmidt K. Chronic subdural hematoma. Surgery or mannitol treatment, Neurosurg 1974;40:639.

28. La Londe AA, Gardner WJ. Chronic subdural hematoma. Expansion of compressed cerebral hemisphere and relief of hypotension by spinal injection of physiological saline solution. N. Eng. J. Med 1948;239:493.

29. Cameron MM. Chronic subdural hematoma: A review of 114 cases. J Neurol Neurosurg Psychiat 1978;41:834.

30. Grisoli F, Graziani N, et al. Perioperative lumbar injection of Ringer's lactate solution in chronic subdural hematomas: A series of 100 cases. Neurosurgery 1988;23:616.

31. D' Arella D, De Blasi F, et al. Intracerebral hematoma following evacuation of chronic subdural hematomas: Report of two cases. J Neurosurg 1986;65:710.

32. Modesti LM, Hodge CJ, et al. Intracerebral hematoma after evacuation of chronic extracerebral fluid collections. Neurosurgery 1982;1:689.

33. Killeffer JA, Killeffer FA, Schochet SS. The outer neomembrane of chronic subdural hematoma. Neurosurg Clin N Am 2000;11:407–12.

34. Haines DE, Harkey HL, Al-Mefty O. The "subdural" space: a new look at an outdated concept. Neurosurgery 1993;32:111–20.

35. Hamilton MG, Frizzell JB, Tranmer BI. Chronic subdural hematoma: the role of craniotomy reevaluated. Neurosurgery 1993;33:67–72.

36. Sambasian M. An overview of chronic subdural hematoma: experience with 2300 cases. Surg Neurol 1997;47:418–22.

37. Lee JY, Ebel H, Ernestus RI, Klug N. Various surgical treatments of chronic subdural hematoma and outcome in 172 patients: is membranectomy necessary? Surg Neurol 2004; 61:523–8.

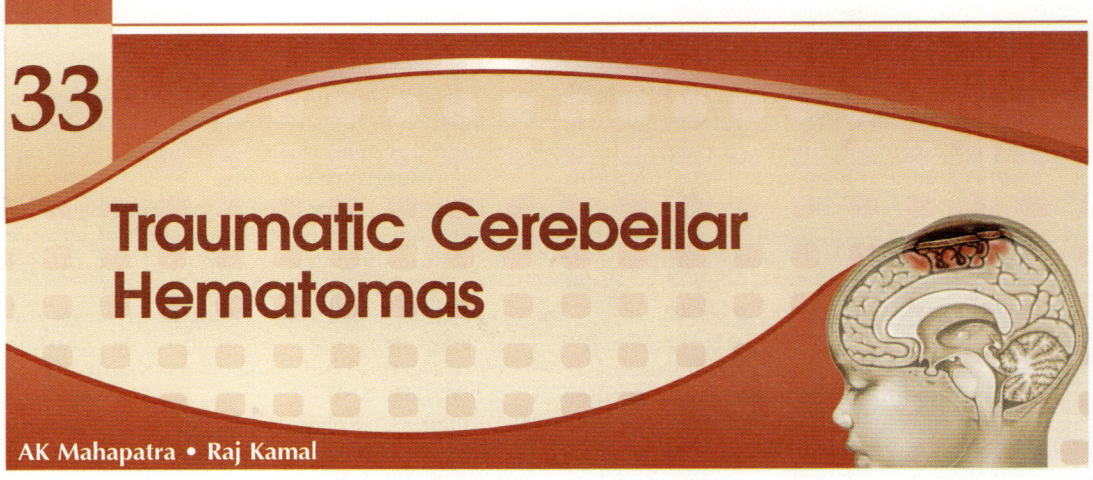

33

Traumatic Cerebellar Hematomas

AK Mahapatra • Raj Kamal

INTRODUCTION

Traumatic posterior fossa lesions are rare[1–3] as compared to supratentorial pathology of any nature. Among the posterior fossa hematomas, extradural hematomas are more frequent.[4–6] Traumatic intracerebellar pathology, be it contusion/hematoma are indeed very rare, and reported as small series, in the literature.[1,7–11] Inspite of being a well recognized clinico-radiological entity, posterior fossa traumatic lesions have received little attention. Because of rarity of lesion, no single series has vast experience. Recently, d'Avella et al[12] published a multicentric study dealing with 81 patients with cerebellar hematoma. Considering the clinical uncertainty and unpredictable course, these lesions require careful evaluation and monitoring. The present chapter is a brief review on the traumatic cerebellar hematoma.

PATHOLOGY OF TRAUMATIC CEREBELLAR LESIONS

Pathologically, traumatic cerebellar lesions could be primary or secondary. **It can be isolated cerebellar lesion or could be a part of diffuse axonal injury (DAI)** (Table 33.1). Posterior fossa lesions can result from both high velocity motor vehicular accidents or low energy[12,15,16] injury, due to fall from the height. Patients can also have coup or contrecoup lesions.[17] Hemorrhagic contusion of the cerebellum constitutes a fourth of the all traumatic lesions of the posterior fossa.[13]

Traumatic cerebellar hematoma is a rare condition and exact incidence is not known. Except the multicentric study published by d'Avella et al[12] no other large series is published in the literature (Table 33.2). The above authors could collect 81 cases over a three years period and provided detailed clinico-radiological profile. Overall, cerebellar pathology is **noticed in three percent** all head injury.[13,14]

Various mechanisms are hypothesized contributing to the formation of traumatic posterior fossa lesion (TPFL). **Most common**

Table 33.1: Classification of traumatic cerebellar lesion

A. Primary cerebellar hematoma
  • Hemispheric
  • Vermian
  • Both

B. Primary cerebellar hematoma associated with
  a. Supratentorial pathology
  b. Posterior fossa hematoma
    i. EDH
    ii. SDH

C. Cerebellar hematoma as a part of diffuse axonal injury

D. Cerebellar contusion/laceration
  • Part of compound injury
  • In closed head injury

mechanism is direct injury or coup injury over the occipital region.[3,16] This type of injury is more frequent due to fall, leading to low energy trauma.[12] **Contrecoup** injury is relatively rarer phenomenon.[15,18]

Other mechanism which produce cerebellar hematoma is the shearing strain. First rotational propulsion of the brain within cranial cavity leads to widespread axonal injury and scattered foci of hemorrhage at the junction of white and grey matter junctional area, in both cerebrum and cerebellum.[19] Thus, in 25% of DAI cerebellum may be involved. This type of injury results from high velocity vehicular injury with rotational force. Fifty percent patients reportedly d'Avella[12] had high velocity injury.

Rarely, cerebellar hematomas could be delayed in onset.[12,20,21] Cerebellar contusions are prone to increase in size. Hematoma may develop at site of previous contusion or even in area which looked normal on the first CT scan.[22] The delayed hematoma may be the result of coagulopathy.[22] Hemorrhagic contusion can slowly grow in size upto 4 days, as noticed by d'Avella et al.[12] While posterior fossa EDH is more common in children, cerebellar hematomas are very rare in pediatric age group.[23] Surprisingly, d'Avella et al[12] reported uniform incidence in all age groups.

Clinical Presentations

Clinical presentations of patients with cerebellar hematomas are varied. It depends on the size and the location of hematoma.[2,12,25]

The associated supratentorial pathology and DAI also influence the clinical presentation. Overall, 50% patients are admitted in coma.[12] As in some cases hematomas may grow in size over a period of time, there is a high possibility of deterioration of conscious state and development of raised ICP due to hydrocephalus. When a patient is in coma from the beginning, it is natural to think a high velocity impact and higher chance of having DAI. In the series presented by d'Avella, et al[12] 81% of patients in coma had an associated supratentorial lesion and 19 of 34 had DAI. A total of nine patients out of 81 had evolving clinical course, which suggest progressive deterioration. In conscious patients, headache, confusional state and presence of cerebellar signs would raise the possibility of posterior fossa mass lesion. A significant number of patients may have occipital scalp hematoma or scalp laceration.

Investigations

As usual CT scan is the investigation of choice.[12,25] In significant number of patients X-ray skull may show occipital bone fracture. In CT scan posterior fossa lesions are reported in 3% cases.[13,14,25] CT scan also delineate the presence of associated supratentorial pathology, DAI and development of hydrocephalus. According to CT scan findings, hematomas can be classified as midline or hemispheric, and small or large depending on the size more than 3 cm in diameter or less. In small percentage of patient may have initial normal

Table 33.2: Few recent series of traumatic cerebellar lesion			
Series authors	*Year*	*Number of patients*	*Other lesions*
1. Pozzati et al[9]	1982	7	Nil
2. Zuccarello et al[23]	1982	5	Nil
3. St. John and French[3]	1986	3	One EDH, one SDH
4. Karasawa et al[13]	1997	53	12 had acute hydrocephalus, Acute EDH in 9 patients and intracerebellar hematoma in 3
5. d'Avella et al[12]	2002	81	—

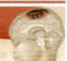

CT and when repeated may show delayed development of cerebellar hematoma,[12,21,22,25] Hence, d'Avella et al[12] suggested repeated CT scan daily for first 4 days, depending on need (Figs 33.1a and b, 33.2).

Management Policy (Table 33.3)

Surgical treatment of cerebellar hematoma is still a topic of considerable controversy. As the clinical course is unpredictable, and there is a possibility of rapid clinical deterioration, some authors advocate early surgery in traumatic cerebellar hematoma to prevent sudden deterioration and death.[13,14] However, few of the above studies are pre CT scan era. Recently, with accumulating evidence, it is convincing that large number of patients do run a benign course, which was not appre-

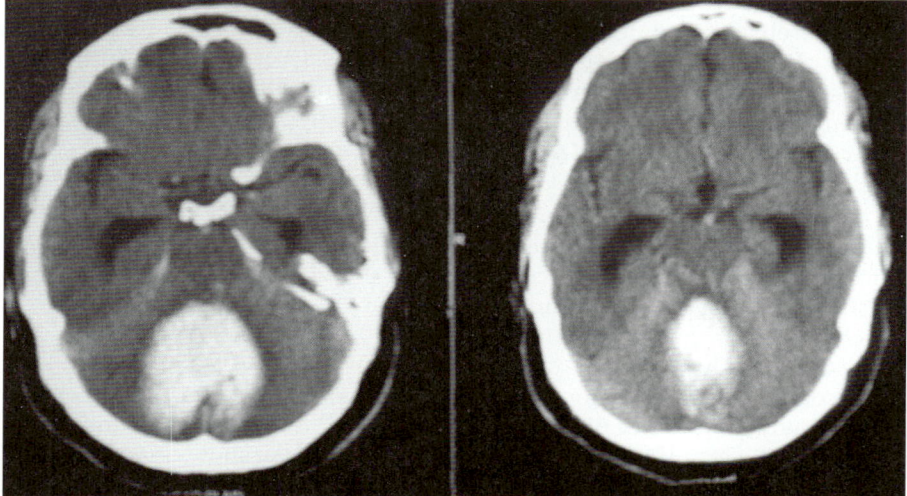

Fig. 33.1a: Non-contrast CT head showing midline post-traumatic cerebellar hematoma

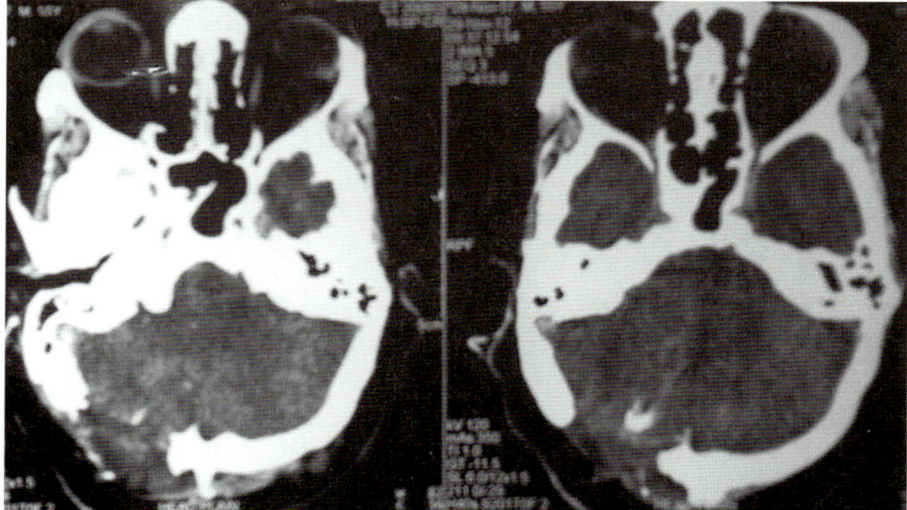

Fig. 33.1b: Postoperative CT head showing adequate evacuation of hematoma

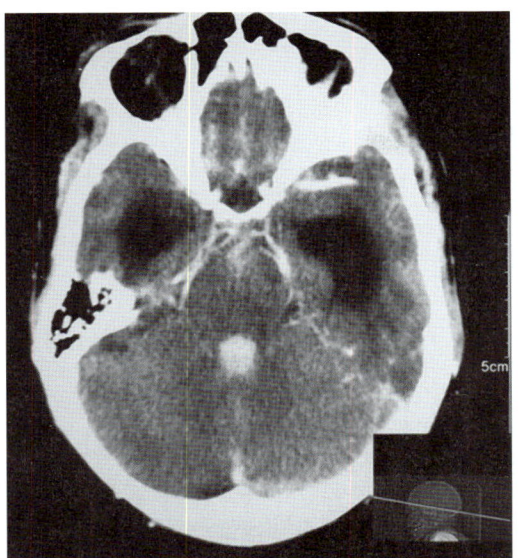

Fig. 33.2: Non-contrast CT head showing small traumatic cerebellar hematoma with dilated temporal horns

Size and site of the cerebellar hematomas are two major radiological parameters help for surgical decision. Clinical criterial state and raised ICP are also important (Table 33.3). There is a general consensus that conservative treatment is a logical option for the non-comatose patients with clots less than 3 cm in diameter, when there is no associated EDH or SDH in posterior fossa. Surgery is indicated in all patients with clot larger than 3 cm in diameter. Large number of patients do need EVD or VP shunt to reduce the ICP, in those patients who develop hydrocephalus,[12,13] which is noticed in 20% cases.

ICP monitoring helps in decision-making for the surgical evacuation. In conscious patients with large hematoma or in unconscious patients with small hematoma it acts as a good indicator. Associated supratentorial hematomas need management according to their own merit.

ciated earlier.[8,9,24,26] Not all hematomas of the cerebellum require surgery.[12,24,26] Surprisingly, no clear-cuts guidelines are available, however, there are several points which favor surgical evacuation. In 1994, Kobayashi, et al[27] had laid down the criteria for surgical treatment of hypertensive cerebellar hematoma. In absence of clear-cut guidelines for traumatic cerebellar hematoma, criteria laid down by Kobayshi,[27] et al can serve as a guideline.

Outcome

Overall poor outcome is reported in around 60% cases (Table 33.4). However, poor outcome is reported between 42 and 85%.[9,12,13,25] d'Avella et al[12] in a multicentric study of 81 cases of cerebellar hematoma reported 44.6% mortality. Mortality is low in patients with hematomas smaller than 3 cm and patients who are not in coma. He divided patients into two groups according to their admission

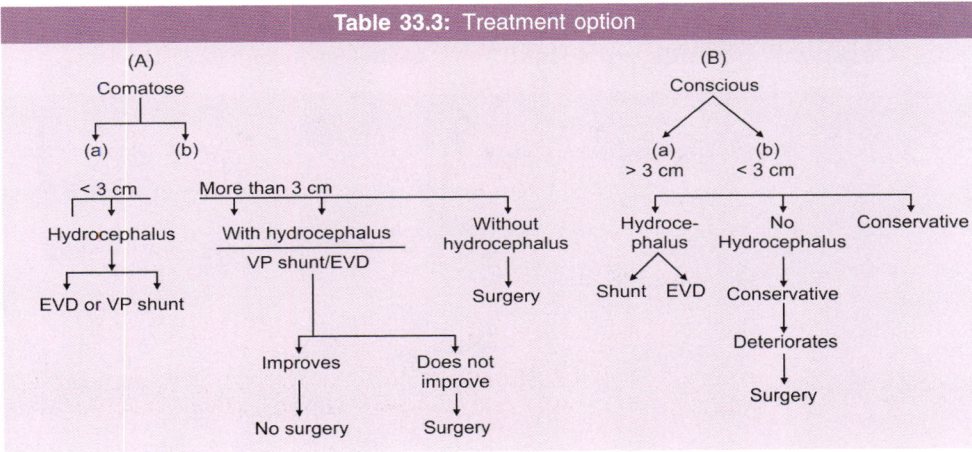

Table 33.3: Treatment option

Glasgow Coma Scale (GCS) scores. In Group 1 (39/81 cases; GCS score, > or = 8), the outcome was favorable in 95% of cases. In Group 2 (42/81 cases; GCS score, <8), the outcome was poor in 81% of cases. In conscious patients favorable result is reported in as high as 85% patients.[2] Patients with brainstem signs, obliteration of basal cistern in CT and with associated supratentorial lesion also have poor prognosis. Thus, large number of factors influences the overall outcome (Table 33.5).

CONCLUSIONS

Traumatic cerebellar hematomas are rare and probably occur in less than 1% of head injury patients. Often, this lesion is associated with other lesions in posterior fossa, supratentorial pathology and with DAI. Significant number of cases may have small hematoma and patients are conscious and neurologically static. This group of patients run a benign course and only a small percentage of patients may deteriorate if hematoma is vermian and there is associated hydrocephalus. By and large cerebellar hematoma patients in coma have hematoma larger than 3 cm in diameter or have associated injury. Small per cent of patients have delayed development of cerebellar hematoma and deteriorate 3–4 days following injury. CT scan is still the investigation of choice, and required repeatedly in first 3–4 days to assess the progression of hematoma or development of the hydrocephalus. Conscious patients with small

Table 33.4: Overall poor outcome		
Authors	*No. of patients*	*%*
1. Tsai et al[25]	14	85
2. Pozzati et al[9]	7	42
3. Sato et al[24]	8	50
4. Karasawa et al[13]	53	54
5. d'Avella et al[12]	81	44

hematomas by and large managed conservatively, while surgery is indicated in unconscious patients with large hematoma. Management of patients of coma with hematoma less than 3 cm remains debatable. Around 20% patients develop hydrocephalus and need either VP shunt or EVD. Overall the outcome is poor in 50–60% of the patients.

REFERENCES

1. Cassinari V, Dorizzi A, Pauli P, et al. Expansive traumatic lesions of the posterior cranial fossa. On 4 cases cerebellar contusion and laceration. Minerva Neurochir 1967;11:230–39.

2. Servadei F, Staffa G, Vorgoni G, et al. Post-traumatic acute subdural hematoma of the posterior fossa extending towards the cerebellopontine region. Report of a case. J.Neurosurg. Sci 1995;39:187–90.

3. St.John JN, French BN. Traumatic hematomas of the posterior fossa. A clinicopathological spectrum. Surg Neurol 1986;25:457–66.

4. Mahapatra AK, Bhatia R, Banerji AK. Posterior fossa extradural hematoma-A report of 5 cases. Neurology India 1982;30:239–44.

Table 33.5: Factors influencing the outcome		
	Good outcome	*Poor outcome*
1. Age	Less than 50 years	Above 50 years
2. Type of injury	Low velocity injury	High velocity injury
3. Associated hematoma	Nil	Present
4. Size of clot	Less than 3 cm	More than 3 cm
5. GCS	9 or above	8 or below
6. Hydrocephalus	Absent	Present
7. Basal cistern	Normal	Obliterated

5. Gupta PK, Mahapatra AK, Lad SD. Posterior fossa extradural hematomas-a study of 29 cases (In press).

6. Mahapatra AK, Posterior fossa extradural hematoma in children. Indian Pediatric 1990; 27:989–92.

7. d' Avella D, Salpietro FM, Angileri FF, et al. Management of traumatic cerebellar hemorrhagic contusions and hematomas. Acta Neurochir Suppl (Wien) 1998;71:410.

8. Pozzati E, Piazza G. Benign traumatic intracerebellar hematoma. Neurosurg 1981;8:102–3.

9. Pozzati E, Grossi C, Padoveni R: Traumatic intracerebellar hematomas. J Neurosurg 1982;56: 691–4.

10. Yokota H, Nakazawa S, Kobayashi S, et al. Clinical study of two cases of traumatic cerebellar injury (In Japanese) No Shinkei Geka 1990;18:67–70.

11. Sokol JH, Rowed DW. Traumatic intracerebellar hematomas. Surg Neurol 1978;10:340–1.

12. d' Avella D, Servadei F, Scerrati M, et al. Traumatic Intracerebellar Hemorrhage: Clinicoradiological Analysis of 81 patients. Neurosurg 2002;50:16–27.

13. Karasawa H, Furuya H, Naito H, et al. Acute hydrocephalus in posterior fossa injury. J. Neurosurg 1997;86:629–32.

14. Wright RL. Traumatic hematomas of the posterior-cranial fossa. J Neurosurg 1966;25:402–9.

15. Stone JL, Ladenheim E, Wilkinson SB, et al. Hematoma in the posterior fossa secondary to a tangential gunshot wound of the occiput: Case report and discussion. Neurosurgery 1991; 28:603–6.

16. Vrankovic D, Splavski B, Hecimovic I, et al. Anatomical intracerebellar protection of contrecoup hematoma development: Analysis of the mechanism of 30 posterior fossa coup hematomas. Neurosurg Rev 2000;23:156–60.

17. Olin MS, Young HA, Schmidek HH. Contrecoup intracerebellar hemorrhage: Report of a case. Neurosurg 1980;7:271–3.

18. Isla A, Alvarez F, Manrique M, et al. Posterior fossa subdural hematoma. J Neurosurg Sci 1987;31:67–69.

19. Adams JH, Doyle D, Ford I, et al. Diffuse axonal injury in head injury: Definition, diagnosis and grading. Histopathology 1989;15:49–59.

20. Nagata K, Ishikawa T, Shigeno T, et al. Delayed traumatic intracerebellar hematoma: Correlation between the location of the hematoma and the preexisting cerebellar contusion—case report. Neurol Med Chir (Tokyo) 1991;31:792–6.

21. Tibbs PA, Goldstein SJ, Smithson JR. Delayed traumatic intracerebellar hematoma. Surg Neurol 1982;16:309–11.

22. Stein SC, Young GS, Talucci RC, et al. Delayed brain injury following head trauma: Significance of coagulopathy. Neurosurgery 1992;30:160–5.

23. Zuccarello M, Andrioli GC, Fiore DL, et al. Traumatic posterior fossa hemorrhage in children. Acta Neurochir (Wien), 1982;62:79–85.

24. Sato K, Hinokuma H, Matsuzawa Y, et al. Clinical study of traumatic cerebellar contusion (In-Japanese) No Shinkei Geka 1987;15:1285–9.

25. Tsai FY, Teal JS, Itabashi HH, et al. Computed tomography of posterior fossa trauma. J.Comput Assist Tomogr 1980;4:291–305.

26. Koziarski A, Frankiewich E. Medical and surgical treatment of intracerebellar hematomas. Acta Neurochir (Wien) 1991;110:24–28.

27. Kobayashi S, Sato A, Kageyama Y, et al. Treatment of hypertensive cerebellar hemorrhage: Surgical or conservative management? Neurosurgery 1994;34:246–51.

34

Traumatic Basal Ganglia Hematomas and Infarcts

Raj Kamal • P Sarat Chandra • AK Mahapatra

INTRODUCTION

Traumatic basal ganglia hemorrhage (TBGH) is defined as a hemorrhagic lesion located in the basal ganglia or neighboring structures such as internal capsule or thalamus.[1] **Traumatic basal ganglion hematomas (TBGH) are observed in approximately 3–10% of patients admitted to a neurosurgical unit following a closed head injury**[2,3] (Figs 34.1 and 34.2). However, the incidence in autopsy series of closed-head injuries, including the pediatric population, is higher in the range of 10–12%.[3] As these are deeply located hemorrhages developing in the parenchyma between coup and contrecoup injuries, they have been considered as intermediary contusions. Traumatic basal ganglia hematomas account for less than 2% of post-traumatic intracerebral contusions. They are believed to rise from **shearing of the lenticulostriate or anterior choroidal blood vessels caused by acceleration/deceleration forces at the time of injury.** This shearing occurs as a result of high-velocity trauma, thus placing TBGHs into a distinctive category.[4,5]

Mechanism of TBGH

Traumatic basal ganglia hematomas occur mainly in young persons, however, the clinicopathological profile of these lesions is still poorly understood.

The mechanism of formation of TBGH is unique as it involves formation of blood clot within the parenchyma and is also known to increase with time.

Formation of TBGH: Courville and Blomquist believed that TBGHs were small, usually multiple, and located in the zone of the **lenticular nucleus and external capsule, on either one or both the sides**[6] (Fig. 34.1). In contrast, spontaneous hemorrhages in this area were large, usually single, and located in the region of the thalamus and internal capsule. Therefore, solitary deep-seated intracerebral hematomas with mass effect were always deemed spontaneous, and thus, when a patient suffered a head injury it was considered to be the consequence rather than the cause of the hematoma.

The above view was considered true till in 1959. Mosberg and Lindenberg[3] reported on one patient whose clinical condition progressively deteriorated and died following a head injury. In their patient, a massive hematoma in the pallidum and a **ruptured arterial twig of the anterior choroidal artery within the clot was found at autopsy.** After histological examination of the vessel, the arterial tear was found to be traumatic in origin, demonstrating that massive hematomas in the basal ganglia can result following head injury. According to these authors, traumatic hemorrhage in the region of the basal ganglia should be

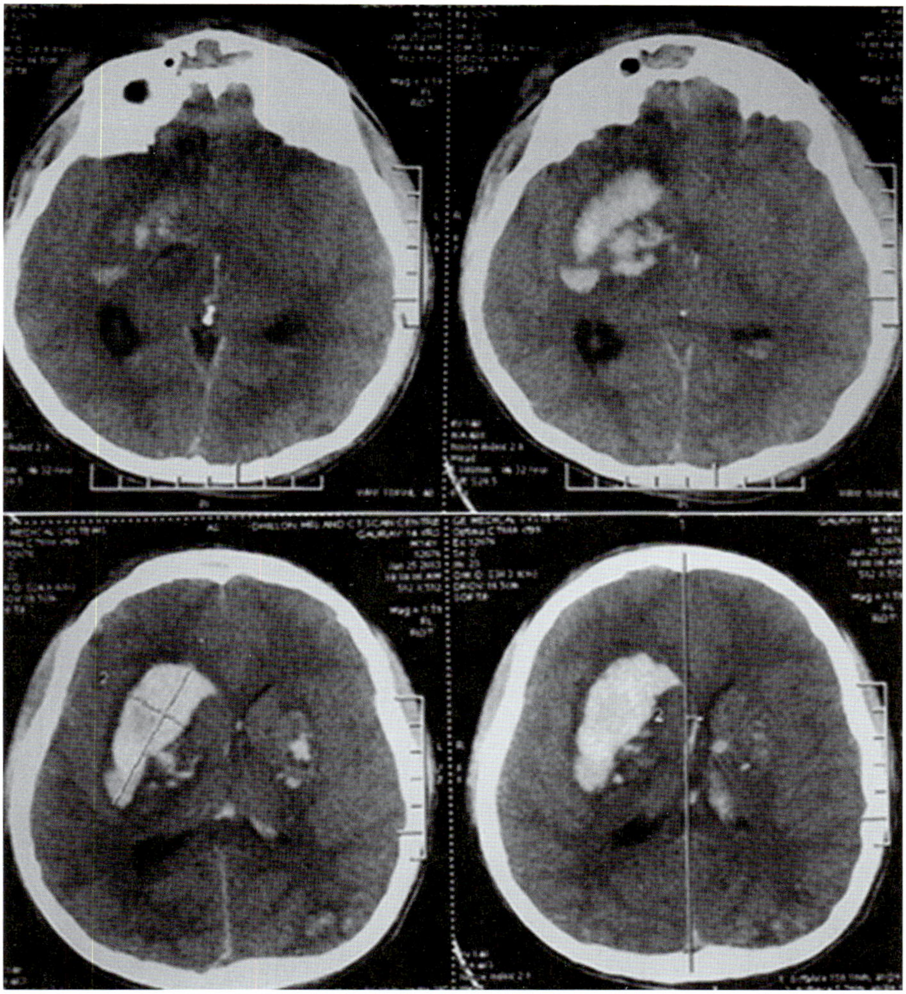

Fig. 34.1: CT scan, non-enhanced, axial section showing evidence of traumatic bilateral basal ganglia hematoma with intraventricular extension and left parietal contusion

diagnosed in cases where trauma occurs while the head is in motion (coup and contrecoup) and the impact, sufficient to deform the skull, is applied to the vertex; forehead, or occipital area and directed toward the tentorium. Under these circumstances, there would be a shift of the brain through the tentorial notch, producing shearing forces among different tissues, which in turn would produce **stretching and tearing of the** *pallidal* **branches** of *the anterior choroidal artery, and*

occasionally, of *the striate branches* of *the* **MCA, resulting in hemorrhages within the basal ganglia region.**[3–6] **Because other brain structures might also be displaced through the tentorial notch, contusions and/or small hemorrhages in areas such as the corpus callosum, thalamus, hypothalamus, hippo-campus, and midbrain** are not uncommonly associated with the TBGH. Thus, previous occurrence of a head injury and the evidence of other typically traumatic lesions in the same

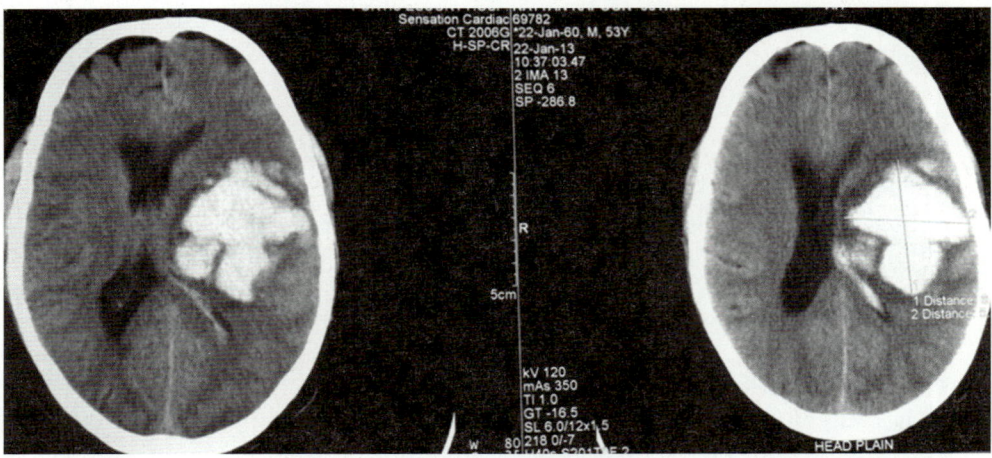

Fig. 34.2a: Plain CT scan showing evidence of traumatic large basal ganglia hematoma

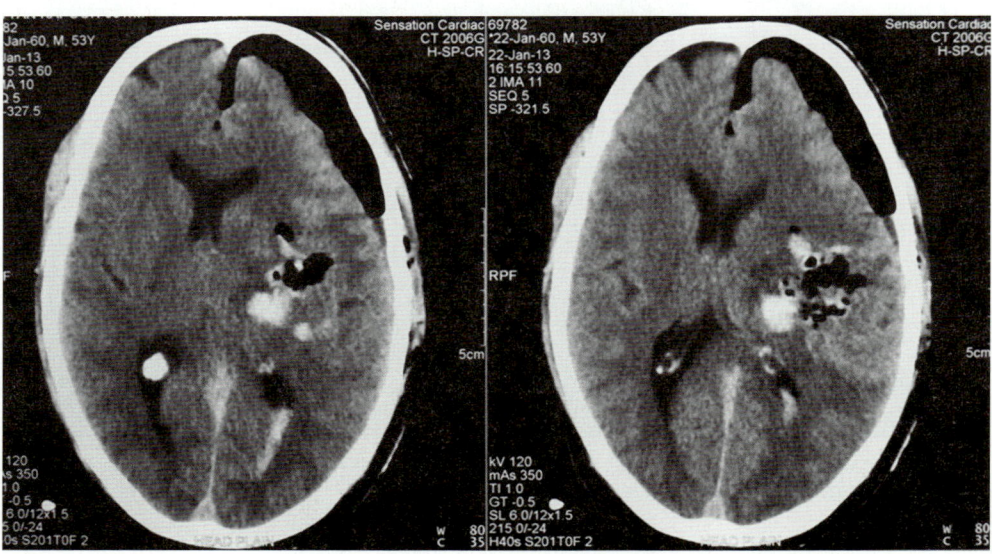

Fig. 34.2b: Postoperative CT scan head showing good evacuation of hematoma

patient would suggest a traumatic origin of the hemorrhage in the basal ganglia. It should also be noted that TBGHs might rarely be accompanied by ventricular hemorrhage, simulating hypertensive intraventricular hematoma.[7,8]

Mosberg and Lindenberg[3] also suggested that the compression of vessels supplying the basal ganglia region might cause not only hemorrhage but also infarcts, and considered the traumatic hemorrhages of the basal ganglia to be hemorrhagic contusions, in contrast to Courville and Blomquist,[6] who labeled them hematomas. Whether TBGHs should be considered contusions or, by contrast, intracerebral hematomas remains a secondary question, and the ultimate mechanisms of these lesions still remain unclear.

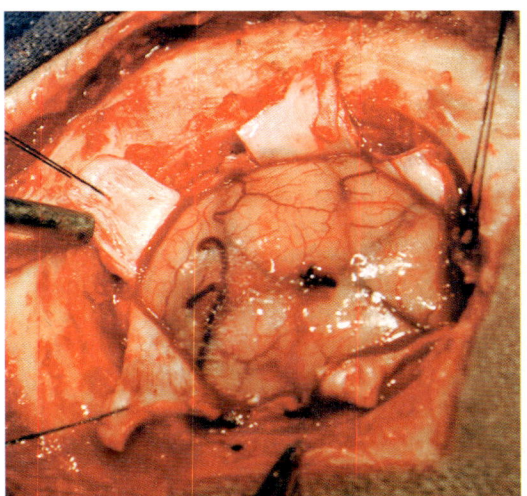

Fig. 34.2c: Peroperative photograph showing bulging of brain

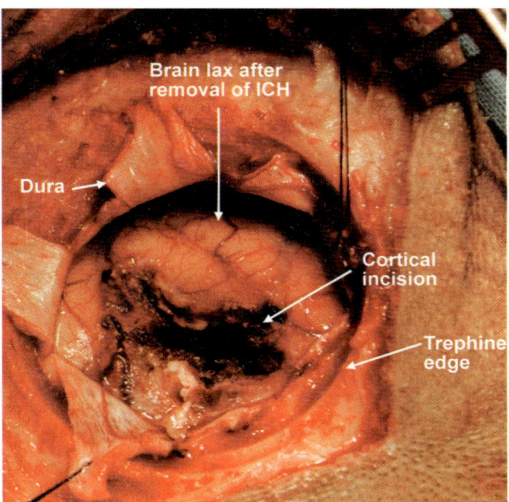

Fig. 34.2d: Lax brain after removal of hematoma (Fig. 34.2a)

Fung et al reported[1] a case of a 30-year-old man with a ruptured lenticulostriate artery after traumatic brain injury that caused the combination of SAH, BGH and ischemic stroke and subsequent cerebral vasospasm. This rupture mimicked the pathophysiology and imaging appearance of aneurysmal SAH.[1] The site of rupture was not secured by any treatment; however, hyperdynamic therapy and percutaneous transluminal angioplasty were feasible in this setting to prevent additional delayed neurological deficit.

In 1980, Maki and Colleagues[9] reported on a 6-year-old girl who after suffering severe head injury presented with a massive unilateral hemorrhage measuring 20 ml and located contralateral to the side of impact; the lesion required surgical aspiration through a craniotomy. The authors postulated that the *anterior stretch of the lateral branch of the perforating vessel of the MCA*, secondary to the opposite direction of rotation of the skull and the brain after injury, plays a major role in the pathogenesis of these lesions. This mechanism could also explain the occurrence of TBGHs located contralateral to the side of impact, which was observed in 76% of the patients in our series. Recently, Fujioka et al[10] have demonstrated that *traumatic dissection of the MCA* produces infarction and hemorrhage in the basal ganglia. Kinoshita et al[11] have also postulated anterior choroidal artery causing basal ganglia bleed. On the other hand, the basal ganglia and the thalamus are the most frequent places in which hypoperfusion is detected using single-photon emission a brain perfusion scanning after mild and moderate head injury.[12] The mechanisms are summarized in Fig. 34.4.

In an autopsy series of 635 fatal non-missile head injuries, Adams et al[4] found 63 patients with basal ganglia hematomas; the lesion was defined as an intracerebral hemorrhage involving the stria turn, pallidum, or thalamus. Most patients were involved in traffic accidents. They rarely experienced a period of lucidity and they exhibited a high incidence of diffuse axonal injuries (DAI), gliding contusions, and large contusions, suggesting that these deep-brain hematomas were a primary event that occurred at the moment of injury and arose from the shear strains elicited by acceleration/deceleration forces[4,13,14] (Fig. 34.3). Patients with this type of injury have a relatively low incidence of skull fractures, in contrast with those suffering falls, in whom TBGHs rarely develop.[2,15] However, it should be noted that TBGHs can occur in the absence of DAI, and not all patients with DAI have TBGHs.

In a recent review of 37 cases of TBGH, in severe head injuries, 73% of the patients had an associated DAI, and skull fracture was present in 43%. This was unlike previous studies where the incidence of skull fractures was quoted quite low.[16]

Enlargement of TBGH

A unique feature of TBGH is that they are known **to expand with time.** They may evolve into large hematomas as early as 30–60 minutes after injury. The rate and extent of volume increase has been related to factors such as the caliber of the injured vessel, the reduction in cerebral blood flow causing secondary ischemia and necrosis in the surrounding white matter leading to hematoma enlargement by coalescence, the occurrence of blood dissection, the presence of hypoxia or systemic arterial hypertension, and a bleeding tendency, which occurs in persons suffering from alcohol abuse.[17] A recent study[16] has shown that 65% of TBGHs enlarged during the acute post traumatic period and 86% of the patients exhibited some type of coagulation disorder that might have contributed to the development of delayed

hematomas or the enlargement of a pre-existing one.

The formation of hematoma has also been shown to have a bimodal peak. In a study by Okada et al[18] reporting 83 cases of traumatic intracerebral hematomas, 49 were delayed; 10 hematomas (four of them delayed) were located in the basal ganglia. According to this author, completion of hematoma formation displays two incidence peaks, the first within 6 hours post-injury and the second between 12 and 24 hours post injury.

Bilateral TBGHs

Another interesting aspect is the occurrence of bilateral TBGHs. Bilateral traumatic basal ganglia hematoma is extremely rare. Descriptions are limited to case reports.[19] Yanaka et al[20] reported on two cases of bilateral TBGHs. Ozgun and Castillo[21] described a case of bilateral TBGH occurring after a lightning strike to the head. Boto et al[16] have shown petechie in the basal ganglia contralateral to the TBGH in three patients.

Basal Ganglionic Infarcts

These are uncommon and more commonly found in children. Maki[9] reported 2 pediatric cases (out of 7 cases of basal ganglia injury) of unilateral basal ganglia infarction.

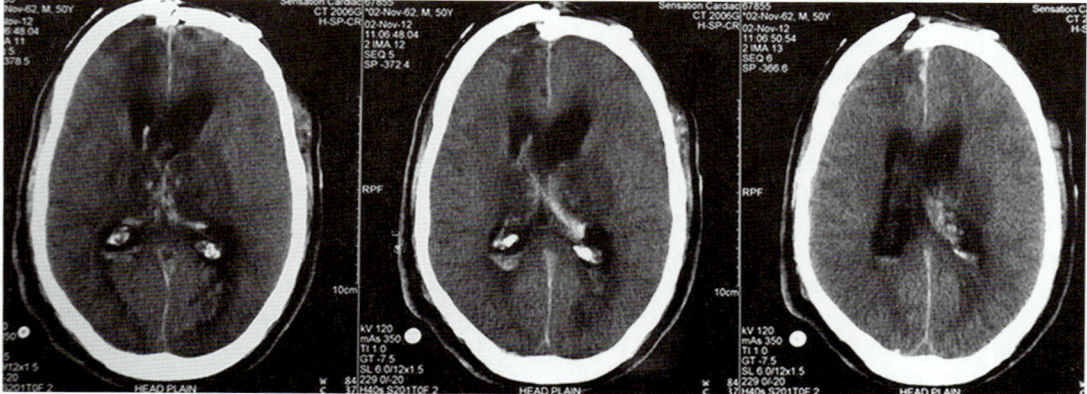

Fig. 34.3: CT scan, non-enhanced, axial section of a patient within severe diffuse axonal injury with a basal ganglia infarct. Frontal bone fracture and frontal contusions are also seen

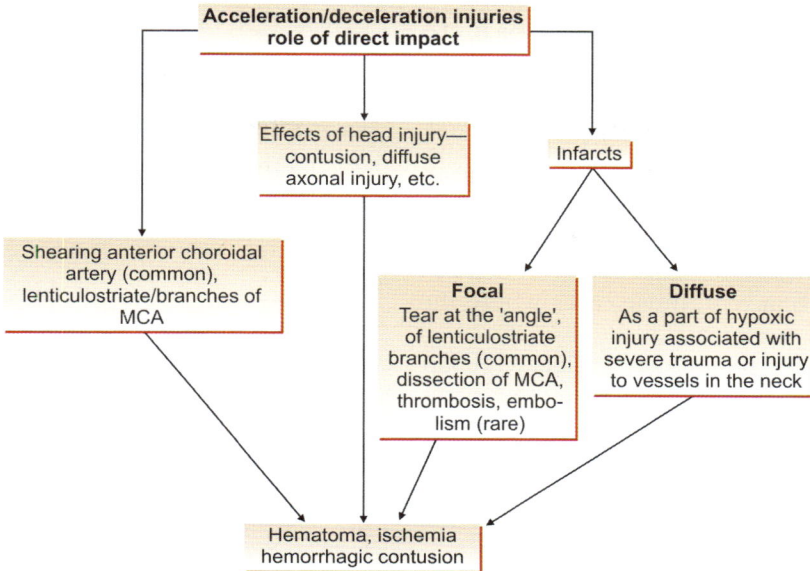

Fig. 34.4: Pathophysiology of basal ganglia injury

Dharker et al[22,23] have described a series of 23 cases that presented with sudden onset of hemiparesis since the time of head injury. Most of the cases were not associated with loss of consciousness. CT scan (Fig. 34.3) showed presence of small infarcts within the region of basal ganglia extending into the posterior limb of internal capsule. They have postulated that head injury could have resulted in damage at the level of the 'angle' of the lenticulostriate branches as they enter the perforating substance leading to shearing, thrombosis or embolism (Fig. 34.4).[22,23] Basal ganglionic infarcts may occur in isolation or they may be associated with diffuse axonal injuries, hematoma or contusions[22,24] or as a part of global ischemia seen in severe head injuries or due to injury to the vessels in the neck.

Management of TBGHs

Mosbeig and Lindenberg[3] first published the case of a severe head injury patient in whom a hematoma located in the region of the pallidum and was successfully aspirated through a brain cannula. Apart from such anecdotal reports, most of cases of TBGH in the past were managed non-operatively. Boto et al[16] showed that in their series only one patient with a TBGH larger than 25 ml survived without surgery and all the other patients with raised ICP as well as 73% of the cases showing hematoma volume enlargement died. This shows that a more aggressive approach should be directed towards patients with TBGH at least in patients in whom ICP is difficult to control. Traumatic basal ganglia hematomas may be evacuated by means of open surgery (Figs 34.2a to d), CT-guided stereotactic aspiration surgery or ultrasound-guided aspiration surgery. **Endoscopic evacuation** is a more recent technique; previously being applied for spontaneous intracerebral hematomas may also be used for TBGH.[25] It has been recently published that early treatment with **citalopram,** a selective serotonin reuptake inhibitor, may have a beneficial effect on the extent of morbidity associated with TBGHs.[26]

Outcome of TBGH

Smaller intermediary contusions of the basal ganglia may cause extrapyramidal signs secondary to changes in the **substantia nigra,** motor paralysis due to involvement of the pyramidal tracts in the internal capsule, visual deficits as well as language and sensory impairments due to injury to the lateral geniculate bodies and the thalamus[9,10,23] respectively, and prolonged unconsciousness due to involvement of the reticular activating system.[26] Lucid intervals have been demonstrated especially in those cases where the hematoma has expanded.[16,27]

Studies have shown that TBGH are generally with a worse prognosis than other types of post-traumatic intracranial hematomas.[2,16,27,28] **However, TBGH** are associated with good recovery especially when they occur in isolation, and their final prognosis is related to the extent of the related DAI.[16]

Some authors have correlated the prognosis with the size and found poorer outcome in massive hematomas,[29] while others have not found any correlation with the size or location.[30] Lee and Wang[15] have shown that advanced patient age (> 60 years), the presence of abnormal pupillary changes, impaired oculocephalic and motor responses, and intraventricular and brainstem hemorrhage correlated with poor prognosis. The prognostic factors are summarized in Table 34.1.

CONCLUSIONS

These are summarized below:

1. TBGH are dynamic lesions and tend to expand in volume during the acute post-traumatic period, hence the importance of serial CT scanning.
2. The pathogenesis and the biomechanics of these lesions is still unclear and further studies are necessary.
3. Surgical intervention is necessary in lesions more than 25 ml. In patients being managed conservatively, a very close monitoring is essential in the ICU and ICP monitoring is mandatory.
4. The overall mortality is high and morbidity considerable in survivors. Some patients with isolated hematomas may do well.

Table 34.1: Summary of the prognostic factory in TBGH

Poor prognostic factors	Good prognostic factors
Age > 60 years	Age < 60 years
Impaired brainstem reflexes	Preserved brainstem reflexes
Poor GCS score	GCS score above 9
Intraventricular/ Brainstem hemorrhage	TBGH in isolation
Associated DAI	Immediate medical surgical intervention
Massive TBGH	

REFERENCES

1. Fung C, Z'Graggen WJ, Beck J, Gralla J, Jakob SM, Schucht P, Raabe A. Traumatic subarachnoid hemorrhage, basal ganglia hematoma and ischemic stroke caused by a torn lenticulostriate artery. Acta Neurochir (Wien). 2012;154(1):59–62. doi: 10.1007/s00701–011–1162–7.
2. Macpherson P, Teasdale E, Dhaker S, et al. The significance of traumatic hematoma in the region of the basal ganglia. J Neurol Neurosurg Psychiatry 1986;49:29–34.
3. Mosberg WH, Lindenberg R. Traumatic hemorrhage from the anterior choroidal artery. J Neurosurg 1959;16:209–21.
4. Adams JH, Doyle D, Graham DI, et al. Deep intracerebral (basal ganglia) hematomas in fatal non-missile head injury in man. J Neurol Neurosurg Psychiatry 1986;49:1039–43.
5. Kimura M, Sobata E, Suzuki S. Traumatic basal ganglion (caudate) with favorable prognosis: Report of two cases. No Shinkei Geka 1994; 22:155–8.
6. Courville CB, Blomquist OA. Traumatic intracerebral hemorrhage with particular reference to its pathogenesis and its relation to "delayed traumatic apoplexy[7] Arch Surg 1940;41:1–28.
7. Lindenberg R. Significance of the tentorium in head injuries from blunt forces. Clin Neurosurg 1964;12:129–42.
8. Kara M, Shiogai T, Tamagawa T, et al. Three cases of traumatic intracerebral hematoma with ventricular hemorrhage. No Shinkei Geka 1980;8:295–9.
9. Maki Y, Akimoto H, Enomoto T. Injuries of basal ganglia following head trauma in children. Childs Brain 1980;7:113–23.

10. Fujioka M, Meda Y, Okuchi K, et al. Secondary change in the substantia nigra induced by incomplete infarct and minor hemorrhage in the basal ganglia due to traumatic middle cerebral arterial dissection. Stroke 1999;30:1975–7.

11. Kinoshita Y, Yasukouchi H, Harada A, Tsuru E, Okudera T. Case report of traumatic hemorrhage from the anterior choroidal artery, No Shinkei Geka 2008;36:891–4.

12. Abdel-Dayem I'M, Abu-Judeh H, Kumar M, et al. SPECT, brain perfusion abnormalities in mild or moderate traumatic brain injury. Clin Nucl Med 1998;23:30–317.

13. Crooks DA. Pathogenesis and biomechanics of traumatic intracranial hemorrhages. Virchows Arch A Pathol Anat Histopathol 1991;418:479–83.

14. Denny-Brown D, Russell WR. Experimental cerebral concussion. Brain 1941;64:93–164.

15. Lee W, Wang ADJ. Post-traumatic basal ganglia hemorrhage: Analysis of 52 patients with emphasis on the final outcome. Trauma 1991;31:376–80.

16. Boto GR, Lobato RD, Rivas JJ, et al. Basal ganglionic hematomas in severely head injuries: Clinicoradiological analysis of 37 cases. J Neurosurg 2001;94:224–32.

17. Lindenberg R. Trauma of meninges and brain. In: Minckler J (ed): Pathology of the Nervous System. New York: McGraw-Hill 1971;2:1705–65.

18. Okada T. (Clinical aspects of traumatic intracerebral hematomas. Pathogenesis of delayed traumatic intracerebral hematomas). Nihon Ika Daigaku Zasshi (Japanese) 1989;56:545–58.

19. Jang KJ, Jwa CS, Kim KH, Kang JK. Bilateral Traumatic Hemorrhage of the Basal Ganglia. J Korean Neurosurg Soc 2007;41:272–4.

20. Yanaka E, Egashira T, Maki Y, et al. Bilateral traumatic hemorrhage in the basal ganglia: Report of two cases. No Shinkei Geka 1991; 19:369–73.

21. Ozgun B, Castillo M. Basal ganglia hemorrhage related to lightning strike. AJNR 1995;16: 1370–1.

22. Dharker SR, Mittal RS, Bhargava N. Ischemic lesions in Basal Ganglia in children after minor head injury. Neurosurgery 1993;33:863–5.

23. Dharker SR. Traumatic ischemic lesions in children. Neurology India (Suppl) 1995;43:61–63.

24. Mahapatra AK, Bhatia R. Basal ganglionic hematomas in head injuries: Review of 26 cases. Neurology India (Abstr) 1986.

25. Auer LM, Deinsberger W, Niederkom K, et al. Endoscopic surgery versus medical treatment for spontaneous intracerebral hematoma: A randomized study. J Neurosurg 1989;70:530–5.

26. Andersen G, Stylsvig M, Sunde N. Citalopram treatment of traumatic brain damage in a 6-year-old boy. J Neurotrauma 1999;16:341–4.

27. Katz DI, Alexander MP, Seliger GM, et al. Traumatic basal ganglia hemorrhage: Clinicopathologic features and outcome. Neurology 1989;39:897–904.

28. Gean AD. Imaging of Head Trauma. New York: Raven Press 1994;165–66.

29. Munemoto S, Komai T, Aizumi S, et al. (Traumatic hemorrhage in the basal ganglia in the child. Five cases). No Shinkei Geka 1985; 13:1027–33.

30. Jayakumar PN, Kolluri VRS, Basavakumar DG, et al. Prognosis in traumatic basal ganglia hematoma. Acta Neurochir 1989;97:114–6.

35

Post-traumatic Meningitis and Brain Abscess

Raj Kamal • AK Mahapatra

INTRODUCTION

Meningitis and brain abscess following trauma constitute the most common infective complications of head injury.[1-8] The rarer ones are subdural empyema, extradural abscess, osteomyelitis and infection in a hematoma.[8] Infective complications not only add to the secondary morbidity of head injury, but also substantially increase the cost associated with its management. Infective complications may affect the ultimate outcome of the patient, and are also known to affect the propensity for developing post-traumatic epilepsy.

The infective complications mostly, but not without exception, affect patients who have sustained compound head injuries. Uncommonly, patients are affected by these complications who have sustained closed injuries.[8,9] Even those patients are affected who have sustained injuries many years ago, even at sites remote from the site of impact. Certainly, closed head injury patients that have been operated can be subject to these complications like any other patient after a neurosurgical procedure.

Over the last decade, methicillin-resistant *Staphylococcus aureus* (MRSA) strains have emerged as serious pathogens. These strains are often multiresistant to several antibiotic classes and are a major cause of serious hospital- and now community-acquired infections and associated morbidity and mortality.[10] As a result of increasing antimicrobial resistance, glycopeptides, such as vancomycin, are widely used as first-line therapy for serious MRSA infections. However, the emergence of glycopeptide tolerance and resistance has complicated treatment and there remains a clinical need for new antibiotics with suitable pharmacokinetic properties with activity against MRSA and other Gram-positive pathogens.[10] Infections caused by MRSA and other bacteria usually respond as well to bacteriostatic agents as to bactericidal ones. Nevertheless, there is evidence that rapid bacterial killing has potential clinical advantages over bacteriostatic therapy in certain infections. Daptomycin, the first of the cyclic lipopeptides, shows rapid bactericidal activity against *S. aureus*, including strains tolerant or resistant to other agents.[10]

Infective complications and their impact have certainly lessened after introduction of effective prophylactic antibiotics, but in most areas of the world these complications are still regularly encountered. Surprisingly, we found that the literature relating to post-traumatic brain abscesses was rather scant. As the incidence of high-velocity vehicular accidents rises, neurosurgeons would more regularly encounter compound injuries with skin, bone and soft-tissue loss and thus the urgent need to be aware of these infections

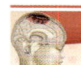

occurring in the background of trauma. The particular aspects of etiopathogenesis of these complications, the latency, the different microbial spectrum and specific issues related to patient investigation and management necessitate separate mention.

A. POST-TRAUMATIC MENINGITIS

Meningitis taking place in the post-traumatic setting is usually bacterial in etiology (Table 35.1 and Fig. 35.1), with incidence widely varying. After an exhaustive review, Kaufman and colleagues[1] arrived at a reported incidence of 0.2–17.8% of head injuries. Kallel et al[11] reported an incidence of 0.96% of patients hospitalized for head injury. The incidence following compound head injury (external or internal) is much higher. For example, the estimated incidence of meningitis after CSF leak is 3–50%.[1,2] A recent study concluded that the presence of a CSF leak increased the probability of meningitis by tenfolds.[3] This risk appears to be greater if the leak persists for more than a week following injury.[4,5] In clinical practice, CSF fistula seems to be the most commonly encountered antecedent of post-traumatic meningitis. A point to note is that the spectrum of causative organisms in the post-traumatic setting is certainly quite distinct from that of community acquired meningitis at different ages of life.[6] One should remember that till recently, the overall case fatality rate for bacterial meningitis is in the range of 25%.[7]

Table 35.1: Common organisms responsible for post-traumatic meningitis

1. Streptococcus *pneumoniae*	CSF fistula or internal compound injuries
2. Other Streptococci	
3. *H. influenzae*	
4. *Neisseria* sp.	
5. *Acinetobacter baumannii*	
6. *Staph. aureus*	Penetrating or external compound injuries
7. Enteric gram-negative bacilli	
8. *Staph. epidermidis*	

Pathogenesis

The pathogenesis of meningitis after head injury may be direct or indirect. The direct course of events follow direct penetrating injury, compound injuries (internal or external) or CSF leaks. The cribriform plate is the commonest site of dural fistula as bone is thin in this region, with the adherent dura predisposing to a dural breach at the time of fracture (Fig. 35.6). Also to be considered in this category are cases of meningitis following neurosurgical procedures in head injury patients. The indirect method involves spread of infection from an adjacent compartment. In this group would be cases of meningitis following skull osteomyelitis, intracranial suppurative phlebitis, and brain abscess. The further sequence of events is the same as for meningitis in general,[8] thus not deserving separate mention here.

Microbiology

In general the common organisms responsible for post-traumatic meningitis are the following[8,9] in the respective clinical settings (Table 35.1). CSF cultures were positive in 15 of 25 (60%) patients (Fig. 35.1) and brain tissue culture was positive in one additional patient.[12]

Acinetobacter meningitis typically occurs following neurosurgery. Patients at risk for post-neurosurgical bacterial meningitis include those with cerebrospinal leakage,[13] concomitant incision infection, prolonged duration of surgery,[13] surgery that enters a sinus, increased severity of illness,[14,15] prolonged external ventricular drainage, and need for repeat surgery.[15]

Sometimes, other unusual organisms may also be isolated, such as Listeria.[9] This emphasizes the importance of using specific culture media according to the organisms expected.

Clinical Features

The onset of meningitis is usually within 3–5 weeks after the head injury, but is well known

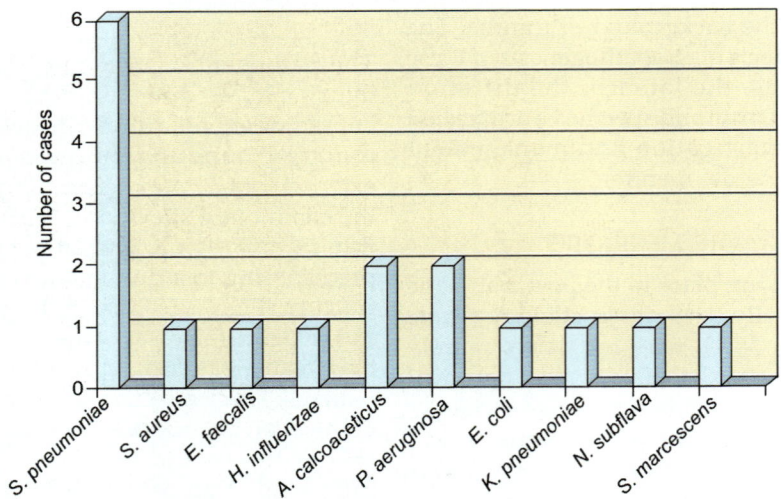

Fig. 35.1: CSF cultures were positive in 15 of 25 (60%) patients and brain tissue culture was positive in one additional patient[12]

to occur even months to years later. This is generally true for those cases associated with initial CSF leak that temporarily stops, only to recur and lead to an attack of meningitis for the first time many months or years later. This underscores the importance of taking a detailed history of events that may have occurred months to years before the patient presents with meningitis. Indeed, the patient may have dismissed the trauma as "trivial" with some minor "nosebleed". Of course, it could occur much earlier in a patient with an external or internal compound injury or in whom the CSF leak persists.[4,5]

For the patient presenting in the acute phase after trauma, the diagnosis is usually straightforward. In addition to an obvious CSF leak from nose/ear often admixed with blood, other evidence of a basilar fracture may be present, such as anosmia, periorbital and retroauricular ecchymoses. Petrous compound fractures are notorious in that they may result in facial nerve paresis, meningitis and at times present with paradoxical rhinorrhea.

Reccurent episodes of meningitis in a patient should always warn against the possibility of a dural fistula (of whatever etiology); recurrent pneumococcal meningitis

is extremely suggestive of an otherwise occult dural fistula.[16]

CSF Analysis

The important objective is to establish that the leaking fluid is, in fact, CSF. Routine bedside estimation of glucose in the fluid may be helpful in confirming that the fluid is CSF, but a negative test may not rule out the possibility. Glucose concentration of more than 30 mg/dl is usually considered confirmatory, whereas concentrations below that may be occasionally observed in lacrimal fluid or mucus.[11] beta-2-transferrin (beta-2 trf) is a specific indicator of the presence of CSF in the leaking fluid.[17]

Usual microscopic and biochemical analysis of CSF is mandatory as soon as meningitis is suspected. Of course, in the acute post-traumatic setting, one must ensure absence of significant mass effect prior to perform a lumbar puncture. Also, the presence of traumatic subarachnoid hemorrhage may confound interpretation of CSF findings due to presence of pleocytosis and hypoglycorrhachia. In this context, gramstain and rapid diagnostic modalities for bacterial detection and isolation are quite useful.[18,19] These are also quite useful in patients who have partially treated meningitis.

Culture of the CSF (bacterial and fungal) should be routinely carried out in consultation with a microbiologist to ensure that proper media are available for plating. A sample of CSF should always be obtained prior to start any antibiotic therapy.

Radiological Evaluation (Table 35.2)

Plain radiographs do not provide any substantive information, hence do not serve any useful purpose in this setting. However, the presence of intracranial air, air-fluid levels or even opacity in the paranasal sinuses are the common findings (Fig. 35.2).

Contrast CT (Fig. 35.3) remains the mainstay of radiological evaluation of patients having post-traumatic meningitis. It provides useful information depending on the clinical situation:

1. *In the acute post-traumatic setting:* CT (Figs 35.2 and 35.4) provides valuable information regarding the presence of fracture, injury to underlying brain and presence of internal or external compounding. Fluid or blood in the sinuses indicates the presence of otherwise occult basilar fractures. Thin-slice axial and coronal studies of the skull base (with bone window) may be required in some cases to demonstrate basilar fractures.[16,20]

Table 35.2: What to look for in contrast CT study for post-traumatic brain abscess

1. Location
2. Size of the abscess
3. Stage of evolution of the abscess
4. Mass effect due to the abscess and the surrounding edema
5. Wall thickness
6. Number of loculi
7. Communication with ventricular system or ventriculitis
8. Hydrocephalus
9. Air in the abscess cavity
10. Presence of foreign body

2. *In the delayed setting:* Routine CT study may show the presence of intracranial air, which is diagnostic. CT with studies of the skull base is required to delineate basilar fractures responsible for CSF leak. In addition, high-resolution CT cisternography using a water-soluble contrast medium should be used to identify the exact site of leak in patients requiring operative closure of the dural fistula (Figs 35.5 and 35.6).

The above studies may also be required in patients presenting with recurrent meningitis (esp. Pneumococcal).[16]

Contrast CT may be necessary on occasion in patients who do not respond or deteriorate

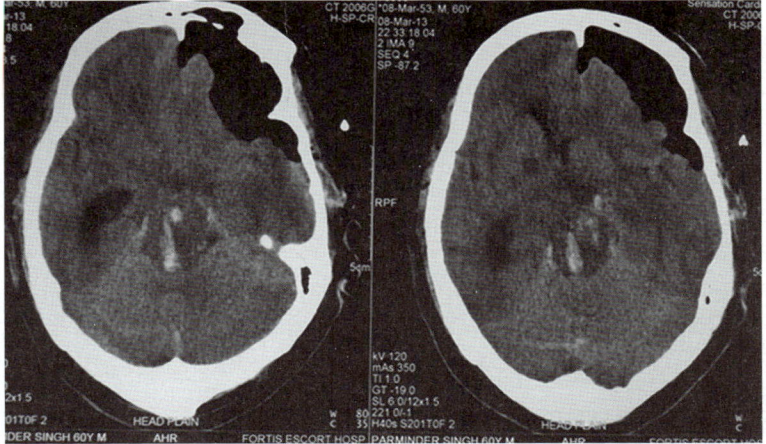

Fig. 35.2: NCCT shows intracranial air following anterior skull base fracture who had CSF leak

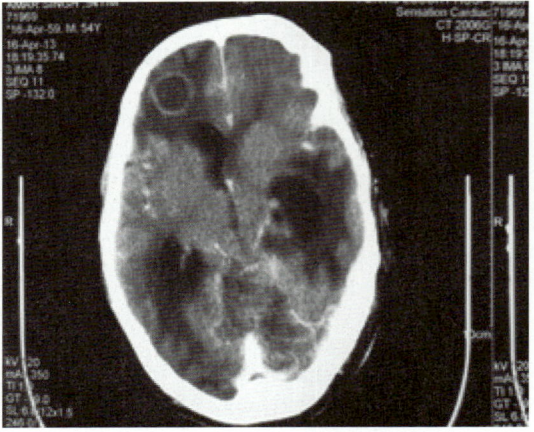

Fig. 35.3: Contrast CT scan head showing left frontal brain abscess with evidence of ventriculitis and periventricular ooze

despite of adequate treatment. In these situations, one may expect to find development of a subdural empyema or even a brain abscess.

MR imaging is also of help, especially in the delayed setting. In the acute setting, blood and blood products may obscure the delineation of dural breach. In the delayed phase, thin-slice coronal imaging is of great value in delineating a dural fistula (Fig. 35.5). This is visualized best in the T_2-weighted images as a continuation of the subarachnoid space reaching exit, durally across a bony gap or fracture. CSF may also be seen in the contiguous air sinuses. An encephalocele may also be seen to accompany this tract in some cases. The advantage of MR imaging here is its non-invasive nature, when compared to the alternative of CT cisternography, which requires intrathecal contrast administration. Brain abscess are very well seen on contrast MRI (Figs 35.6 and 35.7).

Isotope studies at the present time certainly help in documenting a CSF leakage but the poor spatial resolution[1] precludes a useful delineation of the site of leak. Thus, ultimately one has to choose between MR and CT cisternography for identification of the site of CSF leakage.

B. POST-TRAUMATIC BRAIN ABSCESS

The earliest available record of successful drainage of a post-traumatic brain abscess was by Dupuytren in 1839, who opened a compound skull fracture to drain the abscess in a soldier who later survived. Intracranial infections occurring after head injury are among the most dreaded complications.[21] Fortunately, the occurrence of a brain abscess after head injury is a rather uncommon sequel.[22] Most cases, as mentioned, occur following a compound head injury. There are also reports of several cases of post-traumatic abscess following closed head injury,[23–25] including a report from our institution.[27] In a

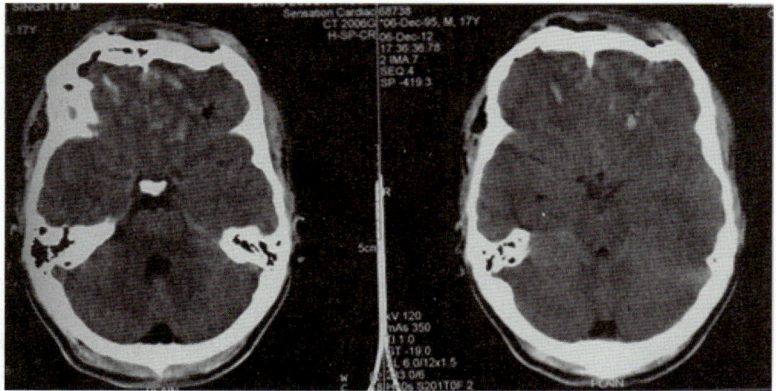

Fig. 35.4: Plain CT showing frontal fracture in patient of compound head injury

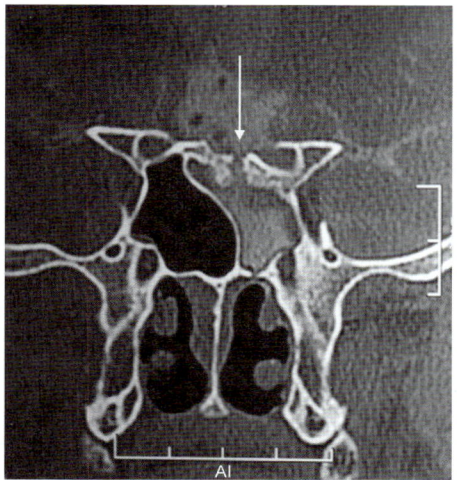

Fig. 35.5: CT cisternography showing bone defect as well as CSF leak

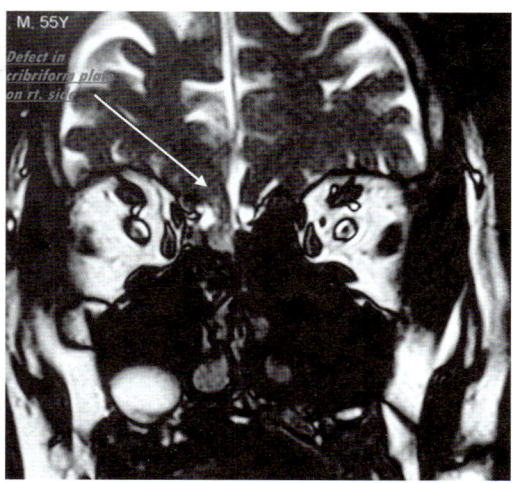

Fig. 35.6: Coronal MRI scan shows CSF filled cavity communicating to nasal cavity

study Carpenter et al[26] found that there was an increase in the number of cases of brain abscess secondary to neurosurgery and trauma compared to earlier series, there was a marked decrease in the number of cases of brain abscess secondary to otitis media and congenital heart disease. They also found that the frontal lobe was the most common site. Streptococcal infection was seen most commonly, but staphylococcal infection predominated in cases following neuro-surgery. Cefotaxime and metronidazole were used most often for empirical therapy.[26]

The reported incidence of abscess following head trauma has ranged from 3% of 203 cases of penetrating head injuries sustained during World War II, to 16.7% of 42 cases of compound brain injuries in various reports.[27–30]

As a percentage of all brain abscesses, traumatic brain abscesses constitute anywhere from 4.1% in an autopsy series[30] to 12–20% in other retrospective series.[31–34] Clearly, this entity cannot be put aside as a rare occurrence. Further, the mortality rate for brain abscesses has declined in the antibiotic era, but still remains high at 10–30%.[8]

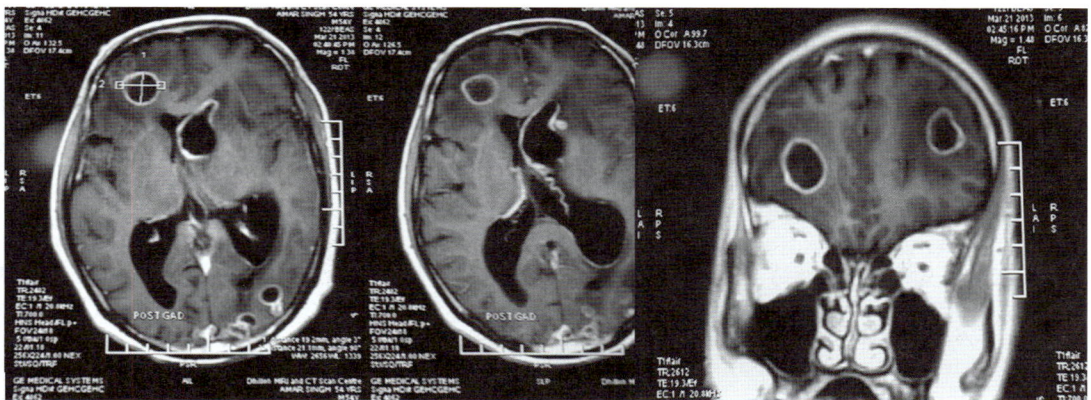

Fig. 35.7: Axial and coronal section of contrast MRI showing typical brain abscess. Also note left-sided ventriculitis

Pathogenesis

The pathogenesis can be conveniently thought of as being direct or indirect. The direct pathway of genesis of a post-traumatic abscess involves direct penetration of the cranial vault and the dura at the time of injury. This results in the following components being present intracranially, all of which individually predispose to formation of the abscess:

1. *Foreign material:* Dust, skin and soft-tissue debris, hair, bone fragments, and metallic or non-metallic fragments of various kinds. These different agents have varying propensity for leading to abscess formation: a high-speed bullet fragment may remain inert for prolonged periods of time, whereas the same is not true of other organic and non-organic fragments such as glass, wood, etc. Furthermore, these non-viable agents lead to the formation of a nidus as described below.

2. *Contused and lacerated brain tissue:* Like the above agents, provide an areas of low oxygen tension and variably low blood supply. This promotes the formation of an infectious nidus.[35]

3. Hematoma around the area of brain injury.

The indirect pathway results in abscess formation after any of the following events have taken place:

1. Meningitis
2. Osteomyelitis
3. Suppurative intracranial phlebitis
4. Hematogenous spread of infective organisms from a focus to a foreign body.

It should be noted that traumatic CSF fistulae also predispose to the development of an abscess,[36] usually as a sequel to meningitis.

The further sequence of events proceeds in much the same way as for any other abscess and the evolution, particularly in a head injury setting may be influenced by various factors such as virulence of the organism, type and duration of the antibiotic therapy apart from others.[8]

At times, organisms may be of low enough virulence or the host reaction may be sufficient to wall these off for prolonged periods, resulting in unusually long latency. An interesting case reported[37] was that of coexistent chronic pyogenic abscess and glioblastoma multiforme developing after 37 years at the site of a metallic splinter injury.

The above discussion would not be complete without commenting on those unusual cases of post-traumatic brain abscesses that occur following supposedly closed injury.[23–25] These abscesses seem to have a predilection for frontal and temporal regions, as was evident from the study from our institution.[26] A review of 3 other cases cited revealed that steroid therapy may have played a role in one patient. In another report,[24] exploration of the abscess that followed supposedly closed head injury revealed a basifrontal fracture. Moreover, the abscess was contiguous and bone splinters were found within the orbitofrontal cortex. This suggests that in many cases of abscess following seemingly "closed" head injury the cause may actually be internally compound head injury. This would also explain the proximity to frontal and temporal regions, where the air sinuses are contiguous.

Microbiology (Table 35.1 and Fig. 35.1)

In one of the earliest reports, Cairns reported that Staphylococci and Streptococci were the commonly isolated organisms.[29] From our institution, the published data revealed that *Staphylococcus aureus* was the commonest organism in 12 (33%) cases.[26] Other microbes isolated were almost equally distributed among the gram-negative enterobacteria (*E. coli, Pseudomonas, Klebsiella* and *Proteus*) and anaerobe groups (*Clostridia, Bacteroides,* and *Bacillus* species). *Streptococcus pneumoniae* (earlier called *Pneumococcus*) is particularly associated with post-traumatic abscesses especially those following CSF rhinorrhea.[36] Gas-containing abscesses, though rare, have been described in other reports, with *Clostridia* being the commonest species responsible for gas containing intracranial abscesses.[38] So far, a total of 38 clostridial abscesses have been described, of which 32 (84%) were related to a penetrating head injury.[38] There are also solitary reports of other unusual organisms such as *Nocardiae*,[39] *Bacillus* species,[40] *Propionibacterium*,[37] among others. As a rare occurrence, fungal organisms may concomitantly be isolated in pus from post-traumatic brain abscess.[38] Only a total of 6 such cases have been reported so far, with *Aspergillus* and *Mucoraceae* being the main offenders.[38]

It is clearly advisable to obtain an adequate pus sample prior to instituting any antimicrobial therapy.[41] However, circumstances may be extenuating, and the patient may already have received broad-spectrum empiric therapy prior to reach neurosurgical attention. Fastidious organisms may still result in a sterile culture despite all above precautions. To prevent this, appropriate culture media should be readily available. For example, specific culture media should be used for plating when suspecting *Haemophilus* or *Clostridia* species as the causative organisms.

Sampling of CSF may be potentially dangerous in the presence of an abscess with mass effect, and should be avoided.[8]

Latency

Post-traumatic abscesses can form as early as 5 weeks after injury. In some cases of penetrating injuries, this may be even sooner. For example, in the case reported by Tekkok et al[38] a gas-containing tract was seen in a CT study 5 days after a penetrating injury with a rusted nail. A well-defined ring-enhancing abscess could be seen 4 weeks post-injury. Despite the occasional exception, 5 weeks seem to be required for the chain of the pathogenetic steps to take place and sequentially result in the formation of an abscess.

The usual latency for a post-traumatic abscess to form is 3–4 months. This seems to be the general experience from various reports, and also in the series reported by

Dinakar and Rao[30] and also from our institution.[26] The latency may at times be unusually long.[37,42,43] The most illustrative example to this effect was the case reported by Robinson et al.[43] They operated a patient suspected to have a meningioma, which turned out at operation to be a chronic abscess containing viable gram-positive cocci even 36 years after sustaining a compound head injury. In the post-antibiotic era, such a delayed presentation is more common, with patients receiving potent antibiotics for suspected compound head injury.

Clinical Features

The affected population seems to be more commonly young males.[26-30] The most important point is the history of penetrating head injury, which is usually present in a majority. One must insist on a thorough description of the events, especially from any witness, as the patient may be amnesic regarding the actual sequence of events. This is important as gauged from numerous reports wherein this information was initially lacking. In children, seemingly innocuous injuries with pencil-tips[44] around the periorbital region have resulted in brain abscesses. This point is to be kept in mind, as the bony walls of the orbit are thin in children (especially the roof), predisposing to penetrate injuries with otherwise harmless objects. A definite subgroup of patients would not have any history of compound or penetrating head injury.[23-37] For example, in the report from our institution,[26] 13 of 36 patients had no evidence of compound head injury (among them 3 had been operated for closed head injury).

Seizures and focal neurological deficits may be seen depending on the severity of the initial injury and location of the developing brain abscess. The other relevant manifestations are that of a wound discharging pus, brain fungus and signs of raised intracranial pressure. In our experience, the signs of raised intracranial pressure were the most common manifestations, followed by seizures. An interesting finding was that patients with closed head injuries seemed to have fresh focal deficits more commonly, which was statistically significant.[26]

Location

By and large, post-traumatic abscesses are confined to the supratentorial compartment. Not only is this because compound injuries and air sinuses usually relate to this compartment, but also because penetrating wounds when occurring in the posterior fossa are commonly fatal.[45] The above observations not withstanding, Webster and Gurdjian[33] encountered one case of abscess in the mid-cerebellar region. Another report by Kepes et al[39] illustrated a fatal case in which the patient survived the trauma but later succumbed to an abscess located in the medulla.

Frontal and parietal regions, favored locations in compound head injuries, are also the leading sites for traumatic brain abscesses.[26,29]

Radiological Evaluation

Plain radiographs at the present time do not seem to much value in the evaluation for a post-traumatic brain abscess. These may demonstrate intracranial air in gas-containing abscesses in 75% of cases,[38] which has important management implications. CT constitutes the mainstay of radiological evaluation.[8] A contrast-enhanced CT study is able to demonstrate brain abscess, with the appearance depending on the evolutionary stage of the abscess (Fig. 35.3). A CT study would be expected to demonstrate important findings related to a post-traumatic brain abscess.

CT serves as a baseline for initial evaluation as well as a medium for objective assessment of the response to the chosen modality of management (medical, aspiration or surgical excision). As mentioned above, in cases supposedly following closed head injury, thin-slice axial and coronal sections should be taken to rule out the basal fractures that may be otherwise missed. In situations wherein a

CSF fistula is thought to result in meningitis leading to brain abscess, a CT cisternography (Fig. 35.5) study after administering intrathecal contrast is often of help.

MR imaging is not of much value in this setting, but may occasionally be required for delineation of rare abscesses (Fig. 35.7), or when the diagnosis itself is in doubt. Pyogenic acute abscesses have fairly striking and specific MR appearances,[46,47] but one should always exclude the possibility of a metallic foreign body prior to MR imaging in a case of post-traumatic brain abscess.

Management

The management of post-traumatic meningitis involves three aspects:
1. Optimal antimicrobial treatment
2. Symptomatic and adjunctive measures
3. Treatment of the cause.

Antibiotic Treatment

In general, it is advisable to start empiric antibiotic treatment with broad-spectrum parenteral antibiotics. The usual recommended combination[36,48,49] is either a third generation cephalosporin with anti-*Pseudomonas* activity plus a penicillinase-resistant penicillin or vancomycin plus an aminoglycoside in proper dosage. If compound injury has involved an air sinus, intravenous metronidazole should be added for the first 3–5 days. The cultures should be expeditiously obtained and specific antibiotic therapy started depending on the sensitivity of the organism isolated. Parenteral antibiotics need to be given for a minimum of 4–6 weeks, and longer in some cases depending on whether aspiration of the abscess has been undertaken or excision.

Infectious Diseases Society of America (IDSA) guideline[50] recommends (Tables 35.3 and 35.4), that, once there is suspicion of acute bacterial meningitis, blood samples must be obtained for culture and a lumbar puncture performed immediately to determine whether the CSF formula is consistent with the clinical diagnosis. In some patients, the clinician may

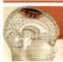

Table 35.3: Recommendations (for grading refer to Table 35.3a) for specific antimicrobial therapy in bacterial meningitis based on isolated pathogen and susceptibility testing[50]

Microorganism, susceptibility	Standard therapy	Alternative therapies
Streptococcus pneumoniae Penicillin MIC		
< 0.1 µg/ml	Penicillin G or ampicillin	Third generation cephalosporin,[a] chloramphenicol
0.1–1.0 µg/ml[b]	Third generation cephalosporin[a]	Cefepime (B-II), meropenem (B-II)
≥ 2.0 µg/ml	Vancomycin plus a third generation cephalosporin[a,c]	Fluoroquinolone[d] (B-II)
Cefotaxime or ceftriaxone MIC ≥ 1.0 µg/ml	Vancomycin plus a third generation cephalosporin[a,c]	Fluoroquinolone[d] (B-II)
Neisseria meningitidis Penicillin MIC		
< 0.1 mg/ml	Penicillin G or ampicillin	Third generation cephalosporin,[a] chloramphenicol
0.1–1.0 µg/ml	Third generation cephalosporin[a]	Chloramphenicol, fluoroquinolone, meropenem
Listeria monocytogenes	Ampicillin or penicillin G[e]	Trimethoprim-sulfamethoxazole, meropenem (B-III)
Streptococcus agalactiae	Ampicillin or penicillin G[e]	Third generation cephalosporin[a] (B-III)
Escherichia coli and other enterobacteriaceae[g]	Third generation cephalosporin (A-II)	Aztreonam, fluoroquinolone, meropenem, trimethoprim-sulfamethoxazole, ampicillin
Pseudomonas aeruginosa[g]	Cefepime[e] or ceftazidime[e] (A-II)	Aztreonam,[e] ciprofloxacin,[e] meropenem[e]
Haemophilus influenzae		
β-Lactamase negative	Ampicillin	Third generation cephalosporin,[a] cefepime, chloramphenicol, fluoroquinolone
β-Lactamase positive	Third generation cephalosporin (A-I)	Cefepime (A-I), chloramphenicol, fluoroquinolone
Staphylococcus aureus		
Methicillin susceptible	Nafcillin or oxacillin	Vancomycin, meropenem (B-III)
Methicillin resistant	Vancomycin[f]	Trimethoprim-sulfamethoxazole, linezolid (B-III)
Staphylococcus epidermidis	Vancomycin[f]	Linezolid (B-III)
Enterococcus species		
Ampicillin susceptible	Ampicillin plus gentamicin	
Ampicillin resistant	Vancomycin plus gentamicin	
Ampicillin and vancomycin resistant	Linezolid (B-III)	

Note. All recommendations are A-III, unless otherwise indicated.
[a] Ceftriaxone or cefotaxime
[b] Ceftriaxone/cefotaxime—susceptible isolates
[c] Consider addition of rifampin if the MIC of ceftriaxone is > 2 µg/ml
[d] Gatifloxacin or moxifloxacin
[e] Addition of an aminoglycoside should be considered
[f] Consider addition of rifampin
[g] Choice of a specific antimicrobial agent must be guided by in vitro susceptibility test results

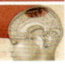

Table 35.3a: Infectious diseases society of America—United States public health service grading system for ranking recommendations in clinical guidelines[50]

Category, grade	Definition
Strength of recommendation	
A	Good evidence to support a recommendation for use; should always be offered
B	Moderate evidence to support a recommendation for use; should generally be offered
C	Poor evidence to support a recommendation; optional
D	Moderate evidence to support a recommendation against use; should generally not be offered
E	Good evidence to support a recommendation against use; should never be offered
Quality of evidence	
I	Evidence from > 1 properly randomized, controlled trial
II	Evidence from > 1 well-designed clinical trial, without randomization; from cohort or case-controlled analytic studies (preferable from > 1 center); from multiple time-series; or from dramatic results from uncontrolled experiments
III	Evidence from opinions of respected authorities, based on clinical experience, descriptive studies, or reports of expert committees

not emergently perform the diagnostic lumbar puncture (e.g., secondary to the inability to obtain CSF), even when the diagnosis of bacterial meningitis is considered to be likely, or the clinician may be concerned that the clinical presentation is consistent with a CNS mass lesion (abscess) or another cause of increased intracranial pressure and will thus order a CT scan of the head prior to lumbar puncture. The Infectious Diseases Society of America (IDSA) guideline recommends meropenem for the treatment of meningitis caused by ESBL-producing GNB, and four of the previous cases were treated with carbapenems.[50–53] It is widely known that meropenem penetrates into the cerebrospinal fluid when there is meningeal inflammation. This guideline recommends a duration of treatment of 21 days for aerobic GNB.[53]

In cases, where the abscess cavity contains gas, the possibility is either an abscess with a coexistent CSF fistula or the causative organism being gas producing. If a CSF fistula can be excluded, the preferred agent in combination is Penicillin G, keeping in mind that the commonest of fenders are usually *Clostridia* species.[38] However, it should be noted that a significant number of clostridial abscesses are polymicrobial,[38] hence the need for other broad-spectrum agents as part of the combination. The use of polyvalent gas gangrene antiserum and hyperbaric oxygen therapy has not shown any clear benefit.[38] In case of a CSF fistula with coexistent brain abscess, the likely organisms to be targeted are as mentioned in the previous section on post-traumatic meningitis.

Treatment with parenteral antibiotics effective against the causative organism in adequate dosage for optimal duration is the key to proper treatment. No time should be lost in initially instituting empirical antibiotic therapy[54] after taking the CSF sample for the various analyses.

The initial empirical antibiotic should fulfil the following criteria:
1. It should have good penetration into the CSF.
2. It should be able to reach a minimum bactericidal concentration (MBC) in the CSF.[54]

Table 35.4: Recommended dosages of antimicrobial therapy in patients with bacterial meningitis (A-III)[50] (for grading refere to Table 35.3a)

Antimicrobial agents	Total daily dose (dosing interval in hours)		Infants and children	Adults
	Neonates, age in days			
	0–7[a]	8–28[a]		
Amikacin[b]	15–20 mg/kg (12)	30 mg/kg (8)	20–30 mg/kg 98)	15 mg/kg (8)
Ampicillin	150 mg/kg (8)	200 mg/kg (6–8)	300 mg/kg (6)	12 g (4)
Aztreonam				6–8 g (6–8)
Cefepime			150 mg/kg (8)	6 g (8)
Cefotaxime	100–150 mg/kg (8–12)	150–200 mg/kg (6–8)	225–300 mg/kg (6–8)	8–12 g (4–6)
Ceftriaxone			80–100 mg/kg (12–24)	4 g (12–24)
Chloramphenicol	25 mg/kg (9–24)	50 mg/kg (12–24)	75–100 mg/kg (6)	4–6 g (6)[c]
Ciprofloxacin				800–1200 mg (8–12)
Gatifloxacin				400 mg (24)[d]
Gentamicin[b]	5 mg/kg (12)	7.5 mg/kg (8)	7.5 mg/kg (8)	5 mg/kg (8)
Meropenem			120 mg/kg (8)	6 g (8)
Moxifloxacin				400 mg (24)[d]
Nafcillin	75 mg/kg (8–12)	100–150 mg/kg (6–8)	200 mg/kg (6)	9–12 g (4)
Oxacillin	75 mg/kg (8–12)	150–200 mg/kg (6–8)	200 mg/kg (6)	9–12 g (4)
Penicillin G	0.15 mU/kg (8–12)	0.2 mU/kg (6–8)	0.3 mU/kg (4–6)	24 mU (4)
Rifampin		10–20 mg/kg (12)	10–20 mg/kg (12–24)[e]	600 mg (24)
Tobramycin[b]	5 mg/kg (12)	7.5 mg/kg (8)	7.5 mg/kg (8)	5 mg/kg (8)
TMP-SMZ[f]			10–20 mg/kg (6–12)	10–20 mg/kg (6–12)
Vancomycin[g]	20–30 mg/kg (8–12)	30–45 mg/kg (6–8)	60 mg/kg (6)	30–45 mg/kg (8–12)

Note. TMP-SMZ: trimethoprim-sulfamethoxazole.

[a] Smaller doses and longer intervals of administration may be advisable for very low birth weight neonates (< 2000 g)

[b] Need to monitor peak and trough serum concentrations

[c] Higher dose recommeded for patients with pneumococcal meningitis

[d] No data on optimal dosage needed in patients with bacterial meningitis

[e] Maximum daily dose of 600 mg

[f] Dosage based on trimethoprim component

[g] Maintain serum trough concentrations of 15–20 µg/ml

3. It should be effective against the probable causative organisms, i.e. must be broad spectrum.

4. The choice should be in accordance with the emerging sensitivities of the expected groups of organisms.

The ideal compound to treat CNS infections is of small molecular size, is moderately lipophilic, has a low level of plasma protein binding, has a volume of distribution of around 1 liter/kg, and is not a strong ligand of an efflux pump at the blood–brain or blood-CSF barrier.[55] When several equally active compounds are available, a drug which comes close to these physicochemical and pharmacokinetic properties should be preferred. Several anti-infectives (e.g. isoniazid, pyrazinamide, linezolid, metronidazole, fluconazole, and some fluoroquinolones) reach a CSF-to-serum ratio of the areas under the curves close to 1.0, and therefore, are extremely valuable for the treatment of CNS infections.[55] For humans, the ratio of the AUCCSF/AUCS (area under the drug concentration) or the CSF-to-serum drug concentration in steady state is the most accurate parameter to characterize drug penetration into the CSF.

Direct injection of drugs, which do not readily penetrate into the CNS, into the ventricular or lumbar CSF is indicated when other effective therapeutic options are unavailable.

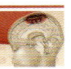

Penetration of Anti-infectives into the CSF and Brain Tissue in the Absence or Presence of Meningeal Inflammation

Drug concentrations measured in the absence of meningeal inflammation represent the minimum concentrations that can be encountered early in the course of a CNS infection or during its resolution. For this reason, it is highly desirable to reach effective drug concentrations in the CNS compartments not only with inflamed but also with uninflamed meninges. In bacterial meningitis, the blood-CSF/blood–brain barrier is becoming leaky by the opening of intercellular tight junctions of the vessel walls particularly within venules.[56] Three mechanisms (increased drug entry into the CSF and delayed removal by a reduction of the CSF bulk flow and by the inhibition of the activity of efflux pumps) synergistically lead to a rise of the CSF concentrations, particularly of drugs that do not enter the CSF readily in the absence of meningeal inflammation.[57,58] Under the conditions of a severe disruption of the blood–brain/blood-CSF barrier, the physicochemical properties of drugs, which govern drug entry into the CNS in the absence of meningeal inflammation, become less important.[58]

β-Lactam Antibiotics

The penetration of all β-lactam antibiotics into the CSF in the absence of meningeal inflammation is relatively poor (Table the AUCCSF/AUCS ratio ~0.15).[55] This class of antibiotics is characterized by a high level of activity against susceptible pathogens and a relatively low toxicity. In the presence of moderately susceptible pathogens, the daily dose of several β-lactam antibiotics can be increased without a high rate of serious side effects, the daily IV dose of ampicillin can be increased to 15 g and beyond for adults with normal renal function.

β-Lactam antibiotics can cause epileptic seizures after intrathecal but also after intravenous administration.[59,60] Epileptic seizures have been observed for up to 33% of children treated with imipenem IV for bacterial meningitis.

Carbapenems

Both imipenem and meropenem have been used in the treatment of meningitis. Lodise and colleagues[61] reported that the penetration of meropenem into the CSF, as measured by the AUCCSF/AUC serum ratio was 4% (2–8%). Additionally, they showed that meropenem 2 g every 8 hours as a 30 min infusion (IDSA recommended dose for bacterial meningitis) had a greater than 80% probability of achieving 50% and 100% T > MIC for MICs of less than or equal to 0.25 µg/ml and 0.125 µg/ml, respectively.

Doripenem has not yet been evaluated in meningitis, although it has *in vitro* activity against many *A. baumannii* strains. Imipenem use appears to be problematic for meningitis due to the possibility of seizures with the high doses needed to adequately treat the infection. Indeed, clinically significant seizure activity was noted in three of 15 patients with *Acinetobacter meningitis* treated with imipenem.[62–64] Meropenem seems to be associated with a very low risk of seizure, even in the presence of meningitis. In animals, doripenem also has minimal epileptogenic activity.[65]

In patients with non-inflammatory occlusive hydrocephalus who had undergone external ventriculostomy, maximal CSF concentrations of meropenem after receiving an initial 2 g meropenem dose, administered over 30 min, were 0.13–1.60 µg/ml (mean concentration 0.63 µg/ml).

After intraventricular injection in rats, cefazolin, imipenem, and aztreonam were most potent in inducing epileptic seizures.[59,60] For this reason, meropenem instead of imipenem is recommended for the therapy of CNS infections.[55]

For the new carbapenems, doripenem and ertapenem, no data concerning their CNS penetrations in humans are available.

Aminoglycosides

Aminoglycosides are hydrophilic compounds with poor CSF penetration; however, based on the AUCCSF/AUCS ratio, their penetration into the CSF in the absence of meningeal inflammation is not lower than those of β-lactam antibiotics and other hydrophilic antibiotics with a similar molecular mass . The therapeutic index of aminoglycosides is low: because of nephro- and ototoxicity. Therefore, they are being used intrathecally. IDSA guidelines recommend daily intraventricular doses of amikacin of 5–50 mg, with 30 mg being the most commonly used daily dose.[66]

Fluoroquinolones

Most fluoroquinolones are moderately lipophilic drugs with penetration into the CSF in the absence of meningeal inflammation is much higher than that of β-lactam antibiotics. Fluoroquinolones are of great value for the treatment of CNS infections by gram-negative aerobic bacilli (ciprofloxacin).[67] Since several fluoroquinolones enter the CNS readily, intrathecal injections of fluoroquinolones are unnecessary.

Chloramphenicol

Chloramphenicol, a small inhibitor of bacterial protein synthesis, is active against a variety of bacteria and readily enters the CSF. It has been used extensively in the last decades for the treatment of bacterial meningitis. In industrialized countries, chloramphenicol is restricted mostly to topical uses because of the risk of induction of aplastic anemia. However, it remains a valuable reserve antibiotic for patients with allergy to β-lactam antibiotics or with CNS infections caused by multiresistant pathogens.

Macrolides

Macrolide antibiotics are basic highly lipophilic compounds. they do not reach sufficient CSF concentrations in the absence of meningeal inflammation. Due to a lack of bactericidal activity in experimental *S. pneumoniae* meningitis, their role in the treatment of CNS infections is limited to *Mycoplasma* sp. and *Legionella pneumophila* encephalitis.

Tetracyclines and Tigecycline

Among tetracyclines, experience for the treatment of CNS infections is greatest with doxycycline. The lipophilic drug doxycycline is readily absorbed after oral application (> 80%). Its protein binding is > 80%, and its elimination half-life is long, ranging from 12 to 25 hours.[55] The CSF penetration is approximately 0.2 in both the absence and the presence of meningeal inflammation. Since daily doses of 200 mg produce CSF concentrations close to the MICs for susceptible bacteria, the daily dose has been increased up to 400 mg. The new glycylcycline tigecycline reaches CSF concentrations of approximately 10% of those found in serum with uninflamed meninges.[69] Penetration of tigecycline into the CSF of patients with uninflamed meninges is minimal, with mean CSF concentrations of about 0.015 µg/ml (concomitant serum concentration 0.306 µg/ml) at 90 min after a single 100 mg intravenous dose.[69]

Oxazolidinones

Linezolid, the first oxazolidinone, which is active against gram-positive bacteria, has amphiphilic properties, has excellent activity against virtually all important gram-positive pathogens, including methicillin-resistant staphylococci, penicillin-resistant pneumo-cocci, macrolide-resistant streptococci, and vancomycin-resistant enterococci.[70] It readily enters the CSF with an AUCCSF/AUCS ratio close to 1. Although primarily bacteriostatic, linezolid has been employed successfully for CNS infections caused by multiresistant organisms.

Metronidazole

Metronidazole is a small lipophilic compound that is active against most anaerobic bacteria penetrating well into most tissues, including abscess contents. In animal studies, metro-nidazole readily penetrated the blood-CSF/

blood–brain barrier, and data regarding the entry into human CSF and brain abscess confirmed this finding. Metronidazole is part of the standard therapy of bacterial brain abscess.

Sulfonamides and Trimethoprim

Sulfonamides and trimethoprim are small lipophilic antibiotics. The penetration of sulfamethoxazole, sulfadiazine, and trimethoprim into the CSF in both the absence and the presence of meningeal inflammation is higher than the penetration of β-lactam antibiotics and aminoglycosides.[55] At high doses, these agents have qualified for the treatment of CNS infections with susceptible bacteria (e.g. *Listeria monocytogenes*, *Nocardia asteroides*, and *Stenotrophomonas maltophilia*) but also with fungi and parasites (e.g. paracoccidioidomycosis and toxoplasmosis).[55] Bone marrow toxicity can limit increases of the daily dose or the duration of treatment.

Glycopeptides

Glycopeptides (vancomycin, teicoplanin) are hydrophilic. Although not as toxic as aminoglycosides on kidneys and the inner ear, toxicity is still high enough to limit an increase of the dose. For patients with good CSF penetration with inflamed meninges, bactericidal CSF concentrations of vancomycin against susceptible pathogens are reached during high intravenous doses. The efficacy of local administration of vancomycin in the treatment of staphylococcal ventriculitis may be attributed to achieving drug concentrations as high as 300 to 800 µg/ml, while by systemic application peak values of 6 µg/ml are not exceeded,[71,72] however, results show that the microbicidal effect reaches a maximum at 5 to 10 µg/ml and cannot be improved by concentrations exceeding that.

Similarly, in adults after severe head trauma receiving for 500 mg doses of vancomycin/day, drug concentrations in the cerebral interstitial space measured by microdialysis 5 to 6 h after dosing were ≤1.2 mg/liter, or approximately 8% of the corresponding serum concentrations, whereas mean subcutaneous tissue levels were 43% of the serum concentrations.[55]

Because of its strong binding to plasma proteins, teicoplanin penetration into the CSF is lower than that of vancomycin. For this reason, it has been administered to treat CNS infections in rare cases only. Successful intrathecal administration of teicoplanin has been reported.

Daptomycin

Daptomycin is the first compound of a new class of antibiotics, the cyclic lipopeptides. In an animal model of meningitis, the mean CSF penetration was 6%, and the compound was rapidly bactericidal. Daptomycin shows activity against a wide range of gram-positive organisms including both drug-susceptible and multidrug-resistant staphylococci and is rapidly bactericidal for these species, both in vitro and *in vivo*.[73–76] Some bactericidal antibiotics, most notably β-lactams, cause bacterial cells to lyse. This can be potentially harmful, as it may release bacterial endotoxins and other inflammatory cell components into the circulation, triggering cytokine cascades and potentially leading to septic shock and multiple organ failure.[76–78] Daptomycin kills bacteria with negligible cell lysis, thereby reducing this risk.[79] Minimizing the release of bacterial cell components may be a means of improving outcome in patients with serious infections.[78] Bactericidal activity *in vitro* in contrast to other classes of bactericidal antibiotics, the rapid bactericidal activity of daptomycin does not require cell division or active metabolism, and daptomycin retains bactericidal activity against non-growing *S. aureus* cells under a variety of physiological conditions.[79] However, the importance of this in clinical therapy requires further investigation. The bactericidal activities of daptomycin, vancomycin, linezolid and quinupristin/dalfopristin against MRSA and VISA have been compared *in vitro* using time-kill studies.[80,81] Daptomycin had bactericidal

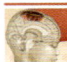
activity equal to or greater than the other agents against all organisms tested, killing 3 log 10 cfu/ml by 8 hours. Cha et al[82] used pharmacodynamic modelling to characterize the relationship between daptomycin exposure and bactericidal activity *in vitro* against MRSA, GISA and VRE isolates. Simulated daptomycin doses of 3–7 mg/kg once daily showed rapid and pronounced bactericidal activity against these multidrug-resistant strains.[83,84] Successful treatment of ventriculitis with intrathecal administration of 10 mg followed by 5 mg daptomycin every third day was reported, and high peak and trough CSF levels were measured.

Polypeptides

Polypeptides consist of large hydrophilic compounds with a high systemic toxicity.[63,64] For the treatment of CNS infections, the majority of data have been gathered with colistin. Colistin is used for the treatment of carbapenem-resistant *Acinetobacter* sp. CNS infections in children and adults. In the absence and presence of ventriculitis, CSF penetration of colistin is poor. The CSF-to-serum concentration ratios were 0.051 to 0.057 and 0.16. Because the relatively high toxicity after IV administration does not allow an increase of the systemic daily dose, colistin is frequently administered intrathecally (Table 35.6).

As indicated in the section on microbiology, one can consider two broad clinical groups in order to determine the effective empirical antibiotic regime.

In the group having meningitis secondary to CSF fistulae or internal compounding, the likely organisms indicated would likely respond to a third generation cephalosporin and an aminoglycoside together with metronidazole. Of these three, metronidazole and the third generation cephalosporin have excellent CSF penetration, and are quite effective.

For the group having penetrating or external compound injuries, a better empiric

choice of antibiotics would be a combination of vancomycin (or a penicillinase resistant penicillin) and a third-generation cephalosporin with good activity even against *Pseudomonas* organisms (such as ceftazidime).[85,86]

The clinical response should be closely monitored and results of CSF cultures obtained as soon as possible. One should convert to the specific antibiotic therapy quickly in adequately high doses. Curtailing the duration of broad-spectrum antibiotics would also help in preventing the rapid development of resistance in these organisms. The duration of the antibiotic therapy should be at least 14 days, and should continue till at least 7 days after defervescence.[54,85] Gram-negative bacillary meningitis requires antibiotics to be continued at least 2 weeks beyond sterilization of CSF.[8]

The Infectious Diseases Society of America (IDSA) guideline recommendations for duration are given in Table 35.5.[50]

Non-responding patients should be evaluated with contrast CT to exclude pus collection elsewhere (such as abscess or subdural empyema). If present, these should be drained. Repeat CSF analysis should also be done, so as to ascertain the response of antibiotics on the cytological and biochemical CSF parameters (decline in cell counts, rise in sugar levels also to repeat CSF cultures and evaluate for other unusual pathogens causing meningitis solely or in combination.

Table 35.5: Duration of antimicrobial therapy for bacterial meningitis based on isolated pathogen (A-III)[50]

Microorganism	Duration of therapy, days
Neisseria meningitidis	7
Haemophilus influenzae	7
Streptococcus pneumoniae	10–14
Streptococcus agalactiae	14–21
Aerobic gram-negative bacilli[a]	21
Listeria monocytogenes	>21

[a] Duration in the neonate is 2 weeks beyond the first sterile CSF culture of > 3 weeks, whichever is longer

Table 35.6: Intraventricular application of antibiotics to reach effective concentrations within the CNS[55]

Antibiotic	Dose for adults	Severe reported side effect(s)
Gentamicin	5 mg every 24 h	Hearing loss (temporary), epileptic seizures, aseptic meningitis, eosinophilic CSF pleocytosis
Tobramycin	5 mg every 24 h	Similar to those of gentamicin
Amikacin	30 mg every 24 h	Similar to those of gentamicin
Streptomycin	Up to 1 mg/kg every (24–48 h)	Hearing loss (temporary), epileptic seizures, radiculitis, transverse myelitis, arachnoiditis, paraplegia
Vancomycin	5–20 mg every 24 h	Hearing loss (temporary)
Colistin (polymyxin E) methane sulfonate (12,500 IU = 1 mg)	10 (1.6–20) mg every 24 h	Meningeal inflammation; with high doses, epileptic seizures, loss of appetite, agitation, eosinophilia, edema, pain, albuminuria
Daptomycin	5–10 mg every 72 h	Fever
Amphotericin B	0.1–0.5 mg every 24 h	Tinnitus, fever, shivering, Parkinson syndrome

Symptomatic and Adjunctive Measures

Antipyretics, analgesics and hydrotherapy may be required for the control of fever. Anticonvulsants are indicated from the point of view of head injury, or if patient has a seizure during the illness.

Corticosteroids have been shown to have a role in preventing the development of sensorineural deafness in children with meningitis due to *H. influenzae*.[87] However, routine use in children is still controversial.[88] Some reports suggest that the use of corticosteroids may be beneficial in adults with pneumococcal meningitis,[89] high CSF bacterial load and in those with high CSF pressure.[20]

Adjunctive surgical measures may be indicated in the following clinical situations:
1. Hydrocephalus (requiring ventricular drainage)
2. Development of subdural empyema or abscess
3. Persistent hydrocephalus after successful treatment of meningitis
4. Treatment of the cause.

Treatment of Cause

The underlying cause if managed optimally would in fact prevent the occurrence of meningitis in the first place. Adequate debridement and removal of foreign material in compound head injuries and proper management of CSF fistulas would certainly help in this regard.

CSF fistulas need specific operative management in case the leak persists more than 7–10 days after injury, or if there is another episode of meningitis. Even a single episode of delayed meningitis is considered an indication for undertaking operative obliteration of the fistula.

The overall management strategy for post-traumatic brain abscesses has undergone changes, but controversies still abound as to the best initial treatment for these patients and whether solely conservative treatment has any role at all.

The best treatment of post-traumatic abscess is still its prevention. Compound injuries need to be treated with adequate debridement, all foreign material must removed and proper dural closure done, together with prophylactic antibiotics.

Treatment with antibiotics is certainly an important part of the overall regime. In fact, Sandermann et al.[90] advocated that as the sole treatment for post-traumatic abscesses. It has been realized that antibiotics in general penetrate the blood–brain barrier poorly. In fact, they may be able to reach therapeutically important levels in the abscess only in the presence of cerebritis and hyperemia.[91–94] In this regard, another finding has been that clinical response may be lacking despite higher-than-MIC concentrations of antibiotics in the abscess pus presumably owing to unfavorable local factors such as local pH and bacterial load.[95]

The first report of successful conservative treatment of brain abscesses was by Heinemann and Braude,[96] who treated 6 patients.[96] However, all the lesions were in the cerebritis stage. Other studies[90–93,97] followed. Sandermann and Colleagues[90] considered surgical options such as aspiration or excision only in extreme situations of raised intracranial pressure. In an analysis of 67 cases of conservatively treated encapsulated abscesses reported in literature, Rosenblum and colleagues[98,99] demonstrated that the mean diameter of abscesses that responded to medical treatment was 1.7 centimeters and no abscess larger than 2.5 centimeters responded to medical treatment alone. Another important result of this study was that in as many as 28% patients, there was no certainty of diagnosis. This fact is important as many lesions can mimic the ring-enhancing appearance of an abscess. Further, a totally conservative approach does not allow us to identify the organism or its particular antibiotic sensitivity. In fact, if a purely medical approach does not yield results, even later conversion to a surgical approach may preclude this identification owing to broad-spectrum empiric antimicrobial therapy.

At the present time, with availability of precise localization techniques and low risk for aspiration performed under local anesthesia, there is little justification for purely medical treatment of an abscess. Possible exceptions are an uncontrolled bleeding diathesis, or a deep seated or small lesion (less than 1.5 cm) in a neurologically intact patient. These situations are rarely encountered in brain abscesses following trauma. For multiple abscesses (rarely seen after trauma), antibiotics can be used for the smaller lesions if a culture has been obtained after aspiration from the larger one or from any of the lesions.[99]

Surgical Treatment

Surgical options seem to have some evident advantages. Indication for surgery are summarized in Table 35.7. Surgery achieves rapid decompression, which may be of crucial importance in patients with raised intracranial pressure. At the same time, it enables us to identify the fending organism and subject it to sensitivity testing. Occasionally, this may completely alter the antibiotic regimen when a typical organisms are cultured such as Nocardiae[39] or Fungi.[38]

Two broad surgical options exist: aspiration of the abscess and excision. With availability of ultrasonic or stereotaxic (frame based or frameless) guidance, aspiration has become even for smaller lesions and those located in functionally dense regions. Additionally, one can target the desired lesion in case there are multiple abscesses or take a biopsy of tissue even in the cerebritis stage (when an open procedure may be more hazardous). Aspiration is likely to succeed if there is no retained foreign body, the pus is of fluid consistency, there is a single locule, and the wall is thin. All these increase the likelihood of the penetration of antibiotics, drainage of a significant amount of purulent material with probability of collapse of abscess walls. With precise

Table 35.7: Indications for surgery
1. Abscess containing foreign material[36]
2. Abscess containing gas (CSF fistula or gas-producing organisms)[35]
3. Abscess with concomitant CSF fistula[35]
4. Abscess following operation for closed head injury[8,27]
5. Cerebellar abscess (failure of decompression may be fatal)[48]
6. Abscess caused by fungi[48]

localization and performance of the procedure under local anesthesia, the surgical risk is quite low.

Excision may entail a slightly higher surgical morbidity, but has definite advantages in many situations. Overall, there is a general opinion that post-traumatic abscesses should more often be subjected to excision rather than aspiration.[8,27] In the study from our institution, 14 patients were initially managed with aspiration of the abscess. This was sufficient in only 3, as 8 patients required excision of the abscess and remaning 3 required repeated aspirations.[27] Excision should be strongly considered as the primary modality of surgical treatment in the following situations:

In addition, abscesses may need to be secondarily excised:

1. No response to antibiotics and aspiration attempts
2. Hematoma following attempted abscess aspiration
3. Non-improvement in clinical condition after aspiration (e.g. after aspiration of a temporal abscess in a comatose patient).

Patients with abscesses rupturing into the ventricular system may require the use of an external ventricular drain till the infection subsides.

Use of Anticonvulsants and Steroids

Majority of the patients would already be on anticonvulsant treatment given the background of prior significant head injury. Some may have uncontrolled seizures, requiring multiple anti-epileptic drugs. In a study by Legg et al[68] 72% of their patients reported seizures when followed up without anticonvulsants. This indicates the rationale of routinely prescribing anticonvulsants to all patients with post-traumatic brain abscesses. There may be a beneficial response as regards seizure frequency after excision, but intractable cases would require formal evaluation to spatially define the epileptogenic focus, and subsequently may have to undergo excision of the focus.

Steroids should be used only in situations where the edema surrounding the abscess poses a danger to the survival of the patient, and then too, for the shortest permissible duration. Though the steroids lessen edema, their effect on lessening both the degree and extent of encapsulation[35] may increase the amount of adjacent tissue destruction.

REFERENCES

1. Kaufman BA, Tunkel AR, Pry or JC, et al. Meningitis in the neurosurgical patient. Inf Dis Clin N Am 1990;4:677–01.
2. Leech PJ, Patterson A. Conservative and operative management for cerebrospinal fluid leakage after closed head injury. Lancet 1973;1013–16.
3. Tenney JH. Bacterial infections of the central nervous system in neurosurgery. Neurol Clin 1986;4:91–114.
4. Mincy JE. Post-traumatic cerebrospinal fluid fistula at the frontal fossa. J trauma 1966;6:618–22.
5. Raaf J. Post-traumatic cerebrospinal fluid leaks. Arch Surg 1967;95:648–51.
6. Durack DT, Perfect JR. Acute bacterial meningitis. In: Rengachary SS and Wilkins RH(eds.): Neurosurgery, Vol. III. New York, McGraw-Hill Book Company 1985;1921–8.
7. Durand ML, Calderwood SB, Weber DJ, et al. Acute bacterial meningitis in adults: A review of 493 episodes. N Engl J Med 1993;328:21–28.
8. Gormley WB, del Busto R, Saravolatz LD, Rosenblum ML. Cranial and intracranial bacterial infections. In: Youmans JR (ed.): Neurological Surgery, Vol. V. Philadelphia, WB Saunders Company, 1996;3195–3220.
9. Hirschmann JV. Bacterial meningitis following closed cranial trauma. In: Sande MA, Smith AL, Root RK (eds.): Bacterial meningitis. New York, Churchill Livingstone 1985;95–103.
10. French GL; Bactericidal agents in the treatment of MRSA infections—the potential role of daptomycin Journal of Antimicrobial Chemotherapy 2006;58:1107–17.
11. Kallel H, Chelly H, Ghorbel M, Bahloul M, Ksibi H, Rekik N, Ben Mansour H, Bouaziz M. Posttraumatic meningitis: incidence, bacteriology, and outcomes, Neurochirurgie. [Article in French] 2006 Nov;52:397–406.

12. BR Plaisier, CJ Yowler, WF Fallon, MJ Likavec, JS Anderson, MA Malangoni: Post-traumatic Meningitis: Risk Factors, Clinical Features, Bacteriology, and Outcome. The Internet Journal of Neurosurgery. 2005 Volume 2 Number 1.

13. Korinek AM, Baugnon T, Golmard JL, van Effenterre R, Coriat P, Puybasset L. Risk factors for adult nosocomial meningitis after craniotomy: role of antibiotic prophylaxis. Neurosurgery. 2006;59:126–33. discussion 126–33. [PubMed]

14. Kourbeti IS, Jacobs AV, Koslow M, Karabetsos D, Holzman RS. Risk factors associated with postcraniotomy meningitis. Neurosurgery. 2007;60:317–25. discussion 325–26. [PubMed]

15. Federico G, Tumbarello M, Spanu T, et al. Risk factors and prognostic indicators of bacterial meningitis in a cohort of 3580 postneurosurgical patients. Scand J Infect Dis 2001;33:533–37.

16. Sponsel C, Park JW. Recurrent pneumococcal meningitis. Search for occult skull fracture. Postgrad Med 1994;95:109–110.

17. Mantur M, Lukaszewicz-Zajac M, Mroczko B, Kulakowska A, Ganslandt O, Kemona H, Szmitkowski M, Drozdowski W, Zimmermann R, Kornhuber J, Lewczuk P. Cerebrospinal fluid leakage—reliable diagnostic methods. Clin Chim Acta. 2011 May 12;412(11–12):837–40.

18. Kaplan SL, Feign RD. Clinical presentations, prognostic factors and diagnosis of bacterial meningitis. In Sande MA, Smith AL, Root RK(eds): Bacterial meaningitis. New York, Churchill Livingstone, 1985;83–94.

19. Wilson CB, Smith AL. Rapid tests for the diagnosis of bacterial meningitis. In : Remington JS, Swartz MN: Current clinical topics in infectious diseases, Vol. 7. New York, McGraw-Hill, 1986;134–56.

20. Rath SA, Knoringer P. Late abscess after severe craniocerebral trauma with fronto-orbital fracture. Childs Nerv Syst 1989;5:121–3.

21. Jennett B, Miller JD. Infection after depressed fractures: Implications for management of non-missile injury. J Neurosurg 1972;36:333–39.

22. deTribolet N, Guiguard G, Zander E. Brain abscess after intracranial penetration of a paint brush. Surg Neurol 1979;11:187–9.

23. Bhatia R. Brain abscesses in children. Ind J Pediat 1983;50:91–597.

24. Rath SA, Knoringer P. Late abscess after severe craniocerebral trauma with fronto-orbital fracture. Childs Nerv Syst 1989;5:121–23.

25. Moskopp D. Septic brain abscess following closed craniocerebral trauma with steroid therapy. Neurochirurgia (Stuttg) 1985;28:147–51.

26. Carpenter J, Stapleton S, Holliman R. Retrospective analysis of 49 cases of brain abscess and review of the literature. Eur J Clin Microbiol Infect Dis. 2007 Jan;26:1–11.

27. Patir R, Sood S, Bhatia R. Post-traumatic brain abscess: Experience of 36 patients. Br J Neurosurg 1995;9:29–35.

28. Gillingham FJ. Neurosurgical experience in Northern Italy. Br J Surg. War Suppl no. 1: Wounds of the head. Bristol, John Wright and Sons, 1947;80–87.

29. Cairns H, Calvert CA, Daniel P, Northcroft GB. Complications of head wounds with special reference to infection. Br J Surg War Suppl no. 1: Wounds of the head. Bristol, John Wright and Sons, 1947;198–243.

30. Dinaker I, Rao B. Post-traumatic brain abscess. J Post Grad Med 1971;17:137–41.

31. Ewans W: Brain abscess, Pathology and Etiology. Lancet 1931;1:1231–5.

32. Kerr FW, King RB, Meagher JN. Brain abscess, a study of 47 consecutive cases. J Am Med Assoc 1958;168:868–72.

33. Webster JE, Gurdjian ES. The surgical management of intracranial suppuration. Surg Gynec Obst 1950;90:209–34.

34. Gurdjian ES, Webster JE. Experiences in the surgical management of intracranial suppuration. Surg Gynec Obst 1957;104:205–14.

35. Young RF, Frazee J. Gas within intracranial abscess cavities: An indication for surgical excision. Ann Neurol 1984;16:35–39.

36. Osenbach RK, Loftus CM. Diagnosis and management of brain abscess. Neurosurg Clin North Am 1992;3:403–20.

37. Sabel M, Felsberg J, Messing-Junger M, Neuen-Jakob E, Piek J. Glioblastoma multiforme at the site of metallic splinter injury: A coincidence? Case report. J Neurosurg 1999;91:1041–4.

38. Tekkok IH, Higgins MJ, Ventureya EC. Post-traumatic gas containing brain abscess caused by Clostridium perfringens with unique simultaneous fungal suppuration by Myceliophthora thermophila: Case report. Neurosurgery 1996;39:1247–51.

39. Kepes JJ, Schoolman A. Post-traumatic abscess of the medulla oblongata containing Nocardia asteroides. J Neurosurg 1965;22:511–4.

40. Bert F, Ouahes O, Lambert-Zechovsky N. Brain abscess due to bacillus macerans following a penetrating periorbital injury. J Clin Microbiol 1995;33:1950–3.

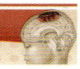

41. Mampalam TJ, Rosenblum ML. Trends in management of bacterial brain abscess: A review of 102 cases over 17 years. Neurosurgery 1988;23:451–8.

42. Marquardt G, Scick W, Moller-Hartmann W. Brain abscess decades after a penetrating shrapnel injury. Br J Neurosurg 1999;13:246–8.

43. Robinson EF, Moiel RH, Gol A. Brain abscess 36 years after head injury. Case report. J Neurosurg. 1968 Feb;28(2):166–168.

44. Foy P, Sharr M. Cerebral abscesses in children after pencil-tip injuries. Lancet 1980.

45. Grant FC. Post-traumatic brain abscess. In: Brock S (ed). Injuries of the brain and spinal cord. London, Cassel, I960, 4 (edn) 187–202.

46. Haimes AB, Zimmerman RD, Morgello S, et al. MR imaging of brain abscesses. AJNR 1989;10:279–91.

47. Sze G, Zimmerman RD. The magnetic resonance imaging of infections and inflammatory diseases. Radiol Clin North Am 1988;26:839–59.

48. Wispelwey B, Scheld WM. Brain abscess. In: Mandell CL, Douglas RG, Bennett JE (eds.): Principles and Practice of infectious disease. New York, Churchill Livingstone, 1990;777–88.

49. Britt RH. Brain abscess. In: Wilkins RH, Rengachary SS (eds.): Neurosurgery. New York, McGraw-Hill, 1985;1928–56.

50. Tunkel AR, Hartman BJ, Kaplan SL, Kaufman BA, Roos KL, Scheld WM, and Whitley RJ;Practice Guidelines for the Management of Bacterial Meningitis Clin Infect Dis. (2004) 39 (9):1267–84.doi: 10.1086/425368

51. Chang WN, Lu CH, Huang CR, et al. Clinical characteristics of post-neurosurgical Klebsiella pneumoniae meningitis in adults and a clinical comparison to the spontaneous form in a Taiwanese population. J Clin Neurosci 2010;17:334–8.

52. de Champs C, Guelon D, Joyon D, Sirot D, Chanal M, Sirot J. Treatment of a meningitis due to an Enterobacter aerogenes producing a derepressed cephalosporinase and a Klebsiella pneumoniae producing an extended-spectrum ?-lactamase. Infection 1991;19:181–3.

53. Tunkel AR, Kaufman BA. Cerebrospinal fluid shunt infections. In: Mandell GL,Bennett JE, Dolin R, editors. Principles and practice of infectious diseases. 6th ed.Philadelphia: Elsevier Science; 2004;1126–32.

54. Roos KL, Tunkel AR, Scheld WM. Acute bacterial meningitis in children and adults. In: Scheld WM, Whitley RJ, Durack DT(eds.): Infections of the central nervous system. New York, Raven Press, 1991;335–410.

55. Roland Nau,Fritz Sörgel, and Helmut Eiffert; Penetration of Drugs through the Blood-Cerebrospinal Fluid/Blood-Brain Barrier for Treatment of Central Nervous System Infections, Clin Microbiol Rev. 2010;23:858–83.

56. Quagliarello VJ, A. Ma, H. Stukenbrok, and G. E. Palade. 1991. Ultrastructural localization of albumin transport across the cerebral microvasculature during experimental meningitis in the rat. J. Exp. Med 174;657–672.

57. Roberts JA, and J Lipman. 2009. Pharmacokinetic issues for antibiotics in the critically ill patient. Crit Care Med 37;840–851, 859.

58. Scheld WM, RG Dacey, HR Winn, JE Welsh, JA Jane, and M. A. Sande. 1980. Cerebrospinal fluid outflow resistance in rabbits with experimental meningitis. Alterations with penicillin and methylprednisolone. J. Clin. Invest. 66;243–53. Kim BN, MD,1,3 Peleg AY, Lodise TP, Lipman J, Jian Li, Nation R and Paterson DL, Management of meningitis due to antibiotic-resistant Acinetobacterspecies, Lancet Infect Dis 2009;9: 245–55.

59. Maganti R, Jolin D, Rishi D, Biswas A. Nonconvulsive status epilepticus due to cefepime in a patient with normal renal function. Epilepsy Behav. 2006;8:312–14. [PubMed]

60. Martinez-Rodriguez JE, Barriga FJ, Santamaria J, et al. Nonconvulsive status epilepticus associated with cephalosporins in patients with renal failure. Am J Med. 2001;111:115–9.

61. Lodise TP, Nau R, Kinzig M, Drusano GL, Jones RN, Sorgel F. Pharmacodynamics of ceftazidime and meropenem in cerebrospinal fluid: results of population pharmacokinetic modelling and Monte Carlo simulation. J Antimicrob Chemother. 2007;60:1038–44. [PubMed].

62. Kendirli T, Aydin HI, Hacihamdioglu D, et al. Meningitis with multidrug-resistant Acinetobacter baumannii treated with ampicillin/sulbactam. J Hosp Infect 2004;56:328. [PubMed]

63. Bukhary Z, Mahmood W, Al-Khani A, Al-Abdely HM. Treatment of nosocomial meningitis due to a multidrug resistant *Acinetobacter* baumannii with intraventricular colistin. Saudi Med J 2005;26:656–58. [PubMed]

64. deFreitas DJ, McCabe JP. *Acinetobacter baumannii* meningitis: a rare complication of incidental durotomy. J Spinal Disord Tech. 2004;17:115–6. [PubMed]

65. Horiuchi M, Kimura M, Tokumura M, Hasebe N, Arai T, Abe K. Absence of convulsive liability of doripenem, a new carbapenem antibiotic, in

comparison with beta-lactam antibiotics. Toxicology 2006;222:114–24. [PubMed]

66. Tunkel AR, Hartman BJ, Kaplan SL, et al. Practice guidelines for the management of bacterial meningitis. Clin Infect Dis 2004;39:1267–84. [PubMed]

67. Sinner SW, Tunkel AR. Antimicrobial agents in the treatment of bacterial meningitis. Infect Dis Clin North Am. 2004;18:581-602. ix. [PubMed]. Lipman J, Allworth A, Wallis SC. Cerebrospinal fluid penetration of high doses of intravenous ciprofloxacin in meningitis. Clin Infect Dis. 2000;31:1131–3. [PubMed]

68. Legg NJ, Gupta PC, Scott OF. Epilepsy following cerebral abscess: A clinical and EEC study of 70 patients. Brain 1973;96:259–68.

69. Rodvold KA, Gotfried MH, Cwik M, Korth-Bradley JM, Dukart G, Ellis-Grosse EJ. Serum, tissue and body fluid concentrations of tigecycline after a single 100 mg dose. J Antimicrob Chemother. 2006;58:1221–29. [PubMed]

70. Moellering RC. Linezolid: the first oxazolidinone antimicrobial. Ann Intern Med. 2003;138:135–42.

71. Arroyo J C, Quindlen E A. Accumulation of vancomycin after intraventricular infusions. South Med J.1983;76:1554–5. [PubMed]

72. Bayston R, Hart C A, Barnicoat M. Intraventricular vancomycin in the treatment of ventriculitis associated with cerebrospinal fluid shunting and drainage. J Neurol Neurosurg Psychiatry 1987;50:1419–23.

73. Silverman JA, Oliver N, Andrew T, et al. Resistance studies with daptomycin. Antimicrob Agents Chemother 2001;45:1799–802.

74. Critchley IA, Blosser-Middleton RS, Jones ME et al. Baseline study to determine in vitro activities of daptomycin against gram-positive pathogens isolated in the United States in 2000–2001. Antimicrob Agents Chemother 2003; 47:1689–93.

75. Ginsburg I. The role of bacteriolysis in the pathophysiology of inflammation, infection and post-infectious sequelae. APMIS 2002; 110:753–70.

76. Nau R, Eiffert H. Modulation of release of proinflammatory bacterial compounds by antibacterials: potential impact on course of inflammation and outcome in sepsis and meningitis. Clin Microbiol Rev 2002;15:95–110.

77. Steenbergen JN, Alder J, Thorne GM et al. Daptomycin: a lipopeptide antibiotic for the treatment of serious gram-positive infections. J Antimicrob Chemother 2005;55:283–8.

78. Nau R, Eiffert H. Minimizing the release of proinflammatory and toxic bacterial products within the host: a promising approach to improve outcome in life-threatening infections. FEMS Immunol Med Microbiol 2005;44:1–16.

79. Mascio CTM, Alder J, Silverman JA. Bactericidal action of daptomycin (DAP) against non-dividing Staphylococcus aureus. In: Abstracts of the Forty-fifth Interscience Conference on Antimicrobial Agents and Chemotherapy, Washington, DC, 2005. Abstract E-1743, p. 174. American Society for Microbiology, Washington, DC, USA.

80. Lamp KC, Rybak MJ, Bailey EM et al. In vitro pharmacodynamic effects of concentration, pH, and growth phase on serum bactericidal activities of daptomycin and vancomycin. Antimicrob Agents Chemother 1992;36:2709–14.

81. Rybak MJ, Hershberger E, Moldovan T et al. In vitro activities of daptomycin, vancomycin, linezolid, and quinupristin-dalfopristin against staphylococci and enterococci, including vancomycin-intermediate and - resistant strains. Antimicrob Agents Chemother 2000;44:106–26.

82. Cha R, Grucz RG Jr, Rybak MJ. Daptomycin dose-effect relationship against resistant gram-positive organisms. Antimicrob Agents Chemother 2003;47:1598–603.

83. LaPlante KL, Rybak MJ. Impact of high-inoculum *Staphylococcus aureus* on the activities of nafcillin, vancomycin, linezolid, and daptomycin, alone and in combination with gentamicin, in an *in vitro* pharmacodynamic model. Antimicrob Agents Chemother 2004; 48:4665–72.

84. Lee BL, Sachdeva M, Chambers HF. Effect of protein binding of daptomycin on MIC and antibacterial activity. Antimicrob Agents Chemother 1991;35:2505–8.

85. Overturf GD. Bacterial meningitis. In: Hoeprich PD, Jordan MC, Ronald AR: Infectious diseases. Philadelphia, Lippincott Company, p-1111, 1994.

86. Rodriguez K, Kickinson GM, Greenman RL. Successful treatment of gram-negative bacillary meningitis with imipenem/cilastatin. South Med J 1985;78:731–2.

87. Lebel MH, Freij BJ, Syrogiannopoulos GA, et al. Dexamethasone therapy for bacterial meningitis: Results of two double-blind, placebo-controlled trials. N Engl J Med 1988;319:964–71.

88. Word BM, Klein JO. Therapy of bacterial sepsis and meningitis in infants and children: 1989 poll of directors of programs in pediatric infectious diseases. Ped Inf Dis J 1989;8:635–7.

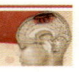

89. Girgis NI, Farid Z, Mikhail IA, et al. Dexamethasone treatment for bacterial meningitis in children and adults. Ped Inf Dis J 1989;8:848–851.

90. Sandermann JE, Harse J, Bartholdy NS, Udison H. Non-surgical treatment of brain abscesses in the child. Childs Nerv Syst 1986;2:49–51.

91. Donald f F, Ispahani P. Use of cefotaxime in brain abscess. Br J Neurosurg 1988;2:539–40.

92. George B, loux F, Pillon M, et al. Relevance of antibiotics in the treatment of brain abscesses: Report of a case with eight brain abscesses simultaneously treated and cured medically. Acta Neurochir (Wien) 1979;47:285–91.

93. Kammin M, Biddle D. Conservative management of focal intracerebral infections. Neurology 1981;31:103–06.

94. Levy RM. Gutin PH, Baskin DS, et al. Vancomycin penetration of a brain abscess: Case report and review of the literature Neurosurgery 1986;18:632–6.

95. Black PM, Graybill JR, Char ache P. Penetration of brain abscess by systemically administered antibiotics. J Neurosurgery 1973;38:705–09.

96. Heinemann HS, Braude Al : Intracranial suppurative disease. JAMA 1971;218:1542–7.

97. Rousseaux M, Lesion F, Destee A, et al. Developments in the treatment and prognosis of multiple cerebral abscesses. Neurosurgery 1985;16:304–08.

98. Rosenblum ML, Mampalam TJ, Pons V. Controversies in the management of brain abscess. Clin Neurosurg 1986;33:603–32.

99. Mamelak AN, Mampalam TJ, Rosenblum ML. Improved management of multiple brain abscesses: A combined surgical approach based on a review of 16 cases. Neurosurgery 1995;36:76–86.

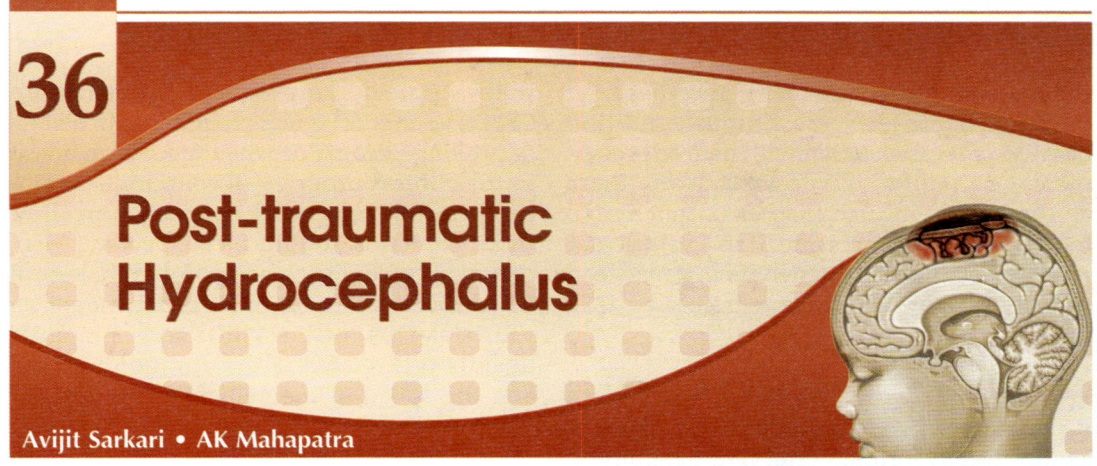

36

Post-traumatic Hydrocephalus

Avijit Sarkari • AK Mahapatra

INTRODUCTION

Post-traumatic hydrocephalus (PTH) is an active and progressive process of excessive intracranial cerebrospinal fluid (CSF) accumulation due to liquorodynamic disturbances following craniocerebral injury.[1]

PTH as a clinicopathologic entity has been recognized since Dandy's report in 1914.[2] It has been described with variable rates of incidence.[3,4] Recognition of PTH is often confounded by attributing the unresolved or added symptoms to the primary or secondary injury inflicted upon the brain by trauma. Established causes of secondary brain injury like cerebral edema, hypoxia, ischemia and infection running in the neurosurgeon's mind surrendering to an unfortunate fatalistic outcome often precludes early identification of this treatable cause of morbidity and mortality. Delayed dilatation of the ventricles may also be due to brain atrophy following head injury, which is of no consequence in long run and merits no specific treatment.

INCIDENCE

Incidence of PTH in world literature is quite variable, ranging from 0.7 to 29 %.[3–7] In many cases, initial brain damage leading to cerebral atrophy with secondary ventriculomegaly (hydrocephalus ex-vacuo) can give a false impression of PTH and if only CT finding of ventriculomegaly is taken into account, then the incidence rises to 30–88%.[8,9] Kishore et al[7] found that only 13.7% of patients with ventriculomegaly had PTH.[7] The incidence is higher after severe head injury (Table 36.1).

INCIDENCE OF PTH IN PEDIATRIC POPULATION

PTH is rare among children and has mainly been published as case reports, except neonatal hydrocephalus secondary to birth

Table 36.1: Incidence of post-traumatic hydrocephalus following severe head injury and outcome after diversion procedures

Study	Incidence of hydrocephalus in severe head injury	Favorable outcome
Cardoso et al (1985)[3]	0.7%	75%
Rodrigues et al (2000)[14]	2.4%	45.4%
Licata et al (2001)[18]	1%	56%
Bhatoe et al (2005)[19]	–	100%
Choi et al (2008)[27]	4%	55.4%
Sarkari et al (2010)[31]	4.9%	79%

trauma and intraventricular hemorrhage.[10,11] PTH in infants is a very serious condition because of its association with neurodevelopmental disability.[11] Hydrocephalus in these children may induce further parenchymal injury due to high pressure. If this ventricular enlargement is not treated in time, it may lead to cerebral damage not reversible by CSF diversion procedures.[11]

Clinical Presentation

PTH may present with various clinical syndromes including obtundation, failure to improve, psychomotor retardation, memory loss, gait ataxia and incontinence.[3,10] Prolonged coma or arrest in clinical progress in conscious patients should arouse suspicion of hydrocephalus. In such patients fundoscopy may reveal papilledema.[3,12] PTH commonly occurs in first year post-trauma and has been described as early as within 7 hours of injury.[3,13,14] Motor disturbances are primarily of gait. Often the patients who following head injury, may be improving slowly in terms of state of consciousness, stop improving or get worse, again becoming drowsy, lethargic or comatose with evidence of increasing intracranial pressure. Sometimes, the patient may be too injured to demonstrate clinical signs and symptoms of PTH, or may present with atypical symptoms.[10] According to Groswasser et al[5] when a patient is in a state of prolonged coma or when there is an arrest in the clinical progress in conscious craniocerebral injured patients, communicating hydrocephalus should be suspected. Also, chronic problem such as neuropsychological deficit in closed head injury is dependent on ventricular brain ratio (VBR)[15] and ventricular dilatation is related to the duration of coma and the speed of the vehicle at the time of injury.

PTH is a rare condition in children with birth trauma.[3,10,11,16] Intraventricular hemorrhage due to birth trauma is a frequent cause of hydrocephalus in preterm infants. Rapid enlargement of head size, inability to thrive and lethargy are the common features. Many of the infants do have evidence of secondary brain damage. However, it is difficult to determine neurological outcome and long-term neurodevelopmental disability.

Investigation

Non-contrast CT scan brain showing ventriculomegaly with periventricular lucencies is taken as radiological criteria of hydrocephalus (Fig. 36.1). This is to exclude ventriculomegaly due to loss of brain volume (hydrocephalus ex-vacuo). There is need for serial CT scan to

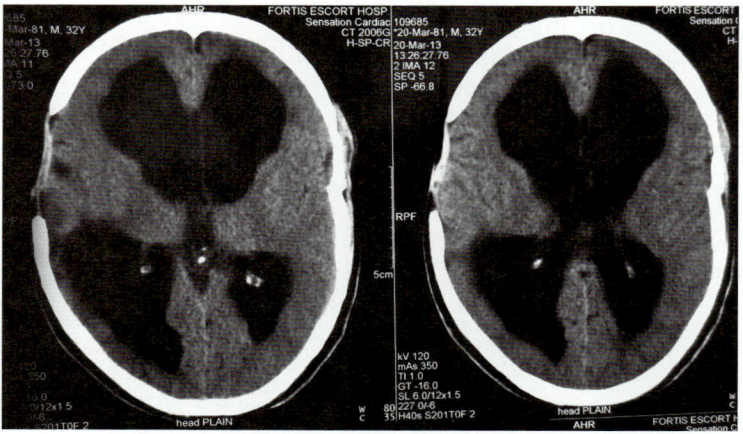

Fig. 36.1: Plain CT head: Development of hydrocephalus after severe head injury. Please note craniectomy of previous surgery

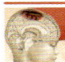

prove not only the progression of the ventricular size or ventricle brain ratio but also the association of periventricular lucency.[3,5,7, 8,11,16] Significant ventricular dilatation may require radionuclide cisternography.[8,10] Overnight intracranial pressure (ICP) recording, lumbar or ventricular infusion tests or even diagnostic lumbar puncture drainage are of importance in diagnosis of PTH especially if CT scan is inconclusive.[3,8,10,12] Some authors have suggested lumbar computerized infusion test to ascertain normal or low resistance to CSF outflow and degree of cerebral compliance.[17] In a study of 22 cases of severe head injury, Rodrigues et al did diagnostic lumbar puncture (LP) in all patients, which revealed an initial pressure of more than 180 cm of H_2O in all the 22 patients.[14]

Pathology

CT scan findings at time of initial trauma have been described with variable rates of incidence of findings.[3,8,14,18–21] (Table 36.2) Subarachnoid hemorrhage (SAH) has been cited as the most important pathology leading to development of PTH.[3,10,20–22] Increase in outflow resistance and CSF pressure in experimental rats

following subarachnoid infusion of plasma or whole blood has been found.[22] Subarachnoid spaces in patients dying after head injury and hydrocephalus are obliterated with fibrosis. Ependymal destruction and presence of subependymal gliosis together with loss of white matter especially around the ventricles are also found. In patients dying soon after subarachnoid hemorrhage, RBCs but little fibrin are visualized in the drainage channel within arachnoid granulations.[23] To what extent fibrosis and obliteration of the subarachnoid granulations[24] or that of the subarachnoid space are contributory factors in the late onset of PTH following subarachnoid hemorrhage is unknown.[25] Obliteration of subarachnoid spaces with fibrous thickening of leptomeninges particularly in sulci of the convexity and base of brain as a result of SAH has been suggested.[26]

Subdural hematoma,[27] intraventricular hemorrhage,[14] diffuse edema and cerebral contusion[19] have been found as the most common CT findings in other studies. In PTH due to subarachnoid and intraventricular blockage, the dilated ventricles cause raised intracranial pressure, which has to be relieved at the earliest to prevent further brain damage.[3] Posterior fossa contusions and blood in the fourth ventricles may also manifest as acute obstructive hydrocephalus.[28,29] Hydrocephalus may be seen acutely in the presence of intracerebral hematoma causing obstruction to CSF flow by mass effect. Communicating hydrocephalus with rapidly enlarging ventricles may develop within hours of severe head injury.[13] Grcevic[29] in 1983, reported an unususal case in whom tear of tela choroidea, followed by intraventricular bleed and SAH

Table 36.2: CT scan findings	
Study	Most common CT scan finding
Black PM et al (1984)[10]	SAH
Rodrigues et al (2000)[14]	IVH
Foroglou et al (1972)[26]	SAH
Bhatoe et al (2005)[19]	Diffuse cerebral edema and contusion
Choi et al (2008)[27]	SDH
Sarkari et al (2010)[31]	Contusion and SAH

Table 36.3: PTH etiology		
Obstructive	Communicative	
A. Acute	• IVH	• SAH
	• Posterior fossa hematomas	
B. Chronic	• Gliosis of aqueduct	• Post-craniectomy
	• Ventriculitis due to EVD	• Meningitis
		• SAH

leading to impairment of CSF absorption and communicating hydrocephalus. Supratentorial clot can lead to acute hydrocephalus of the contralateral ventricle.[3] Meningitis following head injury can lead to communicating hydrocephalus (Table 36.3).

DECOMPRESSIVE CRANIECTOMY AS A CAUSATIVE FACTOR FOR PTH

Decompressive craniectomy (DC) has been found to be associated with development of PTH[3,12,18,20,30] (Figs 36.2a and b) by altering CSF pressure dynamics, mechanical blockage around convexities[26] or inflammation of arachnoid granulations by post-surgical debris.[30] Choi et al found incidence of PTH to be 26% in cases of severe head injury management by decompressive craniectomy as compared to 2.4% in those managed conservatively.[27] In the study by Sarkari et al, PTH was found to occur in 17.7% of cases of decompressive craniectomy as against 4.9% cases managed conservatively.[31] It has been found that decompressive craniectomy leads to flattening of normally dicrotic ICP waveforms due to transmission of pressure pulse through the open cranium.[30] Since arachnoid granulations function as pressure-dependent one-way valves from subarachnoid space to draining venous sinuses, the disruption of pulsatile ICP dynamics results in decreased CSF outflow. Hence, early cranioplasty should lead to restoration of normal intracranial pressure dynamics and spontaneous resolution of hydrocephalus. Higher incidence of PTH has been found with extended DC and re-operation.[27]

Management

In patients with obstructive hydrocephalus, ventriculoperitoneal (VP) shunting is the procedure of choice.[3,14,19,22,32] In these cases, CSF diversion by VP shunt is a simple, cheap and effective therapeutic option. Following the shunting procedure, conscious patients have relief from headache. There is improvement in cognitive functions—some show rapid and complete regression of cognitive impairment, while others show slow improvement over a period of weeks or months.

In communicating hydrocephalus, repeated lumber punctures or even lumboperitoneal shunt is a good enough treatment.[14] However, there is higher risk of lumboperitoneal shunt malfunction as compared to VP shunt.

In acute hydrocephalus and in patients suspected of having meningitis, an external ventricular drainage (EVD)[14,28] should be done as a temporizing procedure followed by VP

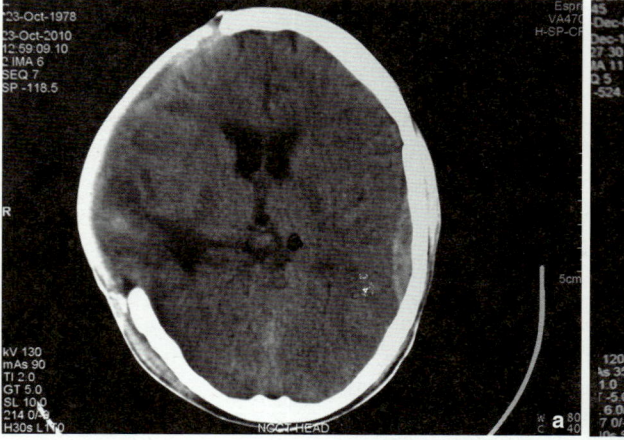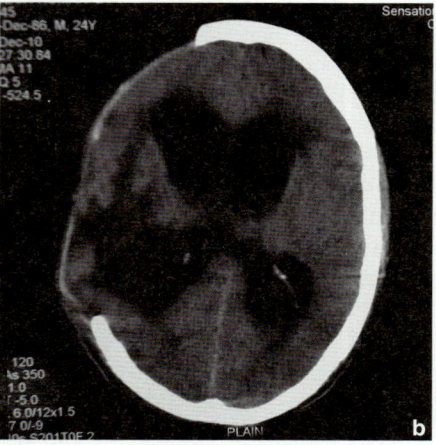

Figs 36.2a and b: CT showing development of severe ventriculomegaly following decompressive craniectomy

shunt. Fleischer et al[28] reported two cases of intraventricular hemorrhage with acute obstructive hydrocephalus, among them ventriculostomy resulted in complete recovery in one patient, while the second patient required ventriculostomy followed by VP shunt after sometime. Placement of Ommaya reservoir is another alternative to ventriculostomy, as there is a higher incidence of ventriculitis in patients with ventriculostomy as compared to insertion of Ommaya reservoir. Both the procedure may ultimately require VP shunt.

In the study by Rodrigues et al,[14] among the 22 patients, 9 (40.9%) underwent medium pressure Codman Medos VP shunts as a primary procedure, 4 patients underwent VP shunt after an initial external ventricular drain (EVD) insertion to clear the blood stained CSF. Five patients with intraventricular hemorrhage had an initial Ommaya reservoir inserted followed by a medium pressure VP shunt insertion. Among the 4 patients with traumatic subarachnoid hemorrhage, 2 of the patients underwent repeated LPs and improved; one had a thecoperitoneal shunt performed. Lumboperitoneal shunt was good enough to relieve raised ICP.

Outcome

Outcome of the treatment for PTH depends upon several factors. Significant factors are age of the patient, cause of hydrocephalus, degree of ventricular dilatation, associated parenchymal damage and condition of the patient. Patients in coma, neonates with intraventricular hemorrhage, and patients with significant brain damage fair badly.[11,16,32] With proper diagnosis and timely performed shunting procedure, good outcome is reported in 45–80% of cases.[3,14,31,33,34] Rarely, ventriculostomy may result in good outcome in patient with acute hydrocephalus due to intraventricular hemorrhage.[28] Overall effectiveness of shunt depends upon evidence of increased ICP. In patients with no raised ICP or asymptomatic ventriculomegaly, shunting procedures are likely to fail.[34]

AIIMS EXPERIENCE

Thirty-eight patients of radiologically diagnosed post-traumatic hydrocephalus underwent ventriculoperitoneal shunting from January 2009 to April 2010.[31] Thirty patients (78%) showed improvement in clinical features after ventriculoperitoneal shunting. Two cases (5%) had no improvement and six (15%) died. The cause of death in 3 patients was uncontrolled septicemia and ventilator associated pneumonia. In other 3 cases, the cause of death was ventriculitis and uncontrolled infection which could not be resolved despite attempts to either revise or exteriorize the shunt or Ommaya reservoir placement. Overall, shunt infection occurred in 5 (12.8%) cases, and blockade in 2 (5%) cases. In these 7 cases (18.4%), shunt revision was done.

CONCLUSIONS

PTH is a treatable complication of head injury with a favorable outcome. It should thus be aggressively sought for and managed. PTH can occur even in mild head injuries. It has a variable period of presentation after initial injury. Clinical features vary widely in individuals and in comatose patients, diagnosis is difficult. Its resemblance with hydrocephalus ex-vacuo can be confounding on CT scans. It is usually lost in oblivion due to other causes of neurological deterioration or lack of progress keeping the neurosurgeon obsessed.

Ventricular dilatation following severe head injury is the result of cerebral atrophy, however, patients do develop PTH, which needs surgical procedure. Baring acute hydrocephalus, due to intraventricular hemorrhage or posterior fossa hematoma, PTH by and large develops three to eight weeks following injury. A careful evaluation is necessary to establish PTH and to determine the need for shunting procedure. When shunt is performed in patients with proper indications, good results are reported in 45–80% cases. Patients with birth trauma, significant primary or secondary damage or patients with coma, do badly, even if shunts are performed with proper indications.

REFERENCES

1. Loshakov VA, Iusef ES, Likhterman LB, Kravchuk AD, Shcherbakova E, Tissen TP, et al. The diagnosis and surgical treatment of post-traumatic hydrocephalus. Zh Vopr Neirokhir Im N N Burdenko 1993;18–22.

2. Dandy W, Blackfan KD. Internal hydrocephalus. An experimental, clinical and pathological study. Am J Dis Child 1914;8:406–82.

3. Cardoso ER, Galbraith S. Post-traumatic hydrocephalus—A retrospective review. Surg Neurol 1985;23:261–4.

4. Hawkins TD, Lloyd AD, Fletcher GI, Hanka R. Ventricular size following head injury : A clinico radiological study. Clin Radiol 1976;27:279–89.

5. Groswasser Z, Cohen M, Reider-Groswasser I, Stern MJ. Incidence, CT findings and rehabilitation outcome of patient with communicative hydrocephalus following severe head injury. Brain Injury 1988;2:267–72.

6. Guyot LL, Micheal DD. Post traumatic hydrocephalus. Neurol Res 2000;22:25–8.

7. Kishore PR, Lipper MH, Miller JD, Giravendulis AK, Becker DP, Vines FS. Post traumatic hydrocephalus in patients with severe head injury. Neuro Radiol 1978;16:261–5.

8. Gudeman SK, Kishore PR, Becker DP, et al. Computed tomography in the evaluation of incidence and significance of post-traumatic hydrocephalus. Radiology 1981;141:397–402.

9. Philippon J, George B, Visot A, Cophignon J. Postoperative hydrocephalus. Neurochirurgie 1976;22:111–7.

10. Beyerl B, Black PM. Post-traumatic hydrocephalus. Neurosurg 1984;15:257–61.

11. Du Plessis AJ. Post hemorrhagic hydrocephalus and brain injury in the preterm infant: dilemma in diagnosis and management. Seminar in Ped Neurol 1998;5:161–79.

12. Phuenpathom N, Ratanalert S, Saeheng S, Sripairojkul B. Post-traumatic hydrocephalus: experience in 17 consecutive cases. J Med Assoc Thai 1999;82:46–53.

13. Takagi H, Tamaki Y, Morii S, Ohwada T. Rapid enlargement of ventricles within seven hours after head injury. Surg Neurol 1981;16:103–5.

14. Rodrigues D, Sharma RR, Sousa J, Pawar SJ, Mahapatra AK, Lad SD. Post-traumatic hydro-cephalus in severe head injuryseries of 22 cases. Pan Arab J Neurosurg 2000;4:63–7.

15. Levin HS, Meyers CA, Grossman RG, Sarwar M. Ventricular enlargement after closed head injury. Arch Neurol 1981;38:623–9.

16. Brye S, Zlomaniec J, Gradzinski S, Kaluzynski F. Post-traumatic hydrocephalus in children in CT image. Ann Univ Manae Curie SK Odowska 1993;48:163–78.

17. Czosnyka M, Copeman J, Czosnyka Z, et al. Post-traumatic hydrocephalus. Influence of craniectomy on the CSF circulation. J. Neurol Neurosurg Psychiat 2000;68:216–8.

18. Licata C, Cristofori L, Gambin R, Vivenza C, Turazzi S. Posttraumatic hydrocephalus. J Neurosurg Sci 2001;45:141–9.

19. Bhatoe HS, Batish VK. Post head injury hydro-cephalus. Ind J Neurotrauma 2005;2:131–3.

20. Jiao QF, Liu Z, Li S, Zhou LX, Li SZ, Tian W, You C. Influencing factors for post-traumatic hydrocephalus in patients suffering from severe traumatic brain injuries. Chinese J Traumatology. 2007;10:159–62.

21. Tian HL, Xu T, Hu J, Cui YH, Chen H, Zhou LF. Risk factors related to hydrocephalus after traumatic subarachnoid hemorrhage. Surg Neurol 2008;69:241–6.

22. Butler AB, Maffeo CJ, Johnson RN, Bass NH. Alteration of CSF outflow in acute subarachnoid hemorrhage; effect of blood components on outflow resistance and vascular transport of CSF in arachnoid villus endothelium. In, Cervos-Navarro J, Fritschka E (eds). Cerebral Micro-circulation and Metabolism. Raven Press, New York (1981):409–14.

23. Upton M, Weller RO. The morphology of human arachnoid granulations. J Neurosurg 1985; 63:867–75.

24. Lorenzo AV, Bresnan MJ, Barlow CF. Cerebrospinal fluid absorption deficit in normal pressure hydrocephalus. Arch Neurol 1974; 30:387–93.

25. DiRocco C, DiTripani G, Maira G, Bentivoglio M, Macchi G, Rossi GF. Anatomoclinical correlation of normotensive hydrocephalus. J Neurol Sci 1977;33:437–52.

26. Foroglou G, Zander E. (Post-traumatic hydro-cephalus and measurement of cerebrospinal fluid pressure). Acta Radiol Diagn (Stockh) 1972; 13:524–30.

27. Choi I, Park H, Chang J, Cho S, Choi S, Byun B. Clinical factors for the development of post-traumatic hydrocephalus after decompressive

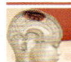

craniectomy. J Korean Neurosurg Soc 2008; 43:227–31.

28. Fleisher AS, Huhn SL, Meislen H: Post traumatic acute obstructive hydrocephalus. Ann Emerg Med 1988;17:165–7.

29. Grcevic N: Traumatic tears of the tela choroidea as an unrecognized cause of post traumatic hydrocephalus. Acta Neurochir (Wien) (Suppl) 1983;32:79–85.

30. Waziri A, Fusco D, Mayer SA, McKhann GM 2nd, Connolly ES Jr: Postoperative hydrocephalus in patients undergoing decompressive hemicraniectomy for ischemic or hemorrhagic stroke. Neurosurgery 2007;61:489–93.

31. Sarkari A, Gupta DK, Sinha S, Kale SS, Mahapatra AK. Post-traumatic hydrocephalus: Presentation, management and outcome—an apex trauma centre experience. Indian Journal of Neurotrauma 2010;7:135–8.

32. Pheupathow N, Ratanalert S, Seheng S, Sripanojkul B. Post-traumatic hydrocephalus: Experience in 17 cases. J Med Ass Thai 1999;82:46–53.

33. Padetti P, Pezzotta S, Spanu G. Diagnosis and treatment of post-traumatic hydrocephalus. J Neurosurg Sci 1983;27:171–5.

34. De Bonis P, Manqiola A, Pompucci A, et al. CSF dynamics analysis in patient with post-traumatic ventriculomegaly. Clin Neurol Neurosurg 2013; 115:49–53.

37

Post-traumatic Epilepsy

Raj Kamal • Vinay Goyal • AK Mahapatra

INTRODUCTION

Post-traumatic epilepsy (PTE) is defined as a recurrent seizure disorder due to injury to the brain following traumatic brain injury (TBI). TBI accounts for 10–20% of symptomatic epilepsy in the general population and 5% of all epilepsy. **After TBI, the occurrence of seizures has been categorized as immediate (< 24 hours), early (1–7 days), or late seizures (> 1 week after TBI).**[1] The immediate and early seizures are considered to reflect the severity of the injury itself, whereas the late seizures result from maturation of epileptogenic pathology. Thus, TBI associated with one unprovoked late seizure qualifies for diagnosis of PTE. The relationship between head injury, early post-traumatic epilepsy and late post-traumatic epilepsy represents perhaps the best studied of all causes of epilepsy. Only specific types of head injury carry a significant risk of post-traumatic epilepsy. The more severe the head injury, greater is the risk of post-traumatic epilepsy.[2–6] Post-traumatic seizures occur clinically in approximately 4% within the first week of head injury. However, continuous EEG monitoring had disclosed incidence as high as 22%.[7] Within the first year after head trauma, the incidence of seizures is 12 times as great as for the population.[4] Patients with severe head trauma and cortical injury with neurologic deficits on physical examination,

but with the dura mater remaining intact, have an incidence of epilepsy from 7 to 39%. Increased severity of trauma, as indicated by dural penetration and neurologic abnormalities, yields a range of epilepsy incidence of 20–57%.[3–6] However, identification of critical molecular, cellular, and network characteristics predicting epileptogenesis with head injury remains a challenge. As epileptogenesis occurs only in a subpopulation of subjects, biomarkers pinpointing individuals at risk for epileptogenesis are urgently needed. As some treatments have shown favorable effects by preventing the development of increased post-TBI seizure susceptibility, their effects on the development of spontaneous seizures, as well as on recovery processes occurring in parallel with epileptogenesis, require further studies.

Jennett classified post-traumatic epilepsy (PTE) into two groups.[3]

1. *Early epilepsy:* Occurring within first week following head trauma.

2. *Late epilepsy:* More than one week after injury.

Seizures occurring during first 24 hours are called immediate seizures.[9]

Risk factors (Tables 37.1 and 37.4); the risk factors for PTE obtained in studies include old age, penetrating injuries, injury severity (GCS < 10), biparietal or multiple contusions, intracranial hemorrhage, frontal or temporal

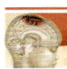

location of the lesion, greater than 5 mm brain midline shift, duration of coma > 24 hours, loss of consciousness > 24 hours, prolonged length of post-traumatic amnesia, multiple intra-cranial procedures, and the occurrence of early post-traumatic seizures.[10–14] Zhao et al[15] retrospectively **reviewed 2826 TBI patients, 141 developed PTE, providing an incidence rate of 5.0%.** Twenty-four cases (0.8%) had post-traumatic seizures (PTS), of which 16 (66.7%) continued to experience after the acute phase of their TBI, accounting for 5.0% of the total PTE cases. A total of 125 cases (88.7%) were diagnosed as presenting with late-stage seizures, occurring from 10 days to three years after TBI, 93/141 (66.0%) presented within six months after the TBI, 14/141 (9.9%) between six and twelve months, 22/141 (15.7%) between one and two years and only 12/141 (8.5%) between two and three years after the TBI. The severity of PTE was rated mild, moderate, and severe in 3.6%, 6.9%, and 17% of the TBI patients. Five parameters contributed to PTE older age, greater severity of brain injury, abnormal neuroimaging, surgical treatment, and early-stage seizures.

Liesemer et al[16] included 275 pediatric patients, 34 had identified early post-traumatic seizures (EPTS) (12%). Risk factors identified on bivariable analysis included **pre-hospital hypoxia, young age, non-accidental trauma (NAT), severe TBI, impact seizure, and subdural hemorrhage, while receiving an AED was protective**. Independent risk factors identified by multivariable analysis were age < 2 years, Glasgow Coma Scale (GCS) score ≥ 8, and NAT as a mechanism of injury. AED treatment was protective against EPTS. Twenty-three (68%) patients developed EPTS within the first 12 hours post-injury.

EARLY POST-TRAUMATIC EPILEPSY

Incidence of early seizures in patients with closed head ranges from 2 to 5%. The presence of risk factors will further increase the incidence of early post-traumatic epilepsy (Table 37.1).

Table 37.1: Risk factors and incidence of early PTE

Risk factors	Incidence of early PTE (Percentage)
1. Severe head injury GCS < 8	– 35%
2. Intracranial hematoma (higher with subdural or intracerebral hematoma)	20–30%
3. Post-traumatic amnesia > 24 hours.	11–14%
4. Depressed fractures	10–11%
5. Children < 5 years	9.8%

Table 37.2: Influence of PTE on incidence of early epilepsy (Jennett[3])

	PTE < 24 hours	PTE 24 hours	Probability
< 16 years	5%	10%	NS
> 16 years depressed	2%	12%	0.001
Fracture	9%	14%	NS
Hematoma	26%	30%	NS
Focal signs	9%	14%	NS
No depressed Fracture or hematoma	2%	9%	0.001

Jennett[3] and others have used post traumatic amnesia as an indicator of severity of injury (Table 37.2). For patients with post-traumatic amnesia of more than 24 hours, a 10% overall incidence of early epilepsy was found in patients under 16 years of age. It was 12% for older patients. Patients with hematomas, focal neurological deficit, and depressed skull fracture were prone to early epilepsy. Of these factors, intracranial hema-toma is the most significant. Intradural hematoma carries more risk than extradural hematoma does[3]. Early seizures are focal in 56% of patients with depressed fracture and in 57% of patients with non-depressed fractures.[2]

LATE POST-TRAUMATIC EPILEPSY

Incidence of late post-traumatic epilepsy in non-missile head injury ranges from 1.85 to 9% (Table 37.3). Late post-traumatic epilepsy

Table 37.3: Incidence of late epilepsy		
Series	*Total cases*	*Epilepsy%*
Jennett (1975)	-	5
Annegers et al (1980)	2747	1.85
De Santis et al (1983)	472	4.44
Zhao et al[15]	2826	5

occurred in 5% of all patients admitted to hospital after non-missile head injury.

Late epilepsy are significantly more common in patients who have suffered early seizures. In Jennett's series.[3] A patient's risk of developing late seizures is 25%, if the patient had an early seizure. Seizures occurring immediately do not necessarily imply a risk of recurrence. However, seizures developing more than 1 hour after injury convey an increased rate of late seizures. Other risk factors for late seizures include focal lesions (hematoma, contusion) focal neurological signs, depressed skull fracture with dural laceration, and prolonged coma or amnesia.[2,3,17,18] With penetrating missile injuries the risk of seizures also increases with the volume of brain tissue destroyed, with lesions located centroparietally, and if metal fragments are retained.[19,20] Important risk factors for late epilepsy are given in Tables 37.4 and 37.5.

After the first late seizure, 86% of patients were reported to develop a second seizure within 2 years, suggesting the establishment of an epileptogenic process.[46]

Data on genetic risk factors for outcome from TBI are emerging but very few studies have assessed the linkage of genes to PTE. Some data are available from genes encoding apolipoprotein E (ApoE) or haptoglobin. The APoE gene, encoding for a cholesterol carrier lipoprotein, exists in three common isoforms: ε2, ε3, and ε4. One study found that ApoE4 allele is associated with a 2.4-fold increased risk of late post-traumatic seizures after moderate to severe TBI.[21] Interestingly, an **ApoE4 allele** has been identified as a susceptibility gene for Alzheimer's disease, which is another condition with increased risk for epilepsy.[22–24]

Fifty percent of patient, having late post-traumatic epilepsy experience, their first seizure within 1 year of head injury and 70–80% within 2 years. Patients with the onset of seizures more than 4 years after injury were more likely to have persistent epilepsy.

The most common type of late PTE was generalized seizures (focal attacks becoming generalized secondarily) found in 60–70% of cases followed by partial seizures in 30–40% of cases.

Hereditary Factors Associated with Early and Late Epilepsy

Heredity plays little influence on risk of post-traumatic seizures. No genetic influence was found by Salazar[20] in a long-term following study of missile injuries incurred in Vietnam. In Jennett's series[3,25] of non-missile injuries,

Table 37.4: Risk factors for late epilepsy (Pagni, 1990)[17]	
	Incidence of Late PTE (%)
1. Penetrating missile head injury	53
2. Intracerebral hematoma	39
3. Focal brain damage on early CT	32
4. Early seizures	25
5. Depressed fracture-torn dura	25
6. Extradural or subdural hemorrhage	20
7. Focal signs	20
8. Depressed skull fracture	15
9. Loss consciousness of 24 hrs	5
10. Linear fracture	5
11. Mild concussion	1

Table 37.5: Factors of late epilepsy[25]			
Factor	*Present*	*n*	*% epilepsy*
Early epilepsy	No	29/868	3
	Yes	59/238	25*
Hematoma	No	27/854	3
	Yes	45/128	35*
Depressed fracture	No	27/832	3
	Yes	76/447	17

*p < .001

hereditary factors did not play any role in early PTE. However, in patients younger than 16 years, a family history played significant role who had late seizure. In adult patient, family history did not play any role in occurrence of late PTE.

In a study by Hanser[26] recurrence of seizure was higher in patients with a family history of seizures or a history of prior neurologic insult. Recently, Suri et al[27] had shown familial incidence of post-traumatic epilepsy.

Pathophysiology

The degree of parenchymal brain damage is related to risk of post-traumatic seizures. Contusional hemorrhage results in deposition of hemoglobin and iron in the brain tissue. Several experimental studies[28–30] have shown hemoglobin and iron to be **epileptogenic** and this has been attributed to free radical formation and lipid peroxidation thus destroying neuronal membranes.[31,32]

Ferric ions decrease the release of **GABA** (gamma-aminobutyric acid) and increase levels of excitatory neurotransmitters such as glutamate and aspartate.[28] Decreased release of GABA and increased release of **excitatory neurotransmitters** result in paroxysmal depolarization shift (PDS) and neuronal synchronization which is necessary for seizure genesis and spread.[33]

Primary injury occurs at the moment of trauma and is accompanied by massive disturbance of the cellular ion homeostasis, release of the excitatory neurotransmitters, and exacerbation of excitotoxicity. The secondary injury occurs in the hours and days following the primary injury, and it is an indirect result of the insult. It includes a complex set of molecular changes and cellular processes, some of which may be relevant also to post-traumatic epileptogenesis. Post-traumatic epileptogenesis refers to a dynamic process that progressively alters neuronal excitability, establishes critical interconnections, and perhaps requires intricate structural changes before the first spontaneous seizure

appears.[34] These changes can include neurodegeneration, neurogenesis, gliosis, axonal damage or sprouting, dendritic plasticity, blood–brain barrier damage, recruitment of inflammatory cells into brain tissue, reorganization of the extracellular matrix, and reorganization of the molecular architecture of individual neuronal cells.[35] Interestingly, all these changes have been reported to occur after experimental TBI.[35] Further, they are not unique for the aftermath of TBI as they have also been described after status epilepticus, which is another common injury type used to trigger epileptogenesis in rodents.[35,36]

Even though data from human PTE is meager, available studies show hippocampal neurodegeneration as well as mossy fiber sprouting.[37,38] Approximately 53% of patients with post-traumatic temporal lobe epilepsy (TLE) have mesial temporal lobe sclerosis on magnetic resonance imaging; in some patients, the MRI abnormalities can be bilateral and associated with multifocal injury.[39,40] Interestingly, a recent study by Vespa et al[40] suggests that hippocampal atrophy detected at the chronic post-injury phase could be caused by (prolonged) seizures at the acute post-TBI phase.

"Recently, many authors have proved the possibility of non-convulsive seizures following head injury.[41,42] The abnormal electrical discharge can be recorded by continuous EEG recording.[41] Towne et al[42] in 2000 had reported non-convulsive status epilepticus in head injury patients."

Prophylaxis of Early and Late Post-traumatic Epilepsy

Drug prophylaxis: Two good randomized double blind placebo-controlled study of phenytoin for the prevention of post-traumatic epilepsy have been done by Young et al[44] (1983) and Tempkin et al 1990.[9,45]

Young et al[44] randomized 204 patients into two groups. One group received phenytoin within 24 hours. of admission and plasma concentration of at least 10 mcg/ml (range 10–20 mcg/ml) was achieved. No significant reduction in the early or late post-traumatic seizures was found between the treated and placebo group.

Tempkin et al[9,45] randomized 404 patients with severe head trauma. Patients were randomly assigned to receive either phenytoin or placebo. Treatment was given for the first year and **phenytoin serum levels** maintained in the optimum therapeutic range in most patients. Patients were followed for 2 years. The results showed that phenytoin was effective in preventing seizures for the first week after cerebral injury (3.6% treated versus 14.2% control) but was no better than placebo in exerting a protective effect during the remainder of the study period. It was, therefore, concluded that phenytoin should be given to patients at risk of post-traumatic seizures during the first week after trauma and then discontinued unless further seizures occur.

Compilation of the available data supports prophylactic administration of phenytoin for prevention of early seizures. A meta-analysis done by Tempkin[45] of the controlled studies found that the phenytoin can prevent early seizures but has no beneficial role in preventing late post-traumatic epilepsy. Other antiepileptic drugs such as sodium valproate, phenobarbital have not been adequately evaluated for their use as prophylactic anticonvulsant in head injury patients.

Cochrane study (2012)[46] concluded that prophylactic anti-epileptics are effective in reducing early seizures, but there is no evidence that treatment with prophylactic anti-epileptics reduces the occurrence of late seizures, or has any effect on death and neurological disability. Insufficient evidence is available to establish the net benefit of prophylactic treatment at any time after injury.

Surgical Prophylaxis

The incidence of post-traumatic seizures has not decreased significantly even with gradual improvement in medical and surgical management of head injury patients.[7]

Depressed fracture and penetrating injuries of head are important risk factors in post-traumatic seizures. No study done till now, shows elevation of depressed fracture decreases the incidence of PTE.

In the study of penetrating injuries by Salazar et al[20] which was done during Vietnam war, the presence of retained intracerebral bone fragments did not correlate with post-traumatic seizures, whereas retained metal fragments did show a relationship to seizure occurrence.

Others

In an experimental study by Atkins et al[47] demonstrated that reductions in seizure susceptibility after TBI are improved with post-traumatic hypothermia and provide a new therapeutic avenue for the treatment of post-traumatic epilepsy.

Treatment of Post-traumatic Seizures

Acute post-traumatic seizures should be treated aggressively with benzodiazepine and a loading dose of phenytoin. Inadequate control of early post-traumatic seizure results in severe hypoxic and secondary metabolic damage of the already injured brain. Uncontrolled seizures should be treated as status epilepticus. **Status epilepticus** is defined as repeated seizures without recovery of consciousness between attack. Post-traumatic status epilepticus if controlled within 1–5 hours is unlikely to cause any significant morbidity, whereas status epilepticus of more than 10 hours has severe morbidity and mortality.[48]

Hypoxia may be the cause and result of seizures. Hypoxia may result from **airway** obstruction or improper ventilation. Seizures also lead to inadequate respiration and ventilation. As metabolic demand of cerebral tissue during seizures is increased, the effects of hypoxia on brain is compounded. Release of excitatory neurotransmitters and decreased level of inhibitory neurotransmitters cause significant neuronal damage.[49]

Hence, during seizures airway patency and ventilation are of prime importance. Patients having multiple fits **(status epilepticus)** with deteriorating level of consciousness, endotracheal intubation and ventilation may be required. Non-convulsive status epilepticus may be missed in comatose patients.[42] **Hyponatremia or hypocalcemia** in such patients should be ruled out.

Post-traumatic seizure should be treated initially with benzodiazepines followed immediately by a loading dose of maintenance anticonvulsant.

For benzodiazepine commonly used are diazepam, lorazepam.

Dose of diazepam: 0.25 mg/kg body given as IV bolus at 2–5 mg/min. This can be repeated after 10 minutes.

IV infusion dose: 8 mg/hour.

Lorazepam: Given as IV bolus 0.1 mg/kg adult usually 4 mg can be repeated after 10 minutes.

Status epilepticus can be divided into following stages:

1. Premonitory stages
2. Early stage
3. Established stage
4. Refractory stage.

Premonitory stage is prodromal period during which there is gradual increase in frequency of seizures. Acute administration of AEDs may stop the progression of status. The initial stage of status epilepticus is called early stage. Once the seizures have continued for 30 min, the stage of established status epilepticus, is entered. Walker and Shorvon[19] suggest the following alternatives at the stage:

1. Diazepam or lorazepam with intravenous phenytoin
2. Phenobarbital.

If the seizures still continue, then the stage of refractory status epilepticus is reached.

A protocol suggested by Walker and Shorvon[50, 51] for the treatment of convulsive status epilepticus in adults is given in Table 37.6. Treatment includes administration and

Table 37.6: Protocol for the treatment of convulsive[50] status epilepticus in adults

Premonitory stage	Diazepam 10 mg rectally repeated once after 15 minutes. Lorazepam 4 mg or alternatively diazepam 10 mg IV repeated after 10 minutes
Established status	Phenytoin 15–18 mg/kg IV at 50 mg/min with lorazepam if not already given and/or phenobarbital 10 mg/kg IV at 100 mg/min
Refractory status	GA with concomitant EEG monitoring continued for 12–24 hours after last clinical seizure/electrographic seizure

intravenous benzodiazepines. Second-line agent include IV phenytoin, phenobarbital, valproate and levetiracetam.[7] Refractory status epilepticus necessitates use of anesthetic agents such as pentobarbital, midazolam or propofol with monitoring of treatment effect by continuous EEG. Non-convulsive status epilepticus should be treated expeditiously but is not as threatening to health as convulsive status epilepticus.[7]

CONCLUSIONS

Post-traumatic epilepsy may occur within first week following head trauma (early epilepsy) or may occur more than one week after injury (late epilepsy). Incidence of early PTE ranges from 2 to 5% and that of late PTE ranges from 2 to 9% of all patients admitted to hospital after non-missile head injury. Risk factors for early PTE are severe head injury, intracranial hematoma, PTA > 24 hours, and depressed fractures. Risk factors for late PTE are more common in patients who have suffered early seizures. Hereditary factor probably does not play any role in PTE. Iron and Hb are epileptogenic as they decrease the release of inhibitory neurotransmitters such as GABA. Phenytoin is most frequently used anticonvulsant which can prevent early seizures but has no beneficial role in preventing late PTE. Auto post-traumatic seizures should be treated with loading dose of phenytoin and benzodiazepines.

Uncontrolled seizures should be treated as status epilepticus. Prevention of early PTE in patients with internal hematoma would prevent rise in ICP and brighten the chance of survival.

REFERENCES

1. Frey LC. Epidemiology of post-traumatic epilepsy: a critical review. Epilepsia 2003;10:11–17.
2. Annegers JF, Grabow JD, Groover RV, Laws ER Jr, Elveback LR, Kurland LT. Seizures after head trauma: a population study. Neurology 1980;30: 683–9.
3. Jennett B. Epilepsy after non-missile head injuries. 2nd edn. Chicago: Heinemann-Year Book, 1975.
4. Caveness WF. Epilepsy, a product of trauma in our time. Epilepsia 1976;17:207–15.
5. Weiss GH, Feeney DM, Caveness WF, et al. Prognostic factors for the occurrence of post-traumatic epilepsy. Arch Neurol 1983;40:7–10.
6. Weiss GH, Salazar AM, Vance SC, et al. Predicting post-traumatic epilepsy in penetrating head injury. Arch Neurol 1986;43:771–3.
7. Shorvon S, Walker M. Status epilepticus in idiopathic generalised epilepsy. Epilepsia 2005;46 (suppl 9):73–9.
8. Annegers JF, Hauser WA, Coan SP, Rocca WA. A population-based study of seizures after traumatic brain injuries. N Engl J Med 1998;338:20–24.
9. Tempkin NR, Dikmen SS, et al. A randomized, double-blind study of phenytoin for the prevention of post-traumatic seizures. N Engl J Med 1990;323:498–502.
10. Brandvold B, Levi L, Feinsod M, George ED. Penetrating craniocerebral injuries in the Israeli involvement in the Lebanese conflict, 1982–1985. Analysis of a less aggressive surgical approach. J Neurosurg 1990;72:15–21.
11. Asikainen I, Kaste M, Sarna S. Early and late posttraumatic seizures in traumatic brain injury rehabilitation patients: brain injury factors causing late seizures and influence of seizures on long-term outcome. Epilepsia 1999;40:584–9.
12. Englander J, Bushnik T, Duong TT, Cifu DX, Zafonte R, Wright J, Hughes R, Bergman W. Analyzing risk factors for late post-traumatic seizures: a prospective, multicenter investigation. Arch Phys Med Rehabil 2003;84:365–73.
13. Messori A, Polonara G, Carle F, Gesuita R, Salvolini U. Predicting posttraumatic epilepsy with MRI: prospective longitudinal morphologic study in adults. Epilepsia 2005;46(9):1472–81.
14. Skandsen T, Ivar Lund T, Fredriksli O, Vik A. Global outcome, productivity and epilepsy 3–8 years after severe head injury. The impact of injury severity. Clin Rehabil 2008;22(7):653–62.
15. Zhao Y, Wu H, Wang X, Li J, Zhang S. Clinical epidemiology of post-traumatic epilepsy in a group of Chinese patients. Seizure 2012;21:322–6.
16. Liesemer K, Bratton SL, Zebrack CM, Brockmeyer D, Statler KD. Early post-traumatic seizures in moderate to severe pediatric traumatic brain injury: rates, risk factors, and clinical features.J Neurotrauma 2011 May;28(5): 755–62.
17. Pagni CA. Post-traumatic epilepsy incidence and (suppl) prophylaxis. Acta Neurosurg 1990;50: 38–47.
18. Weiss GH, Salazar AM, et al. Predicting post-traumatic epilepsy in penetrating head injury. Arch Neurol 1986;43:771–3.
19. Caveners WF, Meirowsky AM, et al. The nature of post-traumatic epilepsy. J Neurosurg 1979;50:545–53.
20. Salazar AM, Jabbari B, et al. Epilepsy after penetrating head injury. Clinical correlates: A report of the Vietnam Head Injury Study. Neurology 1985;35:1406–14.
21. Diaz-Arrastia R, Gong Y, Fair S, Scott KD, Garcia MC, Carlile MC, Agostini MA, Van Ness PC. Increased risk of late post-traumatic seizures associated with inheritance of ApoE4 allele. Arch Neurol 2003;60:818–22.
22. Corder EH, Saunders AM, Strittmatter WJ, Schmechel DE, Gaskell PC, Small GW, Roses AD, Haines JL, Pericak-Vance MA. Gene dose of apolipoprotein E type 4 allele and the risk of Alzheimer's disease in late onset families. Science 1993;261(5123):921–3.
23. Saunders AM, Strittmatter WJ, Schmechel D, George-Hyslop PH, Pericak-Vance MA, Joo SH, Rosi BL, Gusella JF, Crapper-McLachlan DR, Alberts MJ. Association of apolipoprotein E allele epsilon 4 with late-onset familial and sporadic Alzheimer's disease. Neurology 1993; 43:1467–72.
24. Strittmatter WJ, Weisgraber KH, Huang DY, Dong LM, Salvesen GS, Pericak-Vance M, Schmechel D, Saunders AM, Goldgaber D, Roses AD. Binding of human apolipoprotein E to

synthetic amyloid beta peptide: isoform-specific effects and implications for late-onset Alzheimer disease. Proc Natl Acad Sci, USA 1993;90(17): 8098–8102.

25. Jennett B, Teasdale G. Management of Head Injuries. Philadelphia: FA Davis Co 1981;271.

26. Hauser WA, Anderson VE, et al. Seizure recurrence after a first unprovoked seizure. N Engl J Med 1985;307:522–8.

27. Suri A, Mehta TS, Mahaptra AK, Singh VP, Jain S. Factor affecting post-traumatic epilepsy, Neurosurgery 1998;90:20–28.

28. Mori A, Hiramatsu M, et al. Biochemical pathogenesis of post-traumatic epilepsy. Pav J Bid Sci 1982;25:54–62.

29. Rosen AD, Frumin NV. Focal epileptogenesis after intracortical haemoglobin injection. Exp Neurol 1979;66:277–84.

30. William LJ, Hurd RW et al. Epileptiform activity initiated by pial iontophoresis of ferrons and ferric chloride on rat cerebral cortex. Brain Res 1978;152:406–10.

31. Willmore LJ, Hiramatsu M, et al. Formation of superoxide radicals after Fe $C1_3$ Injection into rat isocortex Brain Res 1983;277:393–6.

32. Willmore LJ, Triggs WJ, Gray JD. The role of iron-induced hippocampal peroxidation in acute epileptogenesis. Brain Res 1986;382:422–6.

33. Matsumoto H, et al. Cortical cellular phenomenon in experimental epilepsy. Exp Neurol 1964;9: 305–26.

34. Engel J Jr, Pedley TA. What is epilepsy? Epilepsy: A comprehensive textbook. Philadelphia: Lippincott-Raven 2005;1–11.

35. Pitkänen A, Lukasiuk K. Molecular and cellular basis of epileptogenesis in symptomatic epilepsy. Epilepsy Behav 2009;1:16–25.

36. Pitkänen A, McIntosh TK. Animal models of post-traumatic epilepsy. J Neurotrauma 2006;23:241–61.

37. Swartz BE, Houser CR, Tomiyasu U, Walsh GO, DeSalles A, Rich JR, Delgado-Escueta A. Hippocampal cell loss in posttraumatic human epilepsy. Epilepsia 2006;47:1373–82.

38. Hudak AM, Trivedi K, Harper CR, Booker K, Caesar RR, Agostini M, Van Ness PC, Diaz-Arrastia R. Evaluation of seizure-like episodes in survivors of moderate and severe traumatic brain injury. J Head Trauma Rehabil 2004; 19:290–5.

39. Diaz-Arrastia R, Agostini MA, Frol AB, Mickey B, Fleckenstein J, Bigio E, Van Ness PC. Neurophysiologic and neuroradiologic features of intractable epilepsy after traumatic brain injury in adults. Arch Neurol 2000;57:1611–6.

40. Vespa PM, McArthur DL, Xu Y, Eliseo M, Etchepare M, Dinov I, Alger J, Glenn TP, Hovda D. Nonconvulsive seizures after traumatic brain injury are associated with hippocampal atrophy. Neurology 2010;75:792–8.

41. Vespa PM, Nuwer MR, New V, et al. Increased incidence and impact of non-convulsive and convulsive seizures after traumatic brain injury as detected by continuous electroence phalographic monitoring. J. Neurosurgery 1999;91:50–60.

42. Towne AR, Waterhouse EJ, Boggs JG, et al. Prevalence of non-convulsive states epilepticus in comatose patients. Neurology 2000;25:340–5.

43. Temkin NR, Dikmen SS, Adevsin GD, et al. Valproate therapy for prevention of Post-traumatic seizure: a randamized tricel J. Neurosurgery 1999;91:593–600.

44. Young B, Rapp RP, et al. Failure of prophylactic administered phenytoin to prevent late post-traumatic seizures. J Neurosurg 1983;58:236–41.

45. Tempkin NR, Dikman SS, Winn HR. Management of head injury Post-traumatic seizures. Neurosurg Clin N Am 1991;2:425–35.

46. Schierhout G, Roberts I. WITHDRAWN: Antiepileptic drugs for preventing seizures following acute traumatic brain injury. Cochrane Database Syst Rev 2012 Jun 13;6:CD000173. doi: 10.1002/14651858.CD000173.

47. Atkins CM, Truettner JS, Lotocki G, Sanchez-Molano J, Kang Y, Alonso OF, Sick TJ, Dietrich WD, Bramlett HM. Post-traumatic seizure susceptibility is attenuated by hypothermia therapy. Eur J Neurosci 2010;32:1912–20.

48. Delgado-Escueta AV, Wasterlain C, et al. Management of status-epilepticus. N Engl J Med 1982;306:1337–40.

49. Wasterlain CG, Fujikawa DG, et al. Epilepsia, 34 (suppl 1) 1993;537–53.

50. Walker MC, Shorvon SD. Treatment of status epilepticus and serial seizures. In: The Treatment of Epilepsy. Shorvon SD, Dreifuss F, Fish D, Thomas D (eds), Blackwell Science 1996.

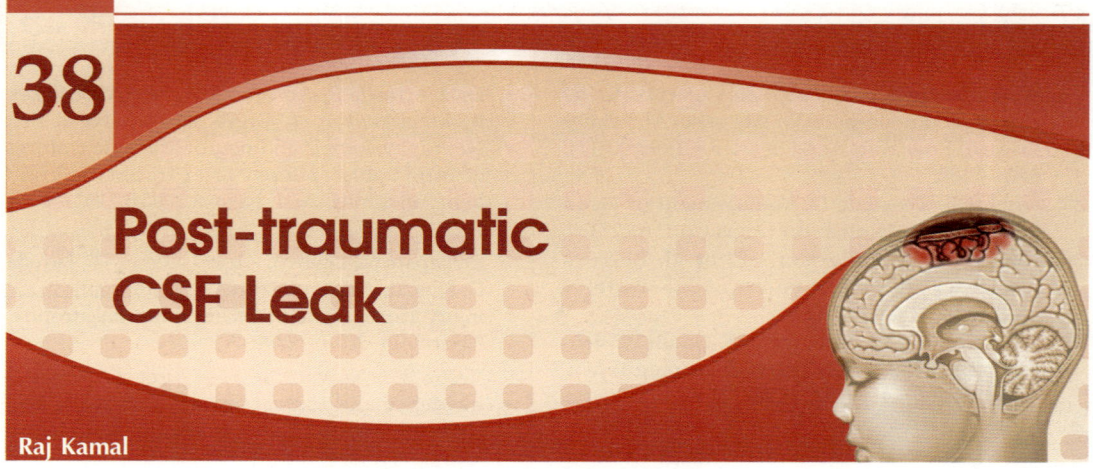

38

Post-traumatic CSF Leak

Raj Kamal

INTRODUCTION

Leakage of **cerebrospinal fluid** from the nose is called **CSF rhinorrhea** and leakage of cerebrospinal fluid from the ear is called **CSF otorrhea.** Blunt trauma to the head is a frequent cause of CSF fistulae, which are diagnosed in 3% of all patients who have a closed head injury and in up to 30% of patients who have fractures of the skull base.[1] Post-traumatic leakage is the evidence that a basal fracture communicates with the subarachnoid space. When rhinorrhea, otorrhea or recurrent meningitis follow a head injury, the causative breach in the duramater and/or skull base may be difficult to identify with enough precision to enable surgical repair. CSF can escape from one nostril, for example, as a result of a dural defect on the same side, anteriorly or posteriorly, on the opposite side or even, via the **eustachian tube,** as the result of a fracture of the petrous bone. The range and number of imaging techniques have been proposed. Thin section CT through the affected region after intrathecal injection of water soluble contrast medium is the technique worth attempting.[2]

INCIDENCE AND ETIOLOGY

According to Lewin,[3] post-traumatic CSF rhinorrhea occurs in 2% of unselected closed head injuries. The risk of CSF leak is higher in penetrating head injuries. Meirowsky, et al.[4] reported 9% patients with penetrating head injuries had CSF leak. Post-traumatic CSF leaks are not related to age and sex. A CSF leak secondary to skull base fracture is reportedly a complication in 1–3% of all closed head injuries.[5–7] The most common sites of injury involve the anterior cranial fossa, with fractures through the frontal sinus or cribriform plates of the ethmoid bones. Central skull base fractures occur at the sphenoid sinus or sella. Lateral skull base fractures occur in the temporal bone, with communication of CSF into the mastoid complex, middle ear cavity, or proximal eustachian tube. These fractures may cause middle ear CSF effusion and drainage into the nasopharynx or result in frank CSF otorrhea if there is a tympanic membrane perforation. The rate is highest in patients with anterior skull base fractures. Brodie and Thompson[8] reported a 14.5% incidence of CSF leaks in a review of 820 cases of temporal bone fractures.

Eighty percent of post-traumatic CSF leaks occur within the first 48 hours after injury, and 95% will manifest within the first 3 months. A small subset of patients will present with rhinorrhea or meningitis decades after the trauma. Most traumatic CSF leaks (up to two-thirds in some reports) close spontaneously, and otorrhea reportedly has a greater chance of spontaneous resolution than does rhinorrhea. However, persistent CSF leaks place the patient at increased risk of meningitis, ranging 4–50%, or less frequently, intracerebral abscess or encephalitis.[5–11] Post-traumatic CSF leaks are uncommon in young children and rare in those younger than 2 years of age.[12–14] The apparent immunity of infants to traumatic CSF leaks likely results from the flexibility of the skull base, especially the cartilaginous nature of the ethmoids, and the poor development of the frontal and sphenoid air sinuses. Beyond the age of 5 years, the frontal air sinuses progressively enlarge reaching adult dimensions by 14 years of age. The rate is highest in patients with anterior skull base fractures. Brodie and Thompson[8] reported a 14.5% incidence of CSF leaks in a review of 820 cases of temporal bone fractures. In patients with facial fractures, the incidence of CSF rhinorrhea is as high as 25%. Beyond the age of 5 years, the frontal air sinuses progressively enlarge reaching adult dimensions by 14 years of age. Interestingly, there is little correlation between the severity of head injury and the occurrence of a CSF leak. Mincy[14] reported that almost 50% of patients with post-traumatic CSF leaks suffered a brief or no loss of consciousness and had no neurological deficits. Of utmost concern with a CSF leak is the potential for meningitis. There seems to be a higher risk in cases of CSF rhinorrhea occurring after accidental trauma and in patients whose CSF leak does not close spontaneously.

Mincy's[14] series of 54 patients with traumatic CSF rhinorrhea demonstrated that meningitis developed in 11% of patients in whom draining stopped spontaneously in 7 days, compared with 88% of patients in whom drainage lasted longer than 7 days. Authors recommend surgical closure of CSF leaks if drainage has not ceased within 1 to 2 weeks. Surgical closure earlier than 1 to 2 weeks is unlikely to prevent meningitis.

Ommaya[15] and McCoy[16] classified CSF leaks into **traumatic** and **non-traumatic** origins (Fig. 38.1). Traumatic is further classified into acute and delayed types. **Non-traumatic CSF leaks** are classified into high pressure and low pressure leaks depending on the etiology (Fig. 38.1). Trauma accounts for 90% of CSF rhinorrhea with approximately 2% of all head injuries and 5% of fractures of the base of the skull demonstrating CSF rhinorrhea. The majority of these occur through the anterior cranial fossa. It is in this area that the dura is tightly adherent to the thin bone of the cribriform plate and roof of the ethmoid. Fortunately, most post-tranmatic leaks resolve spontaneously.

Fifty percent of post-traumatic CSF leaks will cease within one week and almost all stop by 6 months.[15] This occurs due to adhesions or herniation of brain into bony defects and

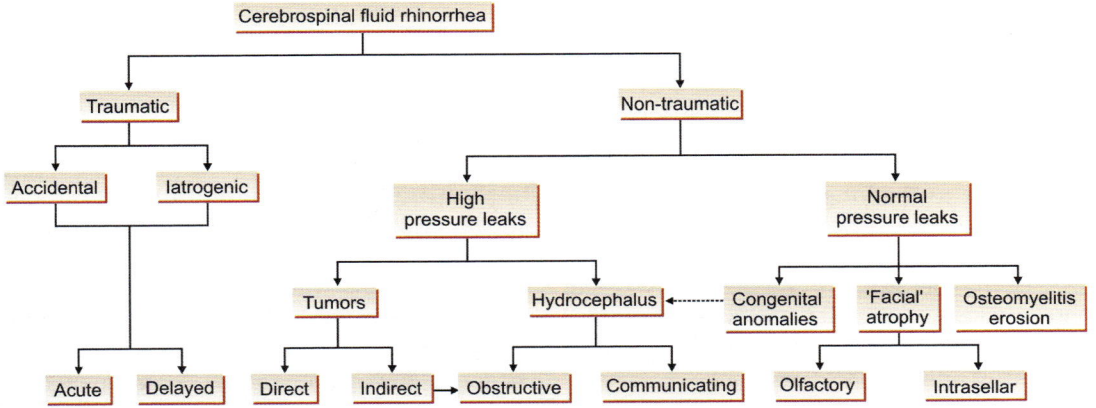

Fig. 38.1: Classification of CSF leaks (from Ommaya AK: Clin Neurosurg 1976;23:363)

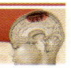

regenerative qualities of meninges. As post-traumatic basal dural tear communicates with paranasal air sinuses, risk of meningitis is considerable even in absence of demonstrable CSF leak.

Most cases of traumatic CSF rhinorrhea are secondary to the fractures involving anterior cranial fossa. The roof of ethmoid, the cribriform plate are the most frequent sites of CSF rhinorrhea because of thin bone and tight adherence of dura to bone in this area.[17] Fracture of frontal sinus are also common sites dural tear leading to CSF rhinorrhea.

The appearance of CSF may be apparent immediately after trauma or days to weeks later. Delayed appearance of CSF leak may be due to delayed elevation of intracranial pressure following trauma, lysis of a clot in an area of bone and dural dehiscence, resolution of soft tissue edema, maturation and contraction of wound edges, or loss of vascularity and necrosis of soft tissue and bone around the wound.[18–20] Also, during or following dural healing, dura may herniate through a fracture line. The constant physiologic changes in CSF pressure may result in progressive dural herniation with its eventual dehiscence and CSF leakage.[17]

CSF otorrhea is defined as leakage of CSF through external auditory canal which requires a pathologic communication between subarachnoid space and the pneumatized areas of the temporal bone. In addition, there must be damage to the tympanic membrane or a defect in the external auditory canal wall. CSF otorrhea results from fracture of middle cranial fossa with damage to tympanic membrane. Fracture can be **longitudinal or transverse** to the long axis of petrous bone. Hicks, et al.[21] studied 40 temporal bone fractures and noted that CSF leak occurred in 29% of the longitudinal fractures and 44% of the transverse. Ghorayeb and Rafie[22] reported a 21% incidence of CSF otorrhea in 123 cases of temporal bone fractures.

If the **tympanic membrane** heals rapidly or if it is not damaged then CSF leaks through

eustachian tube resulting in CSF rhinorrhea. Hence, fracture of middle cranial fossa can result in both CSF otorrhea and rhinorrhea. CSF otorrhea ceases spontaneously in almost all cases. Raaf[23] reported persistent CSF otorrhea in only one case in a series of 79 patients with otorrhea.

Clinical Features

Traumatic CSF rhinorrhea can be present in two ways:

1. Watery fluid discharge from nose
2. Meningitis

In majority of cases they present as watery fluid draining from the nose. CSF leak can be from either nostril but may be ipsilateral to the defect site. Post-traumatic rhinorrhea develops within 48 hours in approximately 55% of all patients who ultimately develop CSF rhinorrhea as a result of trauma. This frequency increases to 70% by the end of the first week as edema, which may be temporarily preventing CSF leakage, resolves.[18]

Sixty percent to eighty percent of patients with CSF rhinorrhea will have **anosmia** and **hyposmia** due to olfactory nerve damage resulting from fracture of cribriform plate. Meningitis can be presenting symptom in about 20% of patients with CSF rhinorrhea.[18] The chances of developing meningitis within first 3 weeks in patients with CSF rhinorrhea following head injury has been reported to be 3–11%.[18] Wehrle reported meningitis in 21% of patients having CSF rhinorrhea following head injury.[4] **Headache** due to presence of intracranial air has been reported in 1/5th of patients with traumatic CSF leakage.[20,24] Post-operative CSF rhinorrhea results from transphenoidal removal of pituitary tumors and anterior skull base surgeries. Incidence of CSF rhinorrhea following **transphenoidal surgery** is approximately 3–6%.

Non-traumatic CSF rhinorrhea have following features.

Age > 30 yrs female preponderance (2:1) insidious at onset. Present for longer duration (in years). Profuse nasal drainage.

Aerocele, anosmia and meningitis are rare. Laun reported that CSF otorrhea occurred immediately in 94% of those who ultimately developed CSF otorrhea following head trauma.[25] CSF rhinorrhea or a sensation of postnasal discharge may occur if the tympanic membrane is intact as the CSF finds its way into nasopharynx through eustachian tube.

Diagnostic Studies

The diagnosis of CSF fistula depends on
1. Demonstration that the leaking fluid is CSF.
2. Localizing the site of leakage. **Demonstration that the leaking fluid is CSF:**
   a. Profuse persistent clear nasal discharge.
   b. *'Halo sign' or 'Target sign'* in which a clear fluid area surrounds a blood stain when CSF mixed with blood is absorbed on a filter paper. This may differentiate between CSF mixed with blood or other nasal secretions and serosanguinous fluids.
   c. *Reservoir sign:* When patient is about to voluntarily produce CSF it will be correct positioning of the head. This is because ethmoid and sphenoid sinus acts as CSF reservoir.
   d. *Glucose content:* If glucose content of discharging fluid is > 30 mg/ml then probably it is CSF. Nasal secretions have glucose content < 10 mg/ml. Glucose detection is not recommended as a confirmatory test. As such, other biomarkers of the CSF leakage, such as beta-2-transferrin (beta-2 trf) and beta-trace protein (betaTP) are necessary to identify and confirm of this condition.[26]
   e. *Immunoelectrophoretic:* Regardless of the presentation or specific etiology, the clinical diagnosis is confirmed by obtaining a sample of the nasal or otologic secretions and measuring the β_2-transferrin activity. β_2-Transferrin, a protein highly specific for human CSF, is an immunohistochemical test that is considered the standard for the clinical diagnosis of a CSF leak.[27–29] At least 0.5 ml

of fluid is necessary, and there may be a false-positive result in the setting of chronic liver disease or inborn errors of metabolism of glycoprotein.[29] A positive β_2-transferrin result confirms an active CSF leak, but cross-sectional imaging is necessary to locate the site of the defect. Some patients experience intermittent leaks, and β_2-transferrin can only be collected when the CSF is actively leaking. Finally, occasionally patients will present with recurrent episodes of meningitis, without symptoms of nasal drainage. This implies an occult CSF fistula, and careful imaging work-up should be performed.[30]

f. *Other techniques to demonstrate CSF leakage:* Injection of colored dyes and radioactive tracer into subarachnoid space be retrieved extracranially for accurate demonstration of CSF leak. It has little localization value. Injection of colored dyes has been abandoned because of morbidity it produces. **Radioactive tracers** are preferred methods because demonstration of even small amount of radioactive tracer is easier. **Isotope cisternography** is performed using in-DTPA (diethylene triamine penta-acetic acid) pledgets placed in anterior roof of nose, middle meatus, posterior roof will be contaminated accordingly. This method is useful in patients with small and intermittent CSF leak.

Localizing the site of leakage: Following investigations may be done to localize the leak and sites of leak.

1. Plain X-ray
2. CT scan
3. MRI

Plain X-ray skull with patient in supine position, the presence of air fluid level in the frontal, ethmoidal and sphenoid sinuses indicate that a fracture exists in anterior cranial fossa.

High-resolution Coronal and Axial CT
(Figs 38.2d, 38.3 to 38.5a and b)

It is the primary imaging modality for localization of cranial vault defects. It often is the only test needed for diagnosis[31-35] however, it is limited to identifying defects in bone. One- to 2 mm sections in coronal and axial planes are recommended to evaluate fully all walls of the sinuses. Thin section (1 to 1.5 mm) through anterior and middle cranial fossa in both axial and coronal planes, fracture of cribriform plate, sella turcica, of ethmoid of frontal sinuses, particularly when associated with an airfluid level in the adjacent sinus, are presumptive evidences of a leak and help to localize subsequent investigation.[31] Partial volume averaging can cause both false-positive and false-negative endings. Plain CT scans have a 9.5% false-positive identification of a bony defect in inactive CSF fistulas.

Metrizamide Computed Tomography Cisternography (MCTC)

CT cisternography was first performed with metrizamide and reported in 1977.[32] High-resolution CT is performed after the intrathecal administration of low osmolar, non-ionic iodine contrast media (Figs 38.5a and b). **Metrizamide,** which is water soluble, non-ionic contrast medium (3–10 ml), is injected by lumbar puncture and positioned in the cranial subarachnoid space by tilting the patient head down (60°) for about a minute. Contiguous 1.5 mm sections in both axial and coronal sections are taken to demonstrate bony defect and site of leak. Maneuvers that provoke an active leak, such as sneezing or head hanging, are performed prior to the CT portion of cisternography. Postcontrast images are then compared with the precontrast images. A positive result involves the presence of a skull base defect and contrast opacification within the sinus, nasal cavity, or middle ear. An increase in Hounsfield units of 50% or greater after CT cisternography is considered a positive study for a CSF leak.[33] In majority of patients with acute leak contrast can be seen passing through the bony defect.[17]

Contrast cisternography followed by CT may provide useful data on CSF flow patterns and dynamics.

Metrizamide showed 92% accuracy in 99 active leaks and 40% accuracy in 15 inactive leaks (review of 325 patients).[33] Moreover, the presence or absence of an active CSF leak at the time of radiologic diagnosis influences the test result.[34] Unlike other cisternographic techniques, magnetic resonance cisternography (MRC) does not require the intrathecal administration of a contrast agent (Figs 38.2a to c and 38.4). MRC takes advantage of the intrinsic contrast generated between CSF and adjacent structures by T_2-weighted sequences (Figs 38.2a and 38.5c). Using T_2-weighted images, MRC localized the site of the CSF fistula in 11 of 11 patients with inactive leaks.[33] MR imaging techniques offer non-invasive methods of imaging a CSF leak and are indicated to assess possible encephalocele or meningoencephalocele. Herniation of brain parenchyma or meninges through the bone defect may be difficult to differentiate from obstructed secretions on CT scans but is obvious on MR images. An MR is always performed in our practice if there is an osseous defect and complete opacification of an adjacent sinus in the patient with a possible CSF leak, as these findings could indicate the presence of a meningocele or encephalocele, particularly if the soft-tissue opacification is lobular or non-dependent. Gadolinium-enhanced images in all three planes help differentiate potential meningocele from sinus secretions and may detect dural enhancement.

The data on MR cisternography are promising, with studies touting sensitivities of 87% and accuracies ranging 78–100%.[35-37] The proponents of MR cisternography state that the non-invasive and nonionizing technique can localize the actual site of a fistulous tract, which may be particularly helpful in patients who have multiple potential fracture sites or osseous defects at CT. While many continue to feel that, similar to CT and radionuclide cisternography, visualization of fistulas is

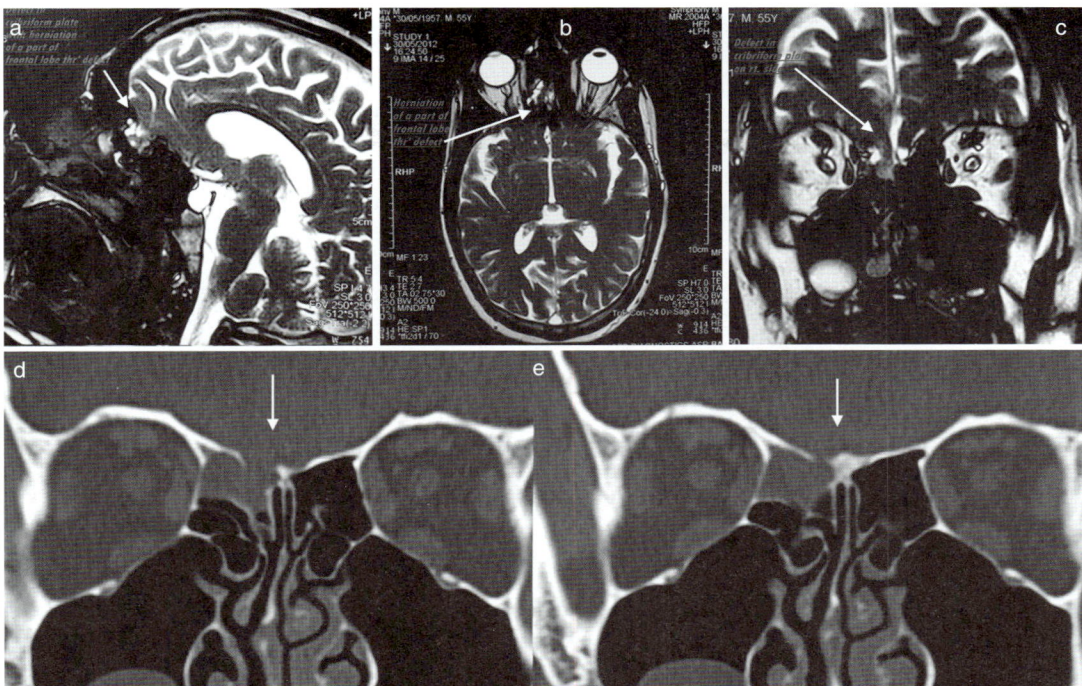

Fig. 38.2a to e: MR cisternography—T_2-weighted images a and b showing defect in cribriform on right side with encephalocele and CSF leak

limited to those actively leaking, other authors have reported success in localizing intermittent or low-flow leaks.[35–37]

A study from 1998[37] reported a sensitivity of 87% and accuracy of 89% for MR cisterno-

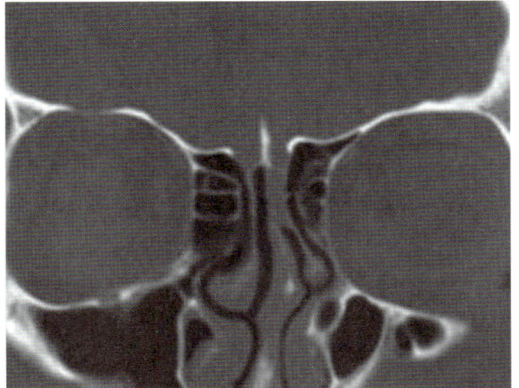

Fig. 38.3: Coronal CT in a patient with a post-traumatic CSF leak

graphy, compared with a sensitivity of 92% and accuracy of 92% for thin-section CT alone, taking into account both active and inactive CSF leaks. Additionally, while MR cisternography showed a high positive predictive value, the negative predictive value for both active and inactive leaks is relatively lower for MR cisternography (58%) compared with CT alone (70%).

MANAGEMENT

The majority of traumatic CSF fistula heal without surgical intervention. Hence, the initial management of CSF leaks should be aimed at supporting the factors which stops CSF leak and prevents meningitis. In nontraumatic CSF rhinorrhea, conservative treatment has no role to play. Following conservative measures can be taken to promote cessation of CSF leak:

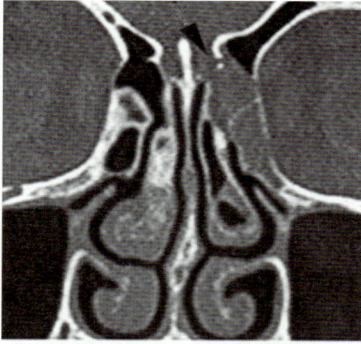

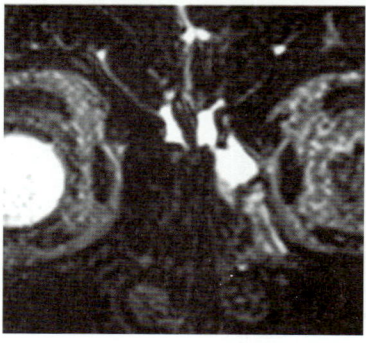

Fig. 38.4: Coronal CT and T$_2$-weighted MRI in a patient with a post-traumatic CSF leak showing defect in cribriform on left side

1. *Position:* Head should be elevated in the range of 30–45° from horizontal. This decreases ICP by improving venous outflow.

2. *Continuous lumbar drainage:* Continuous lumbar drainage reduces the ICP thus reducing the CSF leak. This can be tried for 3–5 days, draining about 150 ml of CSF daily. A19 G catheter is threaded rostrally (–10 cm) percutaneously through 17G **Tuohy needle.** The proximal end of catheter is connected to closed sterile drainage system. Complications of lumbar drainage are infection (meningitis), **pneumocephalus,** headache and vomiting. Headache, vomiting and pneumocephalus results from over drainage.

3. *Drugs:* Drugs which reduces the production of cerebrospinal fluid such as **acetazolamide** (Diamox) may be helpful in reducing CSF leak.

4. *Antibiotics:* Prophylactic antibiotics have not been shown to be effective in the prevention of meningitis and are no longer given for closed **post-traumatic** leaks.[38–41] They are given only postoperatively.

Operative Treatment

Indications for surgery in traumatic CSF leak.

1. Persistent and profuse CSF leak by the end of one week.

2. CSF leaks resulting from penetrating missile injuries, e.g. bullet injury.

3. Recurrent meningitis. Even an attack of meningitis with CSF leak is an indication for operating such patients.

4. The presence of an intracranial aerocele.[43]

Operative approaches can be divided into:

1. Craniotomy, including intracranial intradural and intracranial extradural

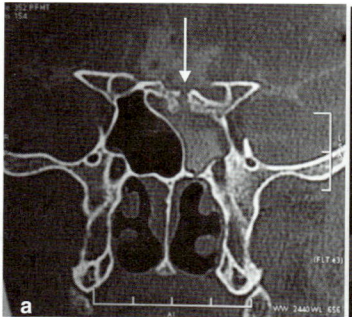
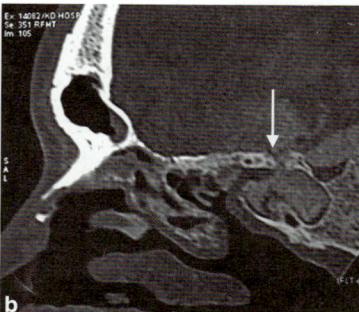
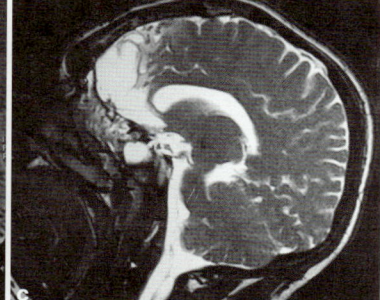

Figs 38.5a to c: (a and b) CT metrizamide cisternography coronal and sagittal sections showing post-traumatic bony defect in posterior part of anterior cranial fossa near sella; (c) MR cisternography of above pateint showing CSF leakage in sella

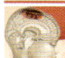

2. Extracranial extradural approach:
   a. Trans-sphenoidal or trans-ethmoidal
   b. Endoscopic
   c. VP shunt

Surgical treatment of CSF rhinorrhea is still problematic. Liu et al[42] evaluated the clinical outcomes of 132 consecutive cases of CSF rhinorrhea treated via transcranial or transnasal endoscopic approaches according to the patient's condition. Of 132 patients with CSF rhinorrhea, a used in 98 to repair cranial base defects in the ethmoid and sphenoid sinuses. A transcranial intradural approach was used in the remaining 34 patients for frontal sinus defects, multiple fractures of the cranial base, or combination injury. CSF rhinorrhea resolved after initial surgery in 124 of 132 patients, giving a success rate of 94%. Of the 8 failures or recurrent cases, 4 were successfully repaired by repeat endoscopic surgery, 2 were cured by transcranial revision surgery, and 2 refused additional surgery (the condition subsequently resolved without treatment in these patients). Postoperative complications included intracranial infection (8 patients) and anosmia (1 patient). No neurological deficits were apparent over the 10 month mean follow-up period. They concluded that transnasal endoscopic repair is a reliable method for CSF rhinorrhea patients

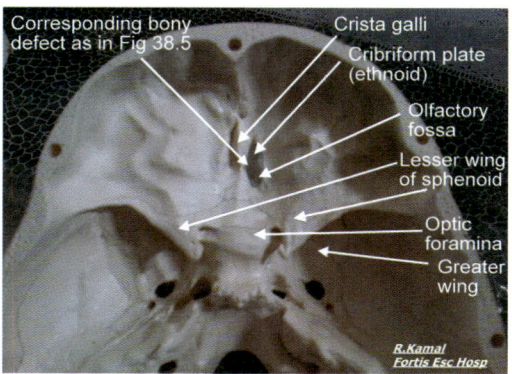

Fig. 38.6: Post-traumatic dural defect corresponding to Fig. 38.5 (anatomy)

whose fistulae are located in the ethmoid and sphenoid sinuses. The transcranial procedure should be the treatment of choice for patients with frontal sinus fracture, multiple or complex anterior cranial base fractures, or nerve injury. A satisfactory surgical outcome depends on exact diagnosis, proper operative approach, and the surgeon's skill and experience.

INTRACRANIAL

The first successful repair of CSF rhinorrhea was done by Dandy in 1926.[43] Dandy described the intracranial approach in detail. For anterior fossa, two approaches have been described: **the intracranial intradural and the intracranial extradural.**

The **intracranial intradural approach is** recommended by many authors as preferred method.[44,45] The intracranial extradural approach allows wide exploration with visualization of both sphenoid wings, both **cribriform fossa,** and both orbital roofs (Figs 38.5 and 38.6). The most important factor is proper **identification and repair of dural defect. The advantage** of intracranial extradural approach is very **little brain retraction** and damage because of intervening dura. The **disadvantages** include inevitable dural tears and areas of cerebral tissue herniation into bony defects cannot be easily visualized.[44] Damage to olfactory nerves is strong possibility in both

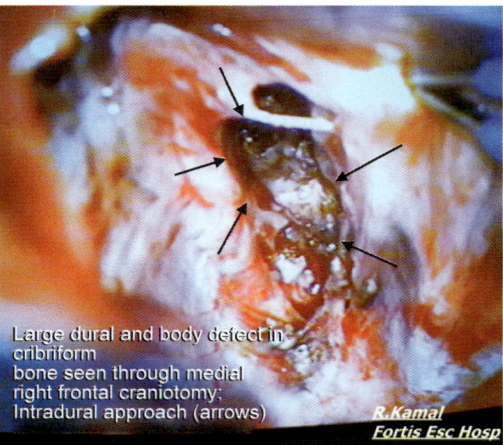

Fig. 38.5: Post-traumatic dural defect from above

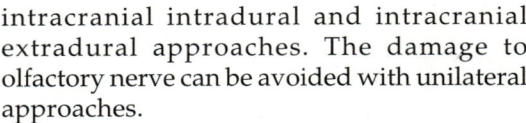

intracranial intradural and intracranial extradural approaches. The damage to olfactory nerve can be avoided with unilateral approaches.

Closure of dural defect can be done by:

i. Autografts of fascia fat and muscles.

ii. Tissue adhesives.

Fascia can be taken from temporalis muscle, pericranium or fascia lata. Tissue adhesives such as **fibrin sealants** [TISSEEL™ Kit (Baxter) consists of a two-component fibrin sealant offers highly concentrated human fibrinogen to seal tissue and stop diffuse bleeding] have been used to achieve water tight closure. Upon mixing sealer protein (human) and thrombin (human), it quickly sets to form a white, elastic mass which firmly adheres to the tissue, i.e. wound surface and achieves hemostasis and sealing or gluing of tissues. Fibrinogen is converted to fibrin strands that join into net-like matrices.[47]

Many common dural closure techniques, such as sutures, autologous grafts, gelatin or collagen sponges, and fibrin glues, are used to achieve watertight closure, although none are US Food and Drug Administration approved for this use. DuraSeal Dural Sealant System is a polyethylene glycol (PEG) hydrogel approved by the US Food and Drug Administration for obtaining watertight dural closure when applied after standard dural suturing. The multicenter, prospective randomized study[46] further evaluated the safety of a PEG hydrogel compared with common dural sealing techniques. The PEG hydrogel dural sealant used in this study has a similar safety profile to commonly used dural sealing techniques when used as dural closure augmentation in cranial surgery. The PEG hydrogel dural sealant demonstrated faster preparation and application times than other commonly used dural sealing techniques.[47]

Recently human fibrin tissue glues is gaining popularity to achieve water tight closure of defect.[48] Large bone defects can be closed by using **methyl methacrylate.**

EXTRACRANIAL

The extracranial approaches which are done in collaboration with ENT surgeons, has less morbidity as compared to craniotomy. The endoscopic endonasal technique for the management of CSF leaks provides a less invasive surgical route to achieve valid dural repair.[49] Extracranial repair of the fistula is the preferred method. In series by Wax et al,[50] the success rate was initially 17 of 18 patients. The patient who releaked 8 months after surgery underwent a second repair and has remained leak free for 2 years. Recent experience with the use of endoscopes in the repair of these leaks has shown that in experienced hands, the success rate is excellent, almost approaching 90% success rate.[50,51]

The morbidity of either approach is minimal. The common extracranial approaches available are:

i. Transnasal trans-sphenoidal for sellar and parasellar leaks.

ii. Transethmoidal trans-sphenoidal approach.

iii. Extranasal approach through frontal and ethmoidal sinuses.

Extracranial approaches are limited to the anterior cranial fossa and paranasal sinuses. Endoscopic techniques have broadened the indications and improved the results associated with the extracranial repair of CSF leaks[53–55] Success rates as high as 90% have been reported. Under direct endoscopic visualization, a leak often can be identified and the sinus into which it drains can be obliterated by packing it with fat or muscle. Other techniques described in conjunction with extracranial techniques include mobilization of mucocutaneous flaps and combinations of autologous tissues with fibrin glue.[56,57] A theoretical disadvantage of extracranial approaches is that the patch is less secure than when it is placed intradurally. Scholsem et al[52] reviewed the 109 patients with an anterior cranial base fracture (having a persistent CSF leak or radiological signs of an unhealed dural tear). All underwent the same surgical procedure, with **combined extradural and intradural closure of the dural tear.** Of the 109 patients, 98 patients (90%) were cured after the first operation. Persistent postoperative CSF rhinorrhea occurred in 11 patients (10%), necessitating an early complementary surgery via a trans-sphenoidal approach (7 patients) or a second-look intracranial approach (4 patients). No postoperative neurological deterioration attributable to increasing frontocerebral edema occurred. During the mean follow-up period of 36 months, recurrence of CSF fistula was observed in five patients and required an additional surgical repair procedure. They cocluded that the closure of CSF fistulae after an anterior cranial base fracture via a combined intracranial extradural and intradural approach, which allows the visualization and repair of the entire anterior base, is safe and effective. It is essentially indicated for patients with extensive bone defects in the cranial base, multiple fractures of the ethmoid bone and the posterior wall of the frontal sinus, cranial nerve involvement, associated lesions necessitating surgery such as intracranial hematomas, and post-traumatic intracranial infection. Rhinorrhea caused by a precisely located small tear may be treated with endoscopy.

With intradural repair the patch is held firmly against the defect by the brain and normal CSF pressure. Wormald and McDonogh[58] recently addressed this concern: They described the endoscopic repair of CSF leaks using a "bath-plug" technique to seal the defect from the intradural side.

Typically, intracranial procedures are reserved for patients with defects that are not amenable to extracranial endoscopic techniques, including patients with extensive skull base fractures, comminuted fractures with displaced fragments that require reduction, and fractures associated with intracranial hemorrhages or contusions that ordinarily would require craniotomy for treatment. A bicoronal incision is usually employed, and

the craniotomy is tailored to the extent of the bony defects and associated intracranial pathology. When bony defects are lateralized to one side, a frontal or pterional craniotomy may be used. The patient's head is positioned to permit gravity to aid in retraction of the frontal lobes. Lumbar drainage of CSF and the intraoperative use of mannitol can further minimize the need for retraction. Depending on the location of the skull base defect, the operative microscope is an invaluable adjunct. Dural defects can be repaired directly by autologous tissue grafts are frequently employed like pericranium, fascia lata or various commercially available dural substitutes can be used. Grafts can be sutured in place, but most surgeons use fibrin glue to reinforce the closure. In clinical and laboratory studies, fibrin glue has been shown to significantly enhance dural closure and to reduce the risk of CSF leakage.[59,60] CSF leakage after transphenoidal surgery initially should be treated with best rest and lumbar drainage of CSF. If the leak persists despite lumbar drainage, repacking of the sphenoid sinus is indicated. The risk of a CSF leak can be minimized by scrupulously packing opened air cells with wax or fat as well as by filling any bony defect with fatty tissue. Bed rest and lumbar drainage are usually sufficient to stop these leaks. Subgaleal collections may respond well to aspiration and a simple compression dressing. A percutaneous technique for aspirating fluid and injecting fibrin glue to close a subgaleal fistula has also been described. Recurrent subgaleal collections should raise suspicion of hydrocephalus.

Lewin[3] and Ommaya[45] did not find any difference in success rate or morbidity between **intracranial and extracranial approaches.** Ommaya recommends that extracranial techniques should be reserved for sellar and parasellar leaks in carefully selected patients. He argued that repair of meninges is more important than closing bone defect which is rarely possible with extracranial approaches except for the lower part of **sella turcica** as

An Algorithm for the Patient with a Definite or Possible CSF Leak (Lloyd et al)[37]

1. When the β_2-transferrin test is positive and multidetector CT scan shows a single osseous defect, no other imaging is necessary to direct the repair. This is the most common scenario in practice.
2. If the β_2-transferrin test is positive and the multidetector CT scan shows more than one osseous defect and an opacified sinus, a CT cisternogram will be obtained to determine which site is actively leaking.
3. If the β_2-transferrin test is positive but the multidetector CT scan does not show an osseous defect, the β_2-transferrin test is repeated in the rare chance the result was a false-positive. If a second sample is positive, CT cisternography or MR cisternography may be performed, preferably when the CSF is actively leaking. This clinical scenario is, in our experience, very rare. If all imaging findings are negative and repeat β_2-transferrin test is positive, the patient is endoscopically examined under anesthesia directed at the side of prior trauma, if applicable, and possibly with the use of intrathecal fluorescein, evaluating for the presence of pulsatile pooling of CSF or fluorescein. This step remains in the algorithm because occasionally osseous defects may be too small to resolve with current imaging techniques.
4. CT cisternography, therefore, is reserved for patients who have a negative multidetector CT scan but in whom the CSF is actively leaking or those with more than one defect.
5. MR cisternography is always performed if multidetector CT reveals an osseous defect with soft-tissue opacification within an adjacent sinus (particularly if it is lobular or nondependent) to exclude the possibility of meningocele or encephalocele. Gadolinium chelate is routinely administered to detect dural enhancement at the site of the leak.
6. Only in the most complex cases is nuclear cisternography with pledgets performed, and then to help document the presence and side of the leak.

exposed through **transphenoidal** route.[45] Hence, leaks through sella turcica are best approached via the trans-sphenoidal route.

CSF Otorrhea

Leaks from posterior fossa dura into the mastoid are approached through **mastoidectomy.** The mastoid approach also allows for obliteration of mastoid cavity and, if necessary, middle ear cleft and eustachian tube orifice. A small extradural craniotomy via the temporal squama, in combination with a mastoidectomy, provides the advantages of limited craniotomy and to those of a mastoidectomy.[61] Herniated brain tissue should be gently excised by means of bipolar coagulation. The dural defect is packed with fat and fascia. A pedicled temporalis muscle flap can be used for further support.

of trauma. In most cases CSF leak stops spontaneously within one week. The roof of ethmoid, the cribriform plate are the most frequent sites of CSF rhinorrhea. CSF otorrhea results from transverse and longitudinal fractures of petrous bone. The risk of meningitis is 3 to 11% in patients who have post traumatic CSF rhinorrhea. Isotope cisternography can be done to demonstrate CSF leak. Metrizamide cisternography and MRI can localize the site of CSF leak in most cases. Most cases of CSF rhinorrhea leak spontaneously in one to two weeks. Indications for surgery are profuse and persistent rhinorrhea, meningitis, and CSF leak following penetrating injuries. Repair of CSF fistula can be done through an intracranial, extracranial or combined approach. Recently, endoscopic repair of CSF rhinorrhea has been reported with good result. In 10% patients there is risk of recurrence of CSF rhinorrhea.

CONCLUSIONS

Post-traumatic CSF rhinorrhea occurs in about 2% of closed head injuries admitted to hospital and in 9% patients with penetrating head injuries. In majority of patients the CSF leak occurs soon after the injury or within 48 hours

REFERENCES

1. Dagi FT, George ED. Management of cerebrospinal fluid leaks. In: Schmidek HH, Sweet WH (eds). *Operative Neurosurgical Techniques: Indications, Methods and Results.* Orlando, FL: Grune & Stratton 1988;49–69.

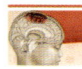

2. Lane B, Moseley IF, Stevens JM. The skull and brain. Methods of examination: Diagnostic approach. In Grainger RG, Allison DJ (eds). Grainger and Allison's Diagnostic Radiology. A Textbook of Medical Imaging (3rd edn). Churchill Livingstone 1997;2039–65.

3. Lewin W. Cerebrospinal fluid rhinorrhea in non-missile head injuries. Clin Neurosurg 1996;12:237–52.

4. Meirowsky AM, Caveness WF, et al. Cerebro-spinal fluid fistulas complicating missile wounds of the brain. J Neurosurg 1981;54:44.

5. Zlab MK, Moore GF, Daly DT, Yonkers AJ. Cerebrospinal fluid rhinorrhea: a review of the literature. Ear Nose Throat J 1992;71:314–7.

6. Schlosser RJ, Bolger WE. Nasal cerebrospinal fluid leaks: critical review and surgical con-siderations. Laryngoscope 2004;114:255–65.

7. Yilmazlar S, Arslan E, Kocaeli H, et al. Cere-brospinal fluid leakage complicating skull base fractures: analysis of 81 cases. Neurosurg Rev 2006;29:64–71.

8. Brodie HA, Thompson TC: Management of complications from 820 temporal bone fractures. Am J Otol 1997;18:188–97.

9. Aarabi B, Leibrock LG. Neurosurgical appro-aches to cerebrospinal fluid rhinorrhea. Ear Nose Throat J 1992;71:300–05.

10. Wax MK, Ramadan HH, Ortiz O, Wetmore SJ. Contemporary management of cerebrospinal fluid rhinorrhea. Otolaryngol Head Neck Surg 1997;116:442–9.

11. Yerkes SA, Thompson DH, Fisher WS. Spon-taneous cerebrospinal fluid rhinorrhea. Ear Nose Throat J 1992;71:318–20.

12. Bergman TA, Rockswold GL: Cerebrospinal fluid fistulae, in Youmans JR (ed): Youmans Neurological Surgery. A Comprehensive Guide to the Diagnosis and Management of Neuro-surgical Problems. Philadelphia: WB Saunders 1996;1840–52.

13. Lescanne E, Bakhos D, Aesch B, Celebi Z, Maheut-Lourmiere J, Cottier JP, Morinière S. Anterior cerebrospinal fluid leaks in children and adults: five years experience. Rev Laryngol Otol Rhinol (Bord). 2008;129(4–5):227–32.

14. Jones ME, Reino T, Gnoy A, et al. Identification of intranasal cerebrospinal fluid leaks by topical application with fluorescein dye. Am J Rhinol 2000;14:93–96.

15. Ommaya AK. Cerebrospinal fluid rhinorrhea. Neurology 1964;14:106.

16. McCoy G. Cerebrospinal fluid rhinorrhea. Laryngoscope 1963;73:1125.

17. Calcaterra TC. Diagnosis and management of ethmoid cerebrospinal rhinorrhea. Otolaryngol Clin North Ame 1985;18:99.

18. Loew F, et al. Traumatic, spontaneous and post-operative CSF rhinorrhea. Adv Tech Stand Neurosurg 1984;11:169.

19. Myers DL. Sataloff RT. Spinal fluid leakage after skull base surgical procedures. Otolaryngo Clin North Am 1984;17:601.

20. Park JI, Strelzow VV, Friedman WH. Current management of cerebrospinal fluid rhinorrhea. Laryngoscope 1983;93:1294–1300.

21. Hicks, GW, Wright WJ Jr, Wright WJ III. Cerebrospinal fluid otorrhea, Laryngoscope 1980;80 (Suppl 25):1–25.

22. Ghorayeb BY, Rafie JJ. Fracture of the temporal bone. Evaluation of 123 cases J Radio (Fr) 1989;70:703–10.

23. Raaf J. Post-traumatic cerebrospinal fluid leaks. Arch Surg 1967;95:648.

24. Ommaya AK. Spinal fluid fistula. Clin Neurosurg 1976;23:363.

25. Laun A. Traumatic cerebrospinal fluid fistulas in the anterior and middle cranial fossa. Acta Neurochir 1982;60:215.

26. Mantur M, Lukaszewicz-Zajac M, Mroczko B, Kulakowska A, Ganslandt O, Kemona H, Szmitkowski M, Drozdowski W, Zimmermann R, Kornhuber J, Lewczuk P. Cerebrospinal leakage—reliable diagnostic methods. Clin Chim Acta 2011;12;412(11–12):837–40.

27. Arrer E, Meco C, Oberascher G, Piotrowski W, Albegger K, Patsch W. Beta-trace protein as a marker for cerebrospinal fluid rhinorrhea. Clin Chem 2002;48:939–41.

28. Meco C, Oberascher G. Comprehensive algorithm for skull base dural lesion and cerebrospinal fistula diagnosis. Laryngoscope 2004;114:991–8.

29. Bachmann G, Nekic M, Michel O. Clinical experience with beta-trace protein as a marker for cerebrospinal fluid. Ann Otol Rhinol Laryngol 2000;109(12 pt 1):1099–1102.

30. Eljamel MS, Pidgeon CN. Localization of inactive cerebrospinal fluid fistulas. J Neurosurg 1995;83:795–8.

31. Douglas A.G. Intracranial trauma, In Puturan CE, Ravin CL (eds). Textbook of diagnostic imaging. Second edn, WB Saunders Company 1994.

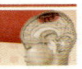
32. Drayer BE Wilkins RH, Boehnke M, Horton JA, Rosenbanm AE. Cerebrospinal fluid rhinorrhea demonstrated by metrizamide CT cisternography. A JR Am J Roentgenol 1977;129:149–51.

33. Eljamel M, Pidgeon C, Toland J, Phillips J, O'Dwyer A. MRI cisternography, and the localization of CSF fistula. Br J Neurosurg 1994;8:433–7.

34. Chow J, Goodman D, Mafee M. Evaluation of CSF rhinorrhea by computerized tomography with metrizamide. Otolaryngol Head Neck Surg 1989;100:99–105.

35. Shetty PG, Shroff MM, Sahani DV, Kirtane MV. Evaluation of high-resolution CT and MR cisternography in the diagnosis of cerebrospinal fluid fistula. AJNR Am J Neuroradiol 1998;19:633–9.

36. El Gammal T, Sobol W, Wadlington VR, et al. Cerebrospinal fluid fistula: detection with MR cisternography. AJNR Am J Neuroradiol 1998; 19:627–31.

37. Lloyd KM, DelGaudio JM, Hudgins PA; Imaging of Skull Base Cerebrospinal Fluid Leaks in Adults, Radiology September 2008;248:3:725–36.

38. Klatersky J, Sadeghi M, et al. Antimicrobial prophylaxis in patients with rhinorrhea or otorrhea: A double blind study. Surg Neurol 1976;6:111.

39. Eden K. Traumatic cerebrospinal rhinorrhea. Repair of a fistula by a transfrontal intradural operation. Br J Surg 1941;29:299–303.

40. Appel baum E. Meningitis following trauma to the head and face. JAMA 1968;173:116–20.

41. Dagi TF, Neyer FB, et al. The incidence and prevention of meningitis after basilar skull fracture. Am J Emerg Med 1983;3:295–8.

42. Liu P, Wu S, Li Z, Wang B. Surgical strategy for cerebrospinal fluid rhinorrhea repair. Neurosurgery 2010;66(6 Suppl Operative):281–5; discussion 285–6.

43. Dandy WE. Pneumocephalus (intracranial pneumatus cele or aerocele). Arch Surg 1926;12: 949–82.

44. Dagi TF, George ED. Surgical Management of cranial cerebrospinal fluid fistulas. In Schmidek HH, Sweet WH (eds). Operative Neurosurgical Techniques, Indications, Methods, and Results, 3rd edn, Volume 1, WB Saunders Company 1995; 117–31.

45. Ommaya AK. Cerebrospinal Fluid Fistula and Pneumocephalus. In Wilkins RH, Rengachargy SS (eds). Neurosurgery, 2nd edn. McGraw-Hill 1996; 2773–82.

46. Osbun JW, Ellenbogen RG, Chesnut RM, Chin LS, Connolly PJ, Cosgrove GR, Delashaw JB Jr, Golfinos JG, Greenlee JD, Haines SJ, Jallo J, Muizelaar JP, Nanda A, Shaffrey M, Shah MV, Tew JM Jr, van Loveren HR, Weinand ME, White JA, Wilberger JE. A multicenter, single-blind, prospective randomized trial to evaluate the safety of a polyethylene glycol hydrogel World Neurosurg 2012;78:498–504.

47. Sierra D, Fibrin sealant adhesive systesm: a review of their chemistry, material properties and clinical applications. J Biomat App 1993;7:309–52.

48. Ferrante L, Palatinsky E, et al. Intradural extracranial repair for cerebrospinal otorrhea with human fibrin glue: Technical note. J Neurol Neurosurg Psychiatry 1988;51:1438.

49. Komatsu M, Komatsu F, Cavallo LM, Solari D, Stagno V, Inoue T, Cappabianca P. Purely endoscopic repair of traumatic cerebrospinal fluid rhinorrhea from the anterior skull base: case report. Neurol Med Chir (Tokyo) 2011;51(3):222–5.

50. Wax MK, Ramadan HH MD, Ortiz O, Wetmore SJ. Contemporary Management of Cerebrospinal Fluid Rhinorrhea to laryngology—Head and Neck Surgery 1997;116:442.

51. Dodson EE, Gross CW, Swerdloff JL, Gustafson LM. Transnasal endoscopic repair of cerebrospinal fluid rhinorrhea and skull base defects: a review of twenty-nine cases. Otolaryngol Head Neck Surg 1994;111(5):600–5.

52. Scholsem M, Scholtes F, Collignon F, Robe P, Dubuisson A, Kaschten B, Lenelle J, Martin D. Surgical management of anterior cranial base fractures with cerebrospinal fluid fistulae: a single-institution experience. Neurosurgery. 2008;62:463–71.

53. Nachtigal D, Frenkiel S, Yoskovitch A, et al. Endoscopic repair of cerebrospinal fluid rhinorrhea: Is it the treatment of choice? J Otolaryngol 1999;28:129–33.

54. Ross IB, Colohan AR, Black MJ: Extracranial repair of cerebrospinal fluid rhinorrhea. Can J Neurol Sci 1990;17:320–23.

55. Tolley NS: A clinical study of spontaneous CSF rhinorrhoea. Rhinology 1991;29:223–30.

56. Citardi MJ, Cox AJ3, Bucholz RD: Acellular dermal allograft for sellar reconstruction after transsphenoidal hypophysectomy. Am J Rhinol 2000;14:69–73.

57. Van Den Abbeele T, Elmaleh M, Herman P, et al. Transnasal endoscopic repair of congenital

defects of the skull base in children. Arch. Otolaryngol Head Neck Surg 1999;125:580–584.

58. Wormald P, McDonogh M. The bath-plug closure of anterior skull base cerebrospinal uidleaks. Am J Rhinol 2003;17:299–305.

59. Hadley MN, Martin NA, Spetzler RF, et al: Comparative transoral dural closure techniques: A canine model. Neurosurgery 1988;22:392–397.

60. Rossitch E Jr, Wilkins RH. Use of fibrin glue in neurosurgery. In Wilkins RH, Rengachary SS (eds): Neurosurgery. New York: McGraw-Hill 1996;623–24

61. Adkins WY, Osguthrope JD. Mini craniotomy for management of CSF otorrhea from tegmen defects. Laryngoscope 1983;93:1038.

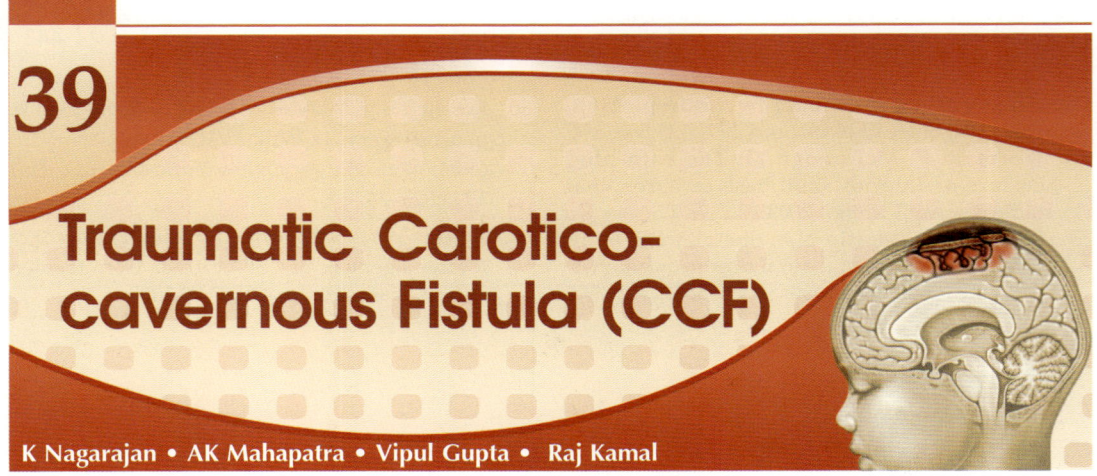

39

Traumatic Carotico-cavernous Fistula (CCF)

K Nagarajan • AK Mahapatra • Vipul Gupta • Raj Kamal

Carotico-cavernous fistulae (CCF) are classified by Barrow et al in 1985 into four types[1]—A, B, C and D with a being direct fistulous communication and B to D are indirect types similar to any other dural arteriovenous fistulae (AVF) (Table 39.1). In other parts of the body, creation of an arteriovenous fistula requires injury to segments of neighboring artery and vein simultaneously, but as cavernous sinus is unique where large artery traverses a venous space, traumatic breach in the internal carotid artery (ICA) alone within the cavernous sinus leads to direct (type A) fistula formation.[2] Indirect types are classified by their feeders Type B from meningeal branches of ICA, type C from branches of external carotid (ECA) and type D from both. Type D is the commoner type of indirect fistulae and is subclassified by Tomsick, et al.[3] into unilateral (D1) and bilateral (D2) types. Indirect CCFs are second common location for dural AVFs after transverse-sigmoid sinuses and they behave like other dural AVFs with similar predisposing factors (sinus thrombosis). They are more common in perimenopausal women.

Type A fistulae are more common in men and are usually due to trauma, mostly motor vehicle accidents, but in children, are due to penetrating injuries and falls.[4] Iatrogenic injuries may occasionally incite fistula formation like—trans-sphenoidal surgery (when ICA located on medial sellar floor), Fogarty catheter manipulation, carotid endarterectomy, gasserian rhizotomy, nasopharyngeal biopsy and recently, following treatment of a cavernous carotid aneurysm using a 'flow-diverter'.[2,4–6] A few cases of indirect, type C fistula between middle meningeal artery and cavernous sinus have been reported after routine craniotomy.[7] Specific disorders leading to defects in arterial wall media predispose to type ACCF formation with trivial or minor injury—Ehlers-Danlos syndrome, pseudoxanthoma elasticum, persistent trigeminal artery, cavernous ICA

		Barrow's	
Direct	High-flow	Type A – Direct	Traumatic
Indirect	Low-flow	Type B – Feeders from ICA	Spontaneous
		Type C – Feeders from ECA	
		Type D – From both ICA & ECA	
		D1 – Unilateral	
		D2 – Bilateral	

Table 39.1: Classification of carotico-cavernous fistulae

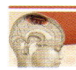

aneurysm and fibromuscular dysplasia and they complicate treatment due to fragility of vessels.[4]

Vascular Anatomy

Cavernous sinuses normally receive blood from intracranially (through spheno-parietal sinuses from superficial middle cerebral veins) and from the orbits (through superior and inferior ophthalmic veins). The outflow is posteriorly into petrosal (superior and inferior) sinuses, clival (basilar) plexus and inferiorly thorough emissary veins into pterygomaxillary plexus. The intercommunication between the cavernous sinuses is the circular (coronary) sinus.

ICA is divided into seven segments by Bouthillier et al[8]—C1 from bifurcation to skull base, C2 petrous segment, C3 lacerum, C4 cavernous, C5 clinoidal, C6 ophthalmic and C7 communicating segments. CCF usually involves the C4 and C5 segments and rarely C6 segment. Debrun et al[9] subclassified cavernous segment into five segments from above downwards (anterior clinoid to petrous canal)—anterior ascending, junction, horizontal segment (corresponding to C4), junction and posterior ascending. The frequency in 54 cases of traumatic CCF in each segment was 10%, 10%, 41%, 28% and 20%, respectively.

The branches of cavernous ICA and ECA branches supplying the dura in cavernous region are potential feeders in indirect CCF. Cavernous ICA gives the following branches—meningio-hypophyseal trunk, inferolateral trunk, McConnell's capsular artery and occasionally the ophthalmic artery. Meningohypophyseal trunk gives three branches—tentorial artery of Bernasconi-Cassinari, inferior hypophyseal artery and dorsal meningeal artery. Inferolateral trunk (ILT, artery of inferior cavernous sinus) gives four branches—superior (tentorial) branch, anteromedial branch, anterolateral branch to foramen rotundum anastomosing with artery of foramen rotundum from distal internal maxillary artery, and posterior branch. ILT

branches have anastomoses with branches of middle meningeal artery and contribute the most to indirect CCF.[10] McConnell's capsular artery arises medially to supply the hypophyseal fossa and anastomose with inferior hypophyseal and contralateral capsular branches. External carotid contribution to vascular network around the cavernous sinus includes accessory meningeal artery and hypoglossal artery. Accessory meningeal artery is a branch of middle meningeal or internal maxillary artery that enters through foramen ovale or Vesalius to anastomose with branches of ILT. Hypoglossal branch of ascending pharyngeal artery anastomoses with medial clival artery.

Clinical and Neuro-ophthalmological Features

The classical presentation of direct CCF is the "**Dandy's triad**"—pulsatile exophthalmos, bruit and conjunctival congestion/chemosis. The clinical manifestations are dependent on the location of fistula and direction of flow. The commoner anterior fistula leads to reversal of flow in the ophthalmic veins with orbital symptoms and signs. The less common posteriorly located fistula opens into the petrosal sinuses, with sixth nerve palsy and post-auricular bruit as the only clinical manifestations (**so-called 'white-eyed' CCF**).[11] In case of cortical venous reflux through the spheno-parietal sinus, venous infarcts or hemorrhage may result.

Orbital congestion due to arterialization of ophthalmic venous system leads to elevation of intraocular pressure (secondary glaucoma), venous stasis retinopathy, weakness and mechanical limitation of extraocular muscles, arterialization and dilatation of conjunctival vessels, conjunctival edema (chemosis), dilatation of veins and edema in the lids, engorged periorbital and facial veins in chronic CCF.[4,12,13] Ophthalmological signs and symptoms include conjunctival congestion and chemosis (edema), proptosis, diplopia, reduced visual acuity, elevated intraocular pressure (IOP), ophthalmoplegia with or without cranial nerve palsies (III, IV & VI) and periorbital bruit.

Ophthalmoplegia results from several mechanisms—proptosis, engorgement of extraocular muscles and cranial nerve palsies. Cranial nerve palsy may be caused by vascular compression or venous ischemia. Direct injury to cranial nerves (III, IV, VI, less commonly V1 and V2) also can occur without appreciable fracture of sphenoid bone and should be differentiated from that of due to CCF itself, as palsy due to trauma is usually present immediately after trauma and is associated with poor outcome, even if CCF development is occasionally delayed. Fifth nerve motor deficits are not due to CCF and are usually due to traumatic neuropathy. Seventh or eighth nerve palsy is due to associated petrous bone fracture and complicates the proptosis-related corneal exposure.

Diminished visual acuity results from many causes—exposure keratitis and corneal ulcer, vitreous hemorrhage, retinal ischemia due to arterial steal or venous congestion, central retinal vein occlusion (rare but irreversible) and retinal detachment. Complete ptosis with involvement of levator is due to third nerve palsy than less common direct levator muscle or aponeurosis damage. Partial ptosis may be due to partial third nerve or sympathetic paresis, local lid edema or combination of all. Pupil may be normal or may be affected due to loss of sympathetic and/or parasympathetic involvement (with loss of light reflex and dilatation in dark). Pupil examination may not be possible if there is iris damage or traumatic uveitis. Afferent pupillary defect is noted (**Marcus-Gunn pupil**) as in any other unilateral optic neuropathy.[2] Optic neuropathy is due to any of the following—ischemia, compression by enlarged cavernous sinus or glaucoma.

Raised intraocular pressure (glaucoma) causes field defect in 20% and retinal artery occlusion in 2% of CCF and is usually unilateral. Gonioscopy can visualize engorgement in **Schlemm's canal** due to raised episcleral venous pressure. The development of glaucoma is multi-factorial—raised episcleral venous pressure, congestion of iris and ciliary apparatus narrowing the trabecular meshwork and shallowing the anterior chamber, choroidal congestion or effusion bowing the lens-iris diaphragm and collapse of intraocular veins.[4,14]

The differential diagnosis for proptosed red eye and congested orbit are cavernous dural AVF, dysthyroid orbitopathy, orbital inflammatory disease or cellulitis, infiltrating neoplasms (e.g. lymphoma) or metastasis, bleeding into orbital tumor (e.g. lymphangioma).[2,4,10,15] Imaging can delineate most of these conditions. If the proptosis is mild, the congestion may be mistaken for conjunctivitis particularly when there is no bruit as in indirect CCF. The conjunctival congestion due to CCF shows as arterialized bright red with limbal loop (**corkscrew**) vessels unlike darker red congestion of conjunctivitis.[4] Chronic CCF reported in older days used to cause iris vessel dilatation, white blood cellular flare in anterior chamber, rarely corneal edema and iris neovascularization (Fig. 39.1).

Fundus may show venous ischemic-hypoxic retinopathy with venous congestion, retinal hemorrhages, disc swelling, retinal edema (macula), cotton-wool spots, choroidal edema/effusion, choroid and serous retinal

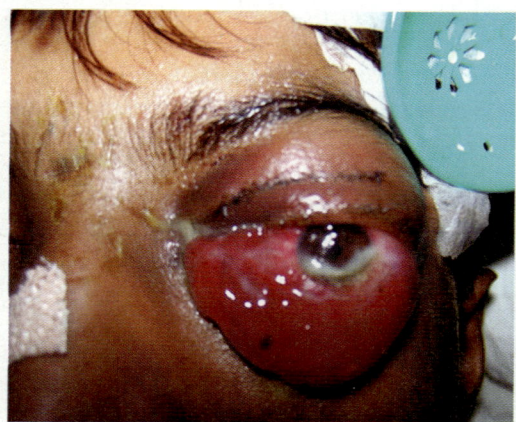

Fig. 39.1: 38-year-old male presenting with gross proptosis, conjunctival congestion and prolapse and anterior chamber 'flare' due to chronicity

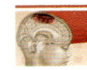

detachments and they have to be differentiated from direct trauma effects.[4]

Though older literature described visible pulsations and thrill (at medial canthus), pulsations are seen or palpated in less than 30% of cases. Pulse-synchronous bruit is heard in most cases of direct CCF and in about 40– 50% of indirect fistulae and it may be positional and responsive to carotid compression in the neck. Differential diagnoses for orbital bruit include vertebral AVF, subclavian occlusion, sphenoid hypoplasia (e.g. neurofibromatosis) due to transmitted CSF pulsations and rarely orbital vascular tumors. Resolution of bruit may be used to follow-up of patency after treatment of direct fistulae.[2]

Enlarged superior ophthalmic vein is seen apart from CCF in:

1. Cavernous sinus thrombosis

2. Orbital AVM due to shunt or mechanical compression

3. Varix due to superior ophthalmic vein thrombosis by direct pressure

4. Inflammatory or neoplastic process in orbital apex or superior orbital fissure

5. Dysthyroid orbitopathy. CT or MR imaging can differentiate most of these causes.

The neuro-ophthalmological signs and symptoms and occasionally their absence depend on location of the fistula in the cavernous sinus (anterior or posterior) and extent of thrombosis of cavernous sinus and draining veins. Even bruit may be heard in contralateral orbit if anterior cavernous sinus or ophthalmic vein is thrombosed. Conversely, orbital congestion may be maximal if there is thrombosis of posterior cavernous sinus and poor communication with contralateral cavernous sinus.[4]

Orbital swelling is more with recumbent and head down position, which decreases with head elevation to 30°. Bilateral orbital signs are noted in 20% of unilateral fistulae and bilateral fistulae are seen in less than 1%. Life-threatening epistaxis is a risk if the CCF drains solely (though rare) inferiorly into pterygomaxillary plexus or with cavernous carotid pseudoaneurysm which is present in 1–2% of all CCF.[10] The details of clinical presentation in our series of 73 cases are given in Table 39.2.

In the acute setting of trauma the more serious injuries to brain parenchyma, orbit and cranial nerves like life-threatening extra-axial hematoma or globe rupture require management prior to CCF apart from extra-cranial injuries to chest, spine, abdomen and extremities. But repair of periorbital fractures is preferably done after the closure of CCF due to increased risk of bleeding from the congested tissues.[4]

Indications for urgent treatment[16] include cortical venous drainage (in hypoplasia or occlusion of cavernous sinus), presence of varix, pseudoaneurysm and ophthalmological deterioration (reducing visual acuity, progressive glaucoma, worsening proptosis).

Total steal with complete absence of distal flow of ICA above the fistula and intracranial vessels occurs in 5% at diagnosis and was previously known as complete carotid transection. It confirms that the fistula is large and of high-flow type and also that the "circle of Willis" is complete, if there are no deficits on opposite side.[10] In such a situation balloon test occlusion is unnecessary if carotid sacrifice is contemplated, as the fistula per se has acted as test occlusion.[2]

Table 39.2: Clinical profile of 73 patients at AIIMS	
Clinical features	*No. of patients*
Proptosis	73
Ocular palsy	50
Chemosis	51
Bruit	43
Tinnitus	17
Visual loss	25
Ptosis	08
Papilledema/optic atrophy	12
Facial hypoesthesia	06
Epistaxis	08
Engorged forehead veins	04

Role of Computed Tomography (CT) and Magnetic Resonance Imaging (MRI)

CT and MRI findings include proptosis, increased attenuation/altered signal changes of intra-orbital fat, extra-ocular muscle enlargement, superior ophthalmic vein enlargement or thrombosis, enlargement of cavernous sinus, enhancing vessels with edema in basifrontotemporal lobes in case of cortical venous reflux and hemorrhages if any (Figs 39.2 and 39.3). Bony erosions may be noted in CT in case of pre-existing cavernous ICA aneurysm.

Digital Subtraction Angiography (DSA)

DSA is the gold standard to rule out a CCF and selective angiography of bilateral ICAs, ECAs and vertebral arteries should be done. The following branches (br) are studied for supply to fistula.

ECA—middle meningeal, accessory meningeal, distal internal maxillary (artery of foramen rotundum, vidian br) and ascending pharyngeal (jugal and hypoglossal br).

ICA—meningohypophyseal, inferolateral artery, McConnell artery.

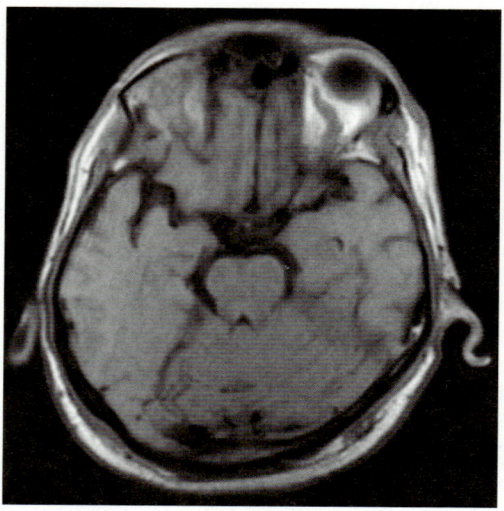

Fig. 39.3: MRI section in a different patient showing partially thrombosed left superior ophthalmic vein

Dangerous anastomoses if any, are noted particularly between:
- ICA and meningeal, vidian, artery of foramen rotundum and ophthalmic
- Ascending pharyngeal with petrous/cavernous ICA
- Occipital artery with ICA or vertebral artery.

The angiographic features in our series are given in Tables 39.3a and b (Figs 39.4a to c).

The complete angiographic evaluation should delineate the following:
- Location and size of fistula
- Differentiation of direct and indirect types
- Specific arterial supply in indirect fistula, dangerous ECA-ICA or ophthalmic connections
- Characterization and mapping of cavernous sinus venous outflow including venous stenosis or thrombosis, patency of inferior petrosal, intercavernous sinuses and superior ophthalmic veins
- Identification of high-risk features—cortical venous reflux, varix, pseudoaneurysm
- Associated vascular injuries (dissection) and displacement due to hematomas

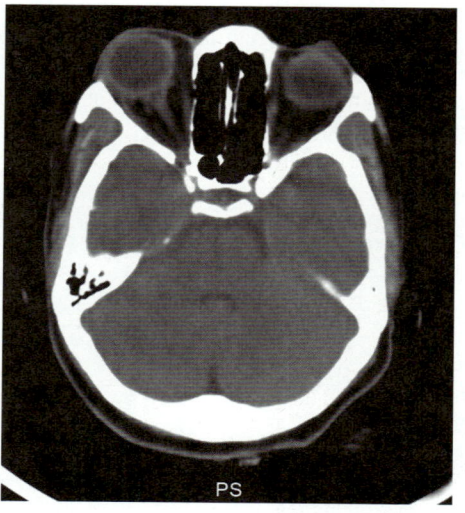

Fig. 39.2: CT sections through the orbit showing right globe proptosis, intra-conal fat stranding and serpiginous vessels

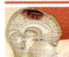
Table 39.3a: Traumatic carotid cavernous fistula	
Radiological features	*No.*
Giant cavernous sinus	20
Intercavernous communications	07
Anterior	34
Posterior	14
Venous drainage	
Inferior	03
Cortical	15
Contralateral	04
Combined	20

Table 39.3b: Traumatic carotid cavernous fistula	
Radiological features	*No.*
ICA segment involved	
C2	02
C2–3	03
C3	05
C3–4	02
C4	05
C4–5	03
C5	19
Steal phenomenon	
Mild	14
Moderate	05
Severe	07

- Predisposing conditions—cavernous aneurysm and fibromuscular dysplasia
- Evaluation of collateral flow and carotid bifurcation (carotid sacrifice or feasibility of manual compression).

The following **maneuvers**[4,17,18] are useful to delineate high-flow fistula apart from high frame rate (> 5 frames/sec) and high contrast volumes (7–8 ml/sec).

Mehringer-Hieshima's maneuver (gentle ipsilateral ICA injection during manual-compression of the ipsilateral carotid artery).

Heuber's maneuver (ipsilateral carotid compression during vertebral artery injection).

Berenstein maneuver (double lumen occlusion balloon catheter in ICA with balloon inflated and slow contrast injection).

Angiography occasionally may not be able to differentiate varix from a pseudoaneurysm. The identification of pseudoaneurysm is important as sudden closure of the fistula may lead to rupture of the pseudoaneurysm.

During diagnostic angiography cross-circulation is tested by ipsilateral carotid compression and contralateral carotid injection and either of the vertebral artery injections. If necessary, balloon test occlusion (BTO) may be done at this time or during the endovascular treatment.[10] BTO is done under monitoring and if available, with imaging (SPECT) and relative hypotensive challenge (nitroprusside). After balloon occlusion of petrous ICA (C2), the following are tested; mental status, speech, visual field, facial movements and motor power in all four extremities. Hypotensive challenge is done by

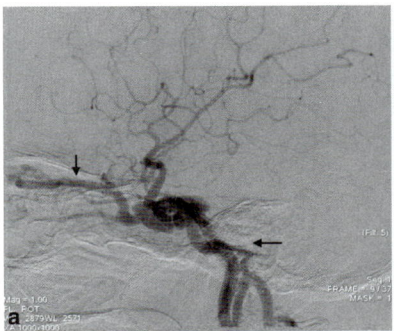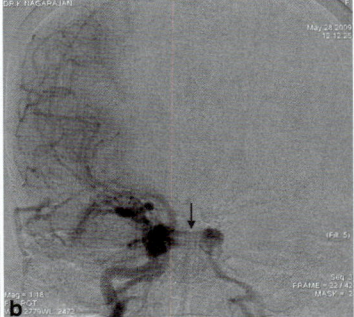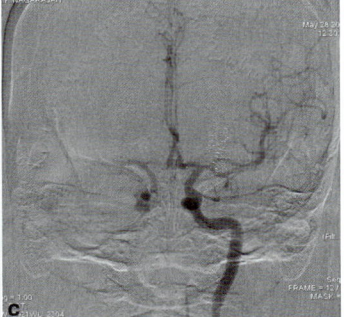

Fig. 39.4: DSA of right ICA (a – lateral, b – frontal) showing direct, high-flow CCF on right side with anterior (ophthalmic), posterior (petrosal) and contralateral cavernous sinus (arrows) drainage. Left ICA (c – frontal) angiograms show no filling of fistula from left side and right ACA filling through anterior communicating artery (Acom)

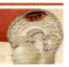

intra-arterial nitroprusside and backup anesthetic support to reach two-thirds of patient's baseline mean arterial pressure. If patient develops neurological signs, the BTO is repeated at the level of fistula or by using double balloons (with ostium of fistula trapped in between).

Management

The goal of therapy is closure of the shunt that will enable to reverse the orbital venous hypertension, normalize ophthalmic blood flow and prevent potential visual loss. All other measures are necessarily compromises and such palliative steps should be considered only if primary goal is not feasible (patient is too old or refuses treatment). Resolution of bruit is a minor or secondary goal of therapy.[4]

Treatment of glaucoma is usually medical, and surgical measures (filtration, canthotomy) are considered only in emergency (when IOP is more than 40 mm Hg) due to precipitation of choroidal effusion/hemorrhage by sudden lowering of IOP. Laser iridotomy or trabeculoplasty may be considered for glaucoma if primary closure of fistula is not done. Similarly, lateral or total tarsorrhaphy is done to protect corneal damage and rarely excision of prolapsed necrotic conjunctiva.[4]

Conservative Treatment

Indirect fistulae of slow flow may be conservatively managed by manual compression provided there is no atherosclerotic disease of the cervical carotid. Manual compression is done only by the patient using his opposite hand so that if there is any cerebral ischemia, the hand drops down with relief of compression. Compression is done for about 10 seconds about 4–6 times per hour. It is not advisable to use ipsilateral hand or be done by anyone other than the patient. Manual compression itself can result in closure of about 30% of slow-flow indirect CCF.[2,5] Complications noted due to manual compression are vasovagal reactions and transient ischemic or thromboembolic events.

Surgical Management

The earliest reports[19,20] of treatment used ligation of carotid artery in the neck, though recanalization was noted subsequently.[21] Trapping was used to occlude ICA both at neck and at ophthalmic or supraclinoid levels along with muscle embolization of ECA.[22] Trapping may lead to ophthalmic artery occlusion or recurrence of fistula with worsening of visual symptoms. Now surgical approach is restricted to provide access to endovascular treatment as in orbitotomy, or for exposure of carotid at bifurcation or in the cavernous sinus. Even parent artery occlusion is done by endovascular means rather than by surgical approach. Surgery is used as last resort or salvage procedure, when endovascular treatment has failed or when proximal access is inaccessible. The surgical approach and technique have been dealt in detail by van Loveren et al.[23]

Stereotactic Radiosurgery

The role of radiation therapy or gamma knife has been reported for indirect CCF, but follow-up of nearly two years is required to confirm the occlusion of the shunt and may not be useful in emergency situations or for direct fistulae.[24–26]

Endovascular Treatment

The earliest endovascular reports involved muscle embolus[27] into the ICA and fistula and the modern detachable balloon treatment started with Prolo and Serbinenko.[28,29] Balloon technology advanced from latex to silicone and gold-valve types and is being replaced by detachable coils and onyx for the direct fistulae.[30–33] For indirect fistulae, various-embolizing agents have been used—initially PVA particles, then liquid embolic agent n-butyl cyanoacrylate (NBCA, glue) and now another liquid agent ethylene vinyl alcohol copolymer admixed with DMSO (onyx). Transvenous route embolization employed coils and occasionally balloons and now being done mainly by using onyx. Anticoagulation

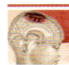

is maintained during endovascular treatment using heparin and maintained by checking the ACT (activated clotting time above 300 seconds).

Detachable Balloon Treatment

Detachable balloon treatment is proven long-standing mode of treatment even today due to its cost-effectiveness particularly in developing countries as coils required to fill a large cavernous sinus may be quite large in number with subsequent cost factor. During the initial days of detachable balloon treatment, balloons matching the fistula ostial size, which is usually between 2 and 6 mm (average 3 mm, corresponds to detachable balloon volume 0.3 cc, equivalent to inflation dimension of 7 × 9 mm) were used.[31]

The types of balloons used for CCF treatment were:
- Latex balloon, Gold valve balloon, Brassal-Ruffenacht, Taki-Handa balloons
- Silicone balloons—Parker, Hieshima

Microcatheters used for mounting balloons have also evolved from stiffer teflon micro-catheters used for hand-tied balloons to polyethylene and silastic catheters that are in use for valved detachable balloons. Depending upon the size of fistula and cavernous sinus, more than one balloon may be necessary for optimal occlusion and double balloon technique may also be used in certain difficult situations.[33]

The advantages of balloon are it can be easily flow-guided to the fistula site, repeated inflation and deflation can be done to see the changes and it is cheap. But balloon treatment had its own set of difficulties. For placement of balloon, the fistula needs to be smaller than an inflated balloon, but must be large enough to allow passage of a deflated or partially inflated balloon. The cavernous sinus should be large enough to accommodate the inflated balloon or balloons.

Failure often occurs when the fistula orifice is too small to allow entry of the balloon catheter, or when a large fistula is combined with a small sinus leading to balloon retraction into the ICA, or sharp margins from bony spicules causing rupture of the balloon during inflation.[33] Further problems are enlarged cavernous sinus that cannot be completely filled by even with multiple balloons leaving empty spaces preventing complete occlusion and cure, and transection of the cavernous internal carotid artery.

Complications following balloon occlusion treatment were unsatisfactory placement of a balloon, rupture of a balloon during manipulation, premature balloon deflation and recurrence of fistula, premature/difficult balloon detachment and displacement or migration of balloon, delayed or partial deflation of balloon resulting in venous pouch, balloon causing cranial nerve compression and arterial or petrosal vein (in transvenous treatment) injury during catheterization/deployment. A tortuous or stenotic ICA or presence of an intimal flap may also involve difficulties in detachable balloon treatment. To avoid premature deflation of balloon, various materials were used to fill the balloon—saline/metrizamide/silicone/hydroxy-ethylmethacrylate (HEMA), but laboratory studies have showed saline-diluted contrast as optimal without any added risk of premature balloon deflation. Xiao-Quan Xu et al[32] in their recent study (2013) of follow-up of 58 cases of CCF embolized with detachable balloon, over a period of seven years, reported 7 cases (12%) ending up with parent artery occlusion, and another 7 (12%) developing recurrence of fistula (3 to 40 days), who subsequently underwent further treatment (4 second balloon treatment, 1-covered stent-graft and 2 parent artery occlusion). At our institute, mainly using detachable balloons, successful fistula closure was achieved in 85% cases and ICA patency was preserved in 85% after embolization.[13] (Tables 39.4a to c). We have also used transcranial Doppler (TCD) to evaluate the fistula closure after embolization and found that TCD velocity increase always accompanied closure and absence of increase

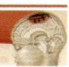

Table 39.4a: Treatment options

1. Conservative—intermittent manual compression
2. Endovascular
   a. Transarterial
   b. Transvenous
   c. Transorbital
   d. Combined
   e. Parent artery occlusion
3. Surgical
   a. Transvenous packing of cavernous sinus
   b. Direct exposure and ligation of CCF under cardiac bypass and deep hypothermia
   c. Carotid ligation

Table 39.4b: Treatment modalities in our series

Treatment modalities	No.
Balloon	30
Coils	02
IBCA	01
Ivalon	01
Balloon + Coil	01
Surgery	01

Table 39.4c: AIIMS experience and results

Results	No.
Complete closure	57
Partial closure	07
Carotid preserved	30
Carotid occluded	05
Spontaneous occlusion	01

in velocity correlated with incomplete or partial embolization observed in angiogram.[34]

After the introduction of Guglielmi detachable coils (GDC) for intracranial aneurysms, coils have been in use for CCF closure either transarterially or by the transvenous route.[35] Balloon protection of the ICA may be used to avoid prolapse of coil into the lumen (balloon-assisted). Newer bioactive coils (hydrocoils, matrix coils) may also be used as similar to their use in aneurysmal obliteration (Fig. 39.5). GDC embolization is reasonably successful with total or near-total fistula obliteration and small or slow residual fistula flow undergoes spontaneous thrombosis on follow-up. Appropriate anticoagulation is maintained to avoid the progression of thrombosis into the parent artery or distal embolic events.

Parent Artery Occlusion

Due to technical difficulties and failure of selective fistula closure, parent artery occlusion may be required, though with current technology of endovascular materials, the need for this becoming less. The cavernous and petrous ICA is occluded preferably sparing the ophthalmic artery origin usually with coils. The material of choice for parent artery occlusion is detachable coils with GDC as first coil distally and may be followed proximally by fibered coils. Though difficult to navigate through tortuous vessels, using **vascular plug (Amplatz)** is another recently developing, cheaper alternative for parent artery occlusion.[36]

Transvenous Access

Transvenous route is more useful for indirect CCF and some of the difficult direct fistulae (Fig. 39.6). Transvenous access is through the femoral vein, venae cavae, jugular vein and inferior petrosal sinus. Less commonly, facial vein, pterygoid plexus, superior petrosal, ophthalmic, even cortical (Sylvian) vein have been tried to access the cavernous sinus.[37] Inferior petrosal sinus (IPS) is fragile with risk of perforation during catheterization. Conversely, even if IPS is thrombosed, guidewire may be passed through the thrombus to enter the cavernous sinus. Transvenous coil embolization in cavernous sinus should preferably start from close to ICA fistula, so that sudden thrombosis of ophthalmic veins or cortical venous reflux does not develop and precipitate worsening of orbital symptoms or intracranial hemorrhage. The transvenous embolization is now done usually with a combination of coils and liquid embolic agents (either NBCA or onyx).

Cavernous sinus can also be accessed through percutaneous transorbital transophthalmic venous route. Transorbital access has been used in difficult situation—either

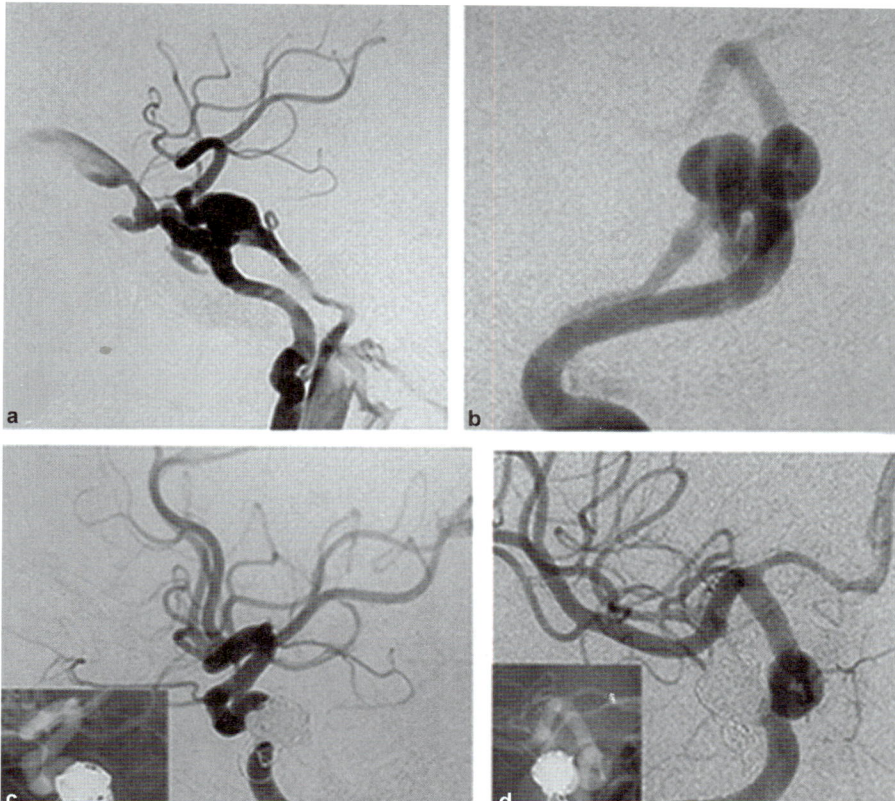

Fig. 39.5: Case of direct CCF treated by coil embolization DSA of internal carotid artery reveals direct CCF arising from cavernous ICA (lateral view–a; anteroposterior view–b). Transarterial embolization was performed with detachable platinum coils resulting in complete occlusion (c, d). Inset in Figs 39.5c and d shows the coil mass

through the ophthalmic vein or rarely through the superior orbital fissure into the cavernous sinus.[38–40] Transorbital treatment has potential complications such as difficulty infinding superior ophthalmic vein, difficulty in determining the direction of flow, orbital hemorrhage due to inadvertent puncture, possible injury to trochlea, sudden orbital congestion due to thrombosis with vision loss and later, infection.[40] Subarachnoid hemorrhage due to dural penetration and vision loss due to direct injury of the optic nerve or ophthalmic artery, or retrobulbar hematoma are other risks associated with transorbital approach.

Indirect CCF Treatment

Indirect fistulae have been treated mainly by transvenous route by obliterating the venous side of the fistula. Transvenous embolization is done using coils and liquid embolic agent (NBCA). If transarterial route is undertaken to embolize the feeders from ECA, PVA particles or NBCA may be used. Both of them have limitations for feeders from the ICA unless there is hypertrophy of feeders. The complication rate is much less with transvenous approach than the arterial feeder embolization. Cranial nerve testing is done before ECA branch arterial feeder embolization to avoid cranial nerve palsies. It is reliably performed

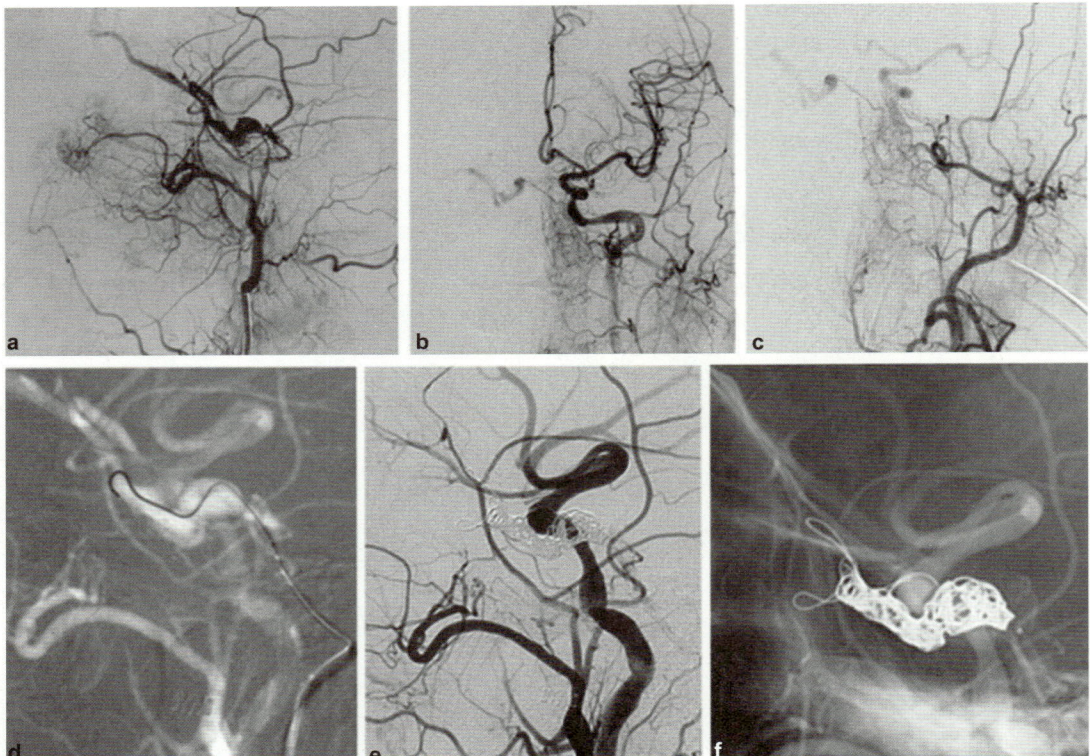

Fig. 39.6: Transvenous embolization of indirect CCF; angiogram of right external carotid artery (a), left internal carotid artery (b) and left external carotid artery (c) reveals a CCF with multiple small feeders draining into the ophthalmic vein. Notice that the ipsilateral petrosal sinus is not opacified, indicating occlusion. Transvenous embolization was performed. A guiding catheter was placed in jugular vein and a microcatheter was placed through the occluded petrosal sinus into the right cavernous sinus (d). Thereafter, the fistula was embolized with detachable coils resulting in complete occlusion (e, f)

by lidocaine (1% solution, 2.5–5.0 ml) followed by the relevant cranial nerve examination.[10]

Covered Stent (Stent-graft) Reconstruction

Polyethylene-covered stent grafts are seemingly attractive alternative for closure of fistula with ICA preservation, but their poor navigability through intracranial vessels introduces technical difficulties apart from thromboembolic complications later.[41–43] Patients are on anticoagulant therapy for 48 hours and double anti-platelet therapy for 3 months followed by single drug (aspirin) probably for life. The long-term results are yet to be ascertained.

The indications for stent-grafts are large tears of the ICA preventing stable positioning and detachment of balloons, and large cavernous sinuses that need large number of coils. However, to navigate a stent-graft, the ICA should not have significant tortuosity and no critical side branches should be present close to the fistula site. The stent-graft also requires extra support to navigate like a long sheath and guide catheter, and stiff exchange wire. Recent reports of stent-graft treatment of CCF in 8 and 7 patients[42, 43] with follow-up showed obliteration of fistula in all with one case of asymptomatic carotid occlusion in each series due to interruption of anti-platelet therapy by the patient and another case of mild intimal hyperplasia.

Onyx Embolization

Onyx is a combination of ethylene vinyl alcohol copolymer (EVAL) dissolved in dimethyl sulfoxide (DMSO) and suspended micronized tantalum powder for opacification and is available in three formulations (onyx 18, 34, 500). It is non-adhesive and polymerizes slowly and this gives the advantages of non-sticking to microcatheter (unlike NBCA) and better penetration as the injection involves 'plug and push' technique allowing reflux and subsequent filling of all compartments and crevices of vascular spaces in the malformation/fistulae.[44] Onyx is used in both direct and indirect CCF, either transarterially or transvenously and with or without balloon assistance.[44,45] Balloon assistance, particularly in direct CCF helps to identify the fistulous point, acts as support for coils, protects from inadvertent arterial embolization, and prevents onyx and coils from obscuring the ICA during the treatment.[46] Complications such as brady-cardia or even asystole have been reported due to onyx possibly due to toxic effect on DMSO on trigeminal nerve or branches (vagal response of trigemino-cardiac reflex) particularly in low-flow/low-volume compartments/malformations and are usually reversible with stopping the onyx injection and administration of atropine.[47] Prophylactic treatment is suggested either with atropine, or transvenous pacemaker in those with heart block or with atropine contraindication. Other complications reported include catheter rupture, angio-toxicity (due to DMSO) and reflux into normal branches.

Post-procedure Follow-up

Though ocular manifestation resolve rapidly in many patients, there is 'paradoxical worsening' in some patients—either orbital congestion or cranial nerve palsy—probably due to extension of thrombosis.[5] This may follow any of the modes of treatment— radiosurgery, endovascular or even conservative manual compression. Anti-inflammatory medications (steroids) are of help for some, but in almost all cases these symptoms resolve within a short span of time.

However, persistence or recurrence of bruit or raised intraocular pressure may be a manifestation of incomplete closure of fistula or recurrence of the shunt and warrants follow-up angiography.[4] Those who have undergone parent artery occlusion and placement of covered stent-graft are also candidates for follow-up with angiography usually after 3–6 months for monitoring the hemodynamic changes.

CONCLUSIONS

- All head injury patients with skull base fractures with or without orbital congestion/proptosis should be considered for possibility of traumatic CCF, more so if they develop orbital symptoms and signs or cranial nerve palsies.
- Those with orbital congestion/proptosis, neuroimaging should be evaluated for enlarged superior ophthalmic vein and prominent/enhancing vessels in the vicinity.
- DSA is the modality of choice to rule out the fistula and it should include the external carotid and if necessary, maneuvers for the fistula delineation.
- Endovascular treatment with detachable balloons or GDC coils is the mainstay of treatment for direct CCF.
- Onyx has become the agent of choice for indirect type of CCF either transarterial or transvenous route, or rarely transorbital access.
- Role of newer devices, like vascular plug and stent-graft, are evolving and to be ascertained for long-term stability.

REFERENCES

1. Barrow D, Spector R, Landman J, et al. Classification and treatment of spontaneous carotid cavernous fistulas. J Neurosurg 1985; 62: 248–56.

2. Phatouros CC, Meyers PM, Dowd CF, Halbach VV, Malek AM, Higashida HT. Carotid artery cavernous fistulas. Neurosurg Clin of North Am 2000;11:67–84.

3. Tomsick TA. Types B, C & D (dural) CCF: Etiology, prevalence and natural history. In Tomsick TA (Ed) Carotid cavernous fistula. Cincinnati, Digital Education Publishing 1997; pp. 59–73.

4. Kuppersmith MJ, Berenstein A. Chap 2: Carotico-cavernous fistulas. In Neurovascular Neuro-ophthalmology. Springer-Verlag, Berlin Heidelberg 1993; pp 69–108.

5. Korkmazer B, Kocak B, Tureci E, Islak C, Kocer N, Kizilkilic O. Endovascular treatment of carotid cavernous sinus fistula: A systematic review. World J Radiol 2013;5:143–55.

6. Mustafa W, Kadziolka K, Anxionnat R, Pierot L. Direct carotid-cavernous fistula following intracavernous carotid aneurysm treatment with a flow-diverter stent: A case report. Interven Neuroradiol 2010;16:447–50.

7. Wantanabe A, Takahara Y, Ibuchi Y, et al. Two cases of dural arteriovenous malformations occurring after intracranial surgery. Neuroradiology 1984;26:375–80.

8. Bouthillier A, van Loveren HR, Keller JT. Segments of the internal carotid artery: a new classification. Neurosurgery 1996;38:425–32.

9. Debrun G, Lacour P, Vinuela F, et al. Treatment of 54 carotid-cavernous fistulas. J Neurosurg 1981;55:678–92.

10. Ringer AJ, Salud L, Tomsick TA. Carotid cavernous fistulas: Anatomy, classification and treatment. Neurosurg Clin of North Am 2005;16: 279–95.

11. Kosomorsky GS, Hanson MR, Tomsak RL. Carotid cavernous fistulae presenting as painful ophthalmoplegia without external ocular signs.J Clin Neuroophthalmol 1988;81:131–5.

12. Kurve AS, Mahapatra AK, Mishra NK. Traumatic CCF: A 17-year experience at AIIMS. Annual Neurotrauma conference at Pune, August 2003.

13. Jindal A, Mishra NK, Mehta VS, Mahapatra AK. Clinical profile, radiological findings and results of CCF—a series of 41 cases: Data presented at 6th National Neurotrauma conference at Varanasi, August 1997.

14. Ishijima K, Kashiwagi K, Nakano K, Shibuya T, Tsumura T, Tsukahara S. Ocular manifestations and prognosis of secondary glaucoma in patients with carotid-cavernous fistula. Jpn J Ophthalmol 2003;47:603–8.

15. Pendharkar HS, Gupta AK, Bodhey N, Nair M. Diffusion restriction in thrombosed superior ophthalmic veins: Two cases of diverse etiology and literature review. Radiol Case 2011; 5:8–16.

16. Halbach VV, Hieshima GB, Higashida RT, et al. Carotid cavernous fistulae: Indications for urgent treatment. AJNR 1987;8:627–33.

17. Mehringer C, Hieshima C, Grinnell V, et al. Improved localization of carotid cavernous fistula during angiography. AJNR 1982; 3:82–84.

18. Huber P. A technical contribution to the exact angiographic localization of carotid cavernous fistulas. Neuroradiology 1976;10:239–41.

19. Travers B. A case of aneurysm by anastomosis in the orbit, cured by the ligature of the common carotid artery.Med Chir Trans 1811;2:1–16.

20. Gamgee JS. Stab through the ear, traumatic aneurysm, death after ligature of common carotid artery. Lancet 1875;1:535.

21. Dandy WE. The treatment of carotid cavernous A-V aneurysms.Ann Surg 1935;102:196–210.

22. Hamby WB, Gardner WJ. Treatment of pulsation exophthalmos with report of two cases. Arch Surg 1933;27:676–85.

23. van Loveren HR, Tauber M, Lewis AI, Tew JM. Direct surgical treatment of carotid cevrnous fistula.In Tomsick TA (ed): Carotid cavernous fistula. Cincinnati, Digital Education Publishing 1997;83–94.

24. Hirai T, Korogi Y, Baba Y, et al. Dural carotid cavernous fistulas: role of conventional radiation therapy, long-term results with irradiation, embolization or both. Radiology 1998;207:423–30.

25. Kurata A, Miyasaka Y, Irikura K, Fujii K, Kan S. Stereotactic gamma surgery combined with endovascular surgery for treatment of a spontaneous carotid-cavernous fistula. Neuro-ophthalmology 2000;23:35–41.

26. Koebbe CJ, Singhal D, Sheehan J, et al. Radio-surgery for dural arteriovenous fistulas. Surg Neurol 2005;64:392–8.

27. Brooks B. The treatment of traumatic arteriovenous fistula. Southern Medical Journal 1930;23:100–6.

28. Prolo DJ, Hanberry JW. Intraluminal occlusion of a carotid-cavernous fistula with a balloon catheter: Technical note. J Neurosurg 1971;35:237–42.

29. Serbinenko FA. Balloon catheterization and occlusion of major cerebral vessels. J Neurosurg 1974;41:125–45.

30. Debrun G. Management of carotid-cavernous fistulas. Chapter in Interventional Neuro-

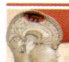
radiology. Endovascular therapy of the central nervous system. Ed Vinuela F, Halbach VV, Dion JE. Raven Press, New York 1992;107–12.

31. Tomsick TA. Carotid cavernous fistulas.Ch in Endovascular and percutaneous therapy of the brain and spine. Marks MP, Do HM (eds). Lippincott, WW, Philadelphia 2002:317–36.

32. Xiao-Quan Xu, Sheng Liu, Qing-Quan Zu, et al. Follow-up of 58 traumatic carotid-cavernous fistulae after endovascular detachable balloon embolization at a single center. J Clin Neurol 2013;9:83–90.

33. Tsai YH, Wong HF, Chen YL, Weng HH. Transarterial embolization of direct carotid-cavernous fistulas with the double-balloon technique. Interven Neuroradiol 2008;14 (Suppl 2):13–17.

34. Arora T. TCD blood flow study before and after embolization of carotico-cavernous fistula: A study at AIIMS. M Ch thesis submitted in 2000.

35. Luo CB, Teng MM, Lin CJ, Chang FC, Chang CY. Transarterial embolization of traumatic carotid-cavernous fistulae by Gugliemi detachable coils: A seven-year experience. Interven Neuroradiol 2008;14 (Suppl 2):5–8.

36. Grala J, Schroth G, Kickuth R, El-Koussy M, Do DD, Brekenfeld C. Closing the gap between coil and balloon in the neurointerventional armamentarium? Initial clinical experience with a nitinol vascular occlusion plug. Neuroradiol 2008;50:709–14.

37. Halbach VV, Higashida RT et al. Transvenous embolization of direct carotid cavernous fistulas. AJNR 1988;9:741–7.

38. Teng MMH, Lirng JF, et al. Embolization of carotid-cavernous fistula by means of direct puncture through the superior orbital fissure. Radiology 1995;194:705–11.

39. Liebovitch I, Modjtahedi S, Duckwiler GR, Goldberg RA. Lessons learned from difficult or unsuccessful cannulations of the superior ophthalmic vein in the treatment of cavernous sinus dural fistulas. Ophthalmology 2006;113:1220–6.

40. Arruabarrena C, Veiga C, Ruiz-Zarate B, Valdes JJ, Rojo P. Massive exophthalmos after traumatic carotid cavernous fistula embolization. Orbit 2007;26:121–4.

41. Weber W, Henkes H, et al. Cure of a carotid cavernous fistula by endovascular stent deployment. Cerebrovasc Dis 2001;12:272–5.

42. Archondakis E, Pero G, Valvassori L, Boccardi E, Scialfa G. Angiographic follow-up of traumatic carotid cavernous fistulas treated with endovascular stent graft placement. AJNR 2007;28:342–7.

43. Gomez F, Escobar W, Gomez AM, Gomez JF, Anaya CA. Treatment of carotid cavernous fistulas using covered stents: midterm results in seven patients. AJNR 2007;28:1762.

44. Saraf R, Shrivastava M, Siddhartha W, Limaye U. Evolution of endovascular management of intracranial dural arteriovenous fistulas: Single center experience. Neurology India 2010;58:62–68.

45. Yu Y, Huang Q, Xu Y, et al. Use of onyx for transarterial balloon-assisted embolization of traumatic carotid cavernous fistulas: a report of 23 cases. AJNR 2012;33:1305–9.

46. Gonzalez LF, Chalouhi N, Tjoumakaris S, Jabbour P, Dumont AS, Rosenwasser RH. Treatment of carotid-cavernous fistulas using intra-arterial balloon assistance: case series and technical note. Neurosurg Focus 2012;32:E14.

47. Amiridze N, Darwish R. Hemodynamic instability during treatment of intracranial duralarteriovenous fistula and carotid cavernous fistula with onyx: Preliminary results and anesthesia considerations. J Neurointer Surg 2009;1:146–50.

40

Traumatic Dural Venous Sinus Thrombosis

Avijit Sarkari • AK Mahapatra

INTRODUCTION

Cerebral dural sinus thrombosis (DST) is an increasingly diagnosed disease with a wide range of symptoms. It was first described by Ribes, in 1825, in a patient with malignancy, headache, seizures and delirium and post-mortem examination revealed DST. DST diagnosis using autopsy or invasive X-ray angiography was difficult until the end of the last century. However, it has been diagnosed more frequently with the availability of better non-invasive diagnostic techniques, such as Computerized tomography (CT) and Magnetic resonance imaging (MRI).[1–3]

Dural sinus thrombosis usually involves the sagittal sinus (70–80%), transverse and sigmoid sinuses (70%), and may extend to the cerebral veins. In approximately one-third of all cases, more than one sinus is involved, and in 30–40% of them, cerebellar and cortical vein thrombosis is associated.[2,3]

EPIDEMIOLOGY AND PATHOPHYSIOLOGY

The annual incidence of DST is estimated to be 1.5 to 3 cases per million in adults and 6.7 per million in children.[3] It is the cause of 1–2% of all strokes in adults.[2] Even though DST may affect all age groups, it is more common in women, particularly in the age group of 20 to 35, due to pregnancy, puerperium, and oral contraceptive use. Other common etiologies are coagulopathies, intracranial infections, infections of the head and neck and head injury.[4] Cranial tumors, deep venous thrombosis, severe dehydration, inflammatory bowel diseases, connective tissue disorders, sarcoidosis, nephrotic syndrome, lumbar puncture, parenteral injections, and neonatal asphyxia have been reported as the causes of DST.[3]

Ecker, in 1946, described the first case of blunt head injury to the skull associated with DST. The incidence of DST after penetrating head trauma is estimated to be about 4%.[5] The incidence in the pediatric age group is about 6.8%.[6] The higher number of children can be explained by the fact that the venous collateral system is not completely mature in their cerebrum.

DST after head injury is usually seen in cases of depressed skull fracture, epidural or subdural hematomas.[7] The pathogenesis of DST in head injury is not well established. Various hypotheses have been proposed. Depressed skull fractures or intracranial hematomas can cause thrombosis either by direct compression of the sinus[8] or by endothelial damage within the sinus, leading to the activation of the coagulation system resulting in sinus occlusion.[9,10] The brain also contains abundant amount of thromboplastin, which is released after injury inducing an abnormal hypercoagulable state[11] leading to

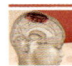

the destruction of platelets and erythrocytes followed by thrombus formation.[4] Intravascular coagulation and microvascular occlusion were exhibited in both experimental models and fatal traumatic brain injury.[12]

Thrombosis may also occur with facture lines crossing over the sinus.[13] Uncommonly, sinus thrombosis can occur after mild closed head injury with sutural diastasis.[4] Intramural hemorrhages caused by the rupture of small sinusoids, extension of the thrombus from injured emissary veins and compression of the sinuses from intracranial edema have been all implicated in the development of DST in closed head injury patients.[5,8] Meningitis and systemic infections like sepsis cause DST by a proposed mechanism of vasculitic destruction of vessel wall.[3,14]

Clinical Features

Clinical symptoms of sinus thrombosis include features of increased intracranial pressure such as headache, papilledema, visual dimunition, and vomiting.[4,8] Headache is present in up to 75% cases. Severe symptoms may arise with progression of the disease and include progressive neurological deficit, deterioration of consciousness, progressive coma and death related to intracranial hemorrhagic infarction and increased intracranial pressure.[1,3]

Radiological Investigations

The confirmation of the diagnosis relies on the demonstration of thrombus by neuroimaging techniques. Non-contrast CT scan may be normal in 10–20% cases. It shows the clot as a high density in the affected sinus or vein in the setting of acute thrombosis. The characteristic CT findings of sinus thrombosis include the cord sign (presence of high density clot within the cortical veins) and dense vein sign (clots within dural sinus) on non-contrast scan and empty delta sign following the administration of contrast agents.[4,8–10] "The empty delta or empty triangle sign" has been described as a reliable finding on contrast CT scan cuts slicing perpendicularily across the posterior

aspect of the sinus. It is due to the presence of an isodense clot within the sinus, enclosed by an area of engorged vessels and enhancing dura.[4,10,15]

In addition to above, there may be less specific secondary signs on CT scan such as intraparenchymal petechial flame-shaped hemorrhages, congested cortical veins, cerebral edema, small ventricles and gyral enhancement in region of venous infarcts.[15]

Digital subtraction angiography is the method of choice for diagnosing sinus thrombosis. Angiographic findings include partial or complete non-opacification of venous sinuses and veins, dilated cortical collateral veins and corkscrew appearance, increased cerebral circulation time, and reversal of flow away from the obstructed sinus or vein. The complete absence of the transverse and sigmoid sinus may be normal anatomic variation and thrombosis involving these areas should be made cautiously.[4,8–10]

In acute phase of thrombus formation, MRI may be extremely valuable to establish the diagnosis.[16] It reveals the thrombus as signal intensities characteristic of oxyhemoglobin. Thus acute blood clot is isointense on T_1-weighted images and hypointense on T_2-weighted images. Post-contrast T_1 coronal images demonstrate a filling defect in the sinus. On T_2-weighted images, there is increased signal from the sinus on MRV due to absence of flow. Though the invasive technique of cerebral angiography is the 'gold standard' for the diagnosis of CVT, the non-invasive magnetic resonance has evolved as the 'technique of choice'. MRV is particularly helpful in children as it does not require contrast medium and can approximately tell the age of thrombus, and the sequential follow-up is also possible.[4,8,10] Lumbar puncture can be performed if there is suspicion of benign intracranial hyper-tension.[10]

Treatment

The treatment of sinus thrombosis is controversial and includes the stabilization of the patient in acute phase and investigations for any known risk factors including prevention and management of deep venous thrombosis, infection, and coagulopathy.[3,8,10,16–18]

There is no consensus on the overall strategy concerning surgical, radiosurgical, or conservative therapy in DST.[3,6,7,18] Firstly, if there is any compression to the dural sinus by depressed fracture or hematoma, it should be removed.[7] If these pathologies were not diagnosed, the priority of treatment in the acute phase is to stabilize the patient's condition. The supportive therapies include hydration, anticonvulsants, steroids, mannitol, acetazolamide and craniectomy for decreasing intracranial pressure. Additionally, the progress of known risk factors, such as deep venous thrombosis, infection and coagulopathy must be prevented.[6,18] Due to a higher fibrinolytic activity in venous walls as compared to that in arterial or capillary walls, the thrombi in the sinuses frequently recanalize with time due to fibrinolysis.[4]

Anticoagulant therapy is the first choice for early partial or propogating dural venous thrombosis, although it remains controversial in traumatic cases.[6,7,18] Low molecular weight heparin (LMWH), which has a longer life than unfractionated heparin, can also be administered since it has a more predictable response at standard doses and lower incidence of thrombocytopenia and hemorrhagic complications.[18] Since the patients have a hemorrhagic lesion related to head injury, anticoagulant therapy should be applied carefully with adequate monitoring for complications such as new bleeding or hemorrhagic infarcts. Urokinase and the recently used recombinant tissue-type plasminogen activator cause thrombolysis and can generally be administered via an endovascular route, but they are limited to case reports in head injury patients.[18]

The recanalization of venous sinuses may be incomplete in some cases. A prospective study found significant functional improvement in 89% cases at 12 month follow-up period but the recanalization rate was determined to be about 60%.[19]

As the recurrence of DST is estimated to occur in approximately 12% and the patients also have an increased risk (14%) of deep venous thrombosis, the anticoagulant therapy should be continued after the patients have been discharged for up to 6–12 months.[3,19]

Some patients deteriorate despite medical therapy. These cases require endovascular thrombolysis or surgical thrombectomy. Initial reports of the use of endovascular treatment of DST have been promising. This aggressive treatment is reserved for those patients with serious neurological sequelae. However, enthusiasm for the use of endovascular thrombolysis and thrombectomy should be tempered by an understanding of possible risks such as intracerebral hemorrhage and/or vessel dissection.[20]

The mortality rate of DST ranges between 4.3 and 30%, and furthermore patients who survive may have permanent neurological deficits with a rate of about 12–25%.[1,3] In the monitored post-traumatic DST cases, better recovery has been observed in right-localized sinus thrombosis than the left-localized ones because generally the left hemisphere is dominant in the population. Moreover, the outcome of patients would be worse if the superior sagittal sinus or deep venous system of the brain has been involved.

CONCLUSIONS

Sinus thrombosis following head injury although considered to be rare is being increasingly recognized. It should be considered as a differential diagnosis especially if cases present with persistent headache, giddiness or vomiting after head injury which seems to be out of proportion to severity of trauma and other obvious contributing intracranial lesions have been excluded. Early detection is important as early management with anticoagulation of this potentially treatable condition results in good outcome.

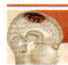

REFERENCES

1. de Bruijn SF, de Haan RJ, Stam J. Clinical features and prognostic factors of cerebral venous sinus thrombosis in a prospective series of 59 patients for The Cerebral Venous Sinus Thrombosis Study Group. J Neurol Neurosurg Psychiatric 2001;70:105–8.

2. Renowden S. Cerebral venous sinus thrombosis. Eur Radiol 2004;14:215–26.

3. Stam J. Thrombosis of the cerebral veins and sinuses. N Engl J Med 2005;352:1791–8.

4. Satoh H, Kumano K, Ogami R, Nishi T, Onda J, Nishimura S. Sigmoid sinus thrombosis after mild closed head injury in an infant: diagnosis by magnetic resonance imaging in the acute phase case report. Neurol Med Chir (Tokyo) 2000;40:361–5.

5. Ochagavia AR, Boque MC, Torre C, Alonso S, Sirvent JJ. Dural venous sinus thrombosis due to cranial trauma. Lancet 1996;347:1564.

6. Stiefel D, Eich G, Sacher P. Posttraumatic dural sinus thrombosis in children. Eur J Pediatr Surg 2000;10:41–44.

7. Yokota H, Eguchi T, Nobayashi M, Nishioka T, Nishimura F, Nikaido Y. Persistent intracranial hypertension caused by superior sagittal sinus stenosis following depressed skull fracture. Case report and review of the literature. J Neurosurg 2006;104:849–52.

8. Yuen HW, Gan BK, Seow WT, Tan HK. Dural sinus thrombosis after minor head injury in a child. Ann Acad Med, Singapore 2005;34:639–41.

9. Carrie AW, Jaffe FA. Thrombosis of superior sagittal sinus caused by trauma without penetrating injury. J Neurosurg 1954;11:173–82.

10. Dalgiç A, Seçer M, Ergüngör F, Okay O, Akdağ R, Ciliz D. Dural sinus thrombosis following head injury: report of two cases and review of the literature. Turk Neurosurg 2008;18:70–7.

11. Hesselbrock R, Sawaya R, Tomsick T, Wadhwa S. Superior sagittal sinus thrombosis after closed head injury. Neurosurgery 1985;16:825–8.

12. Stein SC, Chen XH, Sinson GP, Smith DH: Intravascular coagulation: A major secondary insult in nonfatal traumatic brain injury. J Neurosurg 2002;97:1373–7.

13. Muthukumar N. Uncommon cause of sinus thrombosis following closed mild head injury in a child. Child's Nerv Syst 2005; 21:86–8.

14. Kastenbauer S, Pfister HW. Pneumococcal meningitis in adults: Spectrum of complications and prognostic factors in a series of 87 cases. Brain 2003;126:1015–25.

15. Kumar GS, Chacko AG, Chacko M. Superior sagittal sinus and torcula thrombosis in minor head injury. Neurol, India 2004;52:123–4.

16. Lakhkar B, Lakhkar B, Singh BR, Agrawal A. Traumatic dural sinus thrombosis causing persistent headache in a child. J Emerg Trauma Shock 2010;3:73–5.

17. Barbati G, Dalla Montà G, Coletta R, Blasetti AG. Post-traumatic superior sagittal sinus thrombosis. Case report and analysis of the international literature. Minerva Anestesiol 2003;69:919–25.

18. Stam J. The treatment of cerebral venous sinus thrombosis. Adv Neurol 2003;92:233–40.

19. Stolz E, Trittmacher S, Rahimi A Gerriets T, Rottger C, Siekmann R, Kaps M. Influence of recanalization on outcome in dural sinus thrombosis: a prospective study. Stroke 2004; 35: 544–7.

20. Rahman M, Velat GJ, Hoh BL, Mocco J. Direct thrombolysis for cerebral venous sinus thrombosis. Neurosurg Focus 2009;27:E7.

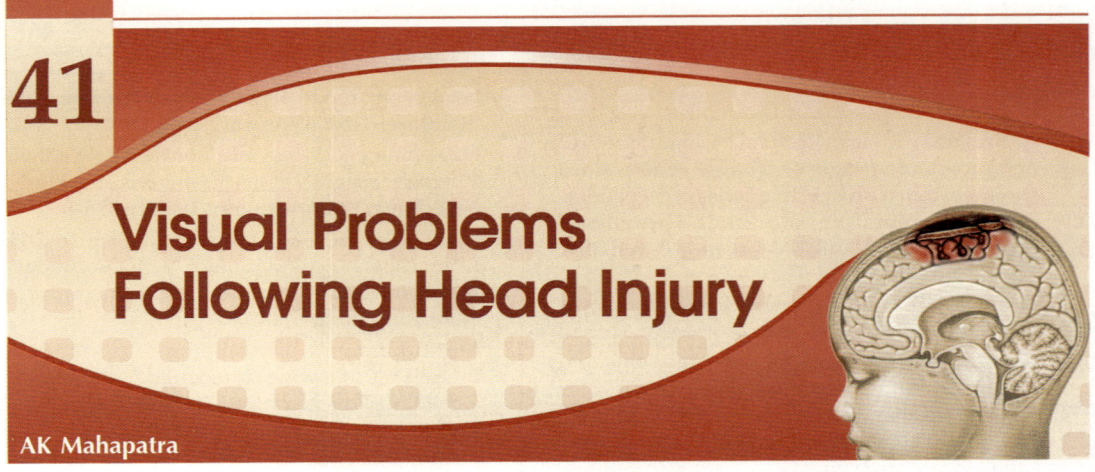

41

Visual Problems Following Head Injury

AK Mahapatra

INTRODUCTION

Visual abnormalities are uncommon findings following closed head injury. Recent epidemiological study over two decades from a largest Canadian adult trauma centerfound about two-thirds of patients with traumatic optic neuropathy (TON) had associated significant head injury, whereas only 2.3% patients with head injury had TON. Mahapatra and Bhatia had reported a figure of 1.5% incidence of optic nerve injury in head injury. However, an incidence as high as 44% was reported by Crompton, among them 24% had bilateral pathology. In a study Mahapatra published 32 cases of bilateral injury. Exact incidence is difficult to determine, as many unconscious patients may die and autopsy is not carried out. In the Canadian study the relative incidence of TON per year has remained variable from 0 to 1.2%.[1] Similarly, a surveillance study from UK revealed a minimum estimated incidence of 1.005 per million. The pathogenesis of optic nerve injuries is by and large not clear and the management is controversial. In the absence of evidence-based guidelines, corticosteroids, surgical decompression of the optic nerve or observation is the advocated line of treatment. Hence, this chapter highlights the etiology, pathophysiology, management and visual outcome of traumatic optic neuropathy (TON).

Anatomical and Pathological Considerations

Visual pathway is divided into anterior and posterior parts. The anterior visual pathway includes, optic nerves and chiasma. The posterior visual pathway includes rest of the visual system distal to the chiasma. Barring the occipital infarction due to herniation, the pathology of posterior visual pathway in head injury is rather rare.

Most important pathology, in optic pathway injury is the optic nerve involvement. Optic nerve extends from the globe to the chiasma and is approximately 5 cm long (Fig. 41.1).

The optic nerve is divided into 4 parts: (a) intraocular part, (b) intraorbital part is the longest around 25–30 mm, (c) intracanalicular part is 4–10 mm long and lies in the optic canal where the nerve is fixed to the periosteum, and (d) the intracranial part, which is 10–15 mm long. Near the intracranial opening to the optic canal there is a strong and sharp dural edge. There is a potential risk of damage to the optic nerve against sharp edge. The blood supply to the nerve is important. The intracanalicular part is relatively avascular and derives blood supply from the centripetal branch of the pial vessels. The small pial vessel of the anterior cerebral and anterior communicating artery supplies the intracranial optic nerve. These small vessels play an important role in optic nerve injury and lead to ischemic neuropathy.

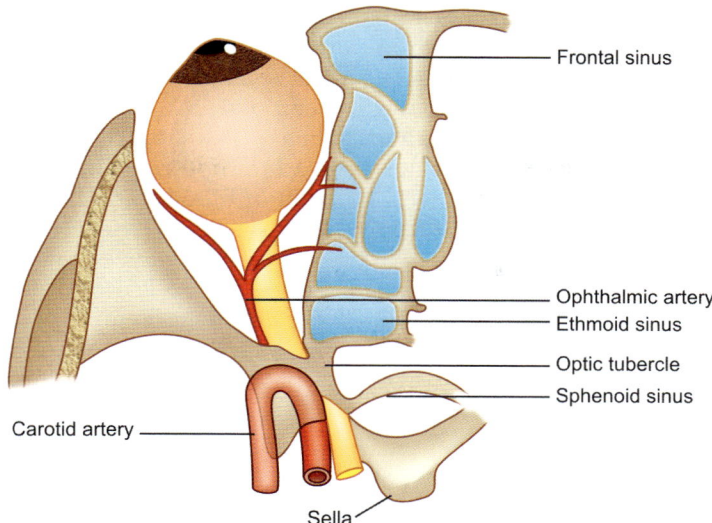

Fig. 41.1: Anatomy of optic nerve and its relation to other structure

Pathology

Visual problem following head injury can involve (a) anterior, and (b) posterior visual pathways. According to the site of injury the lesion can be at various places (Table 41.1).

INDIRECT OPTIC NERVE INJURY

Optic nerve is the most frequent site of visual pathway injury, in head injury. It was first described by "Hippocrates", probably the first case of optic nerve injury was described by Dutonchel in 1822. However, in 1879, Berlin described the optic nerve lesion at autopsy. Battle[10] in 1890 had distinguished the direct optic nerve injury from indirect optic nerve

---

Table 41.1: Sites of visual pathway injury

A. **Anterior visual pathway injury**
   a. *Optic nerve injury*
      1. Anterior marginal tear
      2. Intraorbital optic nerve injury
      3. Intracanalicular injury
      4. Intracranial optic nerve injury
   b. *Chiasmal Injury*
B. **Posterior visual pathway injury**
   a. Optic tract and heniculate lesion
   b. Optic radiation or calcarine lesion

---

injury. Callon[11] in 1892 had postulated the mechanism of optic canal fracture leading to optic nerve injury and reviewed 80 cases of optic nerve injury reported in literature.

Involvement of the optic nerve is reported in 0.6 to 3% of all head injury. The most frequent site of the injury is the optic canal. Hughes in 1962 described the various types of optic nerve injury, depending on the site: (a) anterior marginal tear, (b) anterior optic nerve injury and (c) posterior optic nerve injury, which can be intraorbital, intracanlicular and intracranial.

a. Anterior marginal tear occurs at the optic nerve head in retina. It was first described by Lowenstein in 1943. Hughes reported 13.3% of anterior marginal tear in his patients with optic nerve injury. This type is also associated with retinal and choroidal injury. Ophthalmoscopy reveals hemorrhage and irregular disc margins.

b. Anterior optic nerve injury involves the optic nerve behind the globe till the entry of central retinal artery. An incidence of 12.3% was reported by Hughes.[12] The retinal vessel spasm is reported in 30–35% cases.

c. Posterior optic nerve injury is more frequent. Traumatic orbital apex syndrome is a rare condition occurring in muscle cone. In this situation optic nerve gets involved along with proptosis, III, IV and VI cranial nerve palsy. Intracanalicular optic nerve injury occurs in optic canal, where nerve is relatively fixed as the nerve sheath is firmly adherent to periosteum. This type of injury can occur in anterior cranial fossa fracture. Hughes[12] reported bilateral optic nerve injury in patients with LeForte type III fracture.

Pathophysiology of Optic Nerve Injury

The exact mechanism of optic nerve damage is not understood. However, large number of hypothesis have been put forward. Walsh and Lindenberg in 1963 classified the optic nerve injury into (a) primary and (b) secondary depending on the nature of the pathology, as observed at autopsy (Table 41.2).

The concussion of optic nerve was first described by Walsh in 1979. Secondary involvement of the optic nerve is due to edema and ischemia leading to the infarction of the nerve, as a result of microvascular thrombosis. This hypothesis has been suggested by many authors.[12,14] The most likely mechanism leading to microvascular thrombosis is probably due to shearing strain on the nerve as a result of acceleration and deceleration injury to the orbit. It is also likely that midline forehead injury can produce bilateral optic nerve injury while blow on supraorbital area, temporal area produces unilateral optic nerve injury. The shearing and stretching forces can lead to rupture of optic nerve axons. Disruption of blood brain barrier with associated edema resulting in axonal swelling, disconnection and reorganization resulting in traumatic axonal injury (TAI) of the optic nerve was well demonstrated in an experimental study.

One of the most favored mechanism of optic nerve damage in head injury is vascular insufficiency.[5,6,12] The vascular injury is generally a pial vessel, which could be immediate. Delayed onset of visual involvement is due to edema and ischemia. In patients with irreversible visual loss, the most important cause is probably optic nerve infarction.[12] In two of Hughes's cases, histology of intracanalicular optic nerve revealed infarction. Infarction was also reported by Ramsey,[20] in both intracanalicular and intracranial portion of optic nerve.

The fracture of the anterior cranial fossa, orbital roof, anterior clinoid process and the optic canal can produce optic nerve injury. In the Canadian study traumatic optic neuropathy (TON) was associated with naso-ethmoid complex fracture and significant head injury in multivariate analysis.[1] These fractures can produce tear or compression of the nerve. Contusion of the nerve is a form of primary injury, which results from shearing force to the nerve. Hooper in 1951 had reported contusion of intracranial optic nerve in a patient with anterior clinoid fracture. Rarely, an optic nerve sheath hematoma has also been reported. Intraneural hemorrhage occurs due to the rupture of small veins or capillaries, resulting in a perivascular hematoma. Imachi et al had reported few cases of intraneural hematoma. Mahapatra et al observed one case of optic nerve hematoma among 100 patients. Tandon et al observed a single case among 27 patients subjected to optic nerve decompression.

Table 41.2: Pathology of optic nerve injury

A. Primary pathology
- Concussion
- Avulsion or tear
  - Partial
  - Complete
- Contusion
- Hemorrhage
  - Intraneural
  - Extraneural

B. Secondary pathology
- Edema
- Ischemia
- Microvascular thrombosis
- Infarction of the nerve

Inspite of normal looking optic nerve at surgery or at autopsy histopathological abnormalities are consistently reported.[6,12,21,26] Pathological entities such as degeneration of myelin, loss of axons, chronic inflammation with phagocytosis are found at microscopic examination. Vascular involvement in the form of thrombosis, ischemia and infarction are also seen.

Clinical Features

In conscious patients diagnosis is not difficult. Typical history of unilateral or rarely bilateral visual loss is the main complaint. The visual loss could be immediate or delayed type.[5,6,8,17] In 90% cases, patients do not have history of loss of consciousness. In severe head injury, when a patient is unconscious, unilateral fixed dilated pupil with retained consensual light reflex raised the possibility of unilateral optic nerve injury. This phenomenon is described as 'Marcus Gunn pupil'. By definition eyeball is intact and there is no ocular injury, however, external injury over forehead or temporal region with black eye may be present (Fig. 41.2).

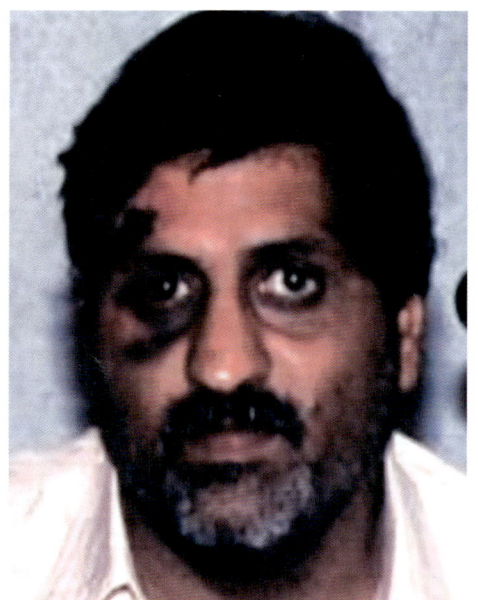

Fig. 41.2: Clinical photograph of a head injury patient with left-sided blindness and right-sided facial palsy

In unconscious patients it is difficult to determine the timing of onset of visual deterioration. In 15–20% patients, visual loss may be partial and patients may also have visual cuts. In patients with optic nerve concussion, patients have transient visual loss. Hence, it may be possible to have some visual recovery by the time patients reach the ophthalmologist or neurosurgeon.[15,19,23]

Examination usually reveals normal cornea, lens and vitreous. In anterior marginal tear, ophthalmoscopy may show retinal hemorrhage.[5,6,12,21] In vast majority of cases fundi reveal no abnormality. Rarely, congestion of the disc may be observed. Optic disc atrophy is observed 4–6 weeks following injury.

Field Defects

Various types of field defects have been reported in patients with optic nerve injury.[5,6,8,12,17] Surprisingly, only few authors have described visual field problem in their patients with optic nerve injury. Traquair et al[27] had reported central or paracentral scotoma and altitudinal field cut. Hughes[12] in 1962 had reported lower field was involved. Mahapatra et al,[8] Mahapatra and Tandon[25] had reported all possible field defects (Figs 41.3a and b) including nasal field.

However, temporal field was most frequently involved. The exact reason is difficult to explain. One of the possible explanation is the selective involvement of nasal fibers as the bone in the medial side of the orbit is thin and is likely to fracture more frequently.

Fundus Finding

Fundus finding varies according to the site of the injury and the degree of damage to the nerve. Except anterior marginal tear, immediate or early examination may not show any abnormality. In anterior marginal tear, fundus examination few hours later usually shows edema and hemorrhage. In anterior optic nerve injury, when the site of damage is nearer to the eyeball, fundus changes occur earlier than distal optic nerve injury. Generally, optic atrophy sets in 3–6 weeks time.[5,12]

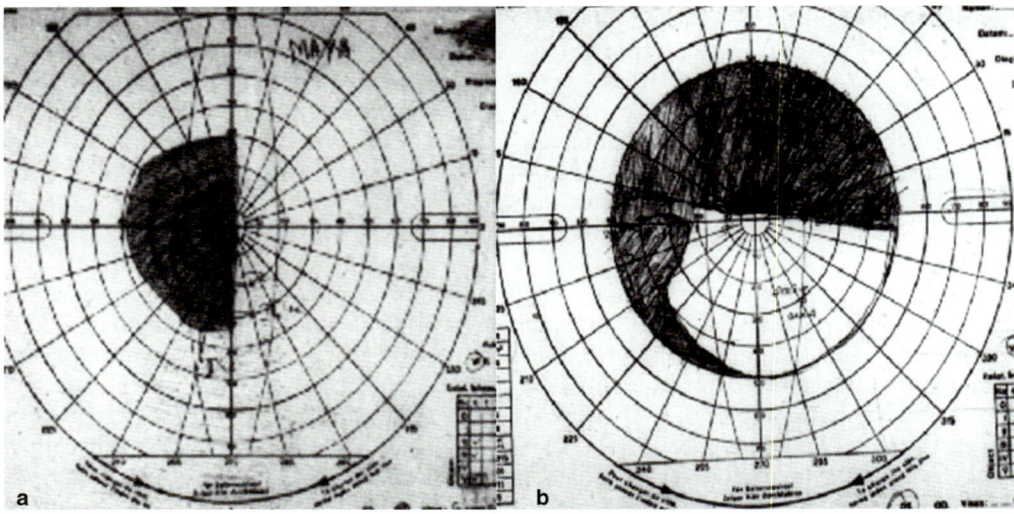

Figs 41.3a and b: Field defects in patients with optic nerve injury

Investigations

X-ray skull, paranasal sinus view and optic canal view are important radiological investigations. Skull fracture are reported in 50–80% patients.[5,6,8,12] A wide variation in the incidence of optic canal fracture has been reported (0–90%). This is basically because of the difference in surgical, radiological and autopsy findings. With the advent of CT scan demonstration of optic canal fracture has become easy. CT cuts with bone window helps in establishing the fracture. Recently, CT scanning is regularly used in suspected cases of optic nerve injury.[8,17] High resolution CT is the procedure of choice (Fig. 41.4).

Manfredi et al[31] reported sphenoid and ethmoid hemorrhage in PNS view and among them 5 had CT scan evidence of optic canal fracture. Grove[30] had pointed out the role of soft tissue injury. We observed optic canal fracture in 8–10% cases, in CT scan.[8,17,25] Tandon et al[26] had observed optic canal fracture in CT scan in 6 patients, among[29] subjected to surgery. CT scan frequently shows fracture in anterior cranial fossa and opacity in ethmoid and sphenoid sinuses. Rarely, CT scan may show optic sheath hematoma. Mahapatra et al[25] reported a single case of optic sheath hematoma among 100 patients.

Recently, MRI scans are freely available. MRI scan is a very good investigation for the orbit. However, there is a limited publication on MRI in optic nerve injury. We have performed MRI over 40 patients and reported our findings.[8,17,25] Nerve swelling and contusion is well visualized in MRI. Surprisingly, I have never seen a real transection of the optic

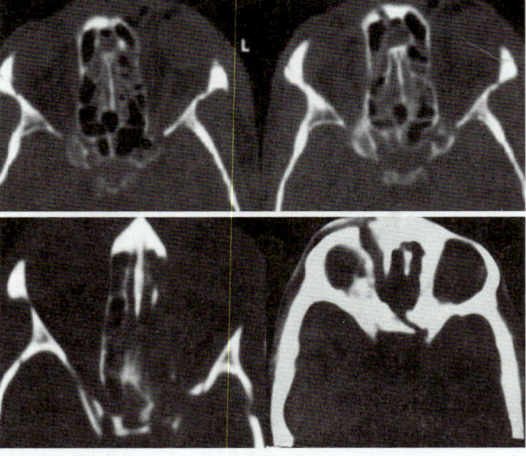

Fig. 41.4: High resolution CT scan showing fracture of optic canal

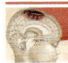

nerve in MRI. A recent study has proposed diffusion tensor imaging (DTI) for evaluating fibers of optic nerve in traumatic optic neuropathy (TON). Bodanapally UK et al proposed that decreased axial diffusivity (AD) and mean diffusivity (ADC) in the posterior segment of the optic nerve as a biomarker of axonal damage in TON. Orbital ultrasound is a very good investigation. It can show thickening of the nerve, orbital hematoma or a bony fragment. In 20 patients repeated ultrasound examination was carried out by us. Initially optic nerves were thickened and after 3–4 weeks, thinning of the optic nerve was observed.

Role of Visual Evoked Potentials

Visual evoked potentials (VEP) is a very good indicator of the integrity of visual pathway. However, till late 80s this test was not frequently used in optic nerve injury. Feinsod and Auerbach in 1973 had retrospectively analysed VEP and electroretinography in 5 patients. Shaked et al 1982 had reported a case and highlighted the value of VEP. Nau et al 1987 reported poor outcome in patients having no VEP waves, however, they did not comment on the role of normal VEP in predicting the good outcome. Prior to our studies there was no prospective study in the world literature on the role of VEP in predicting a good or a poor outcome. Mahapatra and Bhatia, Mahapatra et al[8,25] and Tandon et al[26] have repeatedly shown 85–90% visual recovery in patients with repeated normal or abnormal VEPs (Fig. 41.5).

In their experience none of the patients with repeatedly absent VEP had shown visual recovery. VEP also helps in diagnosis of visual loss in unconscious patients. We have been using Light Emitting Diode (LED) for recording VEP in unconscious patients.[17]

Treatment of Optic Nerve Injury

The treatment of optic nerve injury is controversial, even today. The main controversy, however, centers around the indications for surgery. Large number of studies reported in the world literature show similar results in medically managed and

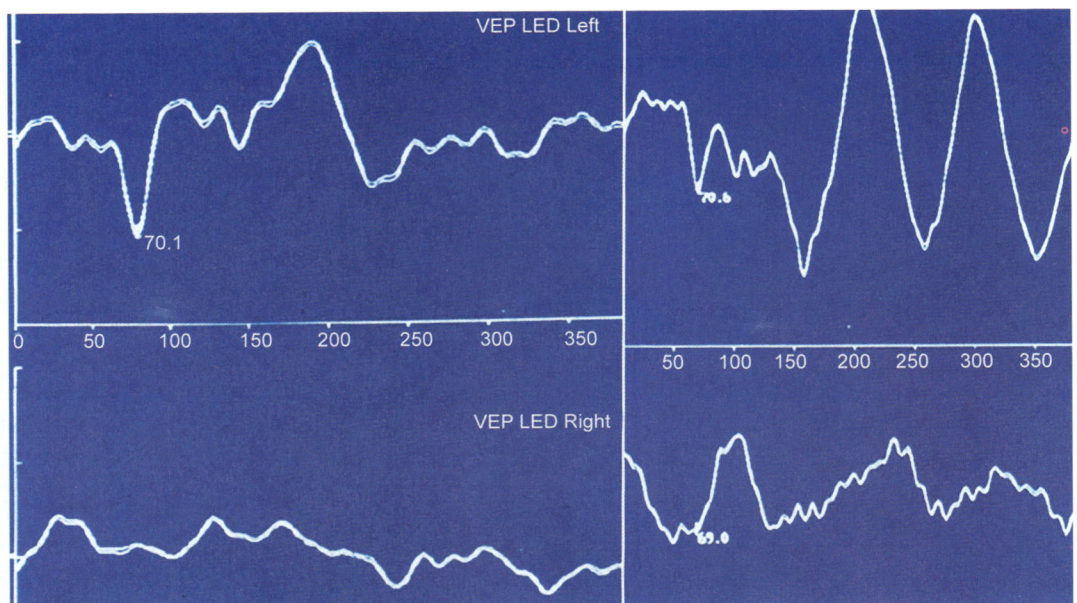

Fig. 41.5: No waves in right eye (below) as compared to left eye (above) in two patients with right traumatic optic neuropathy (TON)

surgically treated group.[5-8,26,32] While many authors from different countries have favored medical management, the Japanese authors have popularized and favored the surgical treatment.[7]

Medical Management (Flow chart 41.1)

There is scanty literature on the medical treatment of optic nerve injury[33,39-42] (Table 41.3).

Many authors who did not believe in surgical management, offered no treatment. Walsh (1966) stated that the "cortisone and mannitol may be helpful in patients in whom optic nerve swelling is a feature." However, establishing the swelling of the optic nerve is difficult. With the advent of ultrasound and MRI scan optic nerve swelling can be diagnosed. Delayed onset of visual deterioration also suggests swelling or edema of the optic nerve. Not much literature is available on the role of steroid in the management of optic nerve injury. Matsuzaki et al[41] 1982 treated 22 patients with a combination of prednisolone, 20% mannitol, urokinase and vit B$_{12}$. He reported 58.8% recovery in this group. Anderson et al[29] used high dose of steroid in 6 patients and 3 had shown improvement. In our study, over all improvement was observed in 53–58% patients.[8,25,26,39,40] I believe steroid must be given for a period of 3–4 weeks following injury (Flow chart 41.1). I found no significant difference using dexamethasone or methylprednisolone. A recent Cochrane database review concluded no additional benefit of steroids over observation and cautioned about its potential detrimental effects. The corticosteroid randomization for acute head trauma (CRASH) trial found increased mortality among patients of acute head trauma treated with high dose corticosteroid as compared to placebo. As most of the patients with traumatic optic nerve (TON) injury have concomitant head injury this is relevant to avoid use of high dose corticosteroid in these patients. Many recent studies have concluded regarding avoiding high dose corticosteroids in TON. Thus in the absence of demonstrable clinical efficacy and potential harmful effects, routine use of high dose corticosteroid for TON should be discouraged. Patient management needs to be individualized till further studies establish clear guidelines. Future treatment concerns include neuroprotective factors, and retinal ganglion cell regenerators.

Optic Nerve Decompression

Decompression of the optic nerve following injury has long been tried[5-7,12,26] (Table 41.4).

Prior to the introduction of transethmoid surgery by Niho et al[43] transcranial route was used for decompression. There is a great deal of controversy regarding the need for surgery and timing of optic nerve decompression. Gjerris[5] in 1976 stated "comparison between two groups of patients treated with and without operation reveals that the prognosis is the same in both groups, that there is no clear cut guidelines for one or the other."

Walsh and Hyot[6] considered immediate visual loss at the time of impact is a contraindication for surgery, as visual recovery is unlikely. Other authors have considered optic canal fractures as one of the indications for surgery.[7,44] Gjerris[5] had suggested against surgery in patients with immediate visual loss, having no sign of visual recovery in next few days. He also suggested conservative management when optic nerve injury is diagnosed in unconscious patients. All our studies had suggested no immediate surgery. Unless there is some spontaneous improvement[8,25,26] surgery is not indicated. Fujitani et al[42] had suggested a trial steroid therapy for 3 weeks. Patients not improving on steroid are unlikely

Table 41.3: Results of conservative management

Author	Year	No. of cases	% of recovery
Hooper	1951	17	29.0
Matsuzaki et al	1982	33	58.8
Mahapatra et al	1992	100	57.0
Mahapatra	2002	800	54.0

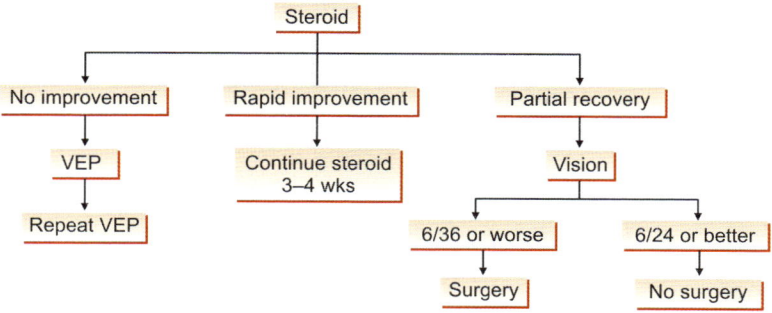
Flow chart 41.1: Our management policy

Table 41.4: Result of surgical decompression			
Author	*Year*	*No. of cases*	*% of recovery*
Niho et al	1961	7	66.0
Impachi et al	1968	61	70.0
Fukado	1981	700	42.0
Matsuzaki et al	1982	11	42.0
Strohim and Jahnkes	1982	15	40.0
Karnik	1986	37	20.0
Tandon et al	1994	39	74

Selected cases

to benefit from surgery. Lessell in 1989 observed that the eyes with total loss of vision at the end of three weeks on steroid are unlikely to respond. Mahapatra in 1992 reported delayed recovery from optic nerve injury. Thakar et al in 2003 reported the results of delayed optic nerve decompression for optic nerve injury.

Indications for Surgery

Till recently, there was no clear cut indication for optic nerve decompression. In fact, in our first study the protocol was ony conservative management.[39] Our subsequent studies showed a limited indication for surgery.[8,25,26,40] Now we manage our cases following Mahapatra's criteria (Table 41.5).

Our protocol offers every patient 3 weeks of corticosteroids. VEPs are repeated and patients are closely followed up for their clinical state. Patients progressively improving or not showing any improvement, are not subjected to surgery. A group of patients those who show minimal improvement and then remain static are subjected to surgery. This situation only suggests that the optic nerve is not completely damaged and given a chance, further improvement may occur. Following the criteria patients are operated. As the group subjected to surgery is highly selective, chances of improvement is also high.[26] Thus the role of surgery in optic nerve injury is limited. A Cochrane review in 2005 concluded that surgical decompression offers no added benefit. There is no class 1 evidence to recommend surgical decompression in TON. A recent review of literature also suggests controversial role of optic nerve decompression in TON. The International Optic Nerve Trauma Study (IONTS), comparing visual

Table 41.5: Mahapatra's criteria
a. All the patients are put on corticosteroids
b. VEP and clinical examination repeated every 2–3 days for the first 3 weeks
c. Patients showing good visual recovery do not need surgery
d. Patients in whom visual acuity remains PL negative inspite of corticosteroid at the end of 3 weeks, do not need surgery
e. Surgery is beneficial in those patients in whom visual improvement is marginal and then remains static
f. One emergency indication for surgery, is delayed onset optic nerve injury, when vision rapidly deteriorates inspite of corticosteroids

Table 41.6: Factors affecting outcome	
Significant	*Non-significant*
Presence of vision	Mode of injury
Normal VEP	Optic canal fracture
Negative VEP	X-ray findings
Age	Timing of surgery
Unilateral/bilateral	

Table 41.7: Result of 987 patients with optic nerve injury of AIIMS, New Delhi	
1983–2007	
Complete recovery	10%
Partial recovery	45–48%
No recovery	42–45%

outcome with corticosteroid, optic canal decompression and observation alone remained inconclusive.

Outcome and Factors Influencing Outcome

Visual outcome in patients with optic nerve injury depends on several factors. Age, mode of the injury, unilateral or bilateral involvement, presence or absence of VEP and presence or absence of vision play important role in visual recovery[5,6,8,17,25,26,39,43,57] (Table 41.6).

In two of our studies in pediatric age group we reported a recovery which was worse than adults. Similarly, presence or absence of VEP waves is of great importance.[8,17,36,38,39] Normal VEP provides a good chance of recovery in all the patients. We found time gap between injury and surgery and presence or absence of optic canal fracture are of very little significance. In one of my study, I reported better outcome in patients with bilateral optic nerve injury.[3,17] Similar observation has not been reported in world literature. In our experience only 10% patients improve to normal vision.[8,17,25] Rest 40–45% patients only have partial visual recovery (Table 41.7).

Rarely, visual recovery may start 8–12 weeks later. I have collected 6 patients in whom vision remained PL negative, surprisingly visual improvement started 8–12 weeks later. Agarwal and Mahapatra reported 23% recovery rate in 100 patients with PL only vision following optic nerve injury.

CHIASMAL INJURY

Introduction

Chiasmal injury is a rare condition. Except for case reports no large series is published.[27]

Only over 100 cases have been reported in the literature. Nieden in 1833 was the first to report chiasmal injury (quoted by Walsh & Hoyt 1969). Till 1935 only 30 cases were reported, and till 1971 the number increased to 89.[27,64] I have collected one of the largest series of chiasmal injury in the literature. Hughes[12] in 1962 reported 4.4% chiasmal injury and 7.8% opto-chiasmal injury. Elisevich et al[63] reported 5 cases of chiasmal injury while Savino et al reported 11 cases.

Pathogenesis

Pathogenesis of chiasmal injury is not clear. However, chiasmal injury can be primary or secondary as observed at operation or at autopsy. Primary involvement can be tear, contusion or laceration.[2,5,6,21,27] In most of these patients, there is evidence of fracture in anterior cranial fossa. In closed head injury, due to forehead impact, there is anterior-posterior distortion of the skull, which leads to midline chiasmal tear.[21,22] In one of the Hooper's[21] cases the chiasma looked normal at surgery, subsequently, when the patient died, the autopsy showed atrophy of the central part of the chiasma. Crompton[2] in 1970 in an autopsy study demonstrated interstitial hemorrhage and necrosis in 5 and 11 cases, respectively. The usual site of the chiasmal necrosis is at the site of decussation. Review of the literature shows that the majority patients of chiasmal injury are either direct contusion or chiasmal necrosis at the central part. Chiasma also gets involved secondary to edema, ischemia leading to infarction.

Clinical Findings

Patients are usually adult vehicular accidents victims. In my study[66] there was no children

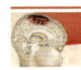

among 15 patients with chiasmal injury. History of unconsciousness is available in 90% patients.

Chiasmal injury is also described as traumatic bitemporal hemianopia, indirect chiasmal injury or post traumatic chiasmal syndrome. History of forehead trauma is available in 100% and loss of consciousness in 90–95%. Head injury is by and large severe.[5,12,21,63] Bleeding from nose or CSF rhinorrhea are commonly associated.[12,63] In my series[66] most of the patients had CSF rhinorrhea.

Bitemporal hemianopia is the most frequent symptom. Laursen[64] reviewed 89 cases of chiasmal injury and found classical bitemporal hemianopia only in 53, while 12 had nasal field cut in one or both the sides. Temporal field cut in one eye and no PL in the other eye suggest opto-chiasmal injury. Rarely, visual deterioration may be possible due to basal meningitis and arachnoiditis. Other unusual symptoms associated with chiasmal injury are anosmia, pituitary insufficiency, diabetes insipidus.[5,6,12] Rarely, there may be cranial nerve deficit, traumatic aneurysm of internal carotid artery (ICA) and carotid cavernous fistula (CCF).

Diagnosis

Clinical diagnosis is difficult in unconscious patients. However, when a patient is conscious, diagnosis is made by the history of bilateral temporal defect, confirmed by field charting. Recently, CT scan and MRI scan have made the diagnosis easy. The series reported by me had MRI demonstration of chiasmal injury in 5 cases.

Treatment

There is no specific treatment for chiasmal injury. As secondary involvement of chiasma can occur due to edema, it is probably rational to prescribe corticosteroid. Ten of my 15 patients with chiasmal injury receive corticosteroid.[66] In the past several authors had explored the chiasma.[12,21,65] However, results were bad. One of Hughe's[12] patients had delayed onset visual loss, patient was operated,

release of adhesion was carried out and the patient's vision improved. Hooper[21] in 1951 had reported swollen chiasma at surgery.

Visual Outcome in Chiasmal Injury

Almost all patients develop varying grade of optic atrophy over a period of time. Walsh and Hoyt[6] reported a patient in whom vision improved. As the central field is retained patients van manage well. Recovery occurs over several weeks and the depth perception is regained. In my study[66] all the patients had some visual recovery. Two of my 3 patients with opto-chiasmal injury remain blind in one eye.

Injury to Posterior Visual Pathway

Posterior visual pathway is the portion distal to optic chiasma. Direct injury to these structures could result due to penetrating injury, either due to bullet or by splinters. However, rarely these structures can be involved in closed head injury. Injury to posterior visual pathway occurs in patients with severe head injury.[5,6,63] Injury to optic tract, optic radiation and calcarine area is well studied in war injured patients. In closed head injury optic tract and optic radiation can get involved in contusion or intracerebral hematoma involving temporal or parietal lobe. In patients with compression of posterior cerebral artery however, many patients with transtentorial herniation may not survive.

The damage to optic tract, optic radiation or geniculate body is difficult to diagnose clinically in unconscious patients. In a statement Walsh and Hoyt[6] in 1969 mentioned that they had not seen clinically any verifiable optic tract lesion following trauma. This was a biblical book in neuro-ophthalmology known as clinical neuro-ophthalmology, 3rd edition. With the availability of CT scan, precise location of contusion and haematoma can be known. The survivors of these lesions do present with various types of homonymous hemianopia. Cortical blindness does occur with head injury and the outcome is unpredictable.

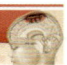

REFERENCES

1. Pirouzmand F. Epidemiological trends of traumatic optic nerve injuries in the largest Canadian adult trauma center. J Craniofac Surg 2012;23:516–20.

2. Crompton MR. Visual lesion in head injury. Brain 1970;93:785–92.

3. Mahapatra AK. Bilateral optic nerve injury. A series of 32 cases. Neurology India 1999;47:92–3.

4. Lee V, Ford RL, Xing W, Bunce C, Foot B. Surveillance of traumatic optic neuropathy in the UK. Eye (Lond) 2010;24:240–50.

5. Gjerris F. Traumatic lesions of visual pathway. In: Vinken PJ and Bruyn GW (eds). Handbook of Clinical Neurology. North Holland Publishing Company, Amsterdam 1976,24:27–57.

6. Walsh FB, Hoyt WF. Involvement of optic nerve in closed head injury. In: Clinical Neuro-ophthalmology, 3rd (edn). Baltimore, William and Wilkins Publishing Company 1969,3:2375–80.

7. Fukado Y. Microsurgical transethmoidal optic nerve decompression. Experience with 700 cases. In: The Cranial Nerve. Samii M and Jenetta P (eds). Springer Verlag 1981:125–8.

8. Mahapatra AK, Tandon DA. Optic nerve injury. A prospective study of 250 patients. In: Skull base anatomy, Radiology and treatment. Samii M (ed) Karger S, Basel 1994:305–9.

9. Berlin R. Uber she storung nach verletzung desschadel dural stample gewalt. Ber Ophthal Ges 1979;2:9–14.

10. Battle WH. Some points relating to injuries of the head. Lancet 1890;11:57–60.

11. Callon DA. Four cases of orbital trauma. J Ame Med Assoc 1892;18:284.

12. Hughes B. Indirect injury to the optic nerve and chiasma. Bull John Hopkin Hos 1962;111:98–126.

13. Lowenstein A. Marginal haemorrhage on the disc. Partial tearing of the optic nerve. Clinical and histological features. Brit J Ophthalmol 1943;27: 208–21.

14. Walsh FB, Lindenberg R. Die Verand ungeh ges schnervan loci indirect trauma, in Entwicklung ng sk urs tur. Augenarzte. Hamburg 1962, Ferdinand Enke, Verlag.

15. Walsh FB. Trauma involving the anterior visual pathways. In: Ocular Trauma. HM Freeman (Eds) Appletion-Century Croft Publication, New York 1979;125–8.

16. Hedge TR, Gragoudas ES. Traumatic anterior ischaemic optic neuropathy. Annal of Ophthalmol v;13:625–8.

17. Mahapatra AK. Some more experience with optic nerve injury. Analysis of last 170 patients. In: Brain protection and Neural trauma. UK Khosla et al (eds), Norosa Publishing House, New Delhi 2000, 269–74.

18. Wang J, Hamm RJ, Povlishock JT. Traumatic axonal injury in the optic nerve: evidence for axonal swelling, disconnection, dieback, and reorganization. J Neurotrauma 2011;28:1185–98.

19. Bodian M. Transient loss of vision following head trauma. New York State J Med 1969;64:916–20.

20. Ramsey JH. Optic nerve injury in fracture of the canal. Brit J. Ophthalmol 1979;63:607–10.

21. Hooper RS. Orbital complications of head injury. Brit J Surg 1951;39:126–38.

22. Pringle JH. Monoocular blindness following differential violence to the skull. Brit J Surg 1917;4: 373.

23. Griffith JF, Dodge PR. Transient blindness following head injury in children. New Eng J Med 1968;278:648–51.

24. Imachi J, Inoue K, Takahashi T. Clinical and Ophthalmogical investigations of optic nerve lesions in cases of head injuries. Jpn J. Ophthalmol 1968;12:70–85.

25. Mahapatra AK, Tandon DA, Bhatia R, Banerji AK. Optic nerve injury: A prospective study of 100 patients. Neurology India 1992;40:17–21.

26. Tandon DA, Thakar A, Mahapatra AK, Ghosh P. Transethmoidal optic nerve decompression. Clin Otolaryngol 1994;19:98–104.

27. Traquir HM, Dott NH, Russeu WR. Traumatic lesion of optic chiasma. Brain 1935;58:398–411.

28. Edmund J Godtfredsen E. Unilateral optic nerve injury. Acta Ophthalmol 1963;41:693–7.

29. Anderson DP, Frod M. Visual abnormality after severe head injuries. Can J Surg 1980;23:163–5.

30. Grove AS Jr. Orbital trauma and computed tomography. Ophthalmology, 1980;89:443–6.

31. Manfredi SJ, Raji MR, Sprinkle PM, et al. Computerized tomographic scan findings in facial fractures associated with blindness. Plast Recurrent 1981;68:479–90.

32. Joseph MP, Lessel S, Rizzo J, Momose KJ. Extracranial optic nerve decompression for traumatic optic neuropathy. Arch Ophthalmol 1990;108:1091–93.

33. Wolin MJ, Lavin PJM. Spontaneous visual recovery from traumatic optic neuropathy after blunt head injury. Ame J Ophthalmol 1990;109:430–5.

34. Yang QT, Fan YP, Zou Y, Kang Z, Hu B, Liu X, Zhang GH, Li Y. Evaluation of traumatic optic

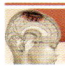
neuropathy in patients with optic canal fracture using diffuse tensor magnetic resonance imaging: a preliminary report. ORL J Otorhinolaryngol Relat Spec 2011;73:301–7.

35. Bodanapally UK, Kathirkamanathan S, Geraymovych E, Mirvis SE, Choi AY, McMillan AB, Zhuo J, Shin RK. Diagnosis of Traumatic Optic Neuropathy: Application of Diffusion Tensor Magnetic Resonance Imaging. J Neuro Ophthalmol 2013 Mar 21. (Epub ahead of print).

36. Feinsod M, Auerbach E. Electrophysiological examination of visual system in the acute phase after head injury. European Neurol 1973;9:56–64.

37. Shaked A, Hadani M, Feinsod M. CT and VER follow up of reversible vision with fracture optic canal. Acta Neurochir (Wien) 1982;62:91–4.

38. Nau, HE Gerhard L, Foerster M, Nacher HCH, Reinhardt V, Joka TH. Optic nerve trauma: Clinical, electrophysiological and histological remarks. Acta Neurochir (Wien) 1987;89:16–27.

39. Mahapatra AK, Bhatia R. Predictive value of visual evoked potential in unilateral optic nerve injury. Surg Neurol 1989;31:339–42.

40. Mahapatra AK. Current management of optic nerve injury. In progress in clinical neurosciences. S Venkataraman & BK Misra (eds), Mediworld Publishing. Delhi 1997;12:241–54.

41. Matsuzaki H, Kunita M, Kawai K. Optic nerve damage in head trauma. Clinical and experimental studies. Jpn J Ophthalmol 1982;26: 447–61.

42. Fuzitani T, Inoue K, Takahashi T, Ikushima K, Asai T. Indirect traumatic optic neuropathy. Visual outcome in operated and non-operated cases. Jpn J Ophthalmol 1986;30:125–34.

43. Niho S, Yasuda K, Sato T, Sugita S, et al. Decompression of the optic canal by the transethmoidal route. Ame J Ophthalmol 1961;51:659–66.

44. Niho S, Niho M, Niho K. Decompression of the optic canal by the transethmoidal route and decompression of superior orbital fissure. Can J Ophthalmol 1970;5:22–40.

45. Yu-Wai-Man P, Griffiths PG. Steroids for traumatic optic neuropathy. Cochrane Database Syst Rev 2011;19:CD006032.

46. Steinsapir KD, Goldberg RA. Traumatic optic neuropathy: an evolving understanding. Am J Ophthalmol 2011;151:928–33.

47. Steinsapir KD. Treatment of traumatic optic neuropathy with high-dose corticosteroid. J Neuroophthalmol 2006;26:65–7.

48. Steinsapir KD. Traumatic optic neuropathy. Curr Opin Ophthalmol 1999;10:340–2.

49. Wu N, Yin ZQ, Wang Y. Traumatic optic neuropathy therapy: an update of clinical and experimental studies. J Int Med Res 2008;36:883–9.

50. Razeghinejad MR, Rahat F, Bagheri M. Levodopa- Carbidopa may improve vision loss in indirect traumatic optic neuropathy. J Neurotrauma 2010;27:1905–9.

51. Wang H, Liu ZL, Zhuang XT, Wang MF, Xu L. Neuroprotective effect of recombinant human erythropoietin on optic nerve injury in rats. Chin Med J (Engl.) 2009:122:2008–12.

52. Benowitz LI, Yin Y. Optic Nerve Regeneration. Arch Ophthalmol 2010;128:1059–64.

53. Naffziger HC. Certain ear and eye affection in association with head injury. Ophthal Rec 1916;25: 502–8.

54. Karnik P. Optic nerve decompression. A new dimension of transethmoid surgery. Ind J Otolaryngol 1986;10:48–51.

55. Sofferman RA. Sphenoethmoid approach to the optic nerve. Laryngoscope 1981;91:184–6.

56. Osguthorpe JD. Transethmoid decompression of the optic nerve. Otolaryngol Clin North Ame 1985;18:125–37.

57. Lessell S. Indirect Optic nerve trauma. Arch Ophthalmol 1989;107:382–6.

58. Mahapatra AK. Delayed recovery from optic nerve injury. Report of two cases. J. Neurosurgical Sciences 1992.

59. Thakar A, Mahapatra AK, Tandon DA. Delayed optic nerve decompression for indirect optic nerve injury. Laryngoscope 2003;113:112–9.

60. Yu-Wai Man P, Griffiths PG. Surgery for traumatic optic neuropathy. Cochrane database Syst Rev 2005;19: CD005024.

61. Warner N, Eggenberger E. Traumatic optic neuropathy: a review of the current literature. Curr opin Ophthalmol 2010;21:459–62.

62. Levin LA, Beck RW, Joseph MP, Seiff S, Kraker R. The treatment of traumatic optic neuropathy: the International Optic Nerve Trauma Study. Ophthalmology 1999;106:1268–77.

63. Elisevich KV, Frod RM, Anderson DP, Strefoed JG, Richardson PM. Visual abnormalities with multiple trauma. Surg Neurol 1984;22:565–75.

64. Laursen AB. Traumatic bitemporal hemianopia. Acta Ophthalmol 1971;49:134–42.

65. Logan WC, Cordon DS. Traumatic lesions of the optic chiasma. Br J Ophthalmol 1973;51:258–60.

66. Mahapatra AK. Chiasmal injury—A study of 15 cases, Neuroscience today 1998;2:114–6.

42

Growing Skull Fractures

AK Mahapatra • Shejoy P Joshua

INTRODUCTION

Skull fractures which widen and appear to be growing with time are called growing skull fractures.[1-3] They occur mainly in 3–8 years age group. They are characterized by progressive diastatic enlargement of fracture line.

They are also called leptomeningeal cyst due to the CSF filled cystic mass associated with the defect in bone. The incidence is around 0.05–1% of childhood skull fractures.

Pathogenesis

Head injury significant to cause a linear fracture with linear dural laceration is the primary starting point in the pathogenesis of growing skull fractures. The continuous pulsatile wedge pressure from the herniating tissue causes the resorption of bone edges at fracture line. This results in the growth of fracture line. It also enlarges the dural gap larger than the fracture line. Both of these together lead to the progressive nature of this condition.

The loss in resistance underlying the bone and dural defect results in the focal dilation of the lateral ventricle which normalises after repair of growing skull fracture. This does not occur with craniotomy without watertight dural closure as the dural laceration does not coincide with the fracture line in this case. The rapidly developing brain in early childhood facilitates the development of growing skull fracture.

Growing skull fractures may be associated with hemorrhagic contusion, loculated CSF collection, post-traumatic aneurysm and subdural hematomas.[3-5] Underlying brain may be gliotic or atrophic, however this is not a prerequisite for the formation of growing skull fractures.[6,7]

A depressed fracture does not become a growing skull fractures. A linear fracture with a diastasis of more than 4 mm is at risk of development of growing skull fractures.[8] Growing skull fractures in older individual occurs in areas of thin bone at the skull base such as orbital roof, ethmoidal plate and frontal sinus. They are often associated with meningoencephalocele.[9]

Clinical Features

Growing skull fractures presents as a progressive pulsatile scalp mass (Fig. 42.1) several months to years after significant head injury sustained in infancy or early childhood. Seizures, hemiparesis and psychomotor retardation. Asymptomatic palpable mass may be the sole sign.

Most common area involved is the parietal bone which could extend to across the suture lines. Skull base growing skull fractures may present with ocular proptosis or CSF rhinorrhea.

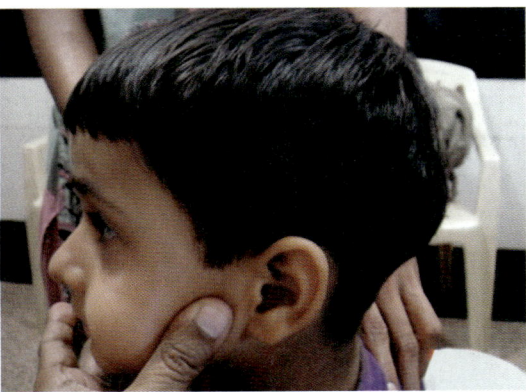

Fig. 42.1: Protrusion seen at left parietal region at the site of growing skull fracture

IMAGING

1. Skull X-ray wide diastasis of fracture line which is progressive on serial X-rays.[10]
2. Computerised tomography shows diastasis of fracture line and often a hypodensity near it (Figs 42.2 to 42.4). These hypo-densities represent encephalomalacia, arachinoid loculation or cortical atrophy. Ipsilateral lateral ventricle may show focal porencephalic dilatation.
3. Magnetic resonance imaging provided further information on pathological process associated with growing skull fractures.

Management

Early recognition and treatment of growing skull fractures prevent further neurological deterioration and development of seizure disorder. Goals of surgery are to repair the dural and cranial defect, to debride the cerebromeningeal cicatrix (gliotic cerebral tissue which is adherent to reactive meningeal and periosteal tissue) and removal of the leptomeningeal cyst.

Surgical Technique

Incision to expose the entire growing skull fractures is given. Scalp flap is turned sub-galeally. Pericranium is incised along the edge of the bone defect. Multiple burr holes at a distance from the defect are made and connected. Dural is freed from the bone and bone flap raised. Cerebromeningeal cicatrix is excised exposing the normal brain parenchyma.

Dural defect is closed with pericranial graft (Figs 42.5a and b). Cranial defect is repaired with split skull graft. If the defect is large and the skull is thin then autologous rib graft is an alternative. If the growing skull fractures crosses the dural sinus perpendicularly the dural sinus edge does not need repair. However, if the defect is parallel with a small dural edge close to the sinus, the pericranial

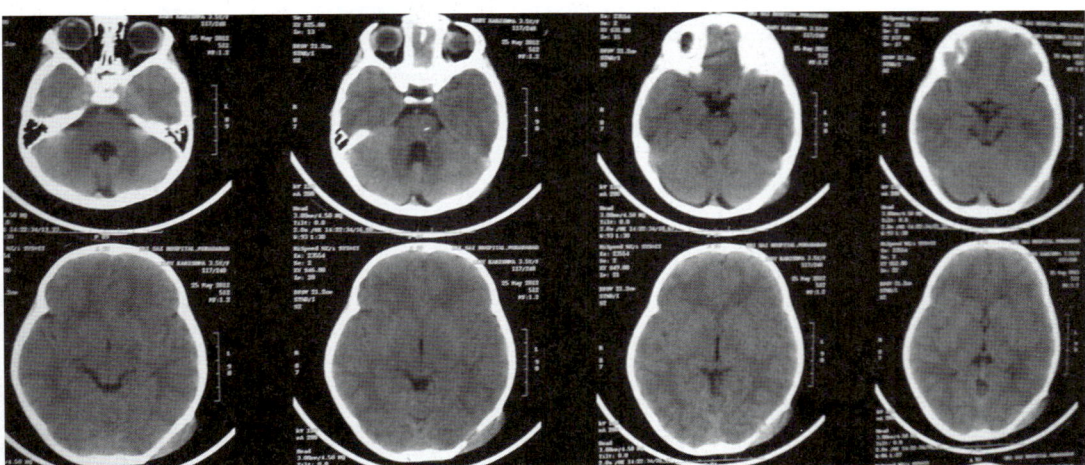

Fig. 42.2: CT scan image of patient in Fig. 42.1 showing growing skull fracture with defect in calvarium and herniation of cortical matter through the defect

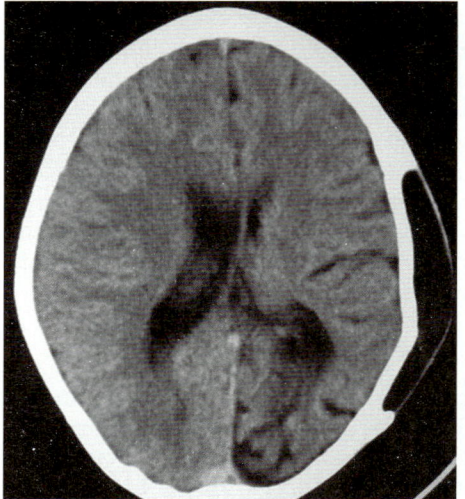

Fig. 42.3: Growing skull fracture with underlying ence-phalomalacic cortical matter

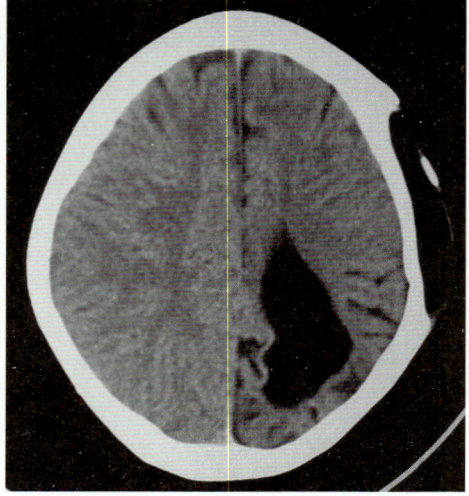

Fig. 42.4: Growing skull fracture with underlying porencephalic cyst

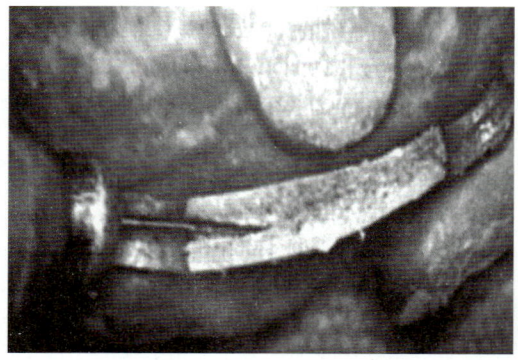

a

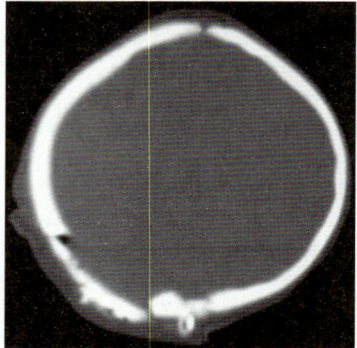

b

Fig. 42.5: Cranial defect repaired with split skull graft after craniotomy and dural repair. (a) Bone flap being split with a Midas Rex Drill (Midas Rex Pneumatic, Fort Worth, TX) using a C-1 bit, (b) Postoperative CT following repair of craniotomy defect with split skull graft

graft can be sutured directly to the skull edge above the sinus or to dura across the sinus. A CSF diversion is recommended for CSF leak or coexisting hydrocephalus.[5,11]

CONCLUSIONS

Growing skull fractures are rare and one noticed less than 2 years of age. It is most frequently situated in parieto-occipital region. There is a progresive brain damage lead to gliosis resulting in epilepsy. Surgical repair is

a must. Repair of dural defect and cranioplasty is sole standard.

REFERENCES

1. Ramamurthi B, Kalyanaraman S. Rationale for surgery in growing skull fractures. J Neurosurg 1970;32:427–30.
2. Goldstein FP, Rosenthal SAE, Garacis JC, et al. Varieties of growing skull fractures in childhood. J Neurosurg 1970;33:25–8.
3. Scarfo GB, Mariottinni A, Tomaccini D Palma L. Growing skull fractures progressive evolution of

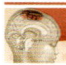

brain damage and effectiveness of surgical treatment. Child Nerv Sys 1989;5:163–7.

4. Bucklingham MJ, Croc KR, Ball WS, et al. Traumatic intracranial aneurysm in childhood: 2 cases and review of literature. Neurosurg 1988; 22:398–408.

5. Locatelli D, Messina AL, Bonfanti N, et al. growing skull fractures an unusual complication of head injury in pediatric patients. Neurochirugia (Stuttg) 1989;32:101–4.

6. Lende RA, Erickson TC. Growing skull fractures of childhood. J Neurosurg 1961;18:479–89.

7. Nemoto S, Hoffman HJ. Leptomeningeal cyst of posterior fossa: case report. J Neurosurg 1986; 65:704–5.

8. Thompson JB, Mason TH, Haines GL, Cassidy RJ. Surgical Management of diastatic linear skull fractures in infants J Neurosurg 1973;39:493–7.

9. Cook PG, Norman PF. Intradiploic leptomeningeal cyst of frontal bone occurring as a complication of head injury in an adult. Clin Rad 1988;39:214–5.

10. Kinsley D, Till K, Hoari R. Growing fracture of skull. J Neurol Neurosurg Psy 1978;41:312–8.

11. Kashigawa S, Akibo S. Aoki H. Growing skull fractures in childhood. A recurrent case treated with shunt operation. Surg Neurol 1986;26: 63–6.

43

Traumatic Subarachnoid Hemorrhage

Raj Kamal • AK Mahapatra

INTRODUCTION

Traumatic subarachnoid hemorrhage (tSAH) was first described by Wilkin in 1859.[1] In his autopsy study, in patients with head injury, he found hemorrhagic CSF, which he described as "Sanguineous meningeal effusion" in subarachnoid space. Surprisingly, however, till recently there have been only a few studies on traumatic SAH. Prior to the advent of CT scan antemortem diagnosis of SAH in head injury was difficult, except lumbar puncture. With the CT scan tSAH emerged as an important issue. Medicolegal reports frequently mention SAH in fatal head injury.[2–7] SAH associated with minor head injuries of medicolegal implication, as it is difficult to establish with certainty that SAH found at autopsy is traumatic and not spontaneous in origin.

Various prognostic factors affect final outcome by minimizing secondary injury. One such variable, traumatic subarachnoid hemorrhage (tSAH), has been the focus of many discussions over the past half century as numerous clinical studies have shown tSAH to be associated with adverse outcome. Whether the relationship of tSAH with poorer outcome in TBI is merely an epiphenomenon or a result of direct cause and effect is unclear.[8] Some investigators believe that tSAH is merely a marker of severer TBI, while others argue that it directly causes deleterious effects such as vasospasm and ischemia. At the present time, no proven treatment regimen aimed specifically at decreasing the detrimental effects of tSAH exists, although calcium channel blockers traditionally thought to target vasospasm have shown some promises. The development of hydrocephalus in patients with head injuries were considered as delayed sequelae of traumatic SAH, due to obstruction of CSF pathways.[9] Similarly, acute blockage of CSF pathways leads to early hydrocephalus which present acutely.[10,11]

Incidence

The incidence of traumatic SAH varies from 11 to 60% in TBI patients.[12–15] Courville[4] in 1950, base of a series of 40,000 autopsies reported SAH as the most common intracranial pathology following head injury. Similar observations were also made by Freytag[16] in 1963, in an autopsy study on 1367 head injury deaths. Wong et al[17] study showed that out of 661 patients admitted with significant head injury 214 patients (32%) had traumatic SAH on admission CT. The mortality rate was significantly greater and a 6-month unfavorable outcome was significantly more frequent in patients with traumatic SAH. Surprisingly, no large clinical study was available prior to 1990, when Eisenberg et al[13] reported a 39% incidence of tSAH, in 753 patients, based on their CT scan finding, Chesnut et al[10] in 1993 reported an incidence as high as 44%. However, a wide range of tSAH is reported in the world literature[10,16–20] (Table 43.1).

Pathology of tSAH

The etiology of subarachnoid hemorrhage is not clear. In autopsy studies of patients with fatal yet relatively minor head or neck injuries, associated with large basal subarachnoid hemorrhage have been attributed, in some cases, to arterial rupture, mostly of intracranial or cervical vertebral arteries.[21–23] tSAH also possibly result from tearing of bridging veins, pial vessels, or from diffusion of blood from cortical contusions into subarachnoid spaces.

Traumatic subarachnoid hemorrhage is known on many occasions to result from a blow on the neck rupturing the vertebral artery within the cervical spine. On some occasions, however, no such damage to the artery in the neck can be found to account for the hemorrhage. Some cases are described in which the source of hemorrhage was rupture of the vertebral artery within the skull close to the basilar artery.[21]

Dowling et al[22] reported postmortem study (of six cases) which showed traumatic ruptures of otherwise normal extra- and intracranial arteries were identified in four cases. Multiple sites of incomplete and complete rupture were found in four cases. Postmortem angiography was used in one case to demonstrate the site of rupture prior to removal of the brain. The site of rupture was not found in one case, and the final case had rupture of a fibrotic intracranial vertebral artery. The characteristic findings exhibited in neck injuries were diastasis of the atlanto-occipital joint with subluxation of the right side of the first cervical vertebra, in the absence of a demonstrable abnormality of the cerebral circulation.[23] A fatal subarachnoid hemorrhage from a ruptured normal intracranial vertebral artery in a 49-year-old male, following a blow to the head, was revealed by a postmortem angiography.[24]

Tatsuno and Lindenberg[25] noted that of the 14 cases in which an identifiable source for the hemorrhage could be found, four cases were noted to have tears in the intracranial internal carotid arteries (28%), four cases revealed lesions in the vertebrobasilar arteries (28%), and two cases showed defects in the stem of the middle cerebral artery (14%). This proximity to the atlanto-occipital joint makes the extracranial portion of the internal carotid artery vulnerable to stretch injury when the head is abruptly hyperextended or rotated. The portion of the internal carotid that is fixed within the sphenoid bone is pulled upwards or laterally, and the portion of the artery that passes close to the atlas and axis is stretched against their lateral masses and can therefore tear.[26,27] It is also by this mechanism that sudden, sharp increases in blood pressure secondary to compression occur in the carotid vessels during abrupt hyperextension or rotation of the head. The intracranial portion of the internal carotid artery is also subject to potentially damaging forces when the head is abruptly hyperextended and/or rotated from a resting position. When the head is suddenly moved, the brain oscillates within the cranial vault due to its inertia.[27] After the head begins to move, the inertia of the brain initially causes it to move in a direction opposite the direction of force of the blow to the head and the head's movement. Then, as the head begins to snap back to its original position, the inertia of the brain has been overcome, and the brain moves

Table 43.1: Incidence of traumatic tSAH			
Authors	*Year*	*No. of cases*	*% tSAH*
1. De Villasante[18] and Taveras	1976	100	2
2. Takizawa et al[25]	1984	197	12
3. Kobayashi et al[28]	1988	414	23
4. Eisenberg et al[13]	1990	753	39
5. Chesnut et al[10]	1993	American Traumatic Data Bank	44
6. Wong et al[17]	2011	661	32

in the direction of the blow as the head moves opposite. This oscillation of the brain is out of phase with the movement of the head, causing the arteries at the base of the brain to be subject to shearing forces. These forces are likely to be greatest when the blow to the head causes it both to be hyperextended and to move laterally.[25–33] Therefore, the intracranial portion of the internal carotid artery, where it is attached to the mobile brain as it joins the circle of Willis above where it is fixed within the sphenoid bone, is subject to these shearing forces during hyperextension and rotation of the head and can sustain a tearing injury. Tatsuno and Lindenberg.[34] identified few possible mechanisms of these tears in fatal traumatic subarachnoid hemorrhage:

1. Rotational acceleration with hyperextension of head.
2. Traumatic subarachnoid hemorrhage vertebroabasilar arterial stretch due to hyperextension.
3. Sudden rise of intra arterial pressure due to the cervical carotid artery.

Alcohol intake prior to injury predisposed SAH. A strong correlation has been reported severe SAH after head injury.[2,18,26,34] In one of the study on tSAH 23% of patients were under the influence of alcohol. An incidence ranging from 23–80%[2,18,35] is reported in tSAH.

It is highly likely that multiple mechanisms are involved in traumatic SAH. Rupture of a coincidental aneurysm is proposed by several authors.[7,27–30] Locksley[30] in 1966 in a co-operative study reported, 3% of aneurysmal SAH had history of head trauma preceding the SAH. Simonsen[31] reported aneurysm in 28% of cases of tSAH. Simonsen[31] could not demonstrate site of bleed in his autopsy study dealing with 430 cases of tSAH.

Traumatic rupture of intracranial arteries and bridging veins, identified at autopsy are also presumed to be the case of tSAH.[5,27,32] Newbarr and Courville[29] hypothesized tearing of superior cerebral veins at their entry point in superior sagittal sinus, as the site or origin of bleeding during displacement of

brain following impact. Rupture of vessel in the pia-arachnoid is thought to occur during brain movement under the dura mater. tSAH is also reported in posterior fossa from rupture of the arteries of the posterior cranial fossa. Freytag[16] in 1963 reported SAH in head-injured patients due to venous rupture. Thin walled veins are more liable to rupture than rupture of thick walled arteries. Overall it looks that tSAH can result in various ways from different sources.

Demographic Aspect of tSAH

Only a few reports are available dealing with demographic pattern of tSAH.[20,31–33] Kakarieka et al[34] in 1994 reported demographic and clinical aspect of both SAH and traumatic SAH. They reported tSAH on average 8 years older than spontaneous SAH. Mean age of their patient was 36 years. Sixty-nine percent of spontaneous SAH were below 40 years of age, women were older than men in tSAH. Incidence of tSAH increases with age[30,32] (Table 43.2). This is probably due to identification of bleed in enlarged subarachnoid space.

Grading of tSAH

The degree of subarachnoid hemorrhage also directly influences the outcome. The Fisher Grade[36] classically classifies the appearance of subarachnoid hemorrhage on CT scan (Table 43.2a). In a study by Greene et al,[12] CT scans from 252 patients with tSAH, treated at a single institution, were reviewed to ascertain thickness of the tSAH; its location; evidence of mass lesion(s); shift of midline structures (≤ 5 vs. > 5 mm); basal cistern effacement; and cortical sulcal effacement. The CT scans were then organized into Grades 1 to 4 with 1 indicating thin tSAH (≤ 5 mm); 2, thick tSAH

Table 43.2: Age in traumatic SAH[34]	
	Mean age in years
1. Mean age	46
2. Extensive SAH	47
3. Moderate SAH	42
4. Mild SAH	38

Table 43.2a: The Fisher Grade classifies the appearance of subarachnoid hemorrhage on CT scan[36]

Grade	Appearance of hemorrhage
1.	None evident
2.	Less than 1 mm thick
3.	More than 1 mm thick
4.	Diffuse or none with intraventricular hemorrhage or parenchymal extension

Table 43.3: Localization of tSAH

Sites	Percent
1. Convexity	65–72
2. Fissures: Sylvian and interhemispheric	40–45
3. Basal cisterns	10–25
4. Tentorial edge	15–20

(> 5 mm); 3, thin tSAH with mass lesion(s); and 4, thick tSAH with mass lesion(s). A stepwise regression analysis of CT features ranked them in descending order of contribution to Glasgow Outcome Scale (GOS) scores at the time of discharge from acute hospitalization as follows: basal cistern effacement, thickness of tSAH, cortical sulcal effacement, presence of mass lesion(s), and location of tSAH. A shift of midline structures was not found to be a significant variable. Further analysis comparing CT grades and admission postresuscitation Glasgow Coma Scale (GCS) scores was highly significant. Patients with lower CT grades had better admission GCS values and discharge GOS scores than those with higher CT grades.

Patients with dilated subarachnoid space tends to collect larger amount of subarachnoid blood. Grading also becomes difficult when 1st CT is performed several days later. Brain swelling and development of contusion or hematomas tends to cause disappearance of SAH (Fig. 43.1). Grading of SAH is done in several ways.[36,37] Hijdra et al[38] scored the SAH 0–48 and average amount of blood seen in CT scan after head injury scores 10 points, while Fisher et al[36] in 1980 classified SAH from Grade 1–4 depending on the amount of blood on CT scan. Most of the patients with tSAH were on Grades 2–3 Fishers grading. Grade 4 tSAH is relatively rare.

Localization of tSAH (Table 43.3)

Convexity is the most frequent site for traumatic SAH (Table 43.3), recorded in 70% in first CT scan followed by Sylvian fissure and interhemispheric fissure in around 40–45% cases (Figs 43.2a and b, 43.3a and b). Basal cisternal blood is recorded less frequently. Bleeding into quadrigeminal cistern is most infrequent. Blood can also be seen around the tentorial edge, which is seen as hyperdense image outlining tentorium area in CT scans, indicating presence of SAH.

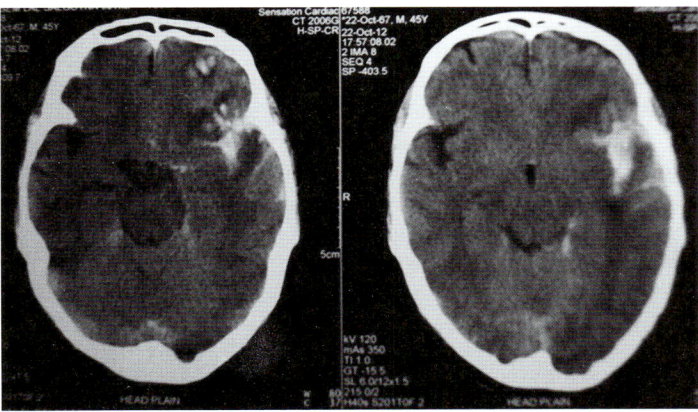

Fig. 43.1: NCCT head of a patient with severe head injury and SAH and frontal contusion

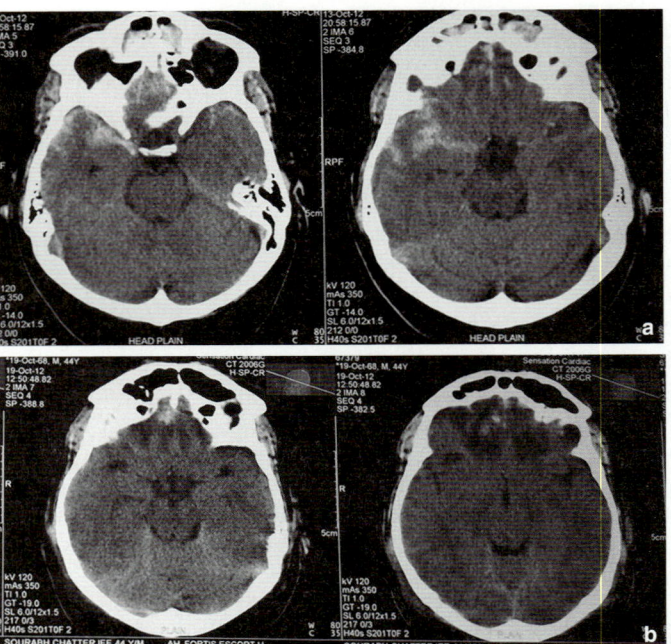

Figs 43.2a and b: CT scan of a head injury. Patient shows SAH in Sylvian fissure (Fig. 43.2a) and clearance of SAH on 6th day

CT has long been considered the first choice in the detection of acute SAH because of its sensitivity, low cost, and wide availability. The sensitivity of CT in detecting SAH is dependent on the resolution of the scanner, the interval after onset, the amount of hemorrhage, and the skills of the radiologist.[39] It has been widely accepted by neuroradiologists that MR imaging is insensitive to acute SAH, and the reason why SAH cannot be seen with MR imaging consistently has been attributed to the complex hemorrhagic signal intensity seen on MR imaging.[40–42] During the past 15 years, new MR imaging sequences have been developed and their application in detecting SAH at high fields have been explored. Some studies have shown that FLAIR is more sensitive than CT in detecting SAH in the acute stage.[43,44] However, hyperintensity in the subarachnoid space on FLAIR can be caused by artifacts such as supplemental oxygen, CSF pulsation, and vascular pulsation rather than SAH[45] on the other hand, gradient-

echo sequences have been used in imaging hyperacute SAH in a small number of patients and some think that it can be reliably used to diagnose SAH at 3T. In a classical paper Wu et al[46] concluded that susceptibility-weighted imaging (SWI) is better than CT in detecting intraventricular hemorrhage. Susceptibility-weighted imaging (SWI) is very sensitive to small amounts of SAH. Aliasing on phase images could be used to help differentiate SAH from veins. However, SWI is not good in detecting basilar cistern SAH. Overall, they concluded that SWI has the potential to provide complementary information to CT in imaging traumatic SAH. SAH can be shown on CT because blood has a higher attenuation coefficient than the surrounding tissue. The attenuation of blood on CT (as measured in HU) decreases as the hemoglobin concentration decreases.[47,48] When the hemoglobin concentration is < 10 g per deciliter, hemorrhage may appear isoattenuated on CT.[49] Overall sensitivity in detecting aneurysmal SAH using

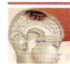

CT is ~92% in the first 24 hours, 85% at 5 days, and 50% after 1 week.[50,51] It is thought that MR imaging is more sensitive than CT in detecting post-traumatic lesions except for skull fractures and SAH. SWI is very sensitive to blood products and has been used to detect parenchymal hemorrhage and was found to be much more sensitive than conventional gradient-echo sequences.[46] The subarachnoid space is between brain parenchyma and arachnoid, and most parts of the arachnoid are in contact with the dura and the skull, where susceptibility artifact occurs, except for those parts that fold into sulci.

Clearance of tSAH

Clearance of tSAH depends on the amount of blood seen in initial scan. In tSAH clearance blood is faster than that described in aneurysmal SAH (Figs 43.2a and b).[29] There are two reasons for the above observations: (a) SAH tends to be moving in aneurysmal bleed, and (b) in aneurysm re-bleed can occur. Rapid clearance of blood in patients of tSAH is reported by Kakarieka 1996.[34] Reduction of subarachnoid blood to 50% was noticed after 2 days of initial CT and 33% after 3 days of initial CT scan.

Vasospasm in Head Injury and tSAH

TCD has allowed the diagnosis of vasospasm at bedside and extended the field of investigation of SAH to head injury in which angiographic studies are seldom performed.[52–60]

These studies showed that post-traumatic vasospasm was more common than previously thought, involving prominently the vertebrobasilar system.[52,53,58] After the comprehensive report of Sloan et al[61] defining TCD criteria for the diagnosis of BA vasospasm, a few studies have provided circumstantial evidence linking elevated FVs in the vertebrobasilar system with poorer neuro-logical outcome in patients suffering from SAH, especially secondary to severe head injury.[52,53,58]

Combining blood flow studies and TCD, Lee et al[53] showed that post-traumatic BA vasospasm correlated significantly with poorer neurological outcome. More recently, Soustiel et al[58] reported on TCD findings in a large cohort of SAH patients and further supported the hypothesis that BA vasospasm may be responsible for secondary brain damage, especially after tSAH. Sixty-two patients (53.4%) had elevated FVs in the BA, among these[34] (29.3%) had FVs above 85 cm/s. Basilar vasospasm was significantly more common in tSAH (59.7%) than in sSAH (40.3%, P = 0.041). In patients with moderate and severe BA vasospasm, FVs in the BA increased on the third day after admission and remained elevated for a week before returning to normal value by the end of the second week. This elevation in BA FVs in patients with BA vasospasm was followed by a significant and progressive worsening in the neurological condition at the end of the first week. Permanent neurological deficit was associated with elevated BA FVs consistent with moderate BA vasospasm whereas patients who remained in persistent vegetative state, had FVs consistent with severe BA vasospasm (P = 0.00019).

Symptomatic vasospasm, or delayed cerebral ischemia associated with arteriographic evidence of arterial constriction, is currently the most important cause of morbidity after acute subarachnoid hemorrhage. The development of vasospasm is directly correlated with the presence of thick blood clots in the basal subarachnoid cisterns, which can be detected by an early computed tomographic scan. Symptomatic vasospasm usually develops between 4 and 12 days after subarachnoid hemorrhage. The onset is gradual, occurring over hours or days. There is typically a gradual deterioration of the level of consciousness, accompanied by focal neurological deficits that are determined by the arterial territories involved. Hyponatremia frequently occurs and may exacerbate the symptoms. The patients are usually volume depleted, and therefore, many authorities now treat them with replenishment and expansion of their intravascular volume with colloid and blood. Taneda et al[63] prospectively studied 130 patients with closed-head trauma, who exhibited subarachnoid blood on admission computerized tomography (CT) scans. Ten (7.7%) of these patients developed delayed ischemic symptoms between days 4 and 16 after the head injury. They consisted of three (3.0%) of 101 patients with small amounts of subarachnoid blood and seven (24.1%) of 29 patients with massive quantities of subarachnoid blood on admission CT scans. In each of the 10 patients, severe vasospasm was demonstrated by angiography performed soon after development of ischemic symptoms. There was a close correlation between the main site of the subarachnoid blood and the location of severe vasospasm. In seven of the patients, follow-up CT scans showed development of focal ischemic areas in the cerebral territories corresponding to the vasospastic arteries.[63]

The correlation between tSAH and arterial spasm was reported in mid 60s.[64–67] Aminmansour et al[68] reported vasospasm in 42.1% patients during the study period and MCA vasospasm was the most common in the first and second weeks (55.5%). The incidence varies from 5 to 90%. Leeds et al[66] in 1966, reported angiographic vasospasm in 31 of 39% head injury patients. Wilkins and Odom[67] reported arterial spasm in 5% of patients with significant head injuries. They also found hemorrhagic CSF in spinal fluid and suggested pathogenesis of ischemia similar to that of spontaneous SAH. Suwanwela and Suwanwela[69] reported 19% incidence of angiographic vasospasm in head-injured patients. Neurological deficit is related to tSAH and vasospasm.[68–71] Hence, tSAH, leading to vasospasm and ischemia play important role in morbidity and mortality in patients with head injury.

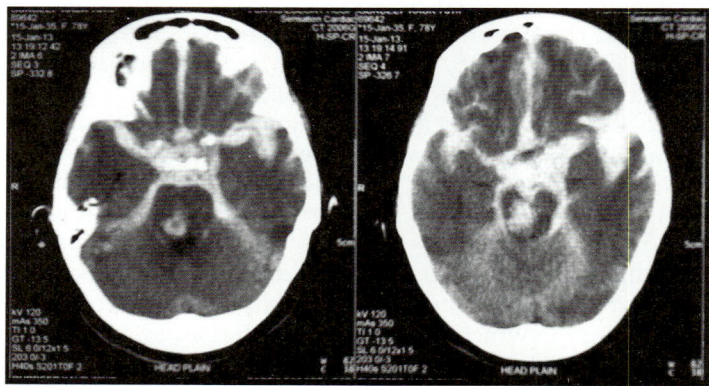

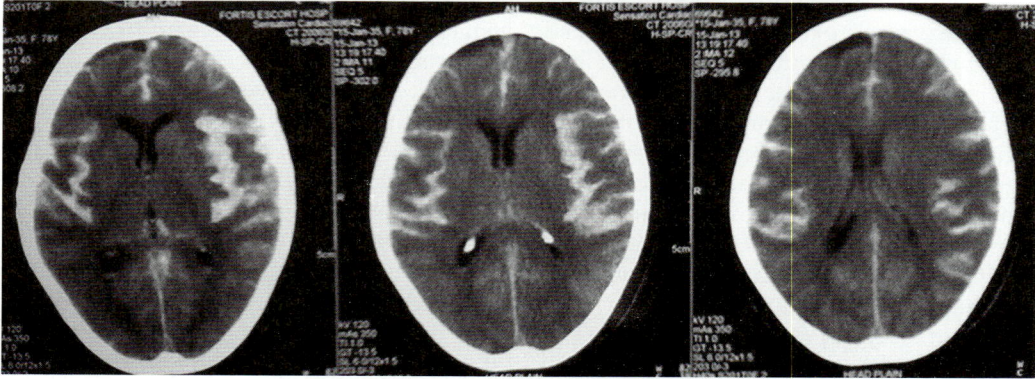

Figs 43.3a and b: CT scan showing thick severe post-traumatic SAH (Fisher's Grade 4)

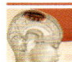

Transcranial Doppler in tSAH

Over last decade, TCD is available for the non-invasive evaluation of cerebral vasospasm. It is also hypothesized that the pathogenesis of vasospasm in SAH and tSAH are same. Vasospasm, as detected by TCD is reported in more than 40–68% of severe head injury patients.[71–73] Comptom and Teddy[72] reported 68% vasospasm in 25 patients with severe head injury. They also reported good correlation between vasospasm and clinical deterioration. Similar correlation was also observed by other authors.[73–75] Dorschb and Zurynski,[76] reported 50% vasospasm in their severe head-injured patients and reported a higher mortality in those patients. However, a varied correlation is reported between degree of subarachnoid blood, BFV (blood flow velocity) and clinical outcome.[73,77–78]

Role of Calcium Channel Blocker in tSAH

Recently, calcium channel blocker has been used as a neuroprotective agent in preventing secondary brain damage. Most extensively tried calcium antagonist is nimodipine. Nimodipine has also been used in severe head injured patients,[80–83] to effectively block calcium channel and prevent ischemic damage. The results of above studies were inconclusive. Nimodipine did not improve the overall outcome in patients with severe head injury. However, in patients with tSAH there was a significantly reduced poor outcome in patients treated with nimodipine.[33,80] In a study reported by Bailey et al,[79] 352 severely injured patients were treated by intravenous nimodipine or placebo for one week. The overall outcome were similar at six months follow-up. In HIT, II-study 852 patients were enrolled. Result did not favor routine use of nimodipine in severe head injured patients. The study showed improvement of favorable outcome from 59 to 61% and reduction of mortality from 24 to 22%.

In a study involving 654 patients, 210 had tSAH, nimodipine in patients with tSAH significantly reduced the mortality and unfavorable outcome. Unfavorable outcome was recorded in 51 and 66% in patients with nimodipine and placebo group, respectively. The incidence of post-traumatic epilepsy was lower in survivors who received nimodipine than in those who did not receive nimodipine[82,83] (13 vs 20%). Overall, nimodipine is safe and is well tolerated in patients. There is a small risk of fall in blood pressure. However, the beneficial role of nimodipine in tSAH outweigh the risk caused by drop in blood pressure. Harders et al[62] did a prospective, randomized, double-blind, placebo-controlled study of nimodipine used to treat traumatic subarachnoid hemorrhage (tSAH) was conducted in 21 German neurosurgical centers. One hundred twenty-three patients with tSAH appearing on initial computerized tomography (CT) scanning were entered into the study. Eligible patients received either a sequential course of intravenous and oral nimodipine or placebo-treatment for 3 weeks. Patients treated with nimodipine had a significantly less unfavorable outcome (death, vegetative survival, or severe disability) at 6 months than placebo-treated patients (25 vs. 46%, P = 0.02).

Traumatic Subarachnoid Hemorrhage and Outcome

Traumatic SAH is one of the important factors influencing the overall outcome in head-injured patients. The mortality is 2–3 times higher in patients with tSAH than those without SAH in CT scan. Eisenberg et al[32] in 1990 reported mortality among tSAH patients twice as high as in no SAH patients. In patients with tSAH unfavorable outcome is reported in 60–70% cases. tSAH patients with mild head injury showed a higher incidence of un-favorable outcome than mild head injury without SAH.[84–87] Demircivi et al[14] in 1993 had shown good outcome in the majority of cases with mild head injury despite of having tSAH in CT scan.

The outcome of patients with tSAH is directly related to clinical state and amount of subarachnoid blood seen on the first CT scan.

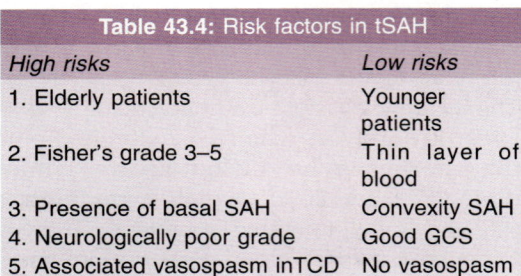

Table 43.4: Risk factors in tSAH

High risks	Low risks
1. Elderly patients	Younger patients
2. Fisher's grade 3–5	Thin layer of blood
3. Presence of basal SAH	Convexity SAH
4. Neurologically poor grade	Good GCS
5. Associated vasospasm inTCD	No vasospasm

The patients with greater amount of subarachnoid blood have a worse outcome. Patients with basal cistern SAH had poorer outcome than those who had blood found over the cerebral hemisphere.

Traumatic SAH and Other Prognostic Factors

tSAH is an important and independent prognostic factor in head injured patients. However, large number of factors in tSAH play important role (Table 43.4). Those include age, amount of blood, site of SAH, alcohol intoxication and associated vasospasm. As already discussed above, there is no relationship between CT findings of tSAH and initial neurological condition when seen at the first time. However, degree of SAH is directly correlated to clinical state.

CONCLUSIONS

Traumatic SAH is an important pathological entity. tSAH more frequent in severe head injury and in the elderly age group, due to wide subarachnoid space. With the advent of CT the diagnosis has become easy and repeated CT scan shows quick resolution. TCD studies have shown vasospasm in 50–60% patients. While nimodipine is not helpful in severe head injury as a whole, it is proved to be beneficial in tSAH. tSAH is an unfavorable factor in head injury, as it increases the mortality and morbidity significantly.

REFERENCES

1. Wilkin S. Sanguineous meningeal effusion. Guy Hosp Rep 1859;5:119–27.

2. Simonsen. Fatal Traumatic Subarachnoid Haemorrhage in alcohol intoxication. J. Forensic Med 1963;8:97–116.

3. Camaron JM, Mant AK. Fatal subarachnoid haemorrhage associated with cervical trauma. Med Sci Law 1972;12:66–70.

4. Courville CB. Pathology of central nervous system. A study based upon a survey of lesions found in a series of forty thousand autopsies, 3rd edn., Pacific Mountain View 1950; p 112.

5. Dowling G, Curry B. Traumatic basal subarachnoid haemorrhage. Report of 6 cases and review of the literature. Am J Forensic Med Pathol 1988;9(1):23–31.

6. Dymock RB. Traumatic basal subarachnoid haemorrhage. Med J Aust 1977;2:216–8.

7. Ford R. Basal subarachnoid haemorrhage and trauma. J Forensic Sci 1956;1:117–26.

8. Armin SS, Colohan AR, Zhang JH. Traumatic subarachnoid hemorrhage: our current understanding and its evolution over the past half century. Neurol Res 2006;28(4):445–52.

9. Fohz EL, Ward AA. Communicating hydrocephalus from subarachnoid bleeding. J Neurosurg 1956;13:564–6.

10. Chesnut RM, Luerssen TG, Van Berkum-Clark M, et al. Post-traumatic ventricular enlargement in Traumatic Coma Data Bank: Incidence, risk factors and influence on outcome. In: Avezaat CJJ van Ejindhover, Mass AIR, Tans JTJ (Eds). Proceedings of 8th International Symposium on Intracranial Pressure. Springer Berlin, Heidelberg, New York 1993;503–6.

11. Javid M. Current Concepts: Head injuries. N Eng J Med 1974;291:890–2.

12. Greene KA, Marciano FF, Johnson BA, Jacobowitz R, Spetzler RF, Harrington TR, Impact of traumatic subarachnoid hemorrhage on outcome in nonpenetrating head injury Part I: A proposed computerized tomography grading scale Journal of Neurosurgery September 1995;83:(3):445–52.

13. Eisenberg HM, Gary HE Jr, Aldrich EF, et al. Initial CT findings in 753 patients with severe head injury: a report from the NIH Traumatic Coma Data Bank. J Neurosurg 1990;73:688–98.

14. Servadei F, Murray GD, Teasdale GM, et al. Traumatic subarachnoid hemorrhage: demographic and clinical study of 750 patients from the European brain injury consortium survey of head injuries. Neurosurgery 2002;50:261–7; discussion 267–69.

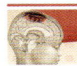
15. Morris GF, Bullock R, Marshall SB, et al. Failure of the competitive N-methyl-D-aspartate antagonist Selfotel (CGS 19755) in the treatment of severe head injury: results of two phase III clinical trials. The Selfotel Investigators. J Neurosurg 1999;91:737–43.

16. Freytag E. Autopsy findings in head injuries from blunt forces. Statistical evaluation of 1367 cases. Arch Pathol 1963;75:402–13.

17. Wong GKC, Yeung JHH, Graham CA, Zhu XL, Rainer TH, Poon WS, Neurological outcome in patients with traumatic brain injury and its relationship with computed tomography patterns of traumatic subarachnoid hemorrhage; Journal of Neurosurgery Jun 2011;114 (6):1510–5.

18. De Villasante JM, Taveras JM. Computerized tomography in acute head trauma. AJR, 1976;126:146–55.

19. Demircivi F, Ozkan N, Buyukkececi J, et al. Traumatic SAH: An analysis of 89 cases. Acta Neurochir (Wien) 1993;122:45–48.

20. Levi L, Guilburd JM, Lemberger A, et al. Diffuse axonal injury: Analysis of 100 patients with radiological signs: Neurosurgery 1996;27:429–32.

21. Coast GC, Gee DJ. Traumatic subarachnoid haemorrhage: an alternative source, J Clin Pathol 1984;37(11):1245–8.

22. Dowling G, Curry B. Traumatic Basal Subarachnoid Hemorrhage: Report of Six Cases and Review of the Literature; American Journal of Forensic Medicine and Pathology 1988;9(1).

23. Dymock RB, Traumatic basal subarachnoid haemorrhage. Med J Aust 1977;13;2(7):216–8.

24. KarhunenPJ, Kauppila R, Penttilä A, vertebral artery rupture in traumatic subarachnoid haemorrhage detected by postmortem angiography.

25. Takizawa T, Matsumoto A, Sato S, Sano A, et al. Traumatic subarachnoid hemorrhage: Neurol Med Chir (Tokyo) 1984 Jun; 24(6):390–5.

26. Wang H, Yu, X., Xu, G., Xu, G., Gao, G., Xu, X. Alcoholism and traumatic subarachnoid hemorrhage: An experimental study on vascular morphology and biomechanics Journal of Trauma—Injury, Infection and Critical Care 70 2011;1:E6-E12.

27. Kindelberger D, Gilmore K, Catanese CA, Armbrustmacher V. Hyperextension and Rotation of Head Causing Internal Carotid Artery Laceration with Basilar Subarachnoid Hematoma, J Forensic Sci 2003;48:(6):1–3.

28. Kobayashi S, Nakazawa S, Hiroyuki Y, et al. Traumatic subarachnoid haemorrhage in acute head injury. Noto Shinkei 1988;40:1131–5.

29. Newbarr FD, Courville CB. Trauma as the possible significant factor in rupture of congenital intracranial aneurysms. Forensic Sci 1958;31:174–99.

30. Locksley HB. Report on the cooperative study of intracranial aneurysm, subarachnoid haemorrhage, and arteriovenous malformations. Based on 638 cases in the cooperative study. J Neurosurg 1966;25:219–39.

31. Simonsen J. Fatal subarachnoid haemorrhage in relation to minor head injuries. J Forensic Sci, 1967;14:146–55.

32. Nakamura N, Taunoda M, Ohwada T, et al. Post-traumatic progressive non-obstructive hydrocephalus report of two cases. No To Shinkei 1971;23:1217–21.

33. Shigemori M, Tokutomi T, Hirohata M, et al. Clinical significance of traumatic subarachnoid haemorrhage. Neurol Med Chir 1990;30:396–400.

34. Kakarieka A, Schakel EH, Fritze J. Clinical significance of the finding of subarachnoid blood on CT scan after head trauma. Acta Neurochir (Wien) 1994;129:1–5.

35. Hillbom M, Kaste M. Does alcohol intoxication precipitate aneurysmal **SAH?** Neurol Neurosurg Psychiat 1981;44:523–6.

36. Fisher CM, Kistler JP, Davis]M. Relation of cerebral vasospasm to SAH visualised by computerized tomographic scanning. Neurosurgery 1980;6:1–9.

37. Tatsun Y, Lindenberg R. Basal subarachnoid haematoma as sole intracranial traumatic lesions. Arch Pathol 1974;97:211–5.

38. Hijdra A, Brouwers PJAM, Verneulen M, et al. Grading the amount of blood on computed tomogram after SAH stroke 1990;21:1156–61.

39. van Gijn J, Kerr RS, Rinkel GJ. Subarachnoid haemorrhage. Lancet 2007;369:306–18.

40. Sipponen JT, Sepponen RE, Sivula A. Nuclear magnetic resonance (NMR) imaging of intracerebral hemorrhage in the acute and resolving phases. J Comput Assist Tomogr 1983;7:954–9.

41. Dooms GC, Uske A, Brant-Zawadzki M, et al. Spin-echo MR imaging of intracranial hemorrhage. Neuroradiology 1986;28:132–8.

42. Bradley WG Jr, Schmidt PG. Effect of methemoglobin formation on the MR appearance of subarachnoid hemorrhage. Radiology 1985;156: 99–103.

43. Noguchi K, Seto H, Kamisaki Y, et al. Comparison of fluid-attenuated inversion-recovery MR imaging with CT in a simulated model of acute subarachnoid hemorrhage. AJNR Am J Neuroradiol 2000;21:923–7.

44. Yuan MK, Lai PH, Chen JY, et al. Detection of subarachnoid hemorrhage at acute and subacute/chronic stages: comparison of four magnetic resonance imaging pulse sequences and computed tomography. J Chin Med Assoc 2005;68:131–7.

45. Stuckey SL, Goh TD, Heffernan T, et al. Hyperintensity in the subarachnoid space on FLAIR MRI. AJR Am J Roentgenol 2007;189:913–21.

46. Wu Z, Li S, Lei J, An D, Haacke EM. Evaluation of traumatic subarachnoid hemorrhage using susceptibility-weighted imaging.

47. Osborn AG, Tong KA. Handbook of Neuroradiology: Brain and Skull, 2nd edn. St Louis: Mosby 1996;25.

48. Fainardi E, Chieregato A, Antonelli V,et al. Time course of CT evolution in traumatic subarachnoid haemorrhage: a study of 141 patients. Acta Neurochir (Wien) 2004;146:257–63; discussion 26.

49. Latchaw RE, Silva P, Falcone SF. The role of CT following aneurysmal rupture. Neuroimaging Clin N Am 1997;7:693–708.

50. Smith WP Jr, Batnitzky S, Rengachary SS. Acute isodense subdural hematomas: a problem in anemic patients. AJR Am J Roentgenol 1981;136:543–6.

51. Sames TA, Storrow AB, Finkelstein JA, et al. Sensitivity of new-generation computed tomography AJNR Am J Neuroradiol 2010;31(7):1302–10. doi: 10.3174/ajnr.A2022. Epub 2010 Feb 25.

52. Hadani M, Bruck B, Ram Z, Knoller N, Bass A. Transiently increased basilar artery flow velocity following severe head injury: a time course transcranial Doppler study. J Neurotrauma 1997;14:629–36.

53. Lee JH, Martin NA, Alsina G, McArthur DL, Zaucha K, Hovda DA, Becker DP. Hemodynamically significant cerebral vasospasm and outcome after head injury: a prospective study. J Neurosurg 1997;87:221–33.

54. Martin NA, Doberstein C, Alexander MJ, Khanna R, Benalcazar H, Alsina G, Zane C, McBride D, Kelly D, Hovda DA, Becker DP. Posttraumatic cerebral arterial spasm. J Neurotrauma 1995;12:897–901.

55. Martin NA, Doberstein C, Zane C, Caron MJ, Thomas K, Becker DP. Posttraumatic cerebral arterial spasm: transcranial Doppler ultrasound, cerebral blood flow, and angiographic findings. J Neurosurg 1992;77:575–83.

56. Martin NA, Patwardhan RV, Alexander MJ, Zane Africk C, Lee JH, Shalmon E, Hovda DA, Becker DP. Characterization of cerebral hemodynamic phases following severe head trauma: hypoperfusion, hyperemia and vasospasm. J Neurosurg 1997;87:9–19.

57. Sander D, Klingelhofer J. Cerebral vasospasm following post-traumatic subarachnoid hemorrhage evaluated by transcranial Doppler ultrasonography.J Neurol Sci 1993;119:1–7.

58. Soustiel JF, Bruk B, Shik B, Hadani M, Feinsod M. Transcranial Doppler in vertebrobasilar vasospasm following subarachnoid hemorrhage. Neurosurgery 1998;43:282–93.

59. Steiger HJ, Aaslid R, Stooss R, Seiler RW. Transcranial Doppler monitoring in head injury: relations between type of injury, flow velocities, vasoreactivity, and outcome. Neurosurgery 1994;34:79–85.

60. Weber M, Grolimund P, Seiler RW. Evaluation of posttraumatic cerebral blood flow velocities by transcranial Doppler ultrasonography. Neurosurgery 1990;27:106–112.

61. Sloan MA, Burch CM, Wozniak MA, Rothman MI, Rigamonti D, Permutt T, Numaguchi Y Transcranial Doppler detection of vertebrobasilar vasospasm following subarachnoid hemorrhage. Stroke 1994;25:2187–97.

62. Harders A, Kakarieka A, Braakman R , Traumatic subarachnoid hemorrhage and its treatment with nimodipine Journal of Neurosurgery July 1996;85:(1):82–89.

63. Taneda M, Kataoka K, Akai F, Asai T, Sakata I,. Journal of Neurosurgery Traumatic subarachnoid hemorrhage as a predictable indicator of delayed ischemic symptoms, May 1996;84(5):762–8.

64. Kakarieka A. Analysis of CT findings in tSAH. In: Traumatic Subarachnoid Haemorrhage. A Kakarieka (ed), Springer Verlag, Berlin, Heidelberg 1997;21–34.

65. Collumella F, Delzano GB, Gaist G, et al. Angiographical in traumatic cerebral laceration with special regard to some less common aspect. Acta Radiol 1963;1:239.

66. Leeds N, Reid ND, Rosen LM. Angiographic changes in cerebral contusions and intracranial Haematomas. Acta Radio Diag 1966;5:320–7.

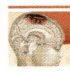

67. Wilkins RH, Odom GL. Intracranial arterial spasm associated with craniocerebral trauma. J Neurosurg 1970;32:626–33.

68. Aminmansour B, Abbas Ghorbani A, Sharifi D, Shemshaki H, Ahmadi A, Cerebral vasospasm following traumatic subarachnoid hemorrhageJ Res Med Sci 2009;14(6):343–8. Forensic Science International 1990;44(2–3):107–15.

69. Suwanwela C, Suwanwela N. Intracranial arterial narrowing and spasm in acute head injury. J Neurosurg 1972;36:314–23.

70. Macpherson P, Graham DI. Correlation between angiographic findings and the ischaemic of head injury. J Neurol Neurosurg Psychiat 1978;41:122–7.

71. Pasqualin A, vivenza C, Rosta L, et al. Cerebral vasospasm after head injury. Neurosurgery 1984;15:855–8.

72. Compton JS, Teddy. Cerebral arterial vasospasm following severe head injury: A transcranial Doppler study, Br J Neurosurg 1987;1:435–9.

73. Bakshi A, Mahapatra AK. Basilar artery vasospasm in severe head injury. A preliminary TCD study. NMJI 1998;113:220–1.

74. Weber M, Grolimund P, Seiler RW. Evaluation of post-traumatic cerebral blood flow velocities by transcranial Doppler ultrasound. Neurosurgery 1990;27:106–12.

75. Muttaquin Z, Arita K, Uozumi T, et al. Vasospasm after traumatic subarachnoid haemorrhage: Transcranial Doppler evaluation. Case report. Neurosurg Rev 1991;14:321–5.

76. Zurynski YA, Dorschb N, Pearsona I, Incidence and effects of increased cerebral blood flow velocity after severe head injury: a transcranial Doppler ultrasound study I. Prediction of post-traumatic vasospasm and hyperemia, Journal of the Neurological Sciences 1995;134(1–2):33–40.

77. Lin TK, Tsai HC, Hsieh TC. The impact of traumatic SAH on outcome: a study with grouping of traumatic SAH and transcranial Doppler sonography. J Trauma Acute Care Surg 2012;73(1):131–6.

78. Sander D, Klingelnofer J. Cerebral vasospasm following post-traumatic subarachnoid haemorrhage evaluated by transcranial Doppler ultrasonography. J Neurol Sci 1993;119:1–7.

79. Bailey I, Bell A, Gray J, et al. A trial of the effect of nimodipine on outcome after head injury. Acta Neurochir (Wien) 1991;110:97–105.

80. European study group on Nimodipine in severe head injury. A multicentre trial on the efficacy of nimodipine on outcome after severe head injury. J Neurosurg 1994;80:797–804.

81. Kakarieka A, Harders A, Braakman R, et al. Traumatic subarachnoid haemorrhage: A clinical entity and its treatment with nimodipine. J Neurotrauma 1995;12:375.

82. Cascino GD, Meyer FB, Whisnant JP, et al. Nimodipine as an add-on therapy for intractable seizure. Neurology 1994;44 (Suppl):S775.

83. Hans P, Triffaux M, Bonhomme V, et al. Control of drug-resistant epilepsy after head injury with intravenous nimodipine. Acta Anaesthesiol, Belg 1994;45:175–8.

84. Rimel RW, Giordani B, Barth JT, et al. Moderate head injury: completing the clinical spectrum of head trauma. Neurosurgery 1982;11:344–51.

85. Dacey RG. Alves WA, Rimel RW, et al. Neurosurgical complications after apparently minor head injury. J Neurosurg 1956;65:203–10.

86. Williams DH, Levin HS, Eisenberg HM. Mild head injury classification. Neurosurgery 1990;27:422–8.

87. Stein SC, Ross SE. The value of computed tomographic scans in patients with low risk head injuries. Neurosurgery 1990;26:638–40.

44

Traumatic Brainstem Injury

Raj Kamal • AK Mahapatra

INTRODUCTION

Traumatic brainstem injury (TBSI) occurs in 0.75–3.6% of all patients admitted to hospital with head injury.[1-4] The prognosis of these patients is dismal because of its critical location. Previous studies have shown that the mortality of this patients ranged from 67 to 83%.[1,4] With the advent of CT scan it is possible to visualise and diagnose traumatic brainstem hemorrhage in head injured patients.[5-8] Prior to the CT, diagnosis was made on clinical ground on findings like decerebrate rigidity and an internuclear ophthalmoplegia, however, these findings can also be present due to functional disturbances, and not always necessary to have anatomical changes in brainstem. In fact, brainstem signs are very frequently observed in head injury patients even in absence of brainstem hematoma in CT scan. Two types of traumatic brainstem injury have been reported. Primary type is the result of direct mechanical distortion of the brainstem. Secondary type results from diffuse cerebral edema, hypoxia, post-traumatic vasospasm, and transtentorial herniation.[1,9] Meyer et al[1] reported that the most frequent site of hemorrhage, in 31 (69%) of 45 patients, was the ventral rostral midbrain adjacent to the interpeduncular cistern. Disruption of axonal tracts in the brainstem injured patients occurs as part of the widespread white matter damage. This lesion often coexists with other brain lesions such as acute epidural hematoma, acute subdural hematoma, and hemorrhagic contusion. Neurological deficits of the affected patients are usually considerable, and thus subsumed in the category of those with severe brainstem injuries. In some cases, however, an isolated type without supratentorial lesions has been described with unexpectedly good recovery.[9,10]

INCIDENCE

Incidence of brainstem hemorrhage is difficult to determine Tandon[11] in 1964 reported 69 cases of brainstem hemorrhage among 132 autopsy cases. Mahapatra et al[12] had reported 7 cases of brainstem hematoma among 62 decerebrating head-injured patients (Fig. 44.1). Tasi et al[13] in 1986 reported brainstem lesions in 67 patients among 1600 head-injured patients. However, the data also included indirect evidence of brainstem involvement, such as, obliteration of prepontine and perimesencephalic cisterns. Thus, only 19 patients in their study had brainstem injury and 12 of them had hemorrhage in CT scan. Zuccarello et al[4] in 1983 reported primary brainstem hemorrhage in 36 patients among 1000 patients in whom CT scans were performed. In one of our study[13] analyzing 2500 patients, 48 had brainstem hematoma. With the advent of CT scan the diagnosis has become easy and incidence of brainstem

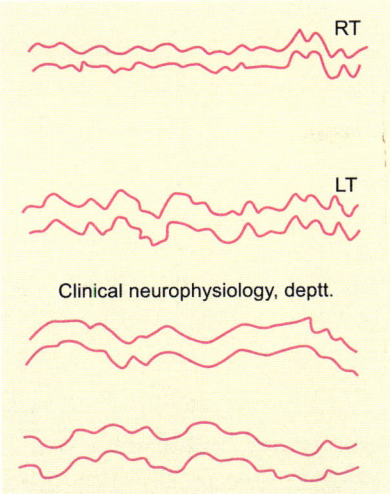

RT

LT

Clinical neurophysiology, deptt.

Fig. 44.1: BAER done twice in a 23 years male with brainstem hematoma shows no wave. Patient expired

hematoma has increased. Kalyanaraman and Ramamurthy[14] reported brainstem in 4.6% of all head injured patients. Recent study by Kim[15] shows an incidence of about 5% (136/2695 patients).

Mechanism of Injury

Since, Duret first described this condition in 1878, there are several pathological studies describing the details of mechanism, location and pathogenesis of brainstem hematoma.[16–19] Acceleration and deceleration injuries involve brainstem to varying degree, depending upon several factors. Mechanical effects of stretching and distortion further aggravate the damage due to vascular injury. Involvement of brainstem can occur due to several mechanisms: (a) damage to the brainstem by direct force of impact, (b) due to flexon and distortion, and (c) vascular involvement. Primary damage is also possible due to brain movement when brainstem get lacerated or contused by the tentorial edge.[11,16,20] While acute flexon is the most frequent cause, rarely hyperextension injury to the head can give rise to brainstem damage.[18] Generally, primary brainstem injury can be in the form of: (a) laceration, (b)

contusion, and (c) brainstem hematoma (Table 44.1). Frequently, brainstem injury is associated with injuries elsewhere in the brain. Isolated brainstem injury/hematoma also occurs rarely.[5,11,16,18,20–22] Very rarely traumatic transection of brainstem has been reported.[18]

Ropper and Miller[2] proposed three mechanisms to cause traumatic brainstem

Table 44.1: Pathology of traumatic brainstem lesions

A. Primary pathology
  i. Laceration
  ii. Contusion
  iii. Primary brainstem hematoma
  iv. Transection of brainstem

B. Secondary pathology
  i. Edema
  ii. Ischemia
  iii. Infarction
  iv. Secondary hemorrhage

C. Combination of primary and secondary pathology

hemorrhage. Brainstem hemorrhage can be caused by primary lesion resulting from either rotational forces, or from transient acceleration-deceleration forces that cause contusion against the tentorium, or secondary to the brainstem compression. However, it is uncertain to define the exact one mechanism because of conflicting neuropathological evidences in brainstem hemorrhage. Some authors described it as a discrete entity attributable to the hyperextension injury of patients who have sustained an impact on the forehead along the rostrocaudal axis.[1,10,14,23] Others have been advocate the acceleration-deceleration injury model in a sagittal plane as the most frequent cause of traumatic brainstem hemorrhage.[16,24]

Secondary damage to the brainstem occurs more frequently as compared to primary damage. Transtentorial herniation is most frequent cause of brainstem damage. Secondary brainstem hemorrhage is more frequent in tegmentum of midbrain and pons.[17,22,25–27]

Multiple subependymal punctate haemorrhage can also occur secondary to transtentorial herniation. Secondary hemorrhage are often bilateral and paramedian in location.[16,18,26–29] Necrosis may occur in distorted area. Secondary medullary lesions are due to longitudinal buckling of medulla.[16] Frequently, both primary and secondary damage in brainstem may coexist. Lesions like ischemic necrosis, small hemorrhage, microhemorrhage and degeneration of axons showing retraction bulb can also be seen.

Subthalamic lesion is prone for microhemorrhage and necrosis. Primary lesions are less common in tegmentum. In medulla, there is selective necrosis of inferior olivary nucleus and vestibular nuclei.[11,16,26] Thus, a widespread pathological lesions can be observed in brainstem, in head injury patients.

Clinical Presentation

Typically, patients with brainstem hematoma are unconscious or in altered sensorium (Table 44.2). However, only on the basis of unconsciousness a clinical diagnosis cannot be made. Rarely, patients may have GCS more than 9.[5,11,26] In our study out of 70 patients, 15 had no response to pain on admission and 35 (50%) were decerebrating. Tandon[11] in 1964 reported that only two-thirds cases were comatose from injury to death, while remaining were unconscious sometime during the period they survived. He also reported lucid interval in 21% and no initial unconsciousness in 9% patients. Mahapatra et al[5] in 1990 reported 5 patients who were conscious at the time of admission. In a series reported by Tandon,[11] 7% patients were conscious at the time of admission.

Decerebrate rigidity is commonly observed in patients with brainstem hematoma.[4,5,26] Rarely, patients can have hypotonicity.[26] However, decerebrate rigidity can occur in absence of brainstem lesion and may only be a manifestation of brainstem dysfunction.[30,31]

Table 44.2: Conscious state in brainstem hematoma (experience at AIIMS)

Responses	Numbers
No response	15
Decerebrating	35
GCS 5–8	15
GCS 9 or better	5
	70

Other clinical findings which are sometime typical to brainstem lesions are respiratory abnormalities pupillary findings and temperature. Varieties of respiratory abnormalities are reported depending on the sites of lesion. It could be classical Cheyne-Stoke breathing, hyperventilation or even shallow breathing. Some patients rapidly deteriorate to brain death with respiratory arrest. Disturbances of temperature regulation lead to hyperpyrexia. In the past, hyperthermia was considered pathognomonic of pontine hematoma. Surprisingly, Tandon[11] in 1964, reported hypothermia in 35% patients with brainstem hemorrhage, as compared to 48% patients with non-hemorrhagic brainstem involvement.

Pupillary abnormalities are well described in brainstem hemorrhage.[11,12,25] Fixed dilated pupils were frequently observed by Tsai et al.[12] Tandon[11] in 1964 described bilateral nonreacting pupils in patients with brainstem hemorrhage, while, amongst 65 nonhemorrhagic cases, 26 had normally reacting pupils. Thus, pupillary changes are nonspecific and not diagnostic of brainstem injury. So called pin-pointed pupils are very rarely observed in patients with brainstem hematomas.[11]

Disturbance of conjugated eye movement is more frequent. This is basically because of involvement of the medial longitudinal fasciculus (MLF). The disconjugated movement and abnormal oculocephalic or doll's eye movement is characteristic findings of brainstem damage.[7,19,33–35]

COLD CALORIC RESPONSE (VESTIBULO-OCULAR REFLEX)

Cold caloric response is an important test assessing the brainstem integrity.[5,8,30,34–38] Its utility in predicting the outcome in severe head injury is well established.[8,30,34–37] It is a simple bedside test. Head is raised by 30 degree and external auditory meatus is irrigated by ice cold saline or water which stimulate semicircular canal. The stimulus is carried by vestibular nerve to vestibular nuclei which is connected to MLF, 3rd and 6th nerve nuclei in brainstem. Thus, stimulating vestibular nuclei, the eye movement and nystagmus are observed. Normally, there is conjugate deviation of eye with nystagmus. Depending on the site of brainstem involvement and the degree of damage there may be absent or abnormal response of varying degree[8,34,36] (Table 44.3). A complete absence of caloric response is indicative of grave prognosis.[4,8] The study must be repeated several times to assess the improvement or deterioration of brainstem function and is more predictive and reliable as compared to brainstem auditory evoked response (BAER).[5]

Table 44.3: Cold caloric response in brainstem hematoma (experience at AIIMS-65 cases)

Responses	Numbers
1. Normal	20
2. Abnormal	24
3. Absent	21
	65

BRAINSTEM AUDITORY EVOKED RESPONSE (BAER)

Brainstem auditory evoked response is a reliable study assessing the auditory nerve and brainstem function. BAER is frequently used as a prognostic test in severe head injury. Patients with normal BAER have a good prognosis, on the contrary, patients with repeatedly absent BAER either die or remain vegetative. Only a few studies have reported the useful value of BAER in brainstem hematoma.[5,8,38–40] Sancesario et al[38] in 1984 reported the BAER findings in 6 patients with brainstem hematomas and most frequent findings, abnormality of wave IV and V and delay in 1—V interpeak latency. In one case BAER was normal. Tsutsui et al[39] reported BAER in one patient with brainstem hematoma, prior to and following hematoma evacuation. BAER normalized following surgery and preceded clinical improvement. Mahapatra et al[5] emphasized the role of BAER in 70 patients with traumatic brainstem hematoma. Patients with repeatedly absent BAER had poor prognosis (Fig. 44.1) on the contrary improvement in BAER finding or repeatedly normal BAER (Fig. 44.2) were associated with favorable outcome.

CT Scan Findings (Table 44.3)

CT scan is a reliable imaging modality for intracranial pathology, because of its ability to demonstrate the extent, sites and nature of brain injury. Hence, today CT is the primary diagnostic method in patients with head injury. There are several reports dealing with CT findings in brainstem hematoma.[4,5,12,38–41] CT scans not only show the hematoma, it can visualize contusion, obliteration of basal cistern and blood in prepontine or perimesencephalic cistern.[5] Tasi et al[3] had considered direct and indirect evidence of brainstem injury. Direct evidence was the presence of hematoma. Among 67 patients diagnosed as cases of brainstem injury, only 12 had hematoma, and rest 55 were diagnosed on indirect evidences.

Indirect signs are obliteration of the pontine, cerebellopontine angle, and perimesencephalic cisterns. Therefore, many cases of TBSI as an indirect evidence were reported where the hematoma were localized along tentorium,[42] for which Kim et al[43] proposed supratentorial impact site as mostly occipital region, midbrain tegmentum, interpedunculoambient cisterns,[44] cisterna magna,[45] and cerebellum[46,47] with or without supratentorial abnormalities. MRI (Figs 44.4a and b) provides a more sophisticated display of brainstem

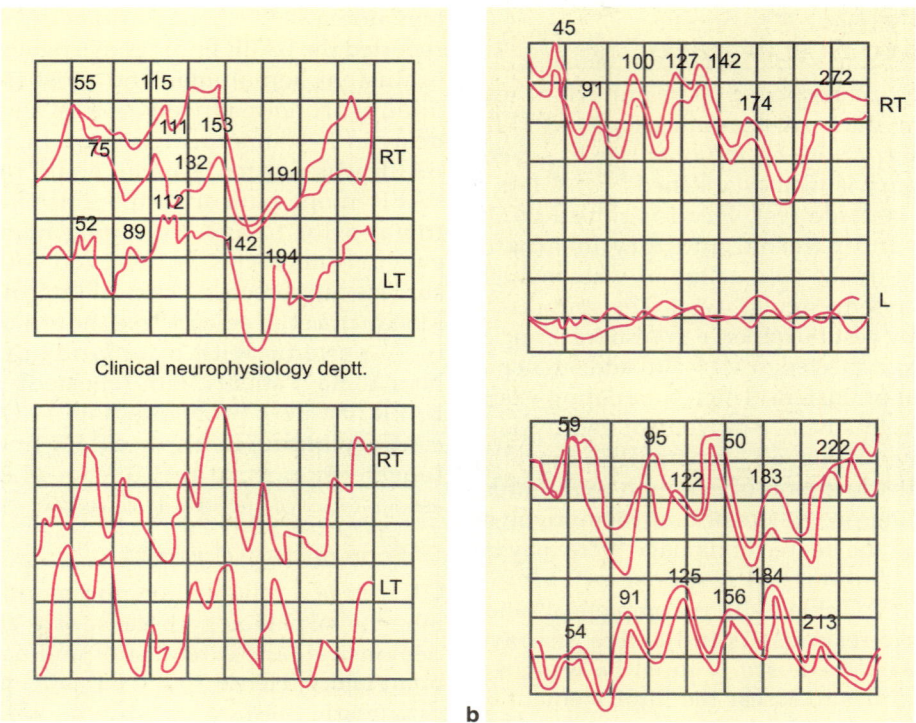

Clinical neurophysiology deptt.

Fig. 44.2: (a) Repeated BAER in a 13-year-old boy with brainstem haematoma shows normal wave pattern. The child had good outcome; (b) BAER findings in a patient with brainstem hematoma show no wave on the left side on 19.10.83, BAER repeated on 26.10.83 shows bilateral normal waves. Patient had good recovery

with improved contrast resolution of structures not appreciated on CT. Therefore, acute stage MRI is used (Figs 44.4a and b) in place of CT or added to CT, because of some limitation of CT in detecting, localizing, and characterizing diffuse injury and posterior fossa lesions; for example, in differentiating between two patterns of TBSI such as ventral or dorsal location.[47,48] Additionally, MRI is more helpful than CT in detecting non-hemorrhagic lesions, cortical contusions, diffuse axonal injury such as supratentorial injury in corpus callosum, and even in normal CT finding when neurological condition could not be explained.[44,46]

Mahapatra et al[5] described their CT finding in 70 patients. Thirty-four patients had midline hematoma and 36 had laterally placed hematoma (Figs 44.4a and b). In 45 patients hematomas were situated in midbrain and in 25 patients hematomas were in pons. Surprisingly, there was no case of medullary hematoma (Table 44.4a). CT scan also demonstrate associate hematoma, elsewhere in brain in a significant number of patients.[4,8] The study reported from our department[4] showed associated focal abnormalities in 25 patients (Fig. 44.5) and 16 of them required surgery (Table 44.4b).

Table 44.4a: CT scan finding in patients with traumatic brainstem hematoma

	Midline	Lateral	Total
Midbrain	20	25	45
Pons	14	11	25
	34	36	70

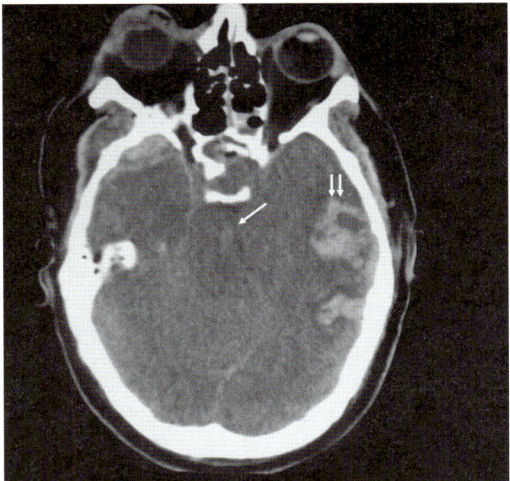

Fig. 44.3: CT scan of a patient with head injury shows brainstem contusion hematoma (single arrow) with left temporal contusion (double arrow) and small right temporal EDH

Treatment

There is no specific treatment for brainstem hematoma. Associated pathology may need surgery,[5,12] depending on size of hematoma and the mass effect they produce. Overall 20% may have sizable hematoma elsewhere in brain needing surgery.

Table 44.4b: Associated abnormalities along with brainstem hematoma, AIIMS experience	
Nature of pathology	Numbers
Extradural hematoma	3*
Cerebral contusion	22 (13*)
Midline shift	15

* Required surgery

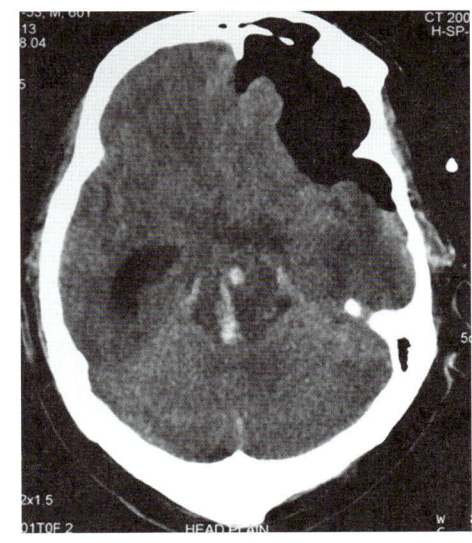

Fig. 44.5: CT scan head showing traumatic brainstem hematoma with pneumocephalous

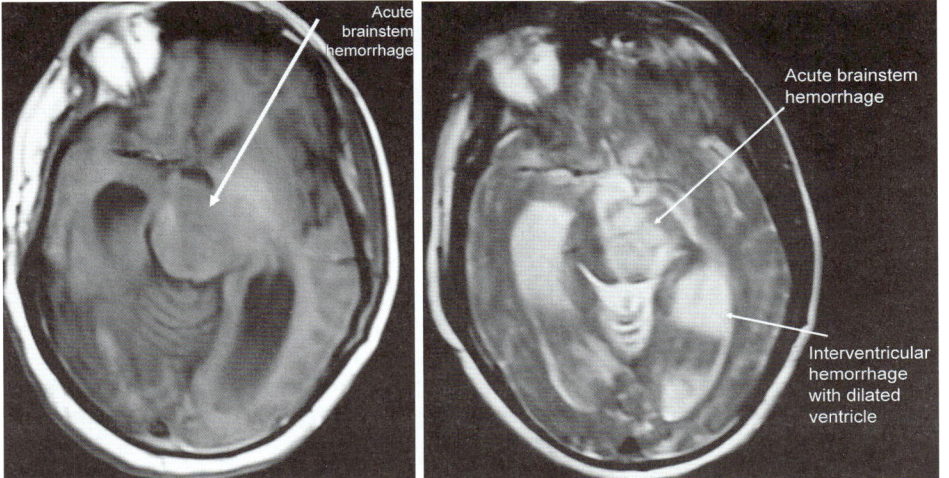

Figs 44.4a and b: MRI brain, T_1 and T_2-weighted images showing acute brainstem hematoma

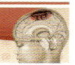

As the patients with brainstem hematoma are very sick and remain unconscious for a longer period, they need longer intensive care management and ventilatory support. Nursing care, management of pulmonary problems and tracheostomy care need a special mention. Moderate hypothermia and control of hyperpyrexia if present, are important factors in survival. Hypothermia definitely enhances the chance of survival.[49]

OUTCOME IN PATIENTS WITH BRAINSTEM HEMATOMA

Outcome of patients with traumatic brainstem hematoma was considered to be grave 2 decades ago. Mostly, definite diagnosis was only made at autopsy.[11,16] With the availability of CT diagnosis and follow-up of these patients has become possible, more reports are available regarding long-term outcome and quality of survival of these patients.[4–6,22,32,38–41,49,50] Mahapatra et al[5] had reported survival in more than 50% cases. Among the 70 patients analysed, 38 survived and 22 patients had a good recovery. Six patients each were severely disabled or remained vegetative (Table 44.5). Stewart et al[50] developed a prognostic model. He also studied many factors and reported age, associated skull fracture and other injuries to be significant factors. Young patients had good outcome (Fig. 44.6). Gilbert and a Thierry[51] reported good recovery in an 8-year-old girl. Kim et al[52] in 1985 reported long-term survival in a patient of brainstem hematoma. In a series reported by Tsai et al[12] mortality rate was 67% in patients with secondary brainstem injury. In another study same authors had reported 27% mortality in patients with transtentorial herniation, without brainstem involvement, and 61% had mild to moderate deficit. The survival rate in transtentorial herniation alone was 73%. Of the 19 patients with primary brainstem injury only 5 patients survived. Thus, in their study patients with primary brainstem hematoma had a survival rate of 25%, which was relatively lower survival rate.

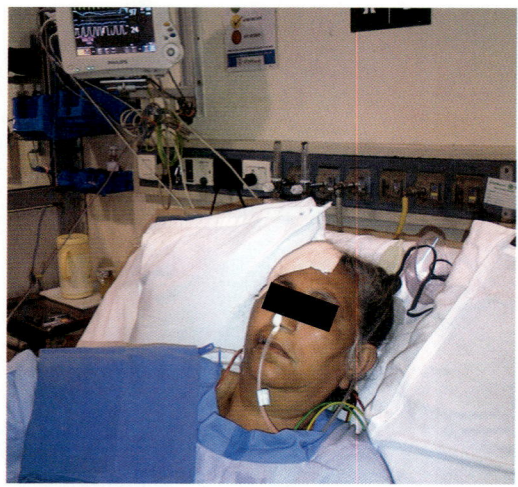

Fig. 44.6: Clinical photograph of a patient with brainstem hematoma who had good outcome at 3 months

Table 44.5: Outcome of patients with brainstem hematoma, 70 patients at AIIMS

Outcome	Numbers	
No deficit	14	
Mild deficit	8	Good recovery
Moderate disability	4	
Severely disabled	6	
Vegetative	6	Poor recovery
Expired	32	
Total	70	

Other significant factors which help in predicting the outcome are, findings of cold caloric response and brainstem auditory evoked potential.[5,8,32,36,39] Absent cold caloric response, in patients with brainstem hemorrhage carries a grave prognosis.[5,8,32] Similarly, when repeated BAER recordings fail to show wave or absence of wave III, IV, V denote a poor outcome[5,38,39] (Table 44.6). Presence of traumatic basal subarachnoid hemorrhage[53] associated with brainstem injury carry a poor prognosis. Thus, outcome of patients with brainstem hematoma is multifactorial, hence, these factors require

Table 44.6: BAER and outcome experience in 32 patients at AIIMS disability

BAER findings	No deficit	Mild deficit	Severe deficit	Vegetative	Dead
A. Normal (8)	4	3	1	–	–
B. Abnormal (16)	4	6	5	–	1
C. Absent (8)	–	–	–	1	7
	8	9	6	1	8

time to time careful observation and documentation.

CONCLUSIONS

Traumatic brainstem hematoma is not a rare condition. With availability of CT scan more cases are diagnosed to have BSH. Com mon sites are pons or midbrain. Around 25% patients are conscious at admission. 50% patients are admitted in a decerebrating state. In more than 30% patients there, are associated hematomas elsewhere in brain. Caloric response and BAER are two good prognostic tests. Repeated normal cold caloric response or BAER indicate good prognosis. Overall survival ranges 30–50% and 25% can have good outcome. Multiple brainstem hematoma and other associated injury reduce the chance of survival and good recovery.

REFERENCES

1. Meyer CA, Mirvis SE, Wolf AL, Thompson RK, Gutierrez MA. Acute traumatic midbrain hemorrhage: experimental and clinical observations with CT. Radiology 1991;179:813–8.
2. Ropper AH, Miller DC. Acute traumatic midbrain hemorrhage. Ann Neurol 1985;18:80–86.
3. Tsai FY, Teal JS, Quinn MF, Itabashi HH, Huprich JE, Ahmadi J, et al. CT of brainstem injury. AJR Am J Roentgenol 1980;134:717–23.
4. Zuccarello M, Fiore DL, Trincia G, De Caro R, Pardatscher K, Andrioli GC. Traumatic primary brain stem haemorrhage: a clinical and experimental study. Acta Neurochir (Wien) 1983; 67:103–13.
5. Mahapatra AK, Tandon PN, Banerji AK. Brainstem haemorrhage. A review of 70 CT ventrical cases. Abstract NSI meeting 1990.
6. Bhutani AK, Singh AK, Prakash B. Posttraumatic brainstem haematoma. Neurology India (Suppl) 1993;41:43.
7. Gentry LR, Godersky JC, Thompson B. Traumatic brainstem injury, MR imaging. Radiology 1989;171:177.
8. Mahapatra AK, Tandon PN. Brainstem auditory evoked response and vestibulo-ocular reflex in severe head injury patients. Acta Neurochir (Wien) 1987;87:40–45.
9. Klintworgh GK. The pathogenesis of secondary brainstem hemorrhages as studied in an experimental model. Am J Pathol 1965;47:525–36. [PMC free article] [PubMed]
10. Hashimoto T, Nakamura N, Richard KE, Frowein RA. Primary brainstem lesions caused by closed head injuries. Neurosurg Rev 1993; 16:291–8.
11. Tandon PN. Brainstem haemorrhage in craniocerebral trauma. Acta Neurol (Scand) 1964;40: 375–80.
12. Mahapatra AK, Tandon PN. Brainstem haematoma study of 48 cases. Annual Conf. of NSI 1988.
13. Tasi FY, Teal JS, Quinn MF, et al. CT of brainstem injury. AJNR 1980;134:717–23.
14. Kalyanaraman S, Ramamurthi B. Analysis of 2000 cases of head injury. Neurology India 1970;18:3.
15. Hun Joo Kim. The Prognostic Factors Related to Traumatic Brain Stem Injury. J Korean Neurosurg Soc 2012;51(1):24–30.
16. Crompton MR. Brainstem lesions after head injury. Lancet 1971;1:669–73.
17. Cooper PR, Maravilla K, Kirkpatrik J, et al. Traumatically induced brainstem haemorrhage and the computerized tomographic scan. Clinical, experimental observations. Neurosurgery 1979;4:115–24.
18. Lindenberg R, Freytag E. Brainstem lesions characteristic of traumatic hyperextension of the head. Acta Pathol 1970;90:509–15.
19. Tomlinson BF. Brainstem lesion after head injury. J Clin Pathol (Suppl) 1970;23:154–65.
20. Hooper R. Patterns of brainstem injury. In: Pattern of acute head injury. R Hooper (ed) Edward Arnold Publisher 1971.
21. Britt RH, Herrick MK, Mason RT, et al. Traumatic lesions of pontomedullary junction. Neurosurgery 1980;6:623–5.

22. Mitchell DE, Adam JH. Primary focal damage to the brainstem in blunt head injuries: does it exist? Lancet 1973;2:215–18.

23. Sganzerla EP, Rampini PM, De Santis A, Tiberio F, Guerra P, Zavanone M, et al. Primary traumatic benign midbrain haematoma in hyperextension injuries of the head. Acta Neurochir Suppl (Wien) 1992;55:29–32.

24. Freytag E. Autopsy findings in head injuries from blunt forces. Statistical evaluation of 1,367 cases. Arch Pathol 1963;75:402–13.

25. Harding B, Erdohazi M. Traumatic transection of the brainstem. J Neurol Neurosurg Psychiat 1981;44:1156–8.

26. Powiertowski H. Results of neurosurgical care in patients with brainstem contusion. In: Head injuries. Proceedings of an International Symposium. Gillingham FJ, Harris P, Shaw JF, Hitchcock ER (eds). Churchill Livingstone, 1971;326.

27. Turazzi S, Bricolo A. Acute pontine syndrome following head injury. Lancet 1977;2:62–64.

28. Courville CB. Effect or closed cranial injuries on midbrain and upper pons. Proc Asso Res Ners Ment Dis 1945;21:131–40.

29. Cohen SI, Aronson SJ. Secondary brainstem haemorrhages. Arch Neurol 1968;19:257–64.

30. Mahapatra AK, Tandon PN, Banerji AK, Bhatia R. Bilateral decerebration in head injury—A study of 62 patients. Surg Neurol 1985;23:536–40.

31. Bricolo A, Turazzi S, Alexander A, et al. Decerebrate rigidity in acute head injury. J Neurosurg 1977;47:680–95.

32. Busch EAV. Brainstem contusion: differential diagnosis, therapy and prognosis. Clin Neurosurg 1963;9:18–25.

33. Mingrino S, Molinari G, Andrioli G, et al. Some observations upon vestibular reaction in acute head injury. Excerpta Medica International Congress Series 1966;110:226.

34. Jadhav WR, Sinha A, Tandon PN, et al. Cold caloric test in unconscious patients. Laryngoscope 1971;31:391.

35. Sinha A, Tandon PN, Kacker SK, et al. Role of vestibular studies in an unconscious patient. In J Otology 1969;21:161.

36. Tandon PN, Bhatia R, Banerji AK. Vestibulo-ocular reflex and brainstem. Neurol (India) 1973;21:193.

37. Nelson JR. The minimal ice water caloric test. Neurology (Minneap) 1969;19:577.

38. Sancesario G, Pozzessere G, Massa R, et al. Prognostic evaluation of brainstem haematoma, the role of CT scan and brainstem auditory evoked potentials. Acta Neurol Scand 1984;70:396–406.

39. Tsutsui T, Ohno M, Symon L, et al. Combined measurement of brainstem auditory and SEP in a surgically treated brainstem haematoma. Surg Neurol 1986;25:575–81.

40. O'Laoire SA, Crockard HA, Thomas DGT, et al. Brainstem haematoma. A report of six surgically treated cases, J Neurosurg 1982;56:222–7.

41. Texier PH, Diebler C, Bruguier A, Ponsot G. Haematoma of brainstem in childhood. Neuroradiology 1984;26:499–502.

42. Moskala M, Polak J, Moskala A, Kleinrok K, Zawiliñski J. Haematoma of the tentorium cerebelli—new pathology or new prognostic factor in neurotraumatology? A preliminary report. Neurol Neurochir Pol 2007;41:234–40.

43. Kim YS, Lim HY, Nah JH, Doh JO, Chang KS. Traumatic tentorial hemorrhage. J Korean Neurosurg Soc 1986;15:439–44.

44. Okuchi K, Fujioka M, Konobu T, Fujikawa A, Nishimura A, Miyamoto S, et al. [Traumatic primary brainstem injury and ambient cistern hematoma evaluated with magnetic resonance imaging] No Shinkei Geka 1993;21:799–804.

45. Kinoshita Y, Tsuru E, Yasukouchi H, Yokota A. [A case of hematoma in cisterna magna after mild head injury]. No To Shinkei 2000;52:320–3.

46. Wong CW. The MRI and CT evidence of primary brain stem injury. Surg Neurol 1993;39:37–40.[PubMed]

47. Park E, Ai J, Baker AJ. Cerebellar injury: clinical relevance and potential in traumatic brain injury research. Prog brain Res 2007;161:327–38.

48. Shibata Y, Matsumura A, Meguro K, Narushima K. Differentiation of mechanism and prognosis of traumatic brain stem lesions detected by magnetic resonance imaging in the acute stage. Clin Neurol Neurosurg 2000;102:124–8.

49. Gruskiewiez J, Doran Y, Peyser E: Recovery from severe craniocerebral injury with brainstem lesions in childhood. Surg Neurol 1973;1:197.

50. Stewart WA, Lilten SP, Sheehe PR. A prognostic model for brainstem injury. Surg Neurol 1973;1:303.

51. Gilbert JJ, Thierry. Unusual brainstem findings following closed head injury. J Paediatr 1972;81:343–5.

52. Kirn RC, Fagin K, Choi BH. Prolonged survival after severe traumatic injury limited to the brainstem. Surg Neurol 1985;23:525–8.

53. Patel F. Traumatic baso-brainstem subarachnoid haemorrhage. Medicine Science and the Law 1996;36:178–81.

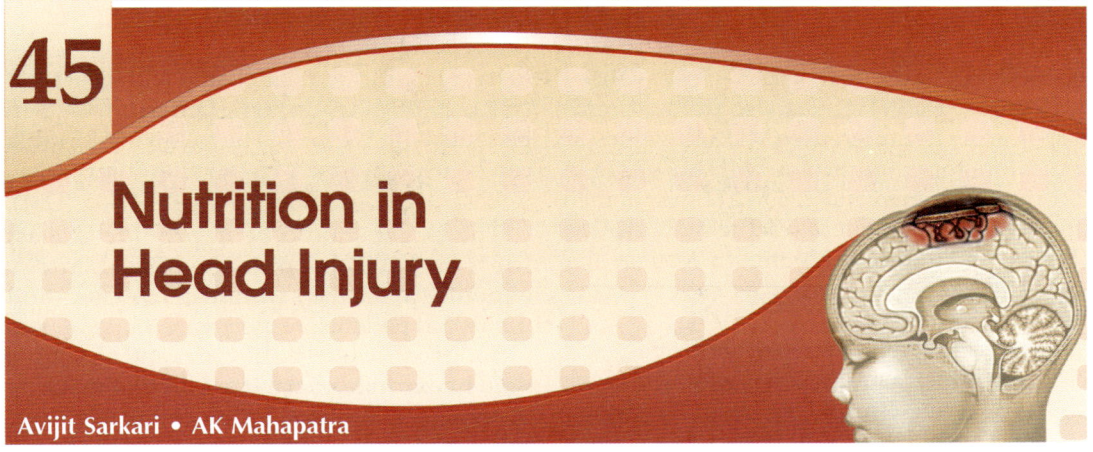

45

Nutrition in Head Injury

Avijit Sarkari • AK Mahapatra

Nutritional support is an integral, though often neglected component of the care of critically injured patient.[1] In a starving human, there is marked decrease in energy requirement and protein utilization. In sharp contrast to this, head injury triggers hypermetabolic and catabolic states, severely impairing nitrogen homeostasis. This hypermetabolic response in TBI has been found to be due to increased release of catecholamines and cortisol.[2] Systematic Cochrane Collaboration reviews have suggested that nutrition therapy may improve mortality and neurological outcomes.[3,4]

METABOLISM IN HEAD INJURY

Nutritional demand in patients with severe TBI is increased due to hypermetabolism and increased protein catabolism.[5,6] The state is characterized by disproportional pro-inflammatory cytokine (e.g. tumor necrosis factor-α, IL-1 and IL-6) production and release that is associated with increased counter-regulatory hormones (e.g. cortisol, glucagon and catecholamines) release. This process leads to increased systemic and cerebral energy needs, even in paralyzed patients.[7] Energy expenditure continues to rise in the first 2 weeks regardless of the neurological course. The increased energy needs can persist for long periods, from weeks to months. Poor nutritional state can result in poor recovery.

NITROGEN METABOLISM

The difference between intake, consumption and excretion of nitrogen in termed nitrogen balance. To measure excretion, 2–3 g (to account for fecal and cutaneous nitrogen loss) is added to the urinary nitrogen. For each gram of nitrogen in urine, 6.25 g protein is catabolized. But there is a lag of 3–8 days in the urinary nitrogen excretion from the metabolic event that influenced it. In head injury patients, protein contributes to 30–45% of total consumed calories as compared to 10–15% in normal state. The urinary nitrogen excretion in severe head injury at 0.36 +/–0.08/kg/day is comparable with other hypercatabolic states like sepsis, severe burns and major surgery.

NUTRITION STATUS INDICATORS

Measures such as body weight, height, body mass index (BMI) and physical constitution including arm muscle circumference, triceps skin fold thickness, etc. should be obtained. Blood values such as serum albumin, prealbumin, transferrin and a lymphocyte count may be used for nutritional status assessment.[8]

Body mass index (BMI) calculated by dividing weight in kilograms by square of body height in meters has been advocated by WHO for assessment.[9] The cut-off BMI for well nourished, mild, moderate and severe

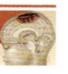

malnutrition are $\geq$ 18.5, < 18.5 – $\geq$ 17, <16.9 – < 15 and < 15. WHO has also defined mid-upper arm circumference (MUAC) values as indicators for malnutrition.[9] MUAC of 214 to 221 mm in women and 224 to 231 mm in men are classified as moderate acute malnutrition (MAM) and values < 214 mm in women and < 224 in men are graded as severe acute malnutrition (SAM).

However by the time these anthropometric changes occur, malnutrition is well advanced, so they have a limited value in the first 3 weeks. A weight loss of 10–15% is not of much significance, 20% increases susceptibility to stress and 30% loss increases morbidity and mortality.

CLINICAL FEATURES OF MALNUTRITION[10,11]

Pedal edema is an indicator of visceral protein or vitamin B1 functional status essential for neuronal function and recovery. Cheilosis indicates riboflavin, vitamin B_6 or niacin deficiency. Skeletal prominence indicates somatic protein depletion. Xerosis occurs due to vitamin A or B complex deficiency. Gum bleeding may either be due to vitamin C or K deficiency.

NUTRITIONAL REQUIREMENTS

A simple 'pocket formula' for energy requirements in normal person is 25 kcal/kg desirable weight/day.

ESTIMATION OF BASAL ENERGY EXPENDITURE (BEE)

Harris Benedict equation[12]

Male

BEE = 66.47 + 113.75 × Weight kgs + 5.0 × Height cm – 6.76 × Age yrs

Female

BEE = 65.51 + 9.56 × Weight kgs + 1.85 × Height cm – 4.68 × Age yrs

Infants

BEE = 22.1 + 31.05 × Weight kgs + 1.16 × Height cm

Resting metabolic expenditure has been assessed with indirect calorimetry and found to have significant relationship with heart rate (HR), days since injury (DSI) and GCS in patients with GCS < 7. The following formula can be used in first 2 weeks after injury.

% RME = 152 – 13 (GCS) + 0.4 (HR) + 7 (DSI).

The target should be to provide at least 140% and 100% of predicted basal energy expenditure (BEE) in non-paralyzed and paralyzed patients, respectively. Latter group includes use of muscle blockers and also those with barbiturate coma. It is said that majority of hypermetabolism is due to muscle tone. However, even with paralysis, energy expenditure remains elevated by 20–30% in some patients.[7] Protein requirement in head injury is 1.5–2 g/kg/day and > 15–20% of caloric replacement should be by proteins.

EARLY NUTRITION AND METHODS OF FEEDING

Mortality is reduced in patients who receive full caloric replacement by 7th day after trauma.[13,14] Early nutritional support reduces the secretion of catabolic hormones, which are already increased in this setting (Table 45.1). It at least partially preserves the previous nutritional conditions, body weight and muscle mass. Level II recommendations from the Brain Trauma Foundation (BTF)[15] are to achieve full caloric replacements by post-trauma day 7. To achieve this goal nutritional replacement should begin within 72 hrs of head injury.

Patients not fed for 5 and 7 days had 2- and 4-fold increased likelihood of dying, respectively.[14] Early nutrition is a significant predictor of death as concluded by Hartl et al,[14] after controlling for factors known to affect mortality including hypotension, age, papillary size, GCS and CT scan findings.

Gastric, jejunal and parenteral are the three ways of early feeding. Better nitrogen retention has been found with jejunal and parenteral methods.[16] Altered gastric emptying, residual, lower esophageal dysfunction and aspiration pneumonia may complicate gastric feeding. Independent risk factors for feeding

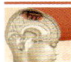

Table 45.1: Recommended range of caloric intake in neurosurgical patients		
Patient state		Caloric replacement kcal/kg
Resting 70 kg male (normal)		26–30
Postoperative craniotomy		26–30
GCS = 4–5	First week	40–50
	Second week	50–60
GCS = 6–7	First week	30–40
	Second week	40–50
GCS = 8–12	First week	30–35

intolerance include use of sucralfate, propofol, pentobarbital, days of mechanical ventilation, older age, admission diagnosis of intracerebral hemorrhage and ischemic stroke.[17] Use of prokinetics has been advocated.

Enteral route is preferred due to reduced risk of hyperglycemia, infection/septicemia and cost. It is associated with less intestinal bacterial proliferation, and therefore, less translocation. The risk of infection from central venous catheters is also overcome.

Parenteral nutrition is started early after injury until enteral feeds are tolerated. The primary advantage of parenteral nutrition is that it is well tolerated. It is preferred if higher nitrogen intake is desired or if there is decreased gastric emptying or there is uncontrolled diarrhea due to antibiotic use. Cerebral edema is a potential contraindication for parenteral alimentation.

No significant difference in serum albumin, weight loss, nitrogen balance or final outcome has been found as far as the route is concerned.[18]

TECHNIQUES TO IMPROVE ENTERAL NUTRITION TOLERANCE

It is critical to adopt protocols with clear target energy intakes and infusion rates, early starting times and specific techniques for measuring gastric residue and infusion frequencies and for detecting cases where the infusion should be discontinued or adjusted.[19] Early enteral nutrition started once patient is stabilized. Some recommend starting as early as within 24 hrs.[20] Complete and isotonic formulas should be initially chosen. Due to their high price, minimally improved tolerance and increased incidence of diarrhea, peptide-based formulas are not recommended.

For intolerant or high-risk patients, continuous infusion is recommended by American Society for Parenteral and Enteral Nutrition (ASPEN).[21] A 10–40 ml/h infusion rate can be used initially. It can be increased by 10 to 20 ml/h every 8–12 hours, as tolerated, until the energy target is reached. Gastric motility disorders may be suggested by symptoms such as nausea, vomiting, abdominal distension, intestinal sounds, flatus and feces elimination and diagnostic techniques such as abdominal radiographs and gastric residue measurements. ASPEN recommends that gastric residue be measured every 4 hours during gastric feeding and recommends avoiding withholding the infusion for residues of less than 500 ml in the absence of other signs of intolerance. There are two ways to measure gastric residue volume: by gravity (leaving a collection bottle below the level of the stomach for 10 minutes) and suctioning with a 50 ml syringe. Use of prokinetic drugs like metoclopramide is recommended if required.

If not medically contraindicated, the head of the bed should be elevated from 30 to 45 degrees. Strict blood glucose control improves survival. It potentially improves tolerance to enteral nutrition as hyperglycemia itself has adverse effects on the gastric emptying and promotes gastroparesis. ASPEN recommends maintaining blood glucose between 110 and 150 mg/dl.[21]

VITAMIN B-COMPLEX

Malnutrition is mostly caused by B_{12} (Cyanocobalamin), B_1 (Thiamine), B_5 (Riboflavin) and B_6 (Pyridoxine) vitamin deficiencies. As they are water soluble and have short half lives; they are easily depleted. Antibiotics may impair their absorption and metabolism.[22] Therefore thiamine, pyridoxine and B_{12} replacement is recommended for polytrauma patients to prevent certain acute neurological syndromes.

ZINC AND MAGNESIUM

Zinc is an important cofactor for substrates associated with metabolism, the immune system and N-methyl-D-aspartate (NMDA) receptor function. Sequestration in liver and increased renal clearance lead to decreased zinc levels in head injury patients. Zinc supplementation for up to one month appears to improve protein metabolism and neurological prognosis.[23] Magnesium also appears to be neuroprotective because it modulates cell energy production and calcium inflow through its effects on NMDA receptors.[24,25]

PROBLEMS WITH OVERFEEDING

Equal attention should be paid to overfeeding, i.e. providing more energy than the patient needs. Excessive or prolonged overfeeding may be harmful. It can result in metabolic issues such as hyperglycemia and a refeeding-type syndrome with electrolytic disorders, liver steatosis, pulmonary issues that complicate ventilator weaning and even obesity in long-term cases.[8] Uremia and increased carbon dioxide production also result from overfeeding.

AIIMS EXPERIENCE[25–27]

In a prospective study of 88 adult severe head injured patients, 76% patients had various clinical features of malnutrition at 3 weeks. Pedal edema was the most frequent sign present in 70% of patients at three weeks, followed by skeletal prominence (19%) and cheilosis (12%). Hypoproteinemia (serum total protein < 5.5 g/dl) at admission and full enteral feeding later than 7 days after admission showed significant association with development of clinical malnutrition. There was significant association of clinical malnutrition with mortality.[26] Another prospective study revealed that >15% fall in serum albumin levels at 3 weeks was an independent risk factor for unfavorable outcome at 6 months.[26]

Parenteral administration of magnesium sulphate within 12 hours of severe closed traumatic brain injury (GCS 5–8) has been found to reduce mortality, intraoperative brain swelling and has favorable influence (73.3% compared to 40% in control group) on outcome at 3 months without any apparently significant adverse effect.[25]

CONCLUSIONS

Management of severe head injury involves adequate devotion to meet nutritional requirements. There should be frequent reassessments, recalculations and tailored readjustments for individual patient. Diet has significant impact on inflammatory responses too. Therefore, taking care of nutrition needs is an active integral component of holistic and global approach of managing severe head injuries.

REFERENCES

1. Jacobs DG, Jacobs DO, Kudsk KA. Nutritional Support in Trauma Patients. J Trauma 2004; 57(3):660–79.

2. Rosner MJ, Newsome HH, Becker DP. Mechanical brain injury: the sympathoadrenal response. J Neurosurg 1984;61:76–86.

3. Perel P, Yanagawa T, Bunn F, Roberts I, Wentz R, Pierro A. Nutritional support for head-injured patients. Cochrane Database Syst Rev 2006;(4): CD001530. Review.

4. Yanagawa T, Bunn F, Roberts I, Wentz R, Pierro A. Nutritional support for head-injured patients. Cochrane Database Syst Rev 2002;(3):CD001530. Review. Update in: Cochrane Database Syst Rev. 2006;(4):CD001530.

5. Clifton GL, Robertson CS, Grossman RG, et al. The metabolic response to severe head injury. J Neurosurg 1984;60:687–96.

6. Deutschman CS, Konstantinides FN, Raup S, et al. Physiological and metabolic response to isolated closed head injury. Part 1: Basal metabolic state: Correlation of metabolic and physiological parameters with fasting and stressed controls. J Neurosurg 1986;64:89–98.

7. Clifton GL, Robertson CS, Choi CS. Assessment of nutritional requirements of head-injured patients. J Neurosurg 1986;64:895–901.

8. Cook AM, Peppard A, Magnuson B. Nutrition considerations in traumatic brain injury. Nutr Clin Pract 2008;23:608–20.

9. WHO. Physical status: the use and interpretation of anthropometry. Report of a WHO Expert Committee. WHO Technical Report Series 854. Geneva: World Health Organization, 1995.

10. Christakis G. How to make a nutritional diagnosis without really trying. J Flor Med Assoc 1979;66:349–56.

11. Mitchell MK. Nutrition across the life span. 2nd ed. Philadelphia: WB Saunders, 2003,44–65.

12. Harris JA, Bendict FG. Biometric studies of basal metabolism in man. Carnegie Institution. Publication no. 279. Washington DC, 1919.

13. Rapp RP, Young B, Twyman D, et al. The favorable effect of early parenteral feeding on survival in severe head injured patients. J Neurosug 1983;58:906–12.

14. Hartl R, Gerber LM, Ni Q, Ghajar J. Effect of early nutrition on deaths due to severe traumatic brain injury. J Neurosurg 2008;109:50–56.

15. Brain Trauma Foundation: Nutrition. J Neurotrauma 2007;24:S77–82.

16. Young B, Ott L, Haack D, et al. The effect of nutritional support on outcome from severe head injury. J Neurosurg 1987;67:668–76.

17. Rhoney DH, Parker D, Formea CM Jr, et al. Tolerability of bolus versus continuous gastric feeding in brain-injured patients. Neurol Res 2002;24:613–620.

18. Hadley MN, Grahm TW, Harrington T, et al. Nutritional support and neurotrauma: A critical review of early nutrition in forty-five acute head injury patients. Neurosurgery 1986;19:367–73.

19. Campos BBNS, Machado FS. Nutrition therapy in severe head trauma patients. Rev Brasil Ter Intensiva 2012;24:97–105.

20. Singer P, Berger MM, van den Berghe G, Biolo G, Calder P, Forbes A, Griffiths R, Kreyman G, Leverve X, Pichard C, ESPEN. ESPEN Guidelines on Parenteral Nutrition: intensive care. Clin Nutr 2009;28:387–400.

21. McClave SA, Martindale RG, Vanek VW, McCarthy M, Roberts P, Taylor B, Ochoa JB, Napolitano L, Cresci G. ASPEN Board of Directors; American College of Critical Care Medicine; Society of Critical Care Medicine. Guidelines for the Provision and Assessment of Nutrition Support Therapy in the Adult Critically Ill Patient: Society of Critical Care Medicine (SCCM) and American Society for Parenteral and Enteral Nutrition (ASPEN). J PEN J Parenter Enteral Nutr 2009;33:277–316.

22. Prelack K, Sheridan RL. Micronutrient supplementation in the critically ill patient: strategies for clinical practice. J Trauma 2001;51:601–20.

23. Young B, Ott L, Kasarkis E, Rapp R, Moles K, Dempsey RJ, et al. Zinc supplementation is associated with improved neurologic recovery rate and visceral protein levels of patients with severe closed head injury. J Neurotrauma 1996;13:25–34.

24. McKee JA, Brewer RP, Macy GE, Phillips-Bute B, Campbell KA, Borel CO, et al. Analysis of the brain bioavailability of peripherally administered magnesium sulfate: a study in humans with acute brain injury undergoing prolonged induced hypermagnesemia. Crit Care Med 2005;33:661–6.

25. Dhandapani SS, Gupta A, Vivekanandhan S, Sharma BS, Mahapatra AK. Randomized controlled trial of magnesium sulphate in severe closed traumatic brain injury. Indian Journal of Neurotrauma 2008;1:27–33.

26. Dhandapani SS, Manju D, Sharma BS, Mahapatra AK. Clinical malnutrition in severe traumatic brain injury: Factors associated and outcome at 6 months. Indian Journal of Neurotrauma. 2007;1:35–39.

27. Dhandapani SS, Manju D, Vivekanandhan S, Agarwal M, Mahapatra AK. Prospective longitudinal study of biochemical changes in critically ill patients with severe traumatic brain injury: Factors associated and outcome at 6 months. Indian Journal of Neurotrauma 2010;1:23–28.

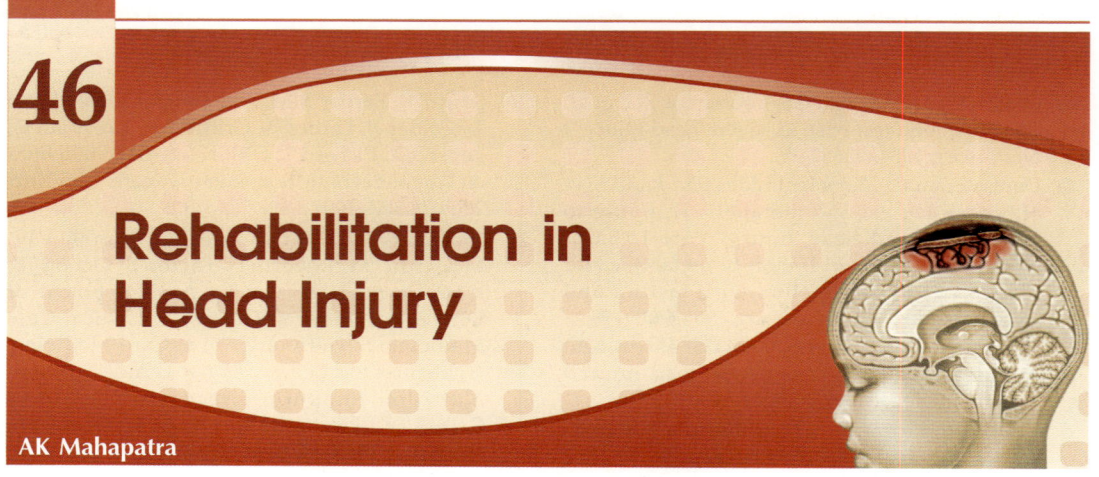

46

Rehabilitation in Head Injury

AK Mahapatra

INTRODUCTION

The overall outcome of patients with severe head injury is bad. A large number of severe head injury patients die or remain vegetative.[1-5] The Glasgow Outcome Scale was developed by Jennett and Bond to grade the outcome of head-injured patients.[6] With the availability of CT scan, ICU care and quick surgery there is a greater number of survivors and many of them do have moderate or severe disability.[7,8] With ever increasing number of head injuries, the cumulative number of disabled and vegetative patients are growing tremendously. Many of our outcome scales do not include cognitive behavioral and professional performance. In fact, to a common garden neurosurgeon or physician, successful recovery means "patient survives, patient can walk and talk". Today, the "walking and talking" are no longer considered as satisfactory measures of good recovery.

Head injury, severe or even minor, leads to large number of behavioral and cognitive problems.[9-16] Over the years, neurosurgeons have tried to bring down mortality and morbidity. Unfortunately, however, adequate attention has not been paid for the proper rehabilitation of head injured patients. Each patient represent, a unique and complex problem, which include, physical, visual, cognitive and behavioral abnormalities

(Table 46.1) due to heterogeneity of neuro-pathology, sociocultural background and educational level. Most frequent and important abnormalities result from frontal lobe function impairment, involving higher level regulatory and problem solving capacities.[9,10]

REHABILITATION OF PHYSICAL DISABILITY

Large number of patients with head injury do have physical disability may be due to paralysis, or weakness of limbs, spasticity, visual or hearing problem and due to speech abnormalities.[16,17] The aim of the treatment is, therefore, to see that the patient returns to a

Table 46.1: Neuropsychological abnormalities following head injury

A. Physical

   Paralysis, spasticity, contractures, visual or hearing problem

B. Cognitive defect
  - Remediation and retraining
  - Defect in arousal and attention
  - Deficit in learning and remembering
  - Communication deficit
  - Executive deficit
  - Anosognosia

C. Behavioral
   a. Aggressive and agitated
   b. Disinhibition
   c. Decreased initiation
   d. Depression

D. Hypothalamic and endocrine dysfunction

productive employment. Overall, the goal of rehabilitation is to reintegrate the patient into a supportive social system and provide a productive and active life.[18]

Weakness can be managed by repeated early mobilization and protocol based exercise. Early ambulation, mobilization in wheel chair is also important. Mackay et al[19] in a large study showed the difference in outcome in patients with formalized protocol based treatment compared to non-formalized treatment in severe head injury.

Prevention of contracture is very important. This can be achieved by various methods such as, casting combined with stretching, different exercises, use of passive positioning with pillows, splints and special bed.[20,21] Once contractures have formed they should be treated if they are progressive by traction and prolonged stretch. Rarely, long-standing severe contracture may need surgery. In severe head injury heterotopic ossification may set in giving rise to contracture.[22–24] Some authors have used different chemicals such as Disodium etidronate, aspirin and indomethacin to prevent ossification.[23,24] Prevention of spasticity is an important part in rehabilitation.[22]

Hypertonia is very common in head injury. Sometimes, spasticity may also be associated with rigidity. Spasticity also helps in development of contracture. More importantly, spasticity hampers skilled movement. Oral medication by dantrolene is the drug of choice in spasticity and it has very a few side effects. Rarely, in severe hypertonia, nerve blocks may be helpful. Head injury patients do have tremor and ataxia (Table 46.2) which also influence in overall motor performance.

Care of Eyes and Prevention of Blindness

In comatose patients, nursing care is important for prevention of bed sore and exposure keratitis. Facial paralysis or damage to corneal sensation can give rise to redness of eyes or even exposure keratitis. Prevention of exposure, proper use of eye drops and

Table 46.2: Physical disabilities

1. Motor weakness
   - Paralysis
   - Spasticity
   - Contractures and deformities
2. Cerebellar dysfunction
   - In co-ordination
   - Ataxia
   - Tremors
3. Speech abnormalities
4. Visual, hearing impairment
5. Bladder dysfunction

ointment can prevent corneal damage. Rarely, a tarsorrhaphy may be necessary to prevent keratitis.

In 2–5% patients can have associated traumatic blindness.[25–29] In unconscious patients dilated fixed pupils are considered as 3rd nerve palsy, while it may be really due to optic nerve injury. Hence, in suspected patients, visual evoked potential (VEP) is necessary to establish the diagnosis.[28,29] Mostly, the blindness is due to ischemic necrosis of the nerve in the optic canal. Timely injection of corticosteroid and if necessary, optic canal decompression can improve the chance of visual recovery and prevent the blindness. Hence, early diagnosis, steroid therapy and, if indicated, surgery is likely to reduce the visual problem in head injured patients.

Cognitive Abnormalities in Head Injury

Cognitive abnormalities are the important factors preventing integration of patients in head injury (Table 46.3). A large number of cognitive abnormalities are encountered in head injury patients.[9,11,14,15,18,30–32] Surprisingly, cognitive function abnormalities are not limited to severe head injury. A significant number of patients with minor head injury do have short-term or long-term cognitive function derangement.[1,13,16,32,33]

In the recent years considerable interest has been generated in remediation of cognitive deficit following head injury (Table 46.3). The mode is by cognitive training and remediation method. However, it is always important to answer whether special education and training skill is enough to correct cognitive deficit? Then the method must be used to improve memory, to perform the work efficiently and to develop skill for better solving of the problems.

The aim of the cognitive rehabilitation is to have a specialized protocol based remedial strategies.[14,17] The specialized strategies must be utilized very early in cognitive rehabilitation. There are evidences that these cognitive defects can improve.[15–16] It is also clear that the recovery of function occurs not by amelioration of damaged function but by adaptation to deficits. Earlier ones adapt to deficit, quicker is the chance of recovery. Hence, it is not absolutely clear whether the attempt to "retrain" memory, attention or problem solving would succeed or not. It is also not clear that a problem is either an additive combination or a component of cognitive process. Many patients with mild but multiple problems may make the entire cognitive deficit more complex and more difficult for correction[15] as compared to severe and single cognitive defect.

Considering above points, it is also important to understand if it is possible to correct the deficit directly. If it is possible, then it is more effective and efficient to remediate a set of deficits independently and then allow the patient to combine them with functional skill or even to educate them in the executive skill. These strategies are only applicable in particular context to each specific task. Hence, the complex cognitive defects leads to dilemma in rehabilitation strategies. Thus, the boundaries between the intelligence, learning, aptitude, achievement, capacity and skill in learning, etc. delineate the complexities of problems in remediation.

Disorder of Arousal, Sleep and Attention

Arousal and attention defect is a most common cognitive abnormality in head injury.

Damage to frontal lobe and reticular activating system play important role in attention. Normal attention requires adequate arousal level throughout the day. The ability to attend particular stimuli in face of potential distractor, provides the ability to maintain prolonged attention. Head injury disrupts the attentional function and reduces the speed of information processing.[34] In head injury there is impaired tonic arousal. Lack of attention is also frequently encountered in patients of minor head injury with post-concussion syndrome. In children, poor attention in classroom is not infrequent. The treatment is basically by behavioral intervention and psychopharmacology. Sometimes, reinforcement of task behavior improves the attentiveness. Rarely, psychostimulants like dextroamphetamine, methylphenidate and pemoline sodium have been used to increase arousal level in lethargic patients.[35–36] However, it is difficult to evaluate the drug response in patients with multiple interacting complex cognitive deficits.

Defects in learning and memory are significant problems in head injury. There is both retrograde and anterograde amnesia. Due to anterograde amnesia, there is considerable difficulty in acquiring new informations. This has tremendous impact in education, professional and vocational point of view.[9,36–38] In head injury, amnesia laterized to both verbal and visuospatial material, and formal testing of memory may be falacious as its validity is limited. Rarely, a certain type of learning is preserved.[36] Chance of improving

Table 46.3: Cognitive abnormalities in head-injured patients

- Disorder or arousal
- Attention abnormality
- Inability to learn and concentrate
- Memory disturbances
- Defective communication
- Executive dysfunction
- Lack of motivation
- Anosognosia (lack of awareness of their problems)

memory by repetition is remote.[37] Sometimes specific memory enhancing exercise such as: (a) drilling patient with a specific piece of information, (b) utilizing memory aid like (diaries, lists and computer, and (c) providing limited context such as name of a few acquaintances. In school, children need specific attention and extra care for learning.[37]

Anosognosia also prevents quick improvement. Rehabilitation requires patient's effort and will, full participation in exercise, and training process. Many patients lack awareness of their deficits, and do not co-operate in learning exercise. Lack of awareness of deficit leads to lack of motivation. Lack of motivation reduces the learning process and prevents or slower the chance of recovery.[39]

Communication abnormalities are not uncommon. It may either be due to speech problem or due to dysarthria.[40] Cognitive based communication deficit needs speech therapy, using various modalities including videotape and feedback. In communication, education status, language and learning abilities help in recovery of speech.

Behavioral Abnormalities and Rehabilitation

Large number of behavioral abnormalities are encountered in head injury patients.[10,12,13,19,31,41-44] The abnormalities can be short-lived or chronic (Table 46.4). These behavioral abnormalities severely limit the reintegration of a head-injured patient into his own family, community and working environment. The differences between behavioral and cognitive deficits are artificial as the cognitive problems often contribute to the genesis of behavioral abnormalities.

Aggressive and "agitated" behavior is one of the most frequent abnormality. These aggressive attitudes can lead to homicidal or suicidal tendency and socially and sexually disinhibited behavior. The aggressive behavior is a reaction to loss of confidence and depression. It should be managed by frequent reassurance, and clear information about what

Table 46.4: Behavioral abnormalities in head injury

A. Problem in adjustment
  - In family
  - At work place
  - In society

B. Aggressive and "agitated behavior"

C. Disinhibited behavior
  - Impulsive
  - Hyper excited
  - Stealing things
  - Making of offensive remarks

D. Decreased initiation

E. Depression—lack of interest, depressed mood, lack of motivation

is about to happen. If the agitated period is prolonged or severe, treatment with amitriptyline or methylphenidate may help.[45,46] It is believed that the extreme aggressive behaviour is due to frontolimbic dysfunction. It may be manifested by epidoside dyscontrol syndrome.[45] Sometimes, carbamazepine is used to increase tolerance to anger. Lithium carbonate and beta-blockers such as propranolol have also been used. Usually, conventional neuroleptics are ineffective in controlling aggressive behavior. Proper training, enforcement of certain social behavior may be of benefit.

Sometimes, patients with head injury lack inhibition. They are more impulsive in their work. Frontal lobe plays an important role in disinhibited behavior. Disinhibited sexual behavior is also rarely noticed. Behaviors such as, sexual fondling of strangers, stealing small things like food and making offensive remarks may be observed in patients with head injury. Attempt should be made to decrease the patient's tendency to react by teaching him to stop and think about the potential consequences.

Decreased Initiation and Depression

Depression and lack of interest are two very important aspects in head injured patients, which make them sceptic about their activity.

Lack of initiation and motivation also hamper in rehabilitation process. These symptoms too, are linked to frontolimbic abnormalities, in which, patient looses link between motivation and action. In some patients there may be only impairment of initiation, but they may have desire to achieve goal and describe the actions required, however, they simply fail to execute them. These patients are benefited from external motivation though structured programmes. Motivation programmes should be focussed on the successful starting on subsequent steps. Sometimes, psychostimulant drugs may also be of some help.

Depression, on the other hand, makes the patient isolated in family and society. In work place, they are unable to mix freely with friends or express freely. Paralysis, fits, other physical disability, and memory disturbances may add to depression. Depression restricts the community involvement and building of new relation, thus making them maladjusted in environment. Confidence building measures, sympathetic hearing to patient's problem and supportive counseling benefit large number of patients. Role of spouse, children and other family members are important, in bringing the patients out of depression.

REHABILITATION OF CHILDREN

Children pose important problem in rehabilitation. In addition to cognitive and behavioral problems, they also have learning and education problems.[47–49] Greenspan and Mackenzie[48] studied 95 children with head injury. They studied: (a) pre-injury status, (b) post-injury status, (c) family economic, and social status. They reported worse outcome in children with poor socioeconomic status, pre-injury ill health and children with lower limb injury. Scott et al[49] studied 43 severely head-injured children. Assessment after 13 months showed 42% had neurological deficits and 35% were identified having a need for special educational support. The score obtained by these children by the parents and teachers showed, significant abnormalities in both

health and habits. Middleton[50] studied cognitive and psychological sequelae in children. They found abnormalities at home and in classroom. Children with head injury are neither sick nor mentally handicapped. However, they need rehabilitation that fits their special need. They often acutely aware of their difficulties and loss of freedom, loss of skill and abilities. There is a sense of fear, anger and frustration. All these parameters must be clearly assessed prior to rehabilitation. In children, parents and teachers play important roles in rehabilitation. Teachers must take extra care and pay a little more attention to these children.

VOCATIONAL REHABILITATION

Gainful re-employment is one of the most difficult aspect in head injury.[16,30,31,51,52] Lack of interest, depression, lack of initiative and motivation hamper their job prospect, in the absence of physical disability. Even, following minor head injury, things are not good. High level of anxiety and stress were noted in 33%[16] of the entire head injury group and in 95% of the group who returned to work. Kraft et al[51] studied Americans suffered head injury during Vietnam war 15 years later, and only 56% gainfully employed and only 64% could complete degree courses.

Dikman et al[52] in 1994 studied type and pattern of employment following head injury. They studied 360 patients and analyzed: (a) pre-injury employment, (b) injury to rest of the body, (c) severity of head injury, and (d) educational status of the patients. In their study 68% had returned to work, 93% were independent. Vocational rehabilitation depends on several factors including cognitive and neuropsychological recovery. In a study, 17% of patients who returned to work had cognitive and personality changes. On the other hand, only 25% patients had cognitive defect, in the group who did not go back to work.

Thus, large number of factors play a role in re-employment of patients. Support of family,

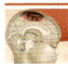

proper rehabilitation, and adjustment of friends at work place are important for patient's confidence building and re-employment.

Post-concussion Syndrome (PCS)

Minor head injury constitutes around 90% of all head injury. Fortunately, mortality, vegetative state and severe physical disability are practically non-existent with minor head injury. Unfortunately, however, association to cognitive and behavioral problems are considerably high. Over 50–60% patients do manifest post-concussion problem.[13,14,16] Postconcussion syndrome is a condition, characterized by the presence of headache, vertigo, lack of concentration, memory disturbance, loss of appetite and slow reaction. Patient remains depressed and less active with slow reaction. Between 50 and 85% patients do have some symptoms and most frequent among them are headache, tiredness and lack of interest to work. In another study 46% complained of poor work performance due to depression, poor memory and lack of motivation. Thus, post-concussion syndrome becomes a major public health problem, considering the magnitude of minor head injury and high incidence of post-concussion syndrome. Recently, physiological studies like P300 and cerebral blood flow by transcranial Doppler have shown abnormalities in minor head injury with post-concussion syndrome.[53,54] In their study, Jain and Mahapatra[54] concluded that the abnormality in blood flow velocities by TCD compared well with P300 abnormalities. Both P300 and blood flow abnormalities indicate a diffuse cerebral involvement. There is also a good correlation of P300 wave abnormalities with severity of vertigo. Patients in whom bilateral P300 abnormalities were detected, CT scan also showed cerebral lesions.

Recently, in a series of study from an department has clearly.[55,56] Show low cerebral perfusion in patients with post-concussion syndrome (PCS) Patient with persistent vertigo do have long-term perfusion defect in temporal lobes. On SPECT study has show this perfusion problems, both in adults and children.

Assurance and confidence building measures are the mainstay of treatment. Relaxation training and reduction of stress level are also important. Deep breathing, autogenic training, mediation and control of emotion are likely to increase the working capability and job prospect. Schwatzberg[57] reported use of audiotape and videotape in rehabilitation of head injury patients. He concluded that it is important to accept head injury group as a separate group with specialized training than other problem focussed group. With proper rehabilitation programme it is possible to provide better job oriented outcome.

Problems of Rehabilitation in Vegetative Patients (Ref Chapter 45)

Around 5–10% of severe head injuries are ultimately remain vegetative (56–58%).[58–60] Persistent vegetative state is a social and economic problem. Treatment of vegetative state is an unsolved problem. Moriya et al.[59] reported useful role of median nerve stimulation, in comatose patients. In another study Ueda and Yana Gida[61] reported music in awakening respect of comatose patient. Recently, dorsal column stimulation (DCS) has shown improvement in some patients[62] since 1st report by Kanno, 133 patients in vegetative state have been treated in Japan and USA,[62] clinical improvement was recorded in 57 cases (42–9%). The favorable factors were: (a) young age, (b) head trauma, (c) coma for less than 3 months and CT scan, which shows no sign of severe damage. Other significant parameters which indicate chance of recovery are EEG and blood flow improvement following dorsal column stimulation. This leads to unresolved issues regarding the grading of vegetative state. There is no scoring system for chronic unconsciousness. Such a classification should include, cerebral blood

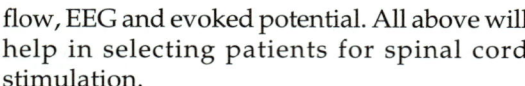

flow, EEG and evoked potential. All above will help in selecting patients for spinal cord stimulation.

Endocrinal Dysfunction (Ref Chapter 20)

All types of endocrinal dysfunction have been reported after severe head injury. In acute head injury with stress, diabetes insipidus and adrenal cortical deficiency may occur. Problem like diabetes insipidus is very obvious and requires judicious management. Chronic endocrinal dysfunctions are by and large of hypothalamic origin.[63-65] Necrosis of pituitary gland and damage to hypothalamus are reported in severe head injury. Amenorrhea or menstrual disorders in females and depressed secretion of testosterone leading the sexual dysfunction are also reported in under hypothyroidism and hypocortisolism require long-term replacement.[63] Hypothalamic disturbances also likely to change sleep cycle.[66]

Driving after Head Injury

Driving skill is impaired following head injury. Several factors are responsible, which include, physical, visual disability, lack of motivation, poor reaction and loss of confidence.[67-69] Shute and Woodhouse[69] discuss the visual problem and driving ability following head injury. They also considered legal points in relation to visual fitness and driving in patients with head injury. Weakness of limbs, contracture, spasticity and more importantly, post-traumatic epilepsy also create problem following head injury. Galski et al[68] in 1993, evaluated driving performance in patients with brain injury. They used combined administration of pre-driver, simulator and behind the wheel evaluation. They analyzed 106 patients and reported that the residual cognitive defects per se did not render a person unfit to drive. They also emphasized that the method used was reliable and relatively sensitive to predict the outcome. Overall, the driving becomes a problem in survivors of both severely and mildly head-injured patients. Disability, spasticity play important role in severe head injury, as compared to loss of confidence, lack of interest and motivation in patients with minor head injury.

CONCLUSIONS

Rehabilitation of head injury has long been neglected. Fortunately, in the recent years things have improved. No doubt rehabilitation is an uphill task in head injury patients due to wide range of involvement, physical, cognitive and behavioral problems. It is a long and tidius process, which needs multi-disciplinary approach, and requires dedicated team work. Co-operation of patients, sympathetic and supportive role of family and friends help in quicker recovery. The rehabilitation process must be well designed and a protocol based treatment must be instituted as early as possible. In minor head injuries, confidence building measures, and reassurance play a vital role. Children need a special care, both at home, and at school. In recovery of the children, teachers play important role, in learning and education. In India, things are much worse as the medical and sociocultural systems are different. Overall, the emphasis is on the development and critical evaluation of community based services like, enhancement of social participation, independent living mode in long-term rehabilitation. As the financial burden is immediate and long-lasting, the impact on family and community is immense. Hence, it is necessary to develop community based rehabilitation facilities and strategy for active participation in productive, recreational and vocational programmes. Thus, knowing the magnitude of the problem, physical, and mental rehabilitation must be considered as an important part in head injury management to improve the overall results.

REFERENCES

1. Jennett B, Teasdale B, Brackman R, et al. Prognosis of patients with severe head injury. Neurosurgery 1979;4:283–9.
2. Langfitt TW. Gennarelli TA. Can the outcome from head injury be improved? J Neurosurg 1982;56:19–23.

3. Becker DP, Miller JD, Ward JD. The outcome from severe head injury with early diagnosis and intensive management (Class II). J Neurosurg 1977;47:491–502.

4. Lennett B, Teasdale G, Galbraith S, et al. Severe head injury in three countries. J Neurol Neurosurg Psychiat 1977;40:291–5.

5. Miller JD, Butterworth JF, Gudeman SK, et al. Further experience in the management of severe head injury. J Neurosurg 1981;54:289–99.

6. Lennett B, Bond M. Assessment of outcome after severe brain damage. A practical scale. Lancet 1975;1:480–9.

7. Narayan RK, Greenburg RP, Miller ID, et al. Improved confidence of outcome prediction in severe head injury. A comparative analysis of the clinical examination, multimodal evoked potential, CT scanning and intracranial pressure. I Neurosurg 1981;54:751–62.

8. Marshall LF. The role of aggressive therapy for head injury: Does it matter? In: Clinical Neurosurgery. William and Wilkin, Baltimore, Md 1986;34:549.

9. Auerbach SH. Neuroanatomical correlation of attention of behavioural subtype I Head Trauma Rehabil 1986;1:1–8.

10. Boll TJ. Behavioural sequelae of head injury. In: Cooper PR (ed), Head injury. William and Wilkin, Baltimore 1982;263.

11. Prigatano GP. Psychiatric aspect of head injury. Problem area and suggested guidelines for research. In: Levin HS, Grafman J, Eisenberg HM (eds). Neurobehavioural Recovery from Head Injury. Oxford University Press. New York 1987;215.

12. Levin HS. The neurobehavioural recovery. In : DP Decker, JT Povlishock (eds). Central Nervous System Trauma Status Report. NIH Bethesda, Med 1985; 251.

13. Levin HS, Mattis S, Ruff R, et al. Neurobehavioural outcome following minor head injury. A three center study. J. Neurosurg 1987;66:234–8.

14. Ben Yishay Y, Diller L. Cognitive defect. In: Rosenthal M, Griffith ER, Bond MR, et al. (eds). Rehabilitation of the head-injured adult. FA Davis Company, Philadelphia 1983;163.

15. Hart T, Hyden ME. The ecological validity of Neuropsychological assessment and Mediation. In: Uzzell BP and Gross Y (eds). Clinical Neuropsychology of Intervention. Martinus Nijhoff Publishing Comp. Boston 1986; 22.

16 Powel TJ, Collin C, Sulton K. A follow up study of patients hospitalized after minor head injury. Disability Rehab 1996;18:231–7.

17. Fearnside MR, Cook RJ, McDougall P, et al. The Westme Head Injury Project. Physical and social outcome following severe head injury. Brit J Neurosurg 1993;7:643–50.

18. Mayer NH, Keating DJ, Rapp D. Skill, routines and activity pattern of daily living. A functional nested approach. In: Uzzell BP, Gross Y (eds). Clinical Psychology of Intervention, Martinus Nijhoff Publishing, Boston 1986;205.

19. Mackay LE, Bernstein BA, Chapman PE, et al. Early intervention in severe head injury: Long-term benefits of a formalized progress. Arch Phys Med Rehabil 1992;73:635–41.

20. Whyte J. Rehabilitation. In. NINS, Head Injury Clinical Management and Research. Elizabeth Frost (ed), AIREN Geneva Switzerland 1990;4: 233–48.

21. Moseley AM. The effect of casting combined with stretching of passive ankle dorsiflexon in adults with traumatic head injuries. Physical Therapy 1997;77:240–7.

22. Glenn M. Rosenthal M. Rehabilitation following severe traumatic brain injury. J Head Trauma Rehabil 1986;1:72.

23. Mital MA, Garber JE, Stinson JJ. Ectopic bone formation in children and adolescents with head injuries, its management. J Ped Ortho 1987;7:83.

24. Spielman G, Gennarelli TA, Rogers CR. Disodium etidronate: Its role in preventory heterotopic ossification in severe head injury. Arch Phys Med Rehabil 1983;64:539.

25. Fukado Y. Microsurgical transethmoidal optic nerve decompression in 700 cases. In: The cranial nerves. M Samii and P Jennetta (eds). Springer-Verlag, New York 1981;125–8.

26. Gjerris F. Traumatic lesions of visual pathway. In: Vinken PJ, Bruyn GW (eds). Handbook of clinical Neurology, North Holland Publishing Company, Amsterdam 1976;24:24–57.

27. Walsh FB. Trauma involving anterior visual pathways. Freeman HM (ed.) Ocular Trauma. Apleton-Century-Craft. New York 1979;335–51.

28. Mahapatra AK, Bhatia R. Predictive value of visual evoked potential in unilateral optic nerve injury. Surg Neurol 1989,31:339–42.

29. Mahapatra AK, Tandon DA. A prospective study of 250 patients with optic nerve injury. In: Majid Samii (ed). Skull base anatomy, radiology and management. S Karger Basel 1994;305–9.

30. Greenwood RJ, McMillan MR, Brooks DN, et al. Effect of case management after severe head injury. BMJ 1994;308:1199–205.

31. Godfrey HP, Bishare SN, Partridze PM, et al. Neuropsychological impairment and return to

work following severe closed head injury, implications for clinical management. New Zealand Medical Jour 1993;106:301–93.

32. Gronwall D, Wrightson P. Delayed recovery of intellectual function after minor head injury. Lancet 1974;2:605.

33. Gronwall D. Advances in the assessment of attention and information processing after head injury. In: Levin HS, Grafman J, Eisenberg HM (eds). Neuro-behavioural recovery from head injury. Oxford University Press, New York, 1987; 335.

34. Van Zomeren AH, Brower WH, Doelman BG. Attention deficit. The riddle of selectivity, special speed and alertness. In: Brook SN (ed). Closed head injury, psychological, social and family consequences. Oxford University Press. Oxford 1984; 84.

35. Evans RW, Gualtieri CT. Psychostimulant Pharmacology in traumatic brain injury. J Head Trauma Rehabil 1987;2:29.

36. Nissen MJ. Neuropsychology of attention and memory. J Head Trauma Rehabil 1986;1:13.

37. Gilsky EL, Schacter DL. Remediation of organic memory disorder. Current status and future prospects. J Head Trauma Rehabil 1986;1:54.

38. Hermann DL. Know the memory. The use of questionnaires to assess and study memory. Psychol, Bulletin 1982;92:434.

39. McGlynm SM. Schacter DL: Unawareness of deficit in neuropsychological syndromes. J Clin Exp Neuropsychol 1989;11:143.

40. Sarno M: The nature of verbal impairment after closed head injury. J Nerv Mental Dis 1980;168: 685.

41. Lezak MD (ed). Assessment of the behavioural consequences of head trauma. In: Frontiers of clinical Neurosciences. Alan R Loss Inc, New York 1980;Vol 7.

42. Logue P, Me Carthy SM: Assessment of Neurological disorder. In: Assessment strategies in behavioural Medicine. Keefe KJ, Blumenthal JA (eds). Grune and Stratton, New York 1982;133.

43. Bond MR. The psychiatry of closed head injury. In Brook N (ed). Closed Head Injury. Psychological, social and family consequences. Oxford University Press. Oxford 1984;148.

44. Benton AL. Behavioural consequences of closed head injury. In GL Odom (ed). Central Nervous System Trauma, Research Status Report, National Institute of Health, NIH, Bethesda Med 1979;220.

45. Glenn MB. A pharmacological approach to aggressive and disruptive behaviour after traumatic brain injury (Part 2). J Head Trauma Rehabil 1987;2:80.

46. Jackson RD, Corrigan JD, Arnett JA. Ami trip tiline for agitation in head injury. Arch Phys Med Rehabil GG 1985;66:180.

47. Appleton R. Head injury rehabilitation for children. Nursing Times 1994;90:29–31.

48. Greenspan Al, Mackenzie EJ. Functional outcome after Pediatric head injury. Pediatrics 1994;94:425–32.

49. Scott JR, Marlow N, Seddon N, et al. Rehabilitation and outcome after severe head injury. Arch Dis Child 1992;67:222–6.

50. Middletn J. Thinking about head injuries in children. J Chil Psychol Psychiat All Discio 1989;30:663–70.

51. Kraft JF, Schwab KK, Salazar AM, et al. Occupational and educational achievements of head injured Vietnam veterans at 15 years follow up. Arch Phys Med Rehabil 1993;74:596–601.

52. Dikman SS, Temkin NR, Machamer JE, et al. Employment following traumatic head injuries. Arch Neurol 1994;51:177–86.

53. Agarwal A, Barua N, Walia BS, Mahapatra AK. P300 wave in patients with post-concussion vertigo: A prospective study of 15 cases. Ind J Otolaryngol Head and Neck Surg 1996;18:121–4.

54. Jain K, Mahapatra AK. P300 and TCD abnormality in minor head injury. A preliminary study. In : Brain protection and neural Trauma, VK Khosla, VK Kak, BS Sharma (eds). Narosa Publisher, New Delhi 2000;298–305.

55. Agrawal D, Naveen K, Bal CS, Mahapatra AK. Post-concussion vertigo. Is the cause Central? Correlation with SPECT and CT. Neuroscience Today 2003;7:33–36.

56. Agrawal D, Naveen K, Bal CS, Mahapatra AV. Post-concussion syndrome in pediatic population. Is medial temporal damage in responsible? Correlation with brain SPECT. A prospective controlled study. Childs Neus Syst 2003;19:628.

57. Schwartzberg SL. Helping factors in a predeveloped support group of persons with head injury. Part I. Participant observer perspective. Ame J Rehabil Occup Therap, 1994;48:297–304.

58. Whyte J. The rehabilitation of the patient in a persistent vegetative state. J Head Trauma Rehabil 1986;1:64.

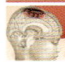
59. Moriya T, Noda E, Sakurai J, et al. Neurological evaluation of unconscious patient with median nerve stimulation. 8th Annual Meeting of Society of Coma, July 1999.

60. Michaud LJ, Rivara FP, Grady MS, et al. Predictors of survival and severity of disability after severe head injury in children. Neurosurg 1992;31:254–64.

61. Ueda K, Yana gida M. Effect of Music on brain in unconscious patient. Paper presented at 8th Annual Meeting of Society for Treatment of Coma, Oita, July 1999.

62. Kanno T, Kamei Y, Yokoyama T. A new treatment for vegetative state after head trauma. Dorsal column stimulation. In: Modern trend in the management of neurotrauma. PS Ramani, A Sharma (eds). Lavanya Printing, Bombay 1994;87–92.

63. Fleischer AS, Rudman DR, Payne NS, et al. Hypothalamic, and hypogonadism in prolonged coma. J Neurosurg 1978;49:550.

64. Hadani M, Findler G, Shaked I, et al. Unusual delayed onset diabetes insipidus following closed head trauma. J Neurosurg 1985;63:456–8.

65. Klingbell GE, Clive P. Anterior hypopituitarysm. A consequence of head injury. Arch Phy Med Rehabil 1985;66:44.

66. Prigantano GB, Stahl ML, Orrwe, et al. Sleep and dreaming disturbances in closed head injury patients. J Neurol Neurosurg Psychiat 1982;45:78.

67. Van Zomeran AH, Brouner WH, Minderhoud JM: Acquired brain damage and driving. A review. Arch Physic Med Rehabil 1987;68:697.

68. Galski T, Bruno RL, Ehle HT. Prediction of behind the wheel driving performance in patients with cerebral brain damage—a discriminent function analysis. Ame J Occup Therapy 1993;47:391–6.

69. Shute RH, Woodhouse JM. Visual fitness to drive after stroke and head injury. Ophthal Physio Optics 1990;10:327–32.

47

Persistent Vegetative State in Head Injury

Raj Kamal • AK Mahapatra

INTRODUCTION

The persistent vegetative state (PVS) in a neurological condition in which a person is in a state of complete unawareness of self, and environment. This clinical state is also associated with sleep and awake cycle with either partial or complete preservation of hypothalamic and brainstem function.[1–5] Frequently, many patients are in vegetative state and over the months they slowly improve. Hence, this condition may be transient (temporary) or permanent.[1,6–9] **After four weeks in a vegetative state (VS), the patient is classified as in a persistent vegetative state. It is classified as a permanent vegetative state (PVS) after approximately one year of being in a vegetative state. Some international studies have reported vegetative state at the end of 6 months.**[5,10,11] However, diagnosis of vegetative state after one year of injury, reflects real clinical state as there is failure to recover from acute or chronic head injury. Approximately 10–14% of all severe head injuries develop into PVS.[6] This chapter highlights some aspects of PVS.

Following coma, some patients will recover wakefulness without signs of consciousness (only showing reflex movements, i.e. the vegetative state) or may show non-reflex movements but remain without functional communication (i.e. the minimally conscious state). [12] Currently, there remains a high rate of misdiagnosis of the vegetative state[13] 55, and the clinical and electrophysiological markers of outcome from the vegetative and minimally conscious states remain unsatisfactory. This should incite clinicians to use multimodal assessment to detect objective signs of consciousness and validate paraclinical prognostic markers in these challenging patients. This review will focus on advanced magnetic resonance imaging (MRI) techniques such as magnetic resonance spectroscopy, diffusion tensor imaging, and functional MRI (fMRI studies in both "activation" and "resting state" conditions) that were recently introduced in the assessment of patients with chronic disorders of consciousness.[11,12]

Despite the importance of diagnostic accuracy and advances in the past 15 years, the rate of misdiagnosis among patients with disorders of consciousness has not substantially changed. Although early detection of signs of consciousness is crucial not only for daily management (particularly, pain treatment), end-of-life decisions[12–14] and prognosis (i.e. patients in minimally conscious state (MCS) but also have significantly more favorable outcomes as compared to those in VS,[14,15] clinicians should recognize that diagnoses established during the acute stage tend to be transitional and may change over time as the injury sequelae resolve. The results of this study suggest that the systematic use of a sensitive standardized neurobehavioral assessment scale may help decrease diagnostic error and limit diagnostic uncertainty. Future studies should investigate other factors influencing diagnostic accuracy.

Minimally conscious state (MCS) is defined as a condition of severely altered consciousness in which minimal but definite behavioral evidence of self-awareness is demonstrated.[15]

CHARACTERIZATION OF VEGETATIVE STATE

Persistent vegetative state (PVS) is a rare condition. Many synonymes have been used by many authors, such as, vegetative state, persistent vegetative state, **apallic syndrome, and coma vigil.**[6,7] The clinical characterization is not always enough to establish the vegetative state hence, Grossman and Hegel,[6] suggested additional criteria to distinguish different subjects of vegetative state. They suggested investigative modalities such as CT, magnetic resonance imaging, SPECT and EEG to assess the brain dysfunction. However, all above parameters are only relative indicators of limited predictive value. The clinical criteria for PVS are given in Table 47.1.[1,2]

The above clinical criterias, when existed for atleast 12 months following injury, the diagnosis of PVS is tenable.[16–18] Large number of patients those who are diagnosed to be in a vegetative state at 6–8 weeks do improve significantly over a period of time.[16,19] Thus,

Table 47.1: Criteria for diagnosis of vegetative state

- No evidence of awareness of self or environment and an inability to interact with others
- No evidence of sustained, reproducible, purposeful, or voluntary behavioral responses to visual, auditory, tactile, or noxious stimuli
- No evidence of language comprehension or expression
- Intermittent wakefulness manifested by the presence of sleep-wake cycles
- Sufficiently preserved hypothalamic and brainstem autonomic functions to permit survival with medical and nursing care
- Bowel and bladder incontinence
- Variably preserved cranial-nerve and spinal reflexes.

From the Multi-Society Task Force on PVS (1994).[16]

diagnosis of PVS is incorrect at 3 or 6 months following trauma.

The persistent vegetative state is the standard usage (except in the UK) for a medical diagnosis, made after numerous neurological and other tests, that due to extensive and irreversible brain damage a patient is *highly unlikely* ever to achieve higher functions above a vegetative state. This diagnosis does not mean that a doctor has diagnosed improvement as impossible, but does open the possibility, in the US, for a judicial request to end life support.[14] Informal guidelines hold that this diagnosis can be made after four weeks in a vegetative state.

In the UK, the term 'persistent vegetative state' is discouraged in favor of two more precisely defined terms that have been strongly recommended by the Royal College of Physicians. These guidelines recommend using a **continuous vegetative state** for patients in a vegetative state for more than four weeks. A medical definition of a **permanent vegetative state** can be made if, after exhaustive testing and a customary 12 months of observation,[20,22] a medical diagnosis that it is *impossible* by any informed medical expectations that the mental condition will ever improve.[21] Hence, a "continuous vegetative state" in the UK may remain the diagnosis in cases that would be called "persistent" in the US or elsewhere.

Pathology in Brain and Pathogenesis of PVS

Earlier it was presumed that the brainstem injury is the commonest cause of PVS. However, neuropathological data do not substantiate the above hypothesis.[23,24] In a MRI study of 42 patients, Kampfl et al[18,19] reported **DAI with lesions in corpus callosum and dorsolateral brainstem to be the key site in post-traumatic PVS.** They also proved that the basal ganglia to be the 2nd common site of injury in patients with PVS. **In there series, all 42 cases there was evidence on MR imaging of diffuse axonal injury, and injury to the corpus callosum was detected in all patients.**

The second most common area of diffuse axonal injury involved the **dorsolateral aspect of the rostral brainstem** (74% of patients). In addition, 65% of these patients exhibited white matter injury in the corona radiata and the frontal and temporal lobes. Lesions to the **basal ganglia or thalamus** were seen in 52 and 40% of patients, respectively. Magnetic resonance imaging showed some evidence of cortical contusion in 48% of patients in this study; the frontal and temporal lobes were most frequently involved. Injury to the parahippocampal gyrus was detected in 45% of patients; in this subgroup there was an 80% incidence of contralateral peduncular lesions in the midbrain. The most common pattern of injury (74% in this series) was the combination of focal lesions of the corpus callosum and the dorsolateral brainstem. In patients with no evidence of diffuse axonal injury in the upper brainstem (26% in this series), callosal lesions were most often associated with basal ganglia lesions. Lesions of the corona radiata and lobar white matter were equally distributed in patients with or without dorsolateral brainstem injury. Moreover, cortical contusions and thalamic, parahippocampal, and cerebral peduncular lesions were also similarly distributed in both groups.

In one of classic case Kinney et al[25] in 1994, suggested **the role of thalamus in a patient with post-traumatic coma.** Other sites which are abnormal leading to vegetative state are the parahippocampal area and the peduncular lesion of the brainstem. Similar observations were also made by other authors on MRI.[26,27] However, lesions of corpus callosum was first identified by Strich in 1956,[28] as a prominent features of DAI. Many of these patients followed by Strich developed severe dementia. In addition to DAI there were deep white matter lesions seen in vegetative patients.[28]

In hypoxic-ischemic injury leading to PVS, damage to basal ganglia and thalamus are reported as prominent pathological features in radiological imaging.[5,23,25] Among the corpus callosum lesions, splenium is the commonest site. Adama et al[29] in 1989, in their neuropathological studies demonstrated corona radiata, white matter of the frontal and the temporal lobe involvement in DAI. Another characteristic feature of DAI is the focal lesion of the dorsolateral part of the midbrain, which was also recorded in 74% of patients of PVS in MRI, reported by Kamfl et al.[19] In addition to above lesions, they reported tegmental lesion in 17 (8-bilateral), periaqueductal injury in 7 patients and ventral midbrain lesions, in 21 patients (bilateral 14). In 32% patients the midbrain lesions had extended into the pons and in 5 patients medullary lesions were noticed, which were exclusively localized in the olives. Thus, neuropathological and neuroradiological studies suggest DAI, involving basal ganglia, midbrain and splenium of corpus callosum, in vast majority of patients with PVS. Overall, histological. Picture reveals a widespread hypoxic and ischemic damage.[5,23,24]

CT and MRI Finding in PVS

Inspite of PVS being a well known (Table 47.2) and common entity not much literature is available dealing with CT finding in PVS.[23] However, study by Levin et al[30] reported only supratentorial swelling and midline shift. In their study brainstem injury was uncommon. MRI is far superior to CT scan in detecting

Table 47.2: Incidence of vegetative state			
	Year 1979	*No. of patients*	*%*
1. Jennett et al[10]	International Coma Data Bank	1000	12
2. Celesia[3]	1996	–	14
3. Heindl and Laub[16]	1996	127	5
4. Kampfl et al[19]	1998	Children 80 in PVS at 6–8 weeks	42 at 1 yr (50%)

DAI, hemorrhagic and non-hemorrhagic contusions in corpus callosum, inferior aspect of frontal and temporal lobes and in the brainstem.[18,19, 27,31,32] Moreover, **MR imaging shows superior sensitivity in detecting post-traumatic shearing injury in subacute stage of head injury.** Due to above reasons, MR considered to be more helpful than CT in localizing and characterizing post-traumatic brain lesions. In PVS, CT and MRI have shown widespread lesions in the brain (Table 47.3). In an MRI study in 42 patients with PSV Kampfl et al[18] **reported DAI as the commonest pathology, followed by brainstem and corpus callosum injury.** Thus, the MR imaging at different intervals has helped in finding out the various brain lesions in patients with PVS, which infact has well correlated with the neuropathological findings. Reider-Groswasser et al[33] correlated finding of third ventricle in CT with poor outcome. They reported poor prognosis in patients having third ventricle width 8 mm and 11 mm distance between septum pellucidum and caudate nucleus (cerebroventricular Index).

Diffusion tensor imaging (DTI)[11,34] to study the neuropathology of 25 vegetative and minimally conscious patients *in vivo* and to identify measures that could potentially distinguish the patients in these two groups. Mean diffusivity (MD) maps of the subcortical white matter, brainstem and thalami were generated. The MCS and VS patients differed significantly in subcortical white matter and thalamic regions, but appeared not to differ in the brainstem.

Table 47.3: Pathological findings reported in MRI and CT in patients with vegetative state

Site of lesion	%
1. Rostral brainstem	75
2. Basal ganglia	52
3. Thalamus	40
4. Hippocampus	21
5. Parahippocampal gyrus	45
6. Cortical contusion	48
7. Corpus callosum	70
8. Corona radiata	56

An improved understanding of variations in neuropathology in the vegetative state (VS) may aid diagnosis, improve prognostication and help refine the selection of patients for particular treatment regimes. Diffusion tensor imaging (DTI) can be useful to characterise the extent and location of white matter loss in VS secondary to traumatic brain injury (TBI) and ischemic-hypoxic injury. DTI demonstrated abnormalities where conventional radiological approaches did not detect lesions in pons, thalamus, ventral midbrain, dorsal midbrain and the corpus callosum.

Nuclear medicine techniques, such as single photon emission tomography (SPECT) and positron emission tomography (PET) have been applied in patients in a vegetative state to investigate brain function in a non-invasive manner.[35] Parameters investigated include glucose metabolism, perfusion at rest, variations of regional perfusion after stimulation, and benzodiazepine receptor density. Compared to controls, patients in a vegetative state show a substantial reduction of glucose metabolism and perfusion. While patients post-anoxia exhibit a rather homogeneous cortical reduction of glucose metabolism, patients after head trauma often show severe cortical and sub-cortical reductions at the site of primary trauma. In acute vegetative state (AVS, duration < 1 month), overall glucose utilization was significantly reduced in comparison with age-matched controls. In a few cases with locked-in syndrome, cortical metabolism was in the normal range. 11C-Flumazenil (FMZ) measures the density of benzodiazepine receptors (BZRs) and thereby furnishes an estimate of neuronal integrity. PET with this tracer demonstrated a considerable reduction in BZRs in cortical areas, but indicated that the cerebellum was spared from neuronal loss. The comparison of FDG- and FMZ-PET findings in AVS demonstrates that alterations of cerebral glucose consumption do not represent mere functional inactivation, but also irreversible structural damage.[35,36]

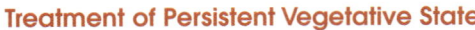
Treatment of Persistent Vegetative State

The patients with early post-traumatic vegetative state can have recovery when they are followed longer period. However, accurate prediction of recovery is not possible, and various clinical and laboratory tests fail to predict the recovery. Treatment with multidisciplinary approach have shown better chance of recovery of patients in vegetative state. No doubt vegetative patients need appropriate medical and nursing care.[33,37] There is also a great role of family and their educational state. Family members also need counseling.

After the acute stage, structured protocol based rehabilitation programme helps in faster recovery. Recently, sensory stimulation have been used, based on hypothesis that these stimulations help in fast recovery.[38–43] Those include electric stimulation of dorsal colum[40–43] and median nerve stimulation.[31] Both Cooper et al[42] and Moriya et al[41] reported improvement in vegetative state following the median nerve stimulation. Recently, deep brain stimulation is also used in patients with PVS.[43,44] Yamamoto et al[44] in 1993 reported changes in CSF levels of PGD2, PGE2 and **monoamines,** following deep brain stimulation, in vegetative patients. Cooper et al[40] studied 25 patients and published the efficacy of median nerve stimulation. Some authors have reported value of musical stimulation in recovery of comatose patients.[45,46]

Pharmacotherapy in Persistent Coma

Pharmacological therapy mainly substances such as tricyclic antidepressants or methylphenidate. Mixed results have been reported using dopaminergic drugs such as amantadine and bromocriptine and stimulants such as dextroamphetamine.

Recently, some drugs have been tried in comatose patients. These include aminergic agents, cholinergic agents[47] and **prostaglandin** E_2.[48] Dopaminergic drugs have also been tried.[49–52] They include L-dopa[49,50] and bromocryptine.[50–53] **Amphetamine**[54] and amantadine have been tried. Some reports are available reporting the effect of bromocryptine. These drugs helps in synaptic transmission of dopamine receptors. A combination of amantadine and bromocriptine has been shown to increase the release of dopamine. Pharmacotherapy must be started much before cerebral atrophy, as PVS more than 3 months have considerably decreased CBF and $CMRO_2$.

The common hypnotic, **zolpidem**, has been reported to temporarily restore consciousness to individuals in the chronic vegetative state.[55,56] Zolpidem is an omega 1 specific indirect GABA agonist that is used for insomnia, but may have efficacy in brain damage.

Overall, outcome[1,2] in patients (Table 47.4) with cerebral atrophy is poor. Overall, there may a role of pharmacotherapy in treatment of prolonged coma.

CONCLUSIONS

Persistent vegetative state is a well-known entity in head injury, by and large caused by DAI. Damage to corpus callosum, brainstem and corona radiata is often reported in MRI. Early physiotherapy, different sensory stimulation, and pharmacological agents can reduce the number of vegetative patients. Recently, spinal cord and deep brain stimulation are under trial and have provided some promising results.

Table 47.4: Outcome one year after insult according to duration of the vegetative state[1,2]				
	Numbers	Dead	Vegetative	Conscious
Vegetative after one month	540	28	18	54
Vegetative after 3 months	268	31	30	39
Vegetative after 6 months	**151**	**28**	**53**	**19**

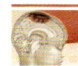

REFERENCES

1. Medical aspects of persistent vegetative state (1). The Multi-Society Task Force on PVS. N Eng J Med 1994;330:1499–1508.
2. The Multi-Society Task Force on PVS. "Medical Aspects of the Persistent Vegetative State—Second of Two Parts". New England Journal of Medicine 1994;330(22):1572–9.
3. Celesia GG. Persistent Vegetative state. Neurology 1993;43:1457–58.
4. Kenard C, Illingworth R. Persistent Vegetative State. J Neurol Neurosurg Psychiat 1995;59:347–55.
5. Doughterty JH, Rawlinson DG, Levy DE, et al. Hypoxic-ischaemic brain injury and vegetative state. Clinical and Neuropathologic correlation. Neurology 1998;34:991–7.
6. Grossman P, Hagel K. Post-traumatic apallic syndrome following head injury. Part 1. Clinical characteristics. Disbil Rehabil 1996;18:1–20.
7. Jellinger 1C, Seitelberger F. Protracted post-traumatic encephalopathy. Pathology, pathogenesis and clinical implication. J. Neurol Sci 1970;10:51–94.
8. Child NC, Mercer WN, Child HW. Accuracy of diagnosis of persistent vegetative state. Neurology 1993;43:1465–67.
9. Andrews K, Murphy L, Munday R, et al. Misdiagnosis of the vegetative state: retrospective study in a rehabilitation unit. BMJ 1996;313:13–16.
10. Jennett B, Teasdale G, Braakman R, et al. Prognosis of patients with severe head injury. Neurosurgery 1979;4:283–9.
11. Newcombe VF, Williams GB, Scoffings D, Cross J, Carpenter TA, Pickard JD, Menon DK., Aetiological differences in neuroanatomy of the vegetative state: insights from diffusion tensor imaging and functional implications. J Neurol Neurosurg Psychiatry 2010;81(5):552–6.
12. Luaba Tshibanda, Audrey Vanhaudenhuyse, Mélanie Boly, Andrea Soddu, Marie-Aurelie Bruno, Gustave Moonen, Steven Laureys, Quentin Noirhomme, Neuroimaging after coma, Neuroradiology 2010;52(1):15–24.
13. Caroline Schnakers, Audrey Vanhaudenhuyse, Joseph Giacino, Manfredi Ventura, Melanie Boly, Steve Majerus, Gustave Moonen and Steven Laureys, Diagnostic accuracy of the vegetative and minimally conscious state: Clinical consensus versus standardized neurobehavioral assessment, BMC Neurology 2009;9:35.
14. Andrews K: Medical decision making in the vegetative state: withdrawal of nutrition and hydration. Neuro Rehabilitation 2004; 19(4): 299–304.
15. Giacino JT: The vegetative and minimally conscious states: consensus-based criteria for establishing diagnosis and prognosis. Neuro Rehabilitation 2004,19(4):293–8.
16. Heindl UT, Laub MC. Outcome of persistent vegetative state following hypoxic or traumatic brain injury in children or adolescents. Neuropediatrics 1996;27:94–100.
17. Wade TD. Misdiagnosis of the vegetative state: Persistent vegetative state should not be diagnosed until 12 months from onset of coma. BMJ 1996;313:943–4.
18. Kampfl A, Franz G, Aichner F, et al. The persistent vegetative state after closed head injury: Clinical magnetic resonance imaging findings in 42 patients. J Neurosurg 1998;88: 809–16.
19. Kampfl A, Schmutzhard E, Franz G, et al. Prediction of recovery from post-traumatic vegetative state with cerebral MRI. Lancet 1998;35:1763–7.
20. Wade DT, Johnston C. "The permanent vegetative state: Practical guidance on diagnosis and management". BMJ (clinical research ed.), 1999; 319(7213):841–4. PMC 1116668. PMID 10496834.
21. Guidance on diagnosis and management: Report of a working party of the Royal College of Physicians. Royal College of Physicians: London, 1996.
22. BMA. Withdrawing and withholding life prolonging medical treatment, 3rd edn. London: BMA, 2007.
23. Kinney HC, Samuels MA. Neuropathology of persistent vegetative state. A review. J. Neuropathol Exp Neurol 1994;53:548–58.
24. Peters G, Rothemund E. Neuropathology of traumatic apallic syndrome. In: Dalle OveG, Gerstenbrand F, Lucking CH (eds). The Apallic Syndrome. Berlin; Springer-Verlag 1977 PV 78–87.
25. Kinney HC, Korein J, Panigraphy A, et al. Neuropathological findings in the brain of Karen Ann Qumlan. The role of the thalamus and the persistent vegetative state. N Eng J Med 1994;330:1469–75.
26. Gentry LR, Thompson B, Godersky JC. Trauma to the corpus callosum: MR features. AJNR 1988;9:1129–38.
27. Mendelsohn BD, Levis HS, Haward H, et al. Corpus callosum lesions after closed head injury in children. MRI, clinical features and outcome. Neuroradiology 1992;34:384–8.

28. Strich SJ. Diffuse degeneration of the cerebral white matter in severe dementia following head injury. J Neurol Neurosurg Psychiat 1956;19:163–85.
29. Adam JH, Doyle D, Ford I, et al. Diffuse axonal injury in head injury: definition, diagnosis and grading. Histopathology 1989;15:49–59.
30. Levin HS, Saydijari C, Eisenberg HM, et al. Vegetative state after closed head injury. A Traumatic Coma Data Bank report. Arch Neurol 1991;48:580–5.
31. Gentry LR. Imaging of closed head injury. Radiology 1994;191:1–17.
32. Gentry LR, Godersky JC, Thompson BH. Traumatic brainstem injury: MR Imaging. Radiology 1989;171:177–87.
33. Reider-Groswasser I, CostefF HB, Sazbon L, et al. CT findings in Persistent vegetative state following blunt traumatic brain injury. Brain Injury 1997;11:865–70.
34. Fernández-Espejo D, Bekinschtein T, Monti MM, Pickard JD, Junque C, Coleman MR, Owen AM. Diffusion weighted imaging distinguishes the vegetative state from the minimally conscious state. Neuroimage 2011;1;54(1):103–12.
35. Heiss WD, PET in coma and in vegetative state. Eur J Neurol 2012;19(2):207–11.
36. Di H, Boly M, Weng X, Ledoux D, Laureys S. Neuroimaging activation studies in the vegetative state: predictors of recovery? Clin Med 2008;8(5):502–7.
37. Grossman P, Hagel K. Post-traumatic apallic syndrome following head injury, Part 2: Treatment Disability and Rehab 1996;18:57–68.
38. Kanno T. Neurostimulation for a case of unconsciousness of chronic stage. Brain and Nerve 1995;47:643–9.
39. Moriya T, Noda E, Sakurai J, et al. Neurological evaluation of unconscious patients with median nerve stimulation 8th Annual meeting of the Society of Treatment of Coma, 1999.
40. Yokoyama T, Kamei Y, Shoda M, et al. Treatment of vegetative status with Dorsal Column stimulation. Neurol Surg (Tokyo) 1990;18:39–45.
41. Moriya T.Hayashi A, Sakurai A, et al. Median nerve stimulation method for severe brain damage with its clinical improvement. In: Proceedings of the 8th Annual meeting of Society of Treatment of coma. Hori S, Kanno T (eds) 1999;111–4.
42. Cooper JB, Jane JA, Alves WM, et al. Right median nerve stimulation to hasten awakening from coma. Brain Injury 1999;13:261–7.
43. Matsui T, Fujiwara S, Takahashi H, et al. Indication of electrical deep brain or dorsal column stimulation and new scoring system for prolonged impaired consciousness. J Neurosurg (Tokyo) 1998;7:14–23.
44. Yamamoto J, Fukuya J Hiramaya T, et al. Deep-brain and spinal stimulation therapy in PVS. Changes in PGD2/PGE2 and monoamine in CSF. Proceedings of 6th Annual meeting of Society of Treatment of Coma. Neuron Publishing Co.Ltd. 1993;6:63–70.
45. Ueda K, Yana gida M. Effect of music on brain in the unconscious patients. Paper presented at 8th Annual meeting of Society for Treatment of Coma. Beppu, Oita, 1999.
46. Ijichi K, Tsutsu A, Maeda T, et al. Musical exercise therapy for patients with persistent disturbance of consciousness. Presented at the 8th Annual meeting of the Society for Treatment of Coma. Beppu, Oita, 1999.
47. Maeda T. Neural mechanism of sleep. Advances in Neurological Sciences (Tokyo) 1995;39:7–15.
48. Matsumura H. Prostaglandins and sleep. Advances in Neurological Science (Tokyo) 1995;39:60–80.
49. Di Rocco C. L-dopa treatment of comatose state due to cerebral lesion. J. Neurosurg Sci 1974;7:169–76.
50. Yoshizawa T, Kikuechi H, Karasawa J, et al. Bromocryptine treatment in patients with prolonged disturbances of consciousness and mentality. Shinryo to Shinnyaku 1984;21:115–25.
51. Saitosh H, Kurisu A, Shinohara Y. Effect of Bromocryptine on patients 7 with aphasia due to cerebrovascular disease. Shinkeinaikachiryo 1991;8:543–7.
52. Nishino K. Facilitated effect of L-dopa on recovery of prolonged consciousness disturbances and motor aphasia in a patient of cerebral stroke. Prog Med 1998;18:1513–20.
53. Sitsu N. A computer assisted EEC study on Psychiatric properties of antiparkinsonian drugs. Seishin Shinkeigaku Zassi 1992;94:238–62.
54. Chrisostomo AD, Duncan PW, Propst MA. Evidence that amphetamine with physical therapy promotes recovery of motor function in stroke patients. Annl Neurol 1988;23:94–97.
55. Whyte J, Myers R. Incidence of clinically significant responses to zolpidem among patients with disorders of consciousness: a preliminary placebo controlled trial. Am J Phys Med Rehabil 2009;88(5):410–8.
56. Clauss R, Nel W. Drug induced arousal from the permanent vegetative state. Neuro Rehabilitation 2006;21(1):23–8.

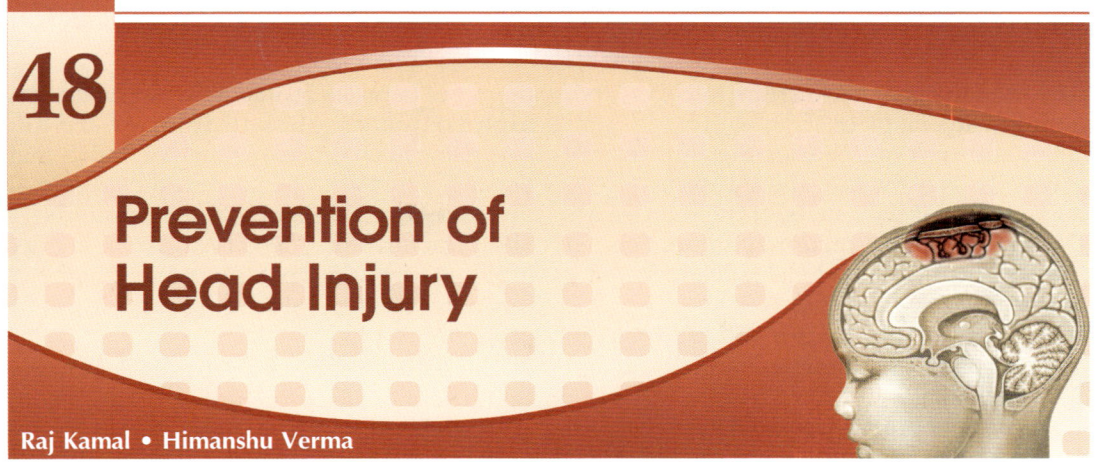

48

Prevention of Head Injury

Raj Kamal • Himanshu Verma

Head injury management places a lot of stress on the managing personnel, on the patients and their attendees. Most of the serious head injuries not only require immediate intensive management, but also long-term physical and cognitive rehabilitation. Even patients with minor head injuries suffer from significant disabling cognitive and somatic symptoms for a considerable period of time. All this causes a lot of drain on personal and national resources, a lot of psychological strain on the immediate family members and cripples the nation's work force. It thus becomes imperative that more importance should be placed at the root level itself, i.e. prevention.

The commonest cause of road traffic accidents is two-wheeler accidents. Motor bike accidents are dangerous and a motorcyclist is eight times more likely to be fatally injured than the occupant of the car on the basis of per unit distance travelled. Delhi, which has one of the heaviest traffic in the world, has recorded a phenomenal growth in the number of accidents. The number of accidents recorded in 1995 were 9216 of which 2000 were fatal in nature. The total number of accidents escalated to a total of 13000 in 1997 of which about 2176 were fatal accidents. The trend of increase in number of transport vehicles is serious and the escalation in the number of accidents places a considerable strain on the already existing meager medical facilities. The

following chapter will deal briefly on safety precautions required for head injury prevention.

CRASH INJURIES— BIOMECHANICAL ASPECTS

As early as 1949, Sergeant Elmer Paul of the Indianapolis, United States made his observations with regard to fatal accidents occurring in rural areas and indicated that many of these fatalities resulted in what he judged to be survivable crashes, and that the deaths were needlessly due to poor automotive design. Paul developed a technique of accident reporting which incorporated three basic principles: vehicle report, medical report, and pictures, a unique accomplishment in the annals of comprehensive police reporting.[1]

Moore in 1953 reported certain observations, which hold well even today.

1. In 50% of the injury producing accidents one or more doors opened during the impact.
2. Thirty percent of the occupants have been ejected, which more than doubles the risk of moderate to fatal head injury. This generally occurs even if there is 9/16 inch separation between the door and the door frame.[2]
3. Cases are hit in front in approximately 51% of the time on the right.

4. Most of the persons are hurt "all over", not simply in one place.
5. Seventy-five percent of the injuries are usually over the face and the neck.
6. Over 56% of the causes of the injuries are contributed by ejection, contact against instrument panel, windshield and steering wheel.

Most of the injuries are still hold true in India, as often the safety regulations are still not followed.

Since there are no "isolated systems" but man-machine pathomechanical combinations, it is appropriate to relate such engineering idioms to man. Several classifications of failure have been described.[2,3]

Rupture: A good example is rupture of a bone.

Buckling: This refers to eccentric compressive force applied to the edges of a plate or column, and is analogous to compression fractures of the anterior margins of the vertebral bodies due to loading applied to it in the forward position.

Excessive deformation: This is related to "whip lashing" injuries of the neck and the back. It is more easily visualized in connection with fractures and dislocations exhibiting marked displacement of fragments; and avulsive injuries of the soft parts, including internal organs and their attachments.

Stress raisers: This term refers to "non uniform surface discontinuities on the member such as screw threads, shoulders, notches, etc". The stress raiser effect is a local affair. It is illustrated by so-called pathological fractures in the bone cysts, bone atrophy and the like. Also, because of pathomechanical behavior of a joint due to disease or other acquired condition, greater forces may be transmitted to other functionally related anatomical structure. This is illustrated in the case of "flexion" fracture of the spine incident to a stiff hip.

CRASH HEAD INJURIES—MECHANISMS

Medical reports place the frequency incidence of crash head injuries of all kinds in round figures at between 50 and 80%. Among these, high frequency of skull injuries are not surprising in view of experimental studies that linear fractures can be produced by minimal input energy levels of 400 inch pounds.[4–6] Skull fractures may also result from energy input as low as 50 inch pounds, if the head impacts an unyielding sharp edge or projection.

The skull is a spheroid structure containing semiliquid contents including brain, blood, and cerebrospinal fluid. This closed cavity feature of the head is a major consideration.[4–6] The cranial dura is intimately attached to the inner aspect of the skull. At the craniospinal junction however, the dura and the bone are not intimately apposed. For this reason, large deformations can occur which tend to prevent a pressure build-up in the spinal canal.

However, a sudden increase in intracranial pressure results in pressure gradients through the regions of the brainstem and cerebellum in the direction of the foramen magnum.[5,6]

Linear fractures produced in the drop tests arise from the failure of the bone because of the tensile strain in the outer surface of the skull. The fracture is initiated some distance from the site of the impact and then propagates both toward and away from the impact site. The fracture line propagates toward the site of impact because at the instant of impact the area of inbending is actually under compression. The rebounding of the bone creates tensile strain with its greatest magnitude at the centre of the impact area. From this centre point onwards the tensile strain decreases rapidly in all directions.[7,8]

Role of Physicians in Accident Prevention

The physician's responsibility becomes very important in evaluating the person's fitness for driving. This medical point of view is significant in view of these three basic propositions.

1. *Human failure overshadows all other factors in the production of highway accidents:* Accident causation is rooted in basic interaction

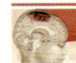

between the driver, highway and the vehicle. Paradoxically enough automation, push button and other inventions designed to offer greater ease of driving do not eliminate the need to exert vigilance and split second timing to manoeuvre these vehicles in traffic with efficiency and safety. On the contrary, the driver must be in proper physical and mental condition to safely control and manoeuvre modern responsive high-speed vehicles. There can be no doubt that poor judgement, lack of physical ability, including impairment of sense organs are responsible for accidents.

2. *Human failure may stem from abnormal physiological states, pathological states, pathological conditions, emotional disturbances and the use of drugs and alcohol.* It is not always easy to ascertain the physical, mental, emotional or physiological impairments of an individual. It is, therefore, not always easy to arrive at a decision in these cases where possible and probable deterrents to safe driving practices may exist. Few patients realise that small amounts of alcohol is required to impair dangerously, the driving ability and almost 50% of fatal motor accidents occur because of alcohol.

3. *The key to ultimate success in motor-vehicle accident prevention lies in the driver.* This means his intelligence, his sense of personal and social responsibility, his reactions to various stimuli in normal conditions and under stress, his ability in good health and in illness. The medical and other implications in regard to driver screening for licensure are obvious, but cannot be overstated, particularly in the domains of his psychosomatic mechanical capabilities. There is a real need to improve the medical and related standards for driver licensing, including civilian, commercial vehicle and public transportation vehicles.

Prevention of Head Injuries in Two-wheeler Occupants

Use of crash helmets is useful in reducing head injury in two-wheeler riders.[9–13] The ICMR head injury study, conducted at AHMS, during 1977–79 showed either lack of use or improper use of helmet leading to head injury.

Motorized two-wheeled vehicles (MTV) constitute a large portion of the vehicle fleet in India.

Fitzharris et al[14] reported the crash characteristics and injury patterns among a cohort of MTV riders and pillions presenting to hospital post-crash. 378 MTV users were enrolled to the study of whom two-thirds were males. The majority (77%) were assessed as having a Glasgow Coma Score (GCS) of 13–15, 12% a GCS of 9–12 and 11% a GCS of 3–8. No difference was seen in the severity distribution of injuries based on GCS among riders and pillions. Open wounds and superficial injuries to the head (69.3%) and upper extremity (27%) and lower extremity (24%) were the most common injuries. Forty-three (11%) sustained an intracranial injury, including 12 (28%) with associated fracture of the bones of the head. There were a few differences in types of injuries sustained by riders and pillions though riders had a significantly lower risk of crush injuries of the lower extremity than pillions (relative risk, RR 0.25, 95% CI 0.08–0.81) and female pillions were at a significantly lower risk of sustaining fractures of the lower extremity than male pillions (RR 0.30, 95% CI 0.09–0.94). Overall, 42 (11%) MTV users died, of which 42.8% died before reaching the hospital.[14] Only 74 (19.6%) MTV users had worn a helmet correctly and failure to wear a helmet was associated with a five times greater risk of intracranial injury (RR 4.99, 95% CI 1.23–20.1). Of the 19 pre-hospital deaths, 16 (84%) had not worn a helmet. Head injuries accounted for the major proportion of injuries sustained in MTV users. **Non-helmet use was associated with increased risk of serious head injuries.** The data presented on the nature and severity of injuries sustained by MTV users can assist with planning to deal with these consequences as well as prevention of these injuries given the high use of MTV in India.[14]

A study from South Australia[12,13] had shown that 38% two-wheeler victims did not use helmet, another 54% used only poorly designed helmets and only 8% victims had used a proper crash helmet. Prospective study at AIIMS during 1981–1982, on two-wheeler accidents had revealed improper use of poorly designed helmets.

Cochrane data base study in 2008[15] concludes that; It seems intuitive that helmets should protect against head injuries but it has been argued that motorcycle helmet use decreases rider vision and increases neck injuries. **Motorcycle helmets reduce the risk of death and head injury in motorcycle riders who crash.** Further well-conducted research is required to determine the effects of helmets and different helmet types on mortality, head, neck and facial injuries. However, the findings suggest that global efforts to reduce road traffic injuries may be facilitated by increasing helmet use by motorcyclists.

Prevention of head injury in two-wheeler accidents is centered on the use of the helmet. In 1970, a Legislation passed in Queensland, Australia made the use of crash helmet compulsory.

In Delhi, the use of helmet was introduced in mid-seventies, which to some extent reduced the severe head injury in two-wheeler riders. Furthermore, with the widespread use of helmets has eventually led to difference in helmet design and production. Vaughan[13] discussed the use of various types of helmets. Original standard helmet (resembled a building site hat) offered much less protection. A jet helmet (resembling a pilot helmet) does not provide facial and lower jaw protection. The newer full-face helmet is more ideal and reduces the chance of facial injury. The use of jet helmet predisposes to facial injury, which not only disfigures the face but also may cause airway impairment.

Use of helmet for the pillion rider must be enforced, as such rules are not yet imposed in most of the cities in India (Fig. 48.2). A large number of pillion riders are exposed to vehicular injury, as they do not use a helmet. Recently, more concern has been placed in the use of helmets in two-wheelers. In the US, 400,000 people are injured due to cycle accidents every year and about 1000 die[20] among the victims, over 70% are children and maximum incidence of bicycle injury has been reported from New York.[21] Although the official figures are not available in India, the figures are expected to be similar, especially in the metropolitan cities.

Cochrane data base study in 2010[17] concludes that riding a motorcycle (a two-wheeled vehicle that is powered by a motor and has no pedals) is associated with a **high risk of fatal crashes, particularly in new riders.** Motorcycle rider training has therefore been suggested as an important means of reducing the number of crashes, and the severity of injuries. The findings suggest that mandatory pre-licence training may be an impediment to completing a motorcycle licensing process, possibly indirectly reducing crashes through a reduction in exposure. It is not clear if training (or what type) reduces the risk of crashes, injuries or offences in motorcyclists, and a best rider training practice can, therefore, not be recommended.

Prevention of Head Injuries in Car Occupants

With the introduction of small, low budget cars and many middle class families are also opting for four-wheelers, it is thus imperative that accidents involving cars and other four-wheelers will also escalate. The use of following measures will lower the incidence of car accidents.

1. Use of Seat Belts for Both Drivers and Passengers

This considerably reduces both the incidences of serious and fatal injuries (Fig. 48.1). Studies have shown that wearing seat belts prevents serious acceleration-deceleration and dashboard injuries like facial injuries, compressive chest injuries, hip joint dislocation and patellar and tibial fractures.[16]

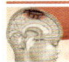

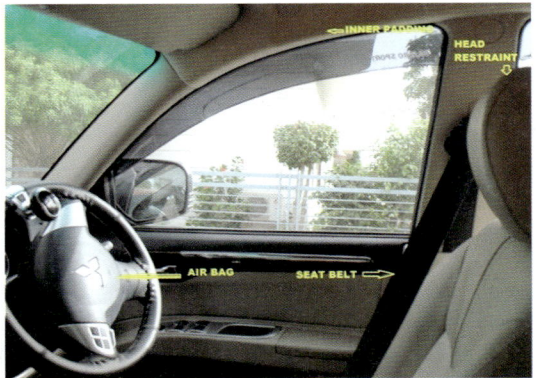

Fig. 48.1: Various measures to lower the severity of head injury for occupants of car

2. *Padding the Upper Interior of the Passenger Compartment*

a. Head injuries to car occupants resulting from crashes on Australian roads are a major cause of death and permanent brain damage. This report by McLean et al[18] **evaluates the benefits that would be likely to accrue from the use of padding materials to reduce the severity of impacts to the head.** A review of the international literature was conducted to examine the range of possible countermeasures, with particular reference to padding the upper interior of the passenger compartment. Three sets of data analyses were then carried out: first, a summary of objects typically struck by the head in a representative sample of crashes; secondly, an examination of actual brain injuries sustained in a sample of crashes, and an assessment of likely outcomes had the objects struck by the head been padded; and finally, a harm analysis to estimate the cost of head injuries and the likely financial benefits from various countermeasures. Harm analysis is a metric which estimates the societal cost of given injury taking into account the frequency with which that injury occurs as well as treatment, rehavilitation, loss of earnings, pain and suffering costs of injury. Results indicate that there is considerable potential for reducing the severity and consequences of impacts to the head by padding the upper interior of the passenger compartment.

b. *Car mechanics.* Use of other modern safety constructs and gadgets in the car, for instance **the presence of crumple zone, high impact side beams, high tensile steel grinders for the passenger cabin, collapsible steering and auto-inflatable balloons significantly reduce the incidence of severe and fatal head injuries.**

c. *Other measures.* These include:
- The use of speed limits near school, institutional and hospital zones.
- The proper placement of speed breakers, and the proper installation of traffic signals.
- **Good quality roads, use of parallel roads for different vehicular speeds, use of road dividers and "on the spot fines for traffic violaters".**
- Enforcement of education at school and college levels for following traffic rules and inducting a sense of moral responsibility in following a safe traffic conduct.

Prevention in Sports

American Medical Society for Sports Medicine[19] concluded that primary prevention of some injuries may be possible with modification and enforcement of the rules and fair play. **Helmets, both hard (football, lacrosse and hockey) and soft (soccer, Rugby) are best suited to prevent impact injuries (fracture, bleeding, laceration, etc.) but have not been shown to reduce the incidence and severity of concussions** (Fig. 48.2). There is no current evidence that mouth guards can reduce the severity of or prevent concussions. Secondary prevention may be possible by appropriate RTP management. Legislative efforts provide a uniform standard for scholastic and non-scholastic sports organizations regarding concussion safety and management.

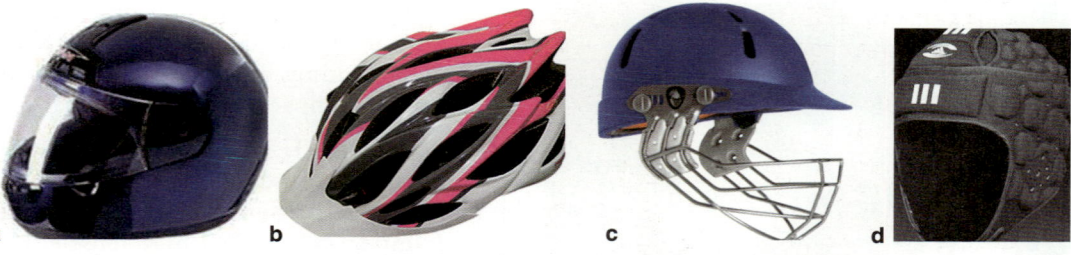

a   b   c   d

Fig. 48.2: Helmets to prevent head injury. (a) Two-wheeler helmet; (b) Bike helmet; (c) Sports helmet (cricket) and (d) Rugby helmet

CONCLUSIONS

Head injuries account for one quarter to one-third of all trauma deaths. But of deaths that occur in patients, who reach hospitals, two-thirds are due to head injuries. Of greater concern is that these head injuries are the commonest cause of lifelong disability after trauma. There is an interesting paradox in the amount of knowledge people have about spinal injuries and how little one tends to hear about permanent disability after head injury, in fact 40 times more common. In a study from UK, about 200 patients arriving in a neuro-surgical unit in coma from head injury, one-third arrived without any care of the airway at all, and lying flat on their backs. This is a common scene in our emergency rooms in India.

In terms of disability, we have lost years of work, not only by the patient but also often by the family, a member of which has often given up work or sold land, property, etc. to support the permanently disabled family member. It is the right time that we focus our attention on **injury prevention.**

REFERENCES

1. Kulowski J. Crash injuries: The integrated medical aspects of automobile injuries and deaths. Illinois, Springfield, 1960.
2. Plant HF. Fractures of the atlas resulting from automobile accidents. Am J Roentgenol 1938; 40:867.
3. Platt FN. Highway transportation problems, organization and evaluation. Traffic Quarterly 1957;64–82.
4. Gurdjian ES, Webster JE. Experiences in the surgical management of intracranial crash injuries. Surg Gyanec and Obst 1957;104:205.
5. Gurdjian ES, Webster JE. Trauma of the Central Nervous System, Baltimore, William and Wilkins, 1945.
6. Gurdjian ES. Acute brain injuries. Surgery 1943;13:333.
7. Evan FG. Stress and Strain in Bones, Springfield, Thomas, 1957.
8. Evans JP. Acute Head injuries, Springfield, Thomas, 1950.
9. Harrington T. Helmet, Head injury and Motorcycles. Ariz Med 1984;41:802–4.
10. Krantz KP. Head and neck injury to motorcycle and moped riders with special regards to effect of protective helmets. Injury 1985;16:253–8.
11. Motorcycle injury and crash helmet (Editorial). Brit Med J 1985;1:1491–2.
12. Jamieson KG, Kelly DA. Med J Aust 1973;2: 806–88.
13. Vaughan RG. Med J Aust 1977;1:125.
14. Fitzharris M, Dandona R, Kumar GA, Dandona L. Crash characteristics and patterns of injury among hospitalized motorised two-wheeled vehicle users in urbanIndia. BMC Public Health 2009;12;9:11.
15. Liu BC, Ivers R, Norton R, Boufous S, Blows S, Lo SK. Helmets for preventing injury in motor-cycle riders. Cochrane Database Syst Rev 2008; (1):CD004333.
16. Callahan D. Legislating Safety—How far one should go? (Editorial). N Eng J Med 1981;320: 1412–3.

17. Kardamanidis K, Martiniuk A, Ivers RQ, Stevenson MR, Thistlethwaite K. Motorcycle rider training for the prevention of road traffic crashes.Cochrane Database Syst Rev 2010 Oct 6;(10):CD005240. doi: 10.1002/14651858. CD005240.pub2.

18. McLean J, Fildes BN, Craig Norman K, Digges KH Anderson, Robert William Gerard, Vivienne Marie M, Simpson, Donald A. Prevention of head injuries to car occupants: an investigation of interior padding options, Federal Office of Road Safety, Transport and Communiations, 1997.

19. Harmon KG, Drezner JA, Gammons M, Guskiewicz KM, Halstead M, Herring SA, Kutcher JS, Pana A, Putukian M, Roberts WO. American Medical Society for Sports Medicine position statement: concussion in sport. Br J Sports Med 2013;47(1):15–26.

20. Fredricks RH. Safety in automotive transportation: Presented to American Association of Motor Vehicle Administrators (AAMVA). Detroit, Mich, June 23rd 1988.

21. Bader M. Helmet for child bicyclists (letter-comments), JAMA 1990;26:1914–5.

49

Newer Trends in Management of Neurotrauma

D Gupta • AK Mahapatra

CEREBRAL MICRODIALYSIS IN TRAUMATIC BRAIN INJURY

Traumatic brain injury is a major cause of mortality and morbidity, with long lasting social and economic consequences. Largely, the prognosis is dependent on the non-modifiable factors such as initial injury severity, Glasgow Coma Score, pupillary response, age and presence of additional physiological derangements such as hypoxia or hypotension. However, secondary insults continue to take place after initial injury and resuscitation. Most commonly, the factors implicated are increased intracranial pressure, reduced cerebral perfusion pressure and derangements in cerebral autoregulation and brain oximetry.[1,2] Various studies have linked the above parameters to outcome in TBI. Recent evidence supports the use of these parameters for guiding neurocritical care and optimization may influence neurological recovery.

Cerebral microdialysis is an established tool for neurochemical research in the neuro-intensive care unit.[3] When combined with various other monitoring methods it provides unique insight into the biochemical and physiological derangements in brain injury. Microdialysis data available at the bedside allows real time assessment of brain bioenergetics, amino acid release and membrane integrity, all of which are implicated in

traumatic brain injury. Many investigators have shown following traumatic brain injury, the tissue at greatest risk of secondary brain injury is the pericontusional tissue. The same tissue, therefore, holds the maximum potential for salvage. Detection and prevention of these secondary injuries are a major target of intensive neuromonitoring. Microdialysis by providing real time data for detection of pathophysiological events should guide targeted therapy and intervention to prevent secondary brain injury. With continuous monitoring, it should also be able to allow assessment of response to therapy.

Like other organs the volume regulation of the brain is mainly determined by mechanisms controlling the fluid exchange across the capillaries. Regarding these mechanisms, the brain differs from other organs in its highly sophisticated semipermeable capillary membrane function: the blood–brain barrier (BBB). In addition to its other physiological functions the BBB is the most important regulator of cerebral volume. Along with volume regulation of the brain tissue, the physiological regulation of cerebrospinal fluid (CSF), CBF, and cerebral blood volume (CBV) determines the intracranial dynamics.[4]

As the brain and its surroundings are enclosed within a rigid shell an increase in volume of one of the components leads to an increase in ICP unless compensated by one of the other constituents. This simple relationship is often referred to as the Monro-Kellie doctrine. All surgical and non-surgical treatments of increased ICP are directed towards a change in volume of one or more of these components. The surgical treatments to decrease the intracranial volumes include evacuation of mass lesions, drainage of CSF or decompressive craniectomy. TBI is frequently exacerbated by secondary events that lead to secondary brain injury, which is a potentially modifiable cause of mortality and morbidity after TBI. Secondary injury to the brain occurs after activation by the primary injury of a cascade of metabolic, immunological and biochemical changes that render the brain more susceptible to secondary physiological insults and ultimately result in irreversible cell damage or death. These pathological processes lead to failing cellular metabolism, calcium overload, and increased production of free

radicals and release of neurotoxic levels of excitatory amino acids. If unchecked, these changes cause cellular swelling, increases in intracranial pressure (ICP) and further neuronal loss resulting in increased mortality and worsened outcome in survivors. Treatment of TBI during neurointensive care is focussed at preventing or minimizing the burden of secondary injury.[2,3]

Clinical microdialysis has been documented to be useful for biochemical monitoring of almost any region of the body tissue namely brain, lung, heart, liver, kidney, intraperitoneal/intrauterine, head and neck , breast tissue, subcutaneous tissue, intestine, intracutaneous, bone tissue (Fig. 49.1).

- *Energy metabolism markers:* Glucose, lactate, pyruvate, glutamate, glyecerol
- *Excitotoxicity markers:* Glutamate (aspartate)
- *Increased ATP utilization markers:* Adenosine, inosine, hypoxanthine

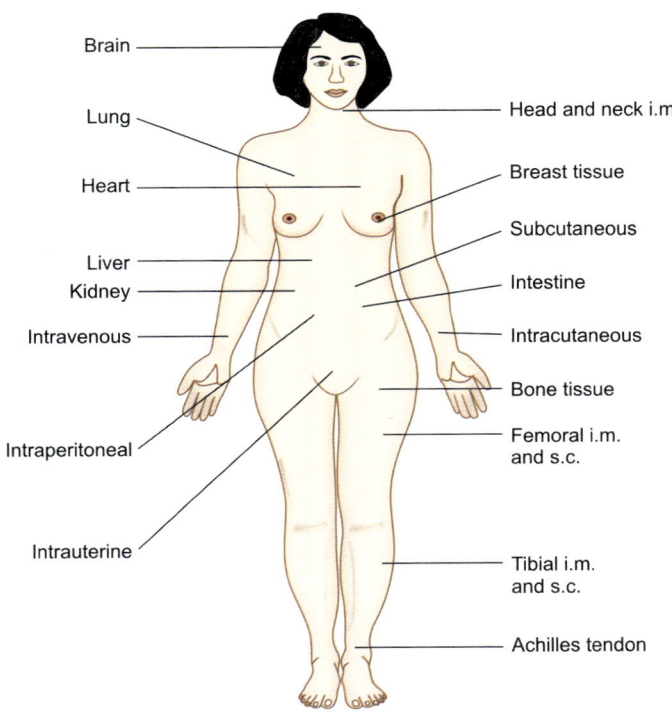

Fig. 49.1: Clinical uses of microdialysis

- *Reactive oxygen species (ROS):* Xanthine, ascorbate, glutathione
- *Nitric oxide (NO) formation:* Nitrite, nitrate, citrulline/arginine
- *Neurotransmitter release:* Glutamate, GABA, glycine, NA, DA, 5HT
- *Cellular swelling:* Taurine, K^+
- *Ionic perturbations:* Sodium, calcium, magnesium
- *Other amino acids/metabolites:* Serine, DOPAC, HVA, 5HIAA
- *BBB leakage:* Alanine, valine, leucine
- *Inflammation/neurotrophins:* IL-1beta, IL-6, GFAP, NGF
- Besides, one can also study drug pharmaco-kinetics with microdialysis technique.

Cerebral microdialysis is a tool for exploring the biochemical changes occurring in the brain leading to secondary brain injury following trauma. It is a technique for continuous sampling of interstitial fluid chemistry of tissue/organ. It commonly measures markers of ischemia, energy breakdown and cell damage. Microdialysis catheters permit recovery of small samples of ECF from vital organs, the samples are diffused over 20 kD dialysis membrane to elimite large molecules. The exact role that cerebral microdialysis plays is currently unclear and this study aims at defining the role. Several studies in the recent past have supported the use of cerebral microdialysis in neurointensive care units as an adjunct for monitoring.

At the focus is bedside monitoring of glucose, lactate, pyruvate, glycerol and glutamate although many other parameters have been studied. Glucose, lactate and pyruvate provide information about the bioenergetics of the brain tissue. Glutamate is measured to gauge the excitatory milieu of the tissue. Glycerol is released from cell membrane breakdown and indicated cellular injury.

Why Monitor Organ Chemistry?

Microdialysis analyses metabolism of specific tissue rather than systemic blood and there is no need to measure organ specific metabolites and so one gets direct measure of tissue damage/ischemia directly from organ itself, continously, bedside instead of one time study (MRI, CT, PET).

There exists a window of opportunity from organ chemistry change to manifestion of clinical signs which varies between organs to organs. The placement of a microdialysis catheter into tissue of an organ at risk allows the physician to monitor bedside the profound biochemical changes that occur before and during an ischemic event.[4-6] In order to make effective use of microdialysis data it is essential to relate them to other data collected bedside. This may be done by software, which allows for integrating data from the microdialysis analyzer, the ICU monitor displaying ICP (intracranial pressure) and CPP (cerebral perfusion pressure), a tissue oxygen analyzer, the ventilator, the infusion pumps, etc. This "multimodal monitoring" allows for the display of all data as trend curves on one computer screen. It creates the framework for individualizing therapy on the basis of clinical status, brain tissue chemistry and the effect of therapeutic interventions.

Principles of Microdialysis

The microdialysis catheter takes up substances delivered by the blood, e.g. glucose and drugs, but also substances released from the cells, e.g. markers of cellular metabolism. The interstitial fluid is the "cross road" of all substances passing between cells and blood capillaries. By monitoring this compartment in the brain it is possible to get crucial information about the biochemistry of neurons and glia and how seriously brain cells are affected by, e.g. ischemia, hyperemia, trauma, hemorrhage, vasospasm as well as various physiological, pharmacological and surgical interventions during intensive care. Although microdialysis samples essentially all small molecular substances present in the interstitial fluid the use of microdialysis in neurointensive care has focused on markers of ischemia, energy break down and cell damage. The reason is that they are of obvious importance for the survival of the tissue, well understood from a biochemical point of view and easy to interpret in the clinical setting of intensive care (Fig. 49.2).

Microdialysis tells us how cells react to an increase or decrease in the supply of oxygen and glucose. However, while normal brain tissue may not suffer when exposed to a moderate decrease in oxygen and glucose, vulnerable cells in the pericontusional penumbra may simply not survive. In this way severe secondary damage to brain tissue may pass unnoticed if microdialysis is not performed in the most vulnerable tissue of the brain.

Microdialysis technique microdialysis probes (molecular weight cut off of 20 kDa, 10 mm membrane, CMA-70, CMA microdialysis) are usually placed in the perilesional tissue (during decompressive craniectomy or by making burr hole percutaneous technique. The probes is perfused with CNS perfusion fluid at 3 μl/minute (P000151, CMA microdialysis), and samples collected every hour. Concentrations of glucose, lactate, pyruvate, glutamate and glycerol in the micro dialysate is analyzed using the CMA-ISCUS flex microdialysis analyzer. Microdialysis catheter is usually kept in place for five days (Figs 49.3 to 49.7).

Microdialysis catheter forms a "biosensor" where samples of the tissue chemistry transported out of body for analysis c.f. traditional biosensor where analysis takes place inside body. The availability of modern analytical techniques has made microdialysis a "universal" biosensor capable of monitoring essentially every small and medium sized molecular compound in the interstitial fluid of endogenous as well as exogenous origin.

Artificial CSF is slowly pumped into the microdialysis probe using a microsyringe pump capable of pumping very low volume of fluids. Probes wall is semipermeable to small molecules which diffuse from extracellular space of the brain into the dialysate fluid. The analyte molecule diffuses through the extracellular space and ultimately the collected analyte can be analyzed.

A microdialysis catheter consists of a fine double lumen probe, lined at its tip with a semipermeable dialysis membrane. The probe tip is placed into biological tissue and perfused via an inlet tube with fluid isotonic to the tissue interstitium. The perfusate passes along the membrane before exiting via outlet tubing into a collecting chamber. Diffusion drives the passage of molecules across the membrane along with their concentration gradient.

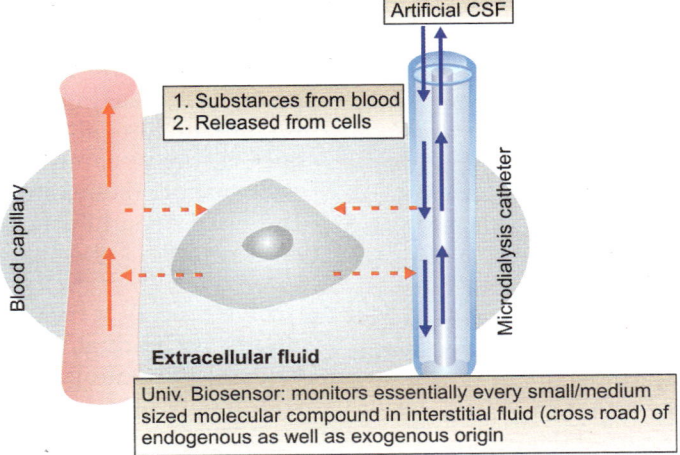

Fig. 49.2: Principle of microdialysis showing artificial CSF being pumped in via MD catheters and substances released in ECF being subsequently collected for analysis by MD catheters

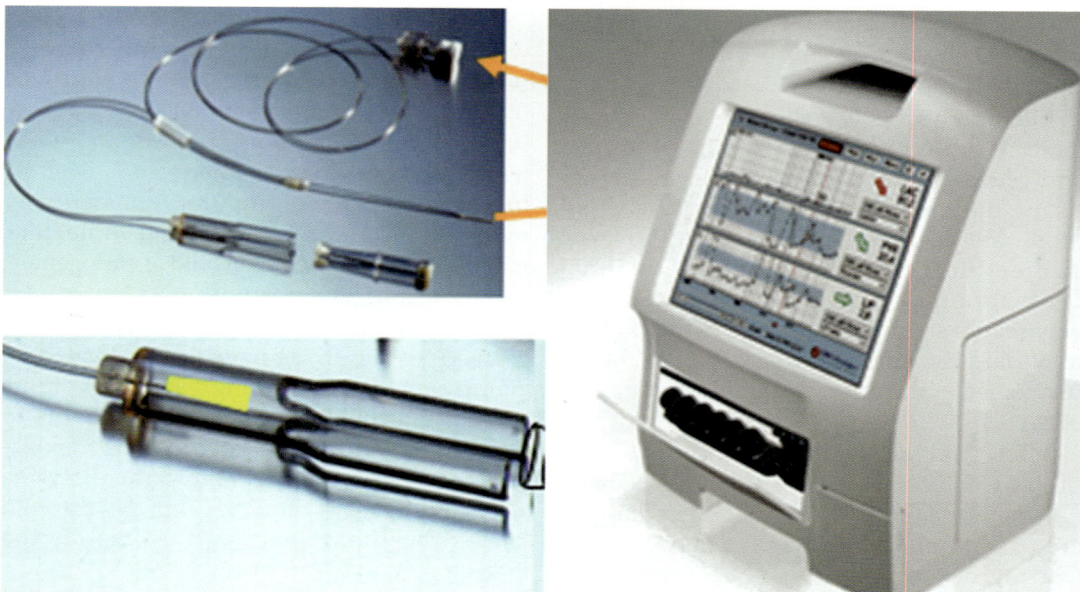

Fig. 49.3: Microdialysis analyzer and catheter assembly with luer-lock system and microvials (yellow arrow head)

Molecules at high concentration in the brain ECF pass into the perfusate with minimum passage of water and, as the perfusate flows and is removed at a constant rate, the concentration gradient is maintained. The MD catheter therefore acts an artificial blood capillary and the concentration of substrate in the collected fluid (microdialysate) will depend in part on the balance between substrate delivery to, and uptake/excretion from, the ECF. The most commonly used system comprises a catheter that is 10 mm in length with a 20 kDa (CMA-70, CMA/microdialysis) or 100 kDa (CMA-71, CMA/microdialysis) molecular weight cutoff, perfused with commercially available perfusate solution (perfusion fluid CNS, CMA/microdialysis) at a rate of 0.3 ml/min. This simple concept provides a powerful technique with many potential applications in which any molecule small enough to pass across the membranecan be sampled (Fig. 49.4).

Data analysis is done at bedside by using TLC method (noting trend, level and comparison of various biochemical variables at differnet sites (penumbra zone and contralateral hemisphere). A graphic plot of these values can be seen and compared in temporal pattern with other parameters (intraparenchymal pressure, cerebral perfusion pressure, mean arterial blood pressure) simultaneously by using special software (ICU pilot, Lab pilot) based on which clinican can easily note a trend and take a decision to target various therapeutics options (increasing cerebral perfusion pressure, minimizing ICP, volume pressure support, using cerebral protectants) in a timely manner (in therapeutic or biochemical window of opportunity) much ahead of ICP rise or neurological deterioration (Fig. 49.5).

Glucose is metabolized aerobically by glycolysis and TCA cycle to produce CO_2 and water in the normal brain tissue. A shift to anaerobic metabolism may occur from hypoxia or ischemia.

Interpretation

Lactate concentration and lactate/pyruvate ratio are good indicators of anaerobic

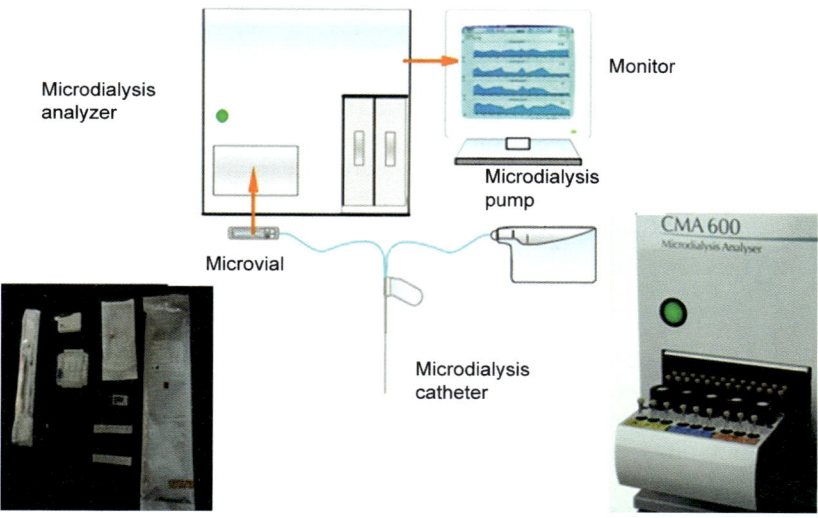

Fig. 49.4: Microdialysis clinical system

metabolism. Episodes of ischemia thus can be well documented using cerebral microdialysis and impact of bioenergetics derangement measured.[7] Recent studies indicate that rise in L/P ratio may not be as specific as thought earlier and increments unrelated to ischemia are common. Two patterns of L/P ratio increased have been thus described. Type I indicating a classical ischemic state with increased lactate and reduced pyruvate. Type II describes a pattern with reduced pyruvate as the predominant feature occurring with limited glucose supply or impairment of glycolysis.

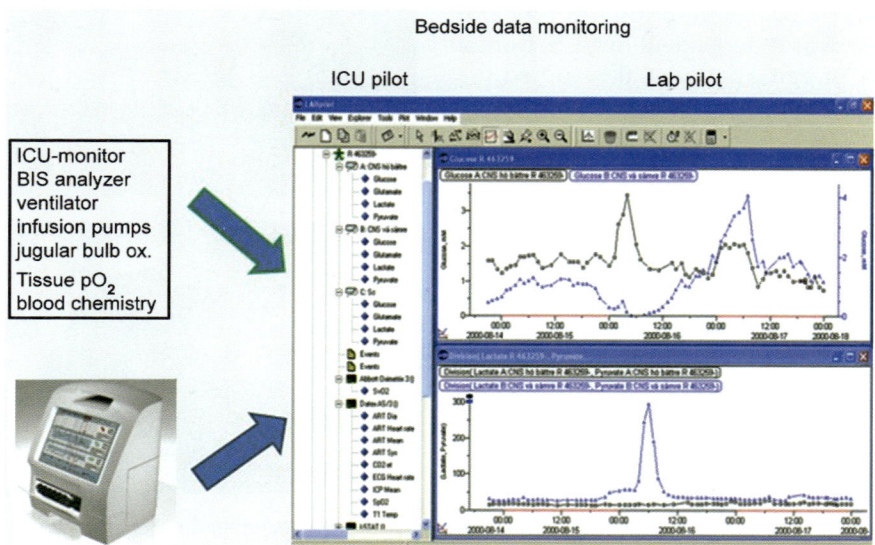

Fig. 49.5: Software used for data analysis in microdialysis (bedside installed in ICU)

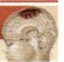

Outcome in Head Injury

Glycerol results from enzymatic degradation of the cell membrane. There is some concern over validity of glycerol as a useful marker due to doubts about formation of glycerol form glucose and spill over from systemic circulation. Recently Clausen et al[8] concluded that glycerol did not provide prognostic significance and more research was needed to validate its use.

Glutamate is a major excitatory amino acid in the brain. Uncontrolled release occurs in TBI, but it is a relatively late indicator of cerebral dysfunction. As astrocyte conversion of glutamate to glutamine is energy dependent, ischemia may lead to low glutamine/glutamate values. Microdialysis has shown good correlation between L/P values and glutamine/glutamate values. Belli et al[9] reported that a L/P ratio >25 and flycerol >100 μ/L were associated with high risk if ICP rise, but glutamate >12 μmol/L was not predictive. These changes occurred before the onset of ICP rise, suggesting that biochemical derangement occurred earlier than other derangements and may act as early warning signs. This may aid in earlier institution of therapy. Marcoux et al[10] reported that L/P ratio in first 4 days following injury was predictive of frontal brain atrophy at 6 months and was independent of GCS, frontal lobe injury or age. Hlatky et al[11] studied the evolution of TBI in 33 patients with severe TBI.

They showed a classical ischemic pattern with markedly raised L/P ratio, glutamate and reduced glucose in patients with fatal refractory intracranial hypertension. Hillered et al suggested a new protocol to inculcate cerebral microdialysis as a clinical tool. It defined a cut off value of L/P ratio > 30 and microdialysis glucose < 0.8 mmol/L for considering a re-assessment of the clinical status and new CT scan (if needed).

Studies have shown that the tissue at greatest risk following TBI is the perilesional tissue. It thereby also holds the potential for greatest salvage. Microdialysis probe placement in this perilesional tissue may thus be of maximum clinical importance (Figs 49.8 and 49.9). Probes placed directly in the contusional tissue shows severe biochemical derangements indicative of irreversible damage. In 2004, a conference for consensus on microdialysis recommended its use along with ICP, CPP monitoring. It advocated the use of glucose, pyruvate, lactate, glycerol and glutamate as markers. The probe placement

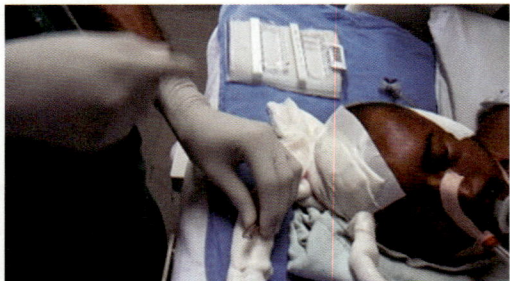

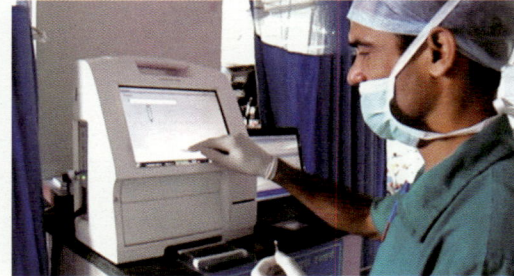

Fig. 49.7: Nursing staff collecting microvial samples from patient and checking for MD values from machine

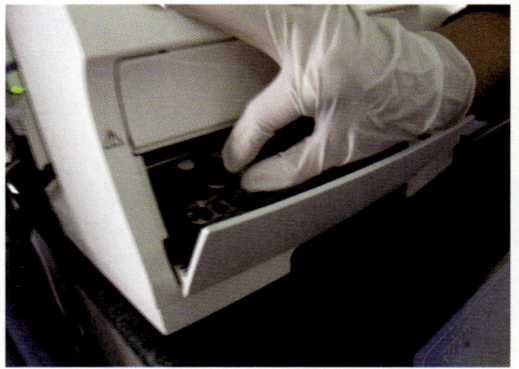

Fig. 49.6: Nursing staff putting the microvials in microdialysis analyzer machine

Focal hemorrhagic contusion

One microdialysis catheter is placed in the contralateral hemisphere

One microdialysis catheter is placed in the penumbra of the contusion

One microdialysis catheter is placed outside the penumbra

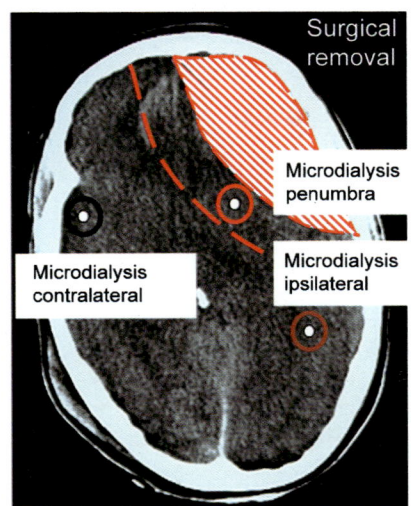

Surgical removal

Microdialysis penumbra

Microdialysis contralateral

Microdialysis ipsilateral

Fig. 49.8: Placement of microdialysis catheters in different regions of brain

was suggested for perilesional tissue and in case of diffuse injury into the right frontal lobe (Bellander et al 2004).[3] In 2008, another conference did not give specific recommendation but acknowledged its scientific validity. The absence of class I trials demonstrating its utility was highlighted (NICEM consensus, 2008).[4]

Experienced at AIIMS, Delhi

In a observational study of 20 cases of severe traumatic brain injury who had microdialysis monitoring at JPNATC (unpublished), we have demonstrated a relationship between cerebral extracellular biochemical markers measured with microdialysis and neurological outcome following TBI. We have observed that in patients with poor outcome (GOS 3 or less), the microdialysis parameters have been consistently abnormal, whereas, in patients with good outcome (GOS 4 or 5), the same parameters have been within normal limits. We also have found correlation of low CPP with abnormal microdialysis parameters and poor outcome (Fig. 49.10).

Lactate/Pyruvate Ratio

The L/P ratio is a balance between lactate and pyruvate reflecting the state of cerebral

oxidative metabolism and is known as a sensitive marker of cerebral ischemia.[3] Microdialysis—L/P ratio has been reported to be an independent positive predictor of poor outcome in a large cohort of TBI patients.[5] In, our study, we have found that those patients, who had poor outcome, in terms of GOS of 1, had persistently high and abnormal values of L/P ratio, as compared to those with more favorable outcome (GOS 3–5). The lactate/pyruvate ratio reflects the metabolic state, and the elevation of lactate/pyruvate ratio may reflect the presence of either mitochondrial dysfunction[6] or lack of tissue level oxygen supply, due to ischemia or hypoxia.[7] Studies have used different L/P ratio threshold levels of cerebral ischemia ranging from 25 to 40.[12–15] However, in our study, we have considered 25 as the cut off value. In the present series, we have seen that elevated L/P ratio is a marker of poor outcome, irrespective of other hitherto usually monitored bedside parameters, like ICP and CPP. However, low CPP had a correlation with elevated L/P ratio.

Glutamate

Glutamate is the main excitatory transmitter of the central nervous system. After glutamate is released from the presynaptic cleft it binds

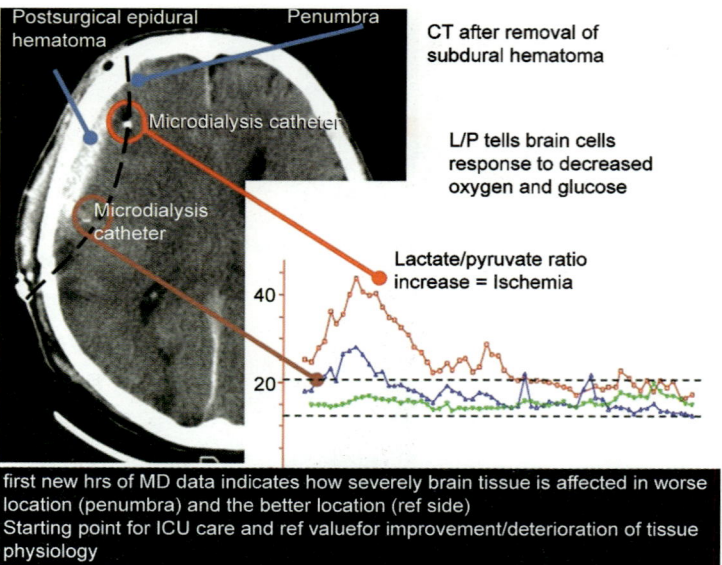

Fig. 49.9: Lab values obtained by microdialysis with a catheter placed in penumbra zone showing high LP ratio suggestive of ischemia

to postsynaptic ligand-gated ion channels which lead to excitation through depolarization. In a healthy brain it is actively taken up by neurons and astrocytes after it is released in the synaptic cleft. Excitatory amino acid transporters and cell membrane bound are responsible for the removal of the glutamate from the interstitial space in order to terminate synaptic transmission and to reduce glutamate levels before it increases to neurotoxic levels. During energy failure or ischemia the transporters responsible for glutamate uptake can be impaired or even reversed, and therefore, can release the glutamate instead of its uptake.[15] If glutamate becomes excessive the target neuron will die and such glutamate induced cell death is called excitotoxicity. Thus, increased interstitial glutamate levels can be used for detection of impaired cerebral metabolism and impending cell damage.[16] Increased brain interstitial MD-glutamate has been reported in TBI studies.[17] A clinical TBI study identified MD-glutamate as a sensitive and early marker of cerebral ischemia.[17] A positive correlation has been demonstrated in TBI patients between high levels of MD-glutamate and increased ICP and poor outcome.[18] The basal interstitial glutamate concentration in humans ranges between 5 and 15 µmol/L.[19,20] In our study, we have considered 10 µmol/L as the normal threshold. We have seen that in those patients with GOS of 1 the glutamate level has been persistently above 10 µmol/L and in those patients with more favorable outcome (GOS 3–5), the same has been well below the threshold level.

CONCLUSION

Extracellular cerebral metabolic markers are independently associated with outcome following TBI with the lactate/pyruvate ratio and glutamate level being consistent predictors at the thresholds of approximately 25 and 10 µmol/L respectively. In future, this may usher a paradigm shift in the line of management of traumatic brain injury from currently practiced ICP-targeted therapy towards achieving cellular metabolic homeostasis, thereby ensuring better outcome. Microdialysis in the ICU allows early and clearly interpretable evidence of changes in organ metabolism to permit better patient management. It

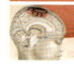

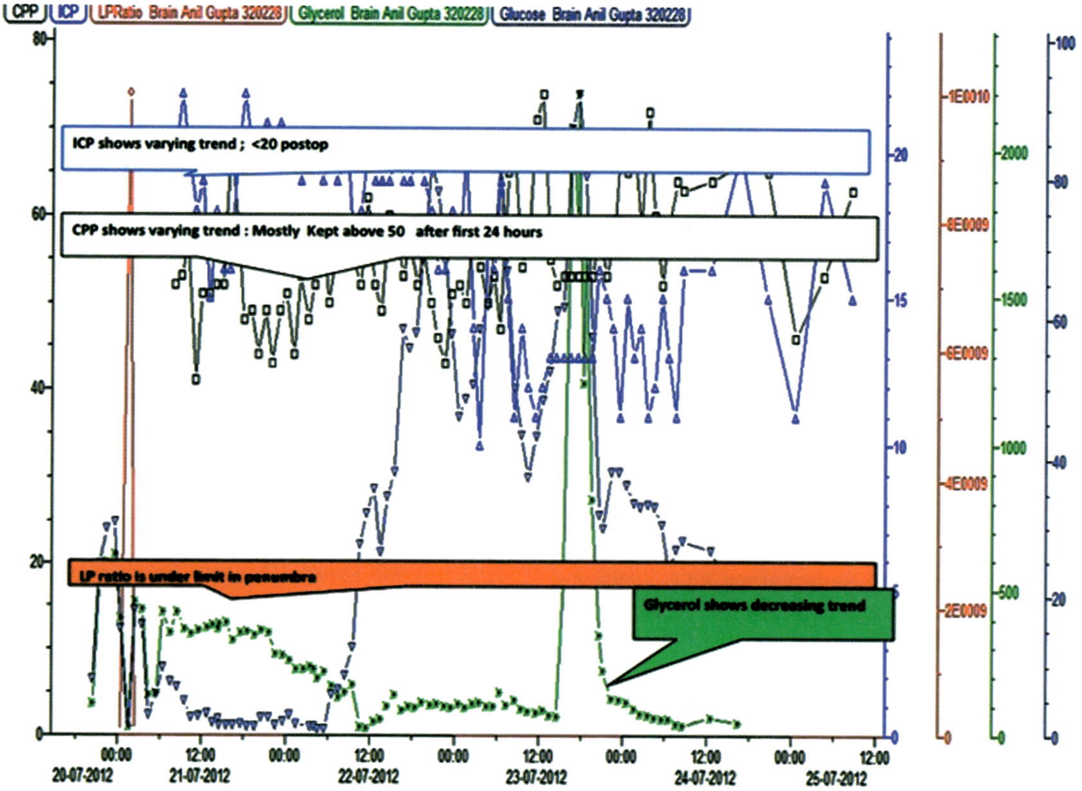

Fig. 49.10: Trend of various biochemical parameters, ICP, CPP all plotted in one single graph

permits an evaluation of the effects of patient treatment changes in ICU. It can also test new drug effectivity. Microdialysis improves tissue outcome. Intracerebral microdialysis with bedside biochemical analysis can be performed safely as a routine procedure.

REFERENCES

1. Bullock MR, Chesnut R, Ghajar J, Gordon D, Hartl R, Newell DW, et al. Surgical management of acute subdural hematomas. Neurosurgery 2006;58:S16-24; discussion Si-iv.

2. Bratton SL, Chestnut RM, Ghajar J, McConnell Hammond FF, Harris OA, Hartl R, et al. Guidelines for the management of severe traumatic brain injury. VI. Indications for intracranial pressure monitoring. J Neurotrauma 24 Suppl 2007;1:S37–44.

3. Bellander BM, Cantais E, Enblad P, Hutchinson P, Nordström CH, Robertson C, et al. Consensus meeting on microdialysis in neurointensive care. Intensive Care Med 2004 Dec;30(12):2166–9. Epub 2004 Nov 10.

4. Andrews PJ, Citerio G, Longhi L, Polderman K, Sahuquillo j, Vajkocz P. Nicem consensus on neurological monitoring in acute neurological disease. Intensive Care Med 2008;34:1362–70.

5. Timofeev I, Carpenter KL, Nortje J, Al-Rawi PG, O'Connell MT, Czosnyka M, et al. Cerebral extracellular chemistry and outcome following traumatic brain injury: A microdialysis study of 223 patients. Brain 2011;134:484–94.

6. Verweij BH, Muizelaar JP, Vinas FC, Peterson PL, Xiong Y, Lee CP. Impaired cerebral mitochondrial function after traumatic brain injury in humans. J Neurosurg 2000;93:815–20.

7. Sarrafzadeh AS, Sakowitz OW, Callsen TA, Lanksch WR, Unterberg AW. Bedside microdialysis for early detection of cerebral hypoxia in traumatic brain injury. Neurosurg Focus 9:e2, 2000.

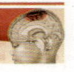

8. Clausen T, Luis Alves O, Reinert M, Doppenberg E, Zauner A, Bullock R. Association between elevated brain tissue glycerol levels and poor outcome following severe traumatic brain injury. Journal of Neurosurgery, August 2005;103(2): 233–8.

9. Belli A, Sen J, Petzold A, Russo S, Kitchen N, Smith M. Metabolic failure precedes intracranial pressure rises in traumatic brain injury: a microdialysis study. Acta Neurochir (Wien) May 2008;150(5):461–9.

10. Marcoux J, McArthur DA, Miller C, Glenn TC, Villablanca P, Martin NA, Hovda DA, et al. Persistent metabolic crisis as measured by elevated cerebral microdialysis lactate/pyruvate ratio predicts chronic frontal lobe brain atrophy after traumatic brain injury. Crit Care Med Oct 2008; 36(10):2871–7.

11. Hlatky R, Valadka AB, Goodman JC, Contant CF, Robertson CS. Patterns of energy substrates during ischemia measured in the brain by microdialysis. J Neurotrauma 2004;21:894–906.

12. Nordstrom CH, Reinstrup P, Xu W, Gardenfors A, Ungerstedt U. Assessment of the lower limit for cerebral perfusion pressure in severe head injuries by bedside monitoring of regional energy metabolism. Anesthesiology 2003;98: 809–14.

13. Purins K, Enblad P, Wiklund L, Lewen A. Brain Tissue Oxygenation and Cerebral Perfusion Pressure Thresholds of Ischemia in a Standardized Pig Brain Death Model. Neurocrit Care 2012;16:462–9.

14. Vespa PM, O'Phelan K, McArthur D, Miller C, Eliseo M, Hirt D, et al. Pericontusional brain tissue exhibits persistent elevation of lactate/pyruvate ratio independent of cerebral perfusion pressure. Crit Care Med 2007;35:1153–60.

15. Trotti D, Danbolt NC, Volterra A. Glutamate transporters are oxidantvulnerable: a molecular link between oxidative and excitotoxic neurodegeneration? Trends Pharmacol Sci 1998;19:328–34.

16. Samuelsson C, Hillered L, Zetterling M, Enblad P, Hesselager G, Ryttlefors M, et al. Cerebral glutamine and glutamate levels in relation to compromised energy metabolism: a microdialysis study in subarachnoid hemorrhage patients. J Cereb Blood Flow Metab 2007;27:1309–17.

17. Chamoun R, Suki D, Gopinath SP, Goodman JC, Robertson C. Role of extracellular glutamate measured by cerebral microdialysis in severe traumatic brain injury. J Neurosurg 2010;113: 564–70.

18. Bullock R, Zauner A, Woodward JJ, Myseros J, Choi SC, Ward JD, et al. Factors affecting excitatory amino acid release following severe human head injury. J Neurosurg 1998;89:507–18.

19. Reinstrup P, Stahl N, Mellergard P, Uski T, Ungerstedt U, Nordstrom CH. Intracerebral microdialysis in clinical practice: baseline values for chemical markers during wakefulness, anesthesia, and neurosurgery. Neurosurgery 2000;47:701–9; discussion 709–710.

20. Schulz MK, Wang LP, Tange M, Bjerre P. Cerebral microdialysis monitoring: determination of normal and ischemic cerebral metabolisms in patients with aneurysmal subarachnoid hemorrhage. J Neurosurg 2000;93:808–14.

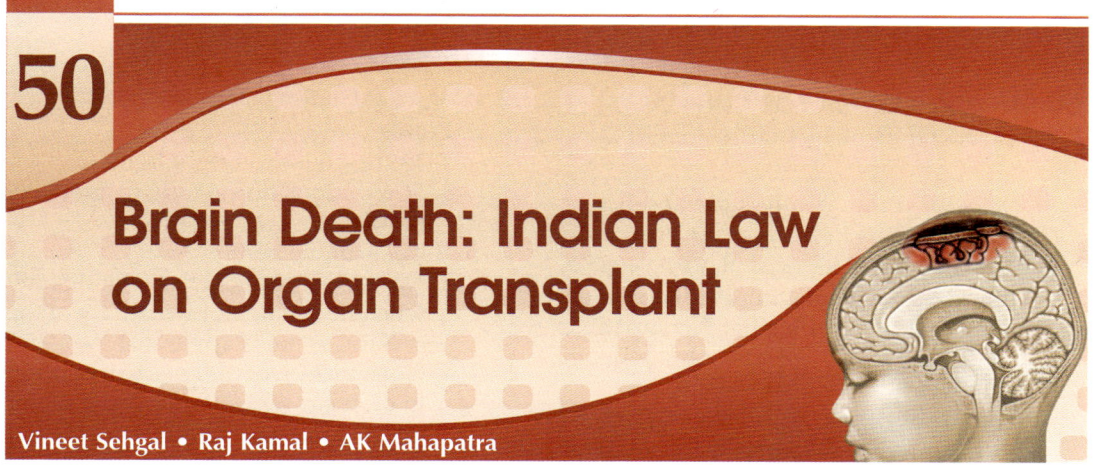

50

Brain Death: Indian Law on Organ Transplant

Vineet Sehgal • Raj Kamal • AK Mahapatra

INTRODUCTION

The concept of **brain death** is now well accepted by the medical professionals. The first description of brain death was given in 1950 by Mollaret and Goulon who identified this condition as coma depassé (a state beyond coma).[1] The sets of criteria which define brain death vary from country to country with one basic aim, that is to demonstrate the absence of all brainstem functions. Therefore, brain death is actually better defined as **brainstem death.** During past two decades, confirmatory paraclinical tests have been progressively abandoned and the clinical examination has become more and more important to establish brain death. A better understanding of brain death has led to increased number of patients in whom the mechanical ventilation has been electively stopped, avoiding excessive amount of money wasted in intensive care on these cases. The concept of brain death became legal issue and in India it was defined in 1995 in "The Transplantation of Human Organ Act, 1995". Variety of criteria used differ around the world. The only controversy is now about the use of EEG/cerebral angiography being used as essential criteria for brain death. As discussed later in the chapter, these tests are useful in difficult situations.

Clinical examination regarding brainstem reflexes is the most important tool for establishing brain death. The other key point is demonstration of significant irreversible damage to brainstem/brain and identifying the cause of death (e.g. severe head injury, etc). Brain death is defined as the irreversible loss of all function of the brain, including the brainstem. The three essential findings in brain death are coma, absence of brainstem reflexes, and apnea. The diagnosis of brain death is primarily clinical.

The Uniform Determination of Death Act[2] indicates that "an individual who has sustained either irreversible cessation of circulatory and respiratory functions, or irreversible cessation of all functions of the entire brain, including the brainstem, is dead," with brain death being determined based on "accepted medical standards." The American Academy of Neurology[3] has published practice guidelines providing medical standards for the determination of brain death. **The most recent American Academy of Neurology[4] guideline update notes that "because of the deficiencies in the evidence base, clinicians must exercise considerable judgment when applying the criteria in specific circumstances" and that "ancillary tests can be used when uncertainty exists about the reliability of parts of the neurologic examination" or when the apnea test cannot be performed.[4] In 2010, the Quality Standards Subcommittee of the American Academy of Neurology provided an update of the 1995 American Academy of Neurology guidelines.[5]**

DIAGNOSTIC CRITERIA FOR CLINICAL DIAGNOSIS OF BRAIN DEATH (AMERICAN ACADEMY OF NEUROLOGY)[3]

A. *Prerequisites.* Brain death is the absence of clinical brain function when the proximate cause is known and demonstrably irreversible.

1. Clinical or neuroimaging evidence of an acute CNS catastrophe that is compatible with the clinical diagnosis of brain death (Fig. 50.1).
2. Exclusion of complicating medical conditions that may confound clinical assessment (no severe electrolyte, acid–base, or endocrine disturbance)
3. No drug intoxication or poisoning
4. Core temperature ≥ 32°C (90°F)

B. *The three cardinal findings* in brain death are coma or unresponsiveness, absence of brainstem reflexes, and apnea.

1. *Coma or unresponsiveness*—no cerebral motor response to pain in all extremities (nail-bed pressure and supraorbital pressure)

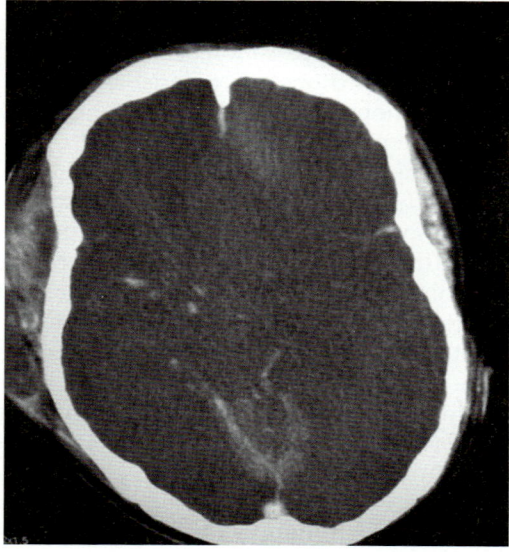

Fig. 50.1: CT scan of a brain dead patient. Gray-white differentiation is lost. Relative sparing of the cerebellum makes vermis appear high density (white cerebellum sign) compared to low density edematous cerebral hemispheres

2. *Absence of brainstem reflexes*
   a. Pupils
      i. No response to bright light
      ii. *Size:* midposition (4 mm) to dilated (9 mm)
   b. Ocular movement
      i. No oculocephalic reflex (testing only when no fracture or instability of the cervical spine is apparent)
      ii. No deviation of the eyes to irrigation in each ear with 50 ml of cold water (allow 1 minute after injection and at least 5 minutes between testing on each side).

ESTABLISHING BRAIN DEATH

Neurological examination is aimed at detecting persisting brainstem function.

a. *Light reflex:* Fixed dilated or intermediate size pupils with absent light reflex is very important criteria. The light and **oculo-cephalic reflexes** can be obtained reliably only after 32 weeks of gestation and hence, caution should be taken in evaluating premature babies.[2]

b. *Absent corneal reflex:* Tested by touching the periphery of cornea with soft cotton. One should look for absence of blinking and related reflexes (oculopupillary, etc.).

c. *Absent oculocephalic reflex:* Cervical spine trauma should be ruled out by X-ray cervical spine before testing this reflex. Tested by rapidly turning the head from side-to-side (also called **Doll's eye response).**

d. *Absent oculovestibular reflex (cold caloric test):* External auditory canal needs to examine for blood, cerumen and perforated drum before performing this test. Ice cold water can be used and if no reaction is obtained with 50 ml water (either a slow deviation of eyes or any **nystagmus)** a larger volume should be used.

e. *Absent gag reflex:* Tested by stimulating posterior pharyngeal wall, tonsils, base of tongue. Both sides need to be tested. Suction catheter through endotracheal tube can be used in intubated patients. The response

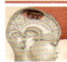

consists of elevation and constriction of pharyngeal muscles with retraction of the tongue.

f. *Apnea test:* Hypoxia must be avoided during apnea test. Different techniques have been used. Continuous oxygenation during the test by placing a cannula into endotracheal tube and giving oxygen[6,7] 6–7 lit/min. The use of a positive end expiratory pressure (PEEP) is an alternative to the cannula technique to prevent hypoxia (but PEEP is not possible in all types of ventilators, e.g. Medisys system used frequently in India). Ideally, first an arterial blood sample is drawn to establish baseline $PaCO_2$ and PaO_2 (150 mm Hg). The oxygen cannula is placed with adequate oxygen flow. ABG samples are repeated every two minutes until $PaCO_2$ reaches 60 mm Hg or and stop condition occurs (arterial oxygen saturation < 80%; PaO_2 < 50 mm Hg or severe cardiac arrhythmias). Spinal respiratory-like movements can be observed during apnea test[8,9] but they are not effective in ventilation and disappear on repeat examination. Total duration of apnea test when serial ABGs are not available is restricted to 5 min.

g. *No reaction to deep central painful stimuli:* No movement should be seen during the painful stimulation. Spontaneous movements of spinal reflex origin do occur in brain dead patients often referred as Lazarus' sign.[10,11] Their origin is supposed to be spinal and they simulate primitive reflexes exhibited by newborns such as Moro reflex. Such movements are more frequent when patient is off the ventilator. The delay in appearance of spinal automatisms usually ranges between 6 and 72 hrs. This delay, longer than the usual observation period for brain death, explains why such movements are not seen in every brain dead patient with intact spinal cord.[12] Another explanation is occurrence of spinal shock concurrent with abrupt rise in intracranial pressure which often occurs during brain death.

h. *Absence of deep tendon reflexes:* Absence of DTK was initially included in brain death criteria, but, since these reflexes are now thought to be of spinal origin, they are irrelevant in the diagnosis of brain death.

i. *Conditions which can interfere with brain death diagnosis*
   Hypothermia (range varies from 32.2°C in USA to 35°C in UK).
   Hypoxia can be ruled out by ABG.
   Drugs, e.g. alcohol, muscle relaxants, sedatives, narcotics, barbiturates (ruled out by toxicology screening).
   Hypotension—(systolic blood pressure <90 mm Hg)
   Metabolic/endocrine disturbances
   In case of any doubt, one should wait and do repeat examinations (never diagnose brain death when in doubt).[13]

j. *Etiology of brain death must be clearly established:* This condition is of crucial importance and must be fulfilled. All relevant investigations (Table 50.1) should be carried out to demonstrate irreversible damage to the brain.
   Irreversible brain damage establishment is more important in children where head injury and intracranial hemorrhage are less common causes of brain death.[14]

Observation Period

The duration of observation is still a matter of controversy. Neurological examination must not be done within 30 minutes of cardiopulmonary resuscitation. It is proposed that if structural brain damage has been established then repeat examination after 6 hours is

Table 50.1: Proposed investigations
1. Brain imaging by CT/MRI
2. Chest X-ray
3. Cervical spine X-ray
4. ECG
5. Electrolytes, blood glucose, renal function test, LFT
6. Arterial blood gas analysis
7. Urine toxicology screening

suffice. Otherwise, the observation period should be prolonged.[11] One should be very careful while evaluating children younger than 5 years of age. Vecchierini et al[6] in 1992 suggested a simple guideline for observation period.

1. 6 hr for children older than 1 year.
2. 24 hr for infants > 3 months.
3. 48 hr for infants < 3 months.

However, such duration is not stated in Indian law and 2 examinations 6 hours apart are suggested for establishing brain death.

Paraclinical Confirmatory Tests

No paraclinical confirmatory test is required if the previous points are fulfilled. EEG, cerebral **angiogram,** cerebral **radionuclide angiogram,** cerebral blood flow using stable xenon, **transcranial Doppler,** ICP monitoring, **evoked potentials,** digital cerebral angiogram with venous injection all have been used to establish low or absent cerebral circulation but none is required in Indian law to diagnose brain death.

Diabetes insipidus is frequently observed finding in brain dead patients. The condition is diagnosed by the presence of **polyuria** (urine output > 7 ml/kg/hr or > 200 ml/hr), serum hyperosmolality (> 310 mOsm/L) hypernatremia (> 150 mEq/lit) and low urine specific gravity (< 1004). Reasons for this conditions are:

i. ADH is no longer produced in dead cells.
ii. Produced ADH is not transported to posterior pituitary.
iii. ADH from posterior pituitary is not released into systemic circulation.

But all patients with brain death do not develop DI. All patients once diagnosed as brain dead go into cardiac asystole within 12 hours to few days time.[16,17] Head injury and intracranial hemorrhage are the two most frequent conditions responsible for brain death. Jennett et al[13] in 1981 found 55% of patients with head injury as primary cause of brain death, whereas intracranial bleed was responsible for 28% cases of brain death.

The Quality Standards Subcommittee of the American Academy of Neurology [5] provided an update of the 1995 American Academy of Neurology guideline with regard to the following questions:

1. Are there patients who fulfill the clinical criteria of brain death who recover brain function?
2. What is an adequate observation period to ensure that cessation of neurologic function is permanent?
3. Are complex motor movements that falsely suggest retained brain function sometimes observed in brain death?
4. What is the comparative safety of techniques for determining apnea?
5. Are there new ancillary tests (MRI and magnetic resonance angiography, CT angiography, somatosensory evoked potentials) that accurately identify patients with brain death?

They concluded that in adults, there are no published reports of recovery of neurologic function after a diagnosis of brain death using the criteria reviewed in the 1995 American Academy of Neurology practice parameter. Complex—spontaneous motor movements and false positive triggering of the ventilator may occur in patients who are brain dead. There is insufficient evidence to determine the minimally acceptable observation period to ensure that neurologic functions have ceased irreversibly. Apneic oxygenation diffusion to determine apnea is safe, but there is insufficient evidence to determine the comparative safety of techniques used for apnea testing. There is insufficient evidence to determine if newer ancillary tests accurately confirm the cessation of function of the entire brain.

Indian Law and Organ Transplantation[18]

The Transplantation of Human Organ Act, 1995 defines the conditions to be fulfilled by the hospitals, medical practitioners and patients before any organ transplantation can be done. Hospitals should be established for at least 2 years, must have obtained a

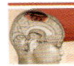
registration under this act, should possess the essential personnels and equipment as specified in the rules.

Brain death certificate includes:

A. *Patient's details:* Name, age, sex, address, hospital number, name and address of next of kin, consent for transplant.

B. *Preconditions:*

1. Diagnosis: Any condition/illness/accident that led to irreversible brain damage:
   - Date and time of accident/onset of illness.
   - Date and time of non-responsive coma.

2. Findings of board of medical experts:
   - Following reversible causes of coma have been excluded—intoxication, CNS depressant drugs, muscle relaxants, primary hypothermia, hypovolemic shock, metabolic/endocrine disorders.
     - First medical examination—date and time.
     - Second medical examination—date and time.
   - Tests for absence of brainstem functions:
     i. Pupillary size.
     ii. Pupillary light reflexes.
     iii. Doll's eye movement.
     iv. Corneal reflexes.
     v. Motor response in any cranial nerve distribution, any response to stimulation of face, limb or trunk.
     vi. Gag reflex.
     vii. Cough reflex.
     viii. Eye movements on caloric testing B/L.
     ix. Any respiratory movements.
     x. Apnea test as specified.

   Date and time of first and second examination to be mentioned.

3. Doctors entitled to certify brain death
   1. Medical administrator I/C of the hospital.
   2. Authorized specialist.
   3. Neurologist/neurosurgeon.
   4. Medical officer treating the patient.

   Minimum time interval between the first and second testing should be six hours.

AMERICAN ACADEMY OF NEUROLOGY[21;] PRACTICE PARAMETERS: DETERMINING BRAIN DEATH IN ADULTS

I. *Diagnostic Criteria for Clinical Diagnosis of Brain Death*

A. Prerequisites: Brain death is the absence of clinical brain function when the proximate cause is known and demonstrably irreversible.
   1. Clinical or neuroimaging evidence of an acute CNS catastrophe that is compatible with the clinical diagnosis of brain death
   2. Exclusion of complicating medical conditions that may confound clinical assessment (no severe electrolyte, acid–base, or endocrine disturbance)
   3. No drug intoxication or poisoning
   4. Core temperature $\geq 32°C$ (90°F)

B. The three cardinal findings in brain death are coma or unresponsiveness, absence of brainstem reflexes, and apnea
   1. Coma or unresponsiveness—no cerebral motor response to pain in all extremities (nail-bed pressure and supraorbital pressure)
   2. Absence of brainstem reflexes
      a. Pupils
         i. No response to bright light
         ii. *Size:* Midposition (4 mm) to dilated (9 mm)
      b. Ocular movement

i. No oculocephalic reflex (testing only when no fracture or instability of the cervical spine is apparent)

    ii. No deviation of the eyes to irrigation in each ear with 50 ml of cold water (allow 1 minute after injection and at least 5 minutes between testing on each side)

  c. Facial sensation and facial motor response

    i. No corneal reflex to touch with a throat swab

    ii. No jaw reflex

    iii. No grimacing to deep pressure on nail-bed, supraorbital ridge, or temporomandibular joint

  d. Pharyngeal and tracheal reflexes

    i. No response after stimulation of the posterior pharynx with tongue blade

    ii. No cough response to bronchial suctioning

3. Apnea—testing performed as follows:

  a. Prerequisites

    i. Core temperature $\geq 36.5°C$ or $97°F$

    ii. Systolic blood pressure ≥ 90 mm Hg

    iii. *Euvolemia option:* Positive fluid balance in the previous 6 hours

    iv. *Normal PCO_2 option:* Arterial $PCO_2 \geq 40$ mm Hg

    v. *Normal PO_2 option:* Preoxygenation to obtain arterial $PO_2 \geq 200$ mm Hg

  b. Connect a pulse oximeter and disconnect the ventilator

  c. Deliver 100% O_2, 6 L/min, into the trachea. Option: place a cannula at the level of the carina.

  d. Look closely for respiratory movements (abdominal or chest excursions that produce adequate tidal volumes)

  e. Measure arterial PO_2, PCO_2, and pH after approximately 8 minutes and reconnect the ventilator

  f. If respiratory movements are absent and arterial PCO_2 is ≥ 60 mm Hg (option: 20 mm Hg increase in PCO_2 over a baseline normal PCO_2), the apnea test result is positive (i.e. it supports the diagnosis of brain death)

  g. If respiratory movements are observed, the apnea test result is negative (i.e. it does not support the clinical diagnosis of brain death), and the test should be repeated.

  h. Connect the ventilator if, during testing, the systolic blood pressure becomes ≥ 90 mm Hg or the pulse oximeter indicates significant oxygen desaturation and cardiac arrhythmias are present; immediately draw an arterial blood sample and analyze arterial blood gas. If PCO_2 is ≥ 60 mm Hg or PCO_2 increase is ≥ 20 mm Hg over baseline normal PCO_2, the apnea test result is positive (it supports the clinical diagnosis of brain death); if PCO_2 is < 60 mm Hg or PCO_2 increase is < 20 mm Hg over baseline normal PCO_2, the result is indeterminate, and an additional confirmatory test can be considered

II. *Pitfalls in the Diagnosis of Brain Death*

The following conditions may interfere with the clinical diagnosis of brain death, so that the diagnosis cannot be made with certainty on clinical grounds alone. Confirmatory tests are recommended

a. Severe facial trauma

b. Pre-existing pupillary abnormalities

c. Toxic levels of any sedative drugs, aminoglycosides, tricyclic antidepressants, anticholinergics, antiepileptic drugs, chemotherapeutic agents, or neuromuscular blocking agents

d. Sleep apnea or severe pulmonary disease resulting in chronic retention of CO_2

III. *Clinical Observations Compatible with the Diagnosis of Brain Death*

These manifestations are occasionally seen and should not be misinterpreted as evidence for brainstem function

a. Spontaneous movements of limbs other than pathologic flexion or extension response
b. Respiratory-like movements (shoulder elevation and adduction, back arching, intercostal expansion without significant tidal volumes)
c. Sweating, blushing, tachycardia
d. Normal blood pressure without pharmacologic support or sudden increases in blood pressure
e. Absence of diabetes insipidus
f. Deep tendon reflexes; superficial abdominal reflexes; triple flexion response
g. Babinski reflex

IV. *Confirmatory Laboratory Tests (Options)*

Brain death is a clinical diagnosis. A repeat clinical evaluation 6 hours later is recommended, but this interval is arbitrary. A confirmatory test is not mandatory but is desirable in patients in whom specific components of clinical testing cannot be reliably performed or evaluated. It should be emphasized that any of the suggested confirmatory tests may produce similar results in patients with catastrophic brain damage who do not (yet) fulfill the clinical criteria of brain death. The following confirmatory test findings are listed in the order of the most sensitive test first.
   Consensus criteria are identified by individual tests

a. *Conventional angiography:* No intracerebral filling at the level of the carotid bifurcation or circle of Willis. The external carotid circulation is patent, and filling of the superior longitudinal sinus may be delayed
b. *Electroencephalography:* No electrical activity during at least 30 minutes of recording that adheres to the minimal technical criteria for EEG recording in suspected brain death as adopted by the American Electroencephalographic Society, including 16-channel EEG instruments.
c. *Transcranial Doppler ultrasonography*
   1. Ten percent of patients may not have temporal insonation windows. Therefore, the initial absence of Doppler signals cannot be interpreted as consistent with brain death
   2. Small systolic peaks in early systole without diastolic flow or reverberating flow, indicating very high vascular resistance associated with greatly increased intracranial pressure
d. Technetium-99m hexamethylpropyleneamine oxime brain scan. No uptake of isotope in brain parenchyma ("hollow skull phenomenon")
e. Somatosensory evoked potentials. Bilateral absence of N20-P22 response with median nerve stimulation
   The recordings should adhere to the minimal technical criteria for somatosensory evoked potential recording in suspected brain death as adopted by the American Electroencephalographic Society

V. *Medical Record Documentation (Standard)*

a. Etiology and irreversibility of condition
b. Absence of brainstem reflexes
c. Absence of motor response to pain
d. Absence of respiration with $PCO_2 \geq 60$ mm Hg
e. Justification for confirmatory test and result of confirmatory test
f. Repeat neurologic examination. Option: The interval is arbitrary, but a 6-hour period is reasonable

CONCLUSIONS

Severe head injury is the most common cause of brain death. All neurosurgeons, neuro-physicians must be well aware of rules and regulations and essential criteria required for the diagnosis of this condition. Each brain dead patient is a potential organ donor. Motivation of family members of brain dead patient is important for cadaveric organ transplantation. Patients with cardiac problem, kidney and liver failure will vastly benefit from cadaver transplant program.

REFERENCES

1. Pallis C. From brain death to brainstem death. Br Med J 1982;285:1487–90.
2. Webb A, Samuels O. Brain death dilemmas and the use of ancillary testing. Continuum (Minneap Minn) 2012;18(3):659–68.
3. Executive Board September 24, 1994. American Academy of Neurology, Published in Neurology 1995;45:1012–1014.
4. Wijdicks EFM, Manno EM, Holets SR. Ventilator selfcycling may falsely suggest patient effort during brain death determination. Neurology 2005;65:774.
5. Wijdicks EFM , Varelas PN, Gronseth GS, Greer DM. Evidence-based guideline update: Deter-mining brain death in adults, Report of the Quality Standards Subcommittee of the American Academy of Neurology. Neurology 2010;74:1911–18.
6. Vecchierini-Blinkeau MF, Moussalli SF. Diagnostic value of neurophysiological tests in the diagnosis of brain: Neurophysiol Clin 1992;22:179–90.
7. Benzel EC, Gross CD, Hadden TA, Kesterson L, et al. The apnoea test for the determination of brain death. J Neurosurg 1989;71:191–4.
8. Marks SJ, Zistein J. Apnoeic oxygenation in apnoea tests for brain death: A control trial. Arch Neurol 1990;47:1066–8.
9. Ropper AH, Kennedy SK, Russel L. Apnoea testing in the diagnosis of brain death: clinical and physiological observation. J Neurosurg 1981;55:942–6.
10. Mandel S, Arenas A, Scasta D. Spinal automation in cerebral death. N Eng J Med 1982;307:501.
11. Ropper AH. Unusual spontaneous movements in brain dead patients. Neurology 1984;34:1089–92.
12. Turmel A, Roux A, Bojanwski MW. Spinal man after declaration of brain death. Neurosurgery 1991;28:298–302.
13. Jennett B, Gleve J, Wilson P. Brain death in three neurosurgical units. Br Med J 1981;282:533–39.
14. Freeman JM, Ferry PC. New brain death guidelines in children: Further confusion. Pediatrics 1988;81:301–3.
15. Black PM, Zervas NT. Declaration of brain death in neurosurgical and neurological practice. Neurosurgery 1984;15:170–4.
16. Black PM. Brain death (Part I of 2). N Eng J Med 1978;299:338–44.
17. Black PM. Brain death (Part II of 2). N Eng J Med 1978;299:393–401.
18. Chaubey PC. Medical ethics and health legislation and patient care in India. Chaubey PC (ed), Saurabh Publishers, New Delhi 1998;258–99.

Index